AN INTRODUCTION

TO THE

HISTORY OF MEDICINE

WITH MEDICAL CHRONOLOGY
BIBLIOGRAPHIC DATA AND TEST QUESTIONS

BY

FIELDING H. GARRISON, A.B., M.D.

PRINCIPAL ASSISTANT LIBRARIAN, SURGEON GENERAL'S OFFICE, WASHINGTON, D. C.

ILLUSTRATED

PHILADELPHIA AND LONDON

W. B. SAUNDERS COMPANY

1913

PRINTED IN AMERICA

PRESS OF
W. B. SAUNDERS COMPANY
PHILADELPHIA

PREFACE

The object of this book is to furnish the medical student or the busy practitioner with a definite outline of the history of medicine, and, at the same time, to place in his hands a large number of important facts which may be of use in his professional work or desirable to know as part of his medical culture. In submitting the volume to the profession, the author is well aware of its limitations. His aim throughout has been to preserve the attitude of an interpreter or expositor of "the best that has been thought and said" upon the subject, rather than to set up as an authority; and, as an outline sketch is not the same thing as a finished painting, so it is to be presumed that a guide-book of these dimensions will not be placed in comparison with the exhaustive handling of a Haeser or a Neuburger. Clarity, concision, and perspicuity have been aimed at, rather than learned or lengthy exposition, and to convey information of value rather than to exploit original investigations. The latter have been confined, in this instance, to the personal verification of facts, dates, and bibliographical references. The publishers and the author have spared no pains and expense to make the volume as accurate and complete as possible; and, if it should realize its practical intention of helping the student or practitioner to pursue his own studies in medical history, the writer will feel much better rewarded for his labors than if a work of this scope should be judged from the dubious viewpoint of originality alone.

My old friend, the late Dr. Robert Fletcher, a man of rare learning, once observed that medical history, and, he might have added, a great deal of medical literature proper, is "mainly repetition, mostly copying." It is in the nature of things that this should be so. The *Postament* (as the Germans say), upon which the subject rests, is the accumulated labor of the past. If we are to have a clear view of the panorama of medical history, we must necessarily stand upon the shoulders of our predecessors. As the historian proper has to do with the deeds of mankind and the motives of their actions, it is the lot of the medical historian to deal rather with information derived from books than with knowledge derived from experience. It is this fact which often makes the subject so distressingly dry and disappointing. As Billings has admirably said: "To attempt to isolate the history of medicine, and to comprehend its curious ebbs and flows of doctrine from medical writings only, is like cutting a narrow strip from the center of a piece of tapestry and speculating upon the origin and purpose of the cut threads of patterns that may be found in it." The history of medicine is, in fact, the history of humanity itself, with its ups and downs, its brave aspirations after truth and finality, its pathetic failures. The subject may be treated variously as a pageant, an array of books, a procession of characters, a succession of theories, an exposition of human ineptitudes, or as the very bone and marrow of cultural history. As Matthew Arnold said of the Acta Sanctorum, "All human life is there." This broader view of medical history has been the special teaching of its ablest modern exponent, Professor Karl Sudhoff, of Leipzig, who has not only made the subject a matter of intensive original research as well as a scientific discipline, but is a medical philologist of the first order and a contributor to *Culturgeschichte* in the widest sense. The same strong human note is the attractive feature of the historical essays of Sir William Osler, which have been a source of inspiration for much of recent work in the United States; and Professor Welch's luminous talks at the Johns Hopkins Hospital Historical Club have gone far to make the delicate appreciation of values in medical history a fine art.

In attempting to treat the subject as a cultural development as well as an important phase in the evolution of inductive science, the obvious lines of the graphic, the biographic, and the bibliographic have been followed, and, at the end of each period, a brief survey of its cultural and social aspects has been appended. The latter have been made purposely sketchy, since any one's own reading will tell him that he is not likely to be stimulated by too exhaustive excursions in this field. For similar reasons, certain passages of detailed exposition have been made available for reference by throwing them into smaller type, without destroying the continuity of the narrative. The pictures are designed to illustrate the costumes as well as the personalities of the leaders of medicine in the different periods and only effective portraits have been chosen. Many of the older copper plates are as valueless and negative as the hideous newspaper woodcuts of not so very long ago. Pictures of some eminent medical worthies, Caspar Friedrich Wolff, John Bell, Stromeyer, James Syme, have been sought for but are apparently not accessible anywhere. Likenesses of living English and American physicians have not been included, for reasons that will suggest themselves, but a few pictures of continental celebrities have been added, as being less

familiar. Of the appendices, which are designed to supplement
the narrative portion, the medical chronology differs from those
of Choulant and Julius Pagel in that, as being more extensive, its
separate items are listed tandem instead of abreast, the advantage
of this arrangement being that a large number of important events
can be brought into correlation, in continuous order, under each
given date. The series of select biographies of important physicians and other bibliographic notes for collateral reading have been
arranged in alphabetic order, for ready reference, and explain
themselves. It was originally proposed to add a series of detailed
histories of important diseases, surgical operations, and therapeutic procedures, but, by reason of the many eponymic expressions and the disputed points of priority, the material soon grew
to proportions which would have made the volume unhandy, and
upon this outgrowth the operation of appendicectomy has, therefore, been charitably performed. Most of these data have been
embodied in the text, with bibliographical references in the foot-
notes. If any exception should be taken to the number of the
latter, it can be testified, from an experience of some twenty years
in a large medical library, that these references, often carelessly
given, even by the most eminent physicians, are exceedingly
difficult to find on the spur of the moment. In mercy to the reader,
many references in the modern period have been omitted, as they
can easily be found (under the names and dates given) in the Index
Catalogue and Index Medicus, or in the catalogue of the historical
collection of the Surgeon General's Library, which was prepared
by the writer at the request of Colonel McCaw, and printed, by
permission of the Surgeon General, in the Index Catalogue (second series, vol. xvii, pp. 89–178).

The "Test Questions" at the end have not been inserted with
any pedagogic designs upon the reader; but it is hoped that they
may be of use as a means of refreshing the memory, in following
up interesting subjects, in setting themes for students, or in quiz-
zing them. It would be idle or pedantic to suppose that one individual reader could be interested in all the points raised. Any
one who has had much to do with medical proof-reading might
multiply such questions indefinitely. In this instance, they have
been carried somewhat beyond "the solemn number, one hundred."

While there are special chairs devoted to medical history in
most of the important European universities, and while we may
some day hope to see an institute for medico-historical research
in the United States, like that of Professor Sudhoff at Leipzig, it
is hardly probable that it would be an advantage to burden the
average American student with a special course of lectures on this
subject. Such a course, given, say, in his graduating year, would

necessarily be superficial and perfunctory, and might defeat its own object by interfering with his work at the most important period of his student life; while his personal interest in medical history will naturally depend upon what he does with himself after graduation. The deficiency can be, and has been, easily supplied in other ways, more especially by occasional demonstrations of books and pictures and by means of the medical history club. The anatomist who can produce some edition of Vesalius, the histologist who is sportsmanlike enough to obtain the original engraving of the Purkinje cells and show it to his students, the pathologist or clinician who can display the fine plates in Bright's or Addison's monographs, will do much more to fix these names in his pupils' minds than by any set course of lectures. The first volume of the Johns Hopkins Hospital Bulletin begins with such a demonstration by the late Dr. John S. Billings, and those published by the late Dr. James Finlayson, of Glasgow, are perfect models of what such things should be—genial, simple, and immensely interesting. Dr. John C. Comrie, lecturer on the history of medicine at the University of Edinburgh, has very cleverly followed up Wunderlich's idea of printing specimen-extracts from the medical classics for advanced students. In such ways as these, the subject can easily be developed, in connection with the different disciplines and specialties, by a sort of "contrapuntal in-weaving," with the advantage of bringing about a closer and more friendly contact between teacher and pupils. The books, facts, and dates are as nothing in comparison with the chance of giving the student an enlarged view of the *humaniora*, the nameless, unremembered things which help to make him a gentleman in his profession. Youth is, or ought to be, the period of generous self-surrender to ideals, and many fine traits, latent in young men, can be brought out by contact with a superior teacher. The example of Pasteur, Ludwig, Henle, Hyrtl, and others, goes to show that the most priceless possession which a medical teacher can acquire is to be held in loving remembrance by his students. Osler's evenings at home with his Johns Hopkins pupils are a case in point, and the general tendency of his teaching, even in the clinic, has been strikingly conveyed by Dr. Arnold Klebs.

"Never can one forget the scenes in the out-patient department, where he stood, surrounded by his boys, helping them as a friend in their struggles with some difficult case. He would go to one, put his arm around his shoulder, and then begin a friendly inquiry, interspersed with humorous remarks and allusions to the work done by special students on a given subject. Urging, encouraging, inspiring, so we saw him, exact always, dogmatic never, and when the humorous and friendly fire kindled in his eyes we could not help but love him and with him the task we had chosen as our lifework. Thus we imagine those *maîtres* of the old French school, a school no longer limited by national boundaries, one of those men who have trodden the paths through the wards of the Salpêtrière, the Charité and Lariboisière, the Necker, the Hôtel Dieu, making apostles and missionaries in the great cause of scientific medicine."

Another pleasant way of studying the history of medicine is by means of the medical history club, which differs from the formal medico-historical society in that the papers read serve as an introduction to a congenial conversazione, with refreshments or otherwise. As the private musical club depends for its success upon the disinterested spirit of the refined amateur, so the law of the history club is that each member must shed all assumption or any trace of the professional jealousy which is common to physicians, musicians, politicians, and those possessed of histrionic or operatic talents. Stevenson said of the Barbizon community of painters that "formal manners being laid aside, essential courtesy was the more rigidly exacted; . . . to a touch of presumption or a word of hectoring these free Barbizonians were as sensitive as a tea party of maiden ladies." The medical history club will never thrive unless each individual member preserves the modest, consistent attitude of a learner. Michael Angelo's cartoon of Father Time in a go-cart, with the legend "*Ancora imparo*," might be its device, if such a club is to be a "going concern."

In preparing this work, I have been mainly indebted to the resources of the Surgeon General's Library, without which it could not have been written; and I desire to express my sincere gratitude to its Librarian, Colonel Walter D. McCaw, for the privileges granted me in connection with the loan of special literature for my private use. Geheimrat Sudhoff (Leipzig) has very kindly permitted me to copy some of his interesting pictures relating to horoscopic medicine and the traditional aspects of anatomic illustration. Similar courtesies have been extended by Professor William Stirling (Manchester, England), Professor William Bateson (London), Dr. Eugen Holländer (Berlin), Dr. Robert Müllerheim (Berlin), Captain Henry J. Nichols, U. S. Army, and others. Dr. Arnold C. Klebs (Lausanne) has placed at my disposal his unique collection of photographs of modern physicians, and has made many valuable suggestions. I am indebted to the editors of the *Journal of the American Medical Association* and the *New York Medical Journal* for the privilege of using certain copyrighted material published by me in these periodicals. Finally, my cordial thanks are due to Dr. Albert Allemann, Assistant Librarian, Surgeon General's Office, and to Dr. Frank J. Stockman, who have very generously given up much of their private leisure to the correction of the proofs.

WASHINGTON, D. C., *December,* 1913.   F. H. G.

CONTENTS

AN INTRODUCTION

TO THE

HISTORY OF MEDICINE

THE IDENTITY OF ALL FORMS OF ANCIENT AND PRIMITIVE MEDICINE

ONE of the best accredited doctrines of recent times is that of the unity or solidarity of folk-lore.[1]   The collective investigations of historians, ethnologists, archeologists, philologists, and sociologists reveal the singular fact that the myths, superstitions, laws, and social customs of primitive peoples all over the earth, as well as the cruder ethnic aspects of religions, converge inevitably to a common point of similarity or identity.   The mind of savage man, in its pathetic efforts to form religious and ethical systems for moral and spiritual guidance, or to beautify the commoner aspects of life with romance and poetry, has unconsciously taken the same lines of least resistance, followed the same planes of cleavage.   The civilized mind differs from the savage mind only in respect of a higher evolutionary development.   Human races and racial customs have changed as they became more highly specialized.   The heart of man remains the same.

It follows that, under different aspects of space and time, all phases of folk-medicine and ancient medicine have been essentially alike in tendency, differing only in unimportant details.   In the light of anthropology, this proposition may be taken as proved. Cuneiform, hieroglyphic, runic, and palm-leaf inscriptions all indicate that the folk-ways of early medicine, whether Accadian or Scandinavian, Slavic or Celtic, Roman or Polynesian, have been the same—in each case an affair of charms and spells, plant-lore and psychotherapy, to stave off the effects of supernatural agencies.

Apart from any theories as to his origin or evolution, we may assume that prehistoric man was not different from what we often find primitive man to be—a savage sunk in his animal instincts.

[1] For a good summary of the matter, see the presidential address of Charlotte S. Burne in Folk-Lore, London, 1911, xxii, 14–41.

At this stage of his existence he killed his food and fought his enemies with sticks and stones, raped his women, hid himself in caves,
and was probably not unaware of certain hygienic precautions
which are instinctive in lower animals. A dog licks its wounds,
hides in holes if sick or injured, limps on three legs if maimed,
tries to destroy parasites on its body, exercises, stretches, and
warms in the sun, assumes a definite posture in sleeping, and seeks
out certain herbs and grasses when sick.[1]   It is not unreasonable
to suppose that actions like these may have been as instinctive
in a grown-up prehistoric man as they are in a primitive child of
his race today. "Man has climbed up from some lower animal
form," says John Burroughs, "but he has, as it were, pulled the
ladder up after him." We do not know when or where, how or
why, this occurred, but we do know the first rung of the ladder.
In the Hall of Anthropology of the National Museum at Washington (or in any other good collection of this kind) there are to
be seen innumerable specimens of a small object in chipped flint
which is the symbol of prehistoric man's uplift, his first step in the
direction of civilization. With this leaf-shaped flint in hand, he
had a new means of protecting himself against enemies, procuring
and preparing food, and of manufacturing other weapons and implements of the same kind or of more highly specialized kinds.
Now the interesting point about these prehistoric flints is that they
are to be found wherever traces of the existence of men are found.
Here cropping up as spear or arrow-point, there as tools or
ceremonial object, these primitive "celts," as they are called, have
been excavated from the river-drifts of England, France, and
North America, in the caverns of Devonshire and the Dordogne, in
the plains of Egypt and Palestine, and the frozen tundra of Siberia
and Alaska, in each case bearing the same identical form.   In
the Early Stone Age (Paleolithic Period) the chipped celts were
little more than the result of a necessary crude flaking of oval or
ovoid stones.   In the Later Stone Age (Neolithic Period) they
were brought to a high point of specialization and polish, but in
shape and intention they have remained the same throughout geologic space and time.   Their employment in surgery by the ancient
Egyptians, or in ritual circumcision by the Hebrews in the desert,
goes to show the unusual veneration in which they were held by
these peoples on account of their great antiquity.   In what is perhaps the most interesting of American contributions to archeology,[2]

---

[1] Usually *Triticum caninum*, *Cynosurus cristatus*, and *Agrostis canina* for
emesis and purgation. Cats have a known fondness for *Valeriana officinalis*
and *Nepta cataria* (catmint).

[2] W. H. Holmes: "Stone Implements of the Potomac-Chesapeake Tide-
water Province," Rep. Bur. Ethnol., 1893–4, Wash., 1897, xv, 1–152.

Professor William H. Holmes has demonstrated inductively (by working out the initial methods of chipping and flaking himself) that even among recent American Indians, like those of the Piney Branch quarries in the District of Columbia, the process of shaping and specializing the leaf-shaped flints was probably not different from that employed by Paleolithic man or even in what seem to be the rude artefacts of Eolithic man. There is apparently no distinction in space and time in the flaking of prehistoric and primitive implements. Similarly, ethnologists, as we have said, find that the folk-lore and other traditions and superstitions of primitive peoples have a strong family likeness at all times and places. The common point of convergence of all medical folk-lore is the notion that spirits or other supernatural agencies are the efficient causes of disease. Primitive medicine is inseparable from primitive modes of religious belief.

Savage man, untutored because inexperienced, first of all confused life with motion. Like Mime in Wagner's "Siegfried," he was puzzled if not awed by the rustling of leaves in the forest, the crash and flash of thunder and lightning, the flicker and play of sunlight and firelight, and he could see no causal relation between a natural object and its moving shadow, a sound and its echo, flowing water and the reflections on its surface. Winds, clouds, storms, earthquakes, and other sights and sounds in nature were to him the outward and visible signs of malevolent gods, demons, spirits or other supernatural agencies. The natural was to him the supernatural, as it still is to many of us. He therefore worshiped the sun, the moon, the stars, trees, rivers, springs, fire, winds, and even serpents, cats, dogs, apes, and oxen; and, as he came to set up carved stocks and stones to represent these, he passed from nature-worship to fetish-worship. Disease, in particular, he was prone to regard at first as an evil spirit or the work of such a spirit, to be placated or cajoled, as with other deities, by burnt offerings and sacrifice. A further association of ideas led him to regard disease as something produced by a human enemy possessing supernatural powers, which he aimed to ward off by appropriate spells and sorcery, similar to those employed by the enemy himself. Again, what he saw in dreams, or in an occasional nightmare from gluttony, suggested the existence of a spirit-world apart from his daily life and of a soul apart from his body, and in this way he hit upon a third way of looking at disease, as the work of offended spirits of the dead, whether of men, animals, or plants. These three views of disease are common beliefs of the lowest grades of human life. Savages, as a rule, cheerfully accept all three, while a lingering belief in human sorcery and the displeasure of the dead is always a trait of the peasant and sometimes of his descendants in "civil-

ized" communities.   Among savages, such beliefs usually go hand
in hand with shamanism, an intermediate stage between polytheism and monotheism, which assumes a Supreme Being or Great
Spirit, with lesser divinities and demons subordinated.   With the
beginnings of shamanism we have everywhere the advent of the
medicine man and the bilbo or witch-doctor, who assumes a solemn
supervisory relation to disease and its cure, not unlike that of the
priest to religion.   The shaman handles disease almost entirely
by psychotherapeutic manœuvers, which serve to awaken a cor-
responsive state of autosuggestion in his patients.   Whether North
American Indian or Asiatic Samoyed, he does his best to frighten
away the demons of disease by assuming a terrifying aspect, covering himself with the skins of animals so as to resemble an enormous
beast walking on its hind legs, resorting to such demonstrations as
shouting, raving, slapping his hands or shaking a rattle, and pretending (or endeavoring) to extract the active principle of the disease by sucking it through a hollow tube.   To prevent future attacks, in other words, to keep the demon away for the future, he
provides his patient with a special fetish or amulet to be worn or
carried about his person.   Furthermore, any fantastic thing he
may elect to do or not to do, such as passing in or out of a door or
stepping over an object with intention, he considers in the light
of "making medicine."   We may smile at these phases of shaman-
istic procedure, but, except for the noise, they are not essentially
different from the mind-medicine or faith-healing of our own day.
Both rely upon psychotherapy and suggestion, and for a sick savage, the fantastic clamor made about him might be conceivably as
effective as the quieter methods of Christian Science to a modern
nervous patient.

Apart from shamanism, the actual medical knowledge of
primitive man, given his limitations, was far from contemptible.
As the folk-lorists point out, the function of the medicine man was
a limited one, and the art of healing, even in its lowest stages, never
progressed very far so long as it was under the sway of priestcraft
and sorcery.   As the savage advanced a little further in the knowledge which is gained from experience, it was natural that some
special talent for herb-doctoring, bone-setting, and rude surgery
should be developed and employed as a special means of livelihood
by certain individuals.   Along with these nature-healers there
went, of course, the inevitable "wise-women," who followed herb-
therapy and midwifery, and such specialists soon perceived that
a number of poisons are also remedies under various conditions.
Medicine, which Huxley has so truly styled the foster-mother of
many sciences, really began with this crude plant-and-poison lore
of primitive peoples.

Primitive man's knowledge of medicinal simples was exactly like the drug phase of our modern therapeutics,—extensive, if not intensive,—and where he made mistakes it was (as in our own case) due to the cause which Kant assigns for all human error—the inveteracy of the *post hoc, propter hoc* tendency in the human mind. Like many physicians today, he tried to treat the disease rather than the patient, not realizing (as we are just beginning to realize) that the dynamic effect of a drug upon the patient's body depends as much upon the delicate chemical adjustments of that body as upon the composition of the drug itself. Whenever many different remedies are proposed for a disease, it usually means that we know very little about treating the disease, and the same thing is true of a drug which is vaunted as a panacea or cure-all for many diseases. "In listening to the praises of these panaceas," said Peter Krukenberg, the old Halle clinician, "we seem to be actually standing before the booth of a mountebank."[1] We are not much better off than early man in this respect. Thus, the hieratic writings of the Egyptian papyri reveal an unusually extensive materia medica, the excellence of which is vouched for in the Homeric poems, and which can today be duplicated, in extent at least, in the materia medica of old civilizations like China or Japan, or even in our own bulky pharmacopeias. We find that savages in different countries know instinctively the most fatal arrow-poisons— curare, ouabain, veratrin, boundou—as well as the virtues of drugs, like opium, hashish, hemp, coca, cinchona, eucalyptus, sarsaparilla, acacia, kousso, copaiba, guaiac, jalap, podophyllin, or quassia. Not to go further than our own country, we find the North American Indians aware that arbutus is "good" for rheumatism; lobelia for coughs and colds; wild sage tea, goldenseal, flowering dogwood, and prickly ash berries for fevers; elder, wild cherry, and sumac for colds and quinsies; wild ginger, ginseng, and euphorbia for digestive disorders; inhalations of pennyroyal for headache; sassafras or violet leaves for wounds and felons; and the roots of sassafras and sarsaparilla for "cooling and purifying the blood." In 1535–36, the Iroquois around Quebec, as Jacques Cartier relates, treated scurvy in his crew very successfully with an infusion of the bark and leaves of the hemlock spruce; and the French at Onondaga in 1657 found the sassafras leaves, recommended by the same tribe, "marvelous" for closing wounds of all kinds.[2] The "Materia Medica Americana" (1780) of the old Anspach-Bayreuth

---

[1] Cited by Baas.

[2] See A. Hrdlička: Bur. Am. Ethnol., Bull. No. 34, 231–253, and Yager: "Medicine in the Forest," Oneonta, N. Y., 1910. Yager notes the infrequency of panaceas and gunshot prescriptions among the North American Indians; each remedy was administered by itself for a given condition.

surgeon Schoepf, who came over with the Hessian troops during the war of the Revolution, shows that the Anglo-Saxon settlers in the New World had already learned many wrinkles in herb-therapy from the red men, in addition to the very rich medical folk-lore which they undoubtedly brought with them from Old England. The plant-lore of rural England included a knowledge of the virtues of camomile-, sage-, and dandelion teas as laxatives; of marjoram and primrose root for headache; of wormwood as a tonic; of valerian for the "nerves"; of agrimony and parsley for jaundice; of meadow-saffron (colchicum) for gout; of fennel, eye-bright (euphrasy), and rue for bad eye-sight; of male fern and peach-leaves for worms; of tansy as a vermifuge and abortifacient; of horehound, marshmallow or candied elecampane for coughs and colds; of foxglove as "the opium of the heart"; and of such "vulnerary plants" as bryony, agrimony, hare's ears, moonwort, alehoof, and goldenrod. English poetry and folk-lore are full of references to thyme and marjoram, rosemary and rue, mistletoe and ash, as well as poisons like hemlock, leopard's bane (aconite), the deadly nightshade (belladonna), "the juice of cursed hebenon" (yew), and henbane (hyoscyamus), which Aretaeus regarded as a cause of insanity and to which Shakespeare refers in the same spirit as

> . . . the insane root
> That takes the reason prisoner.

Asphodel, or dittany, is often mentioned in the Homeric poems as a balm against the pain of newly inflicted wounds, and the same tradition is still current among the country folk of Lancashire, Ireland, and the moors of Scotland. Kipling has summed up the whole matter in a charming verse—

> Alexanders and Marigold,
> Eyebright, Orris and Elecampane,
> Basil, Rocket, Valerian, Rue,
> (Almost singing themselves they run),
> Vervain, Dittany, Call-me-to-you—
> Cowslip, Melilot, Rose of the Sun.
> Anything green that grew out of the mould
> Was an excellent herb to our fathers of old.

In the use of natural or physical means against disease we discover that primitive man, with his well-ventilated habitations and his hardy life in the open air, has advantages which his civilized brother often seeks or finds only on compulsion. The Indian knew, for example, the importance of keeping the skin, bowels, and kidneys open, and, to this end, the geyser, the warm spring, and the sweat-oven were his natural substitutes for a Turkish bath. Emesis or catharsis, followed by a vapor bath and a cold plunge, set off by a dose of willow-bark decoction (salicin), was the North American Indian's successful therapeutic scheme in the case of intermittent and remittent fevers; a vapor bath and cimicifuga were his mainstays against rheumatism. Like the ancient Babylonians, he had his fixed periods for ritual emesis and catharsis (e. g., the green-corn feast), much as our forefathers used zodiacal calendars for blood-letting. Massage was long known and practised by the Indians, Japanese, Malays and East Indians; hypnotism by the Hindus; inoculation against smallpox by the Hindus, Persians and Chinese. Lady Mary Wortley Montagu got her idea of variolation from the East, and it is still employed among the North and Central African tribes and races (Arnold Klebs).[1] The early Japanese employed the moxa as the Chinese did acupuncture. The Chinese of the fifteenth century also knew of the use of spectacles, and snow-spectacles have been employed by polar tribes.

Surgery became a science in recent times, not so much through individual skill or specialization of instruments, as through the introduction of two new factors—anesthesia and antisepsis. Primitive surgery included all the rudiments of the art. The earliest surgical instrument was in all probability not the specialized leaf-shaped flint or "celt," already referred to, but rather some fragment unusually sharpened as to edge and point by accidental flaking,[2] as in the obsidian knives of Peru. By means of these sharpened flints or of fishes' teeth, blood was let, abscesses emptied, tissues scarified, skulls trephined, and, at a later period, ritual operations like circumcision were performed, as we have seen, with the primitive celts themselves. Trephining for epilepsy or other cerebral disorders goes back to prehistoric times, the finds showing that it was often done more than once upon the same person, the bits of skull excised being used as amulets. It is said that trephining is still practised among the Aymaras of Bolivia and the Quichuas of Peru,[3] and another evidence of it is the curious cross-wise mutilation along the lines of the coronal and sagittal sutures, first noticed as a common practice among the Loyalty Islanders by an English missionary, Rev. Samuel Ella, in 1874,[4] and which Manouvrier found afterward in neolithic female crania

---

[1] Klebs: Johns Hopkins Hosp. Bull., Baltimore, 1913, xxiv, 70.

[2] The writer is indebted to Prof. William H. Holmes for this important information.

[3] A. Bandelier: Ueber Trepanieren unter den heutigen Indianern Bolivias (Internat. Cong. Americanists, 1894). Mozans, in his "Along the Andes and down the Amazon" (New York, 1911), pp. 206, 207, is of opinion that the leaves of Erythroxylon coca, when chewed, have anesthetic properties, of which he gives a remarkable instance. This would explain how easily the Peruvians may have accomplished trephining with the aid of a sharp piece of flint or obsidian.

[4] Ella: Med. Times & Gaz., London, 1874, i, 50.

from Seine-et-Oise and called the "sincipital T" (1895).[1]
Primitive man's wounds were dressed with moss or fresh
leaves, ashes or natural balsams, and, when poisoned, treated by
sucking or cauterization. Cupping was performed by means of
animals' horns. The revulsive effects of some accidental wound
or hemorrhage, or the natural and periodic process of menstruation, suggested, no doubt, the advantages of blood-letting, which
was to become a sort of therapeutic sheet-anchor through the ages.
For couching a cataract or opening an abscess, even a sharp thorn
sufficed. The Dayaks of Borneo employ a sharp root (pinjampo).
In the more advanced phases of cultural development, pieces of
hard wood may have been pointed and edged, like the flint knives.
During the Bronze and Iron Ages expert skill in mental work
became accomplished fact, and surgical instrumentation was correspondingly improved. In the excavations of the Swiss Lake
Dwellings, which were discovered in 1853,[2] the different cultural
objects were found in successive layers, from the Stone Age up to
the Bronze and Iron Ages, and of these, the real beginnings of
northern European culture are now held to be the iron implements and objects found at La Tène. The phrase "La Tène"
symbolizes, for anthropologists, the starting-point of the cultural
periods following upon the three Ice Ages, with their two inter-
glacial periods, not because the Lake Dwelling finds are necessarily
the earliest iron objects known, but because they are the most
representative and characteristic. The La Tène finds, of date
about 300 B. C., entirely distinct from Egyptian, Indian or Greek
culture, include iron knives, needles, fibulæ, swords and lances,
with bracelets, necklaces, and ear-rings of Etruscan or West Celtic
pattern, and funeral urns containing human remains, showing that
cremation was the rule among the La Tène people. Some time
later, as, for example, among the Gallo-Roman finds in France, we
trace the evolution of the jointed or articulated surgical instruments like scissors, in which cutting was done by indirect action.[3]
With improved metal instruments, such cosmetic operations as
tattooing, infibulation, boring holes for ear-rings and nose-rings,
or the Mica operation (external urethrotomy), as well as amputation and lithotomy, could be essayed. The ancient Hindus performed almost every major operation except ligation of the ar-

---

[1] L. Manouvrier: Rev. mens. de l'École d'anthrop. de Paris, 1896, vi, 57;
1903, xiii, 431. Manouvrier thinks the sincipital T may have been identical
with the crucial cauterizations of the skull recommended by Avicenna and
others, if not a ritual mutilation. Grön regards it as a mode of judicial torture.
Sudhoff identifies it with a derivative procedure employed by the Alexandrian
surgeons for ocular catarrhs and mentioned by Celsus (vii, cap. xii, sect. 15).

[2] First investigated by Ferdinand Keller in 1853–4.

[3] See, M. Baudouin: Arch. prov. de chir., Paris, 1910, xix, 228–238.

teries; ovariotomy has been done by Indian and Australian natives, and Felkin witnessed a native Cesarean section in Uganda in 1878. Both operations are said to have been performed by German sowgelders in the sixteenth century.

The use of a soporific potion as a substitute for anesthesia goes back to remote antiquity, as symbolized in the twenty-first verse of the second chapter of Genesis: "And the Lord God caused a deep sleep to fall upon Adam, and he slept: and he took one of his ribs, and closed up the flesh instead thereof." From the soothing Egyptian nepenthe of the Odyssey, which Helen casts into the wine for Ulysses, to the "samme de shinta" of the Talmud, the "bhang" of the Arabian Nights, or the "drowsy syrups" of Shakespeare's time, the soporific virtues of opium, Indian hemp (*Cannabis indica*), the mandrake (*Atropa mandragora*), henbane (*Hyoscyamus*), dewtry (*Datura stramonium*), hemlock (*Conium*), and lettuce (*Lactucarium*) appear to have been well known to the Orientals and the Greeks;[1] and, in the thirteenth and fourteenth centuries, a mixture of some of these ingredients ("oleum de lateribus") was formally recommended for surgical anesthesia by the medieval masters, Hugh of Lucca and his son Theodoric.[2] Again, the use of such natural antiseptics as extreme dryness, smoke (creosote), honey, nitre, and wine was long known to early man, and in seeking an "artificial paradise" by means of narcotics and intoxicants like alcohol, opium, hashish, or mescal, priority certainly belongs to primitive man, to whom we also owe such private luxuries as tea,

---

[1] Poppy and Indian hemp were probably known to the Egyptians and consequently to the Greeks; mandragora to the Egyptians, Babylonians, and Hebrews. Theophrastus and Dioscorides were the first to mention the aphrodisiac and soporific properties of *Atropa mandragora*. It is not clear whether the mandrakes which Rachel sought of Leah (Genesis xxx, 14–16) were for the former purpose or to ease the pangs of childbirth. Dioscorides was the first to speak of the employment of mandragora for surgical anesthesia and his recipe was tried out with success by Sir Benjamin Ward Richardson. The mandrake is also mentioned by Celsus, Pliny, Apuleius, Paul of Ægina, and Avicenna, and the legends about the human shape of the root of the plant, its frightful shrieks when uprooted, and the necessity of employing a dog, hitched to it for this purpose, are a common feature of early English and German folk-lore. Drugging with Indian hemp or henbane ("tabannuj") was common among the ancient Hindus and the later Arabs, and Sir Richard Burton adds: "These have been used in surgery throughout the East for centuries before ether and chloroform became the fashion in the civilized West." (Arabian Nights, Denver edition, vol. iv, footnote to p. 71.) According to S. J. Mozans ("Along the Andes and Down the Amazon," New York, 1911, pp. 206, 207), the ancient Peruvian Incas probably utilized the anesthetic properties of the active principle of *Erythroxylon coca* in trephining. He cites a modern instance of a *coquero* (habitual chewer of coca leaves) who was run over by a car and experienced no apparent pain, although his foot had been taken off in the accident.

[2] Theodoric: Cyrurgia, lib. iv, cap. viii, "Confectio soporis," cited by Gurlt: Gesch. d. Chir., Berlin, 1898, i, 753. The reference is: Cyrurgia Guidonis (etc.), Venice, 1498, f. 146, 1 col.

coffee, cocoa, and tobacco. Medicine is curiously indebted to the non-medical man for many of its innovations. As Oliver Wendell Holmes has said:

> It learned from a monk how to use antimony, from a Jesuit how to cure agues, from a friar how to cut for stone, from a soldier how to treat gout, from a sailor how to keep off scurvy, from a postmaster how to sound the Eustachian tube, from a dairy-maid how to prevent smallpox, and from an old market-woman how to catch the itch-insect. It borrowed acupuncture and the moxa from the Japanese heathen, and was taught the use of lobelia by the American savage.[1]

In the field of obstetrics, we find the midwife to be one of the most ancient of professional figures. Engelmann's careful ethnic studies of posture in labor show the universal tendency of primitive and frontier women to assume attitudes[2] best adapted to aid or hasten delivery. The obstetric chair, first mentioned in the Bible and by the Greek writers, appears to be of great antiquity and is still used by some races of the far East.

We now come to a phase of primitive healing which is intimately connected with even the most recent aspects of the subject, namely, the effect of therapeutic superstitions and the actual cure of disease through the influence of the mind upon the body. This is a matter which can be approached in no derisive spirit, especially in the light of modern quackery and its successes. The closer we look into the ways of primitive man, the more liable it is to take down our own conceit. The untutored savage, as we have seen, thought that motion of any kind is equivalent to life. Wherein does he differ from the ultra-mechanistic physiologist who reverses the equation? Simply in this, that the mind of the savage is, as Black says,[3] like a looking-glass, reflecting everything and retaining nothing. As soon as an object passed from his observation its image disappeared from his mental vision and he ceased to hug the fact of its existence, still less to reason about it. The primitive mind is, as Rowland scornfully said of "the ordinary cultivated or legal mind," essentially "discontinuous." The scientific mind at least aims, in its methods, at continuity of thought. The folk-mind, even today, has this inevitable tendency to mix up the *post hoc* with the *propter hoc* and to confuse accidentals with essentials. Almost any one who has lived in the country, for instance, will be familiar with various rural superstitions relating to warts—that killing or handling a toad may cause them and that

---

[1] O. W. Holmes: Medical Essays, Boston, 1883, 289. For a more extensive presentation of this interesting subject, see George M. Gould's essay on "Medical Discoveries by the Non-Medical," in Jour. Amer. Med. Assoc., Chicago, 1903, xl, 1477–1487.

[2] George J. Engelmann: "Labor Among Primitive Peoples," St. Louis, J. H. Chambers & Co., 1882.

[3] W. G. Black: Folk-Medicine, London, 1883, p. 207.

they can be removed by some one touching them with pebbles or muttering charms over them; or with the notion that stump-water is good for freckles, while bad eye-sight can be remedied by the water into which the blacksmith has dipped his red-hot iron. In some parts of Holland, if a boy carrying water-lilies in his hand falls down, it is supposed to render him liable to fits. Readers of Longfellow's "Evangeline" may recall the line which refers to malaria as

> Cured by wearing a spider hung around one's neck in a nutshell.

In Norfolk, England, this spider was tied up in a piece of muslin and pinned over the mantelpiece as a remedy for whooping-cough. In Donegal, a beetle in a bottle was regarded as a cure for the latter disease; in Suffolk, to dip the child, head downward, in a hole dug in a meadow; in northeast Lincolnshire, fried mice; in Yorkshire, owl-broth; in other parts of England, riding the child on a bear; in Scotland, anything that might be suggested by a man riding upon a piebald horse.[1] Compare these fallacies, inept as they seem, with what has happened so often in the history of therapeutics. A patient's cure follows seemingly upon the administration of some new-fangled remedy or drug. Immediately, a causal relation is established and the discoverer rushes into print with the glad tidings. Statistics begin to mount up, until presently the correlation-curve is perceived to have so insignificant a slope that nothing positive can be affirmed of the remedy whatever. It is then speedily consigned to the limbo of forgotten things.[2] Not so with folk-remedies. The superstition becomes, as the derivation of the word implies, a "left-over"; and for a very important reason, namely, that in some cases "Nature cures the disease while the remedy amuses the patient"; in others a cure is, in all probability, brought about by the effect of the mind upon the body.

Black, the leading English authority on medical folk-lore, has made a careful and exhaustive classification of the different superstitions to which average suffering humanity is liable.[3] These include ideas as to the possible transference of disease, sympathetic relationships, the possibility of new-birth or regeneration, the effects of such accidental specific factors as color, number, solar

---

[1] Black: Op. cit., passim.

[2] J. C. Bateson cites a recorded case of a Turkish upholsterer who, during the delirium of typhus fever, drank from a pail of pickled cabbage and recovered, whereupon the Turkish doctors declared cabbage-juice a specific for the disease. The next patient dying under this régime, however, they modified the dogma by saying that cabbage-juice is good for typhus provided the patient be an upholsterer. Dietet. & Hyg. Gaz., N. Y., 1911, xxvii, pp. 297, 298.

[3] Op. cit., pp. 34–177.

and lunar influences, magic writings, rings, precious stones, parts of the lower animals, and charms connected with the names of the saints, the lore of plants, the evil eye, birth, death, and the grave. To look into these is to see clearly that, of all human impulses, "none burn higher and holier than that of mysticism." As the savage "sees God in clouds, or hears him in the wind," so his ancestors saw disease not as a quality or condition of the patient, but as something material and positive inside his body—a view held even by Paracelsus. From this idea arose a notion that disease could be transferred from one body to another, as where Pliny, in his Natural History, claims that abdominal pain can be transferred to a dog or a duck. Touching warts with pebbles, healing snake-bite by clapping the bleeding entrails of a bisected fowl to the wound (natural absorption), and the negro superstition of pegging a hank of the patient's hair into a tree in order to transfer chills and fever to the tree or its owner, are well-known forms of this curious belief. Sir Kenelm Digby proposed the following remedy for fever and ague: "Pare the patient's nails; put the parings in a little bag, and hang the bag around the neck of a live eel, and place him in a tub of water. The eel will die, the patient will recover."[1] Closely connected with this idea of transference was the old tradition of a sympathy existing between parts of bodies separated in space, amusingly illustrated in Sir Kenelm's weapon-salve, which was applied to the weapon instead of the wound, and in the same worthy's

> Strange hermetic powder
> That wounds nine miles point blank would solder,
> By skilful chemist with great cost
> Extracted from a rotten post.

The idea of material regeneration or new-birth is of Hindu (Aryan) origin and sprang from the primitive worship of the generative power in nature, the cult of the lingam and the yoni, the Hellenized form of which is so strikingly set forth in the fourth book of Lucretius. A cleft or hole in a rock or tree was regarded as symbolic of the sacred yoni, and children (even adults) afflicted with scrofula, spinal deformity, or other infirmities, were supposed to be freed from these bodily ills when passed through it. Traces of the Saxon form of this superstition survive in the "holed stone" near Lanyon, Cornwall, through which scrofulous children were passed naked three times, in the "Deil's Needle"[2] in the bed of the

---

[1] Cited by O. W. Holmes, "Medical Essays," Boston and New York, 1883, p. 381.

[2] See "The Stone in Scottish Folk-Medicine," by Dr. David Rorie, in the Caledonian Medical Journal, Glasgow, 1911, viii, pp. 410–415, giving an interesting photograph of the "Deil's Needle."

River Dee (Aberdeenshire) which was held to make barren women fertile if they crept through it, and in the Crick Stone in Morva, Cornwall, passage through which was esteemed a cure for any one with a "crick in the back." It was White of Selborne[1] who described the most recent form of this folk-belief, which consists in passing a child afflicted with hernia through a cleft in an ash-tree. As late as 1895–6, such trees were described as existing for this purpose in Suffolk and Richmond Park,[2] and there was once a similar tree in Burlington County, New Jersey. The Scotch custom of passing a consumptive child through a wreath of woodbine, the English trait of crawling under a bramble bush for rheumatism, and the "eye of the needle tree" on the island of Innisfallen, Killarney, squeezing through which insures long life and safe delivery to women with child, are mentioned by Black as variants of this superstition.

Color is a factor of great moment in folk-healing; in particular, red, which the Chinese and New Zealanders regard as hateful to evil spirits, and other peoples as a heat-producer. Red silken bands, necklaces of coral beads, red pills and red fire, as well as the red coral ring and bells with which the baby cuts its teeth, have all had their superstitious associations, and the virtues of the familiar red flannel cloth worn around the neck for sore throat and whooping-cough were supposed to reside "not in the flannel but in the red color."[3] Finsen's red-light treatment, to prevent pitting in smallpox, was once an ancient folk-belief, known to the Japanese, and employed successfully by John of Gaddesden in the case of the son of Edward II.[4] According to Valescus of Taranta, the rationale of the red-light treatment was the ancient "doctrine of signatures," in virtue of which a remedy was applied on account of some fancied resemblance, in shape or color, to the disease. The red cloth hangings around the smallpox patient were supposed to lower his temperature by drawing the red blood outward.

The idea that certain numerals can be sacred or malignant is of Accadian origin and connected with Chaldean and Babylonian astrology. Of mystic numbers, usually odd, three or a multiple of three is the most popular for luck, good or bad; seven or one of its multiples for supernatural powers. It was not for nothing that there were three Fates, three Furies, nine Muses, twelve months

---

[1] Gilbert White: Natural History of Selborne, 1789, p. 202 (cited by Black).

[2] Folk-Lore, London, 1896, vii, p. 303; 1898, ix, p. 330, with photos.

[3] Black: Folk-Medicine, London, 1883, 111.

[4] Recent investigation by Cholmeley has shown that both Gilbertus Anglicus (1290) and Bernard de Gordon (1305) antedated Gaddesden in references to the red-light treatment. The original reference to Gaddesden's paragraph is folio 51a of his "Rosa Anglica," second column, near the top.

and twelve signs of the zodiac, seven days to the week, twelve hours around the clock, and so on. Three handfuls of earth are always dropped on the coffin at burial. Palmists, fortune-tellers, and others of their kind work assiduously (as their signs read) "from nine to nine," and gamblers usually bet on odd numbers. In Scotland and Portugal, the seventh son of a seventh son is often regarded with horror or veneration, as one possessed of second sight and other uncanny attributes. Such folk-remedies as the West Sussex recipe for ague—"eat fasting seven sage leaves for seven mornings fasting"—are common enough. A reasonable aspect of number-lore in medical literature is the Hippocratic doctrine of crises and critical days, which probably derived from the teaching of Pythagoras, who had assimilated it from the Chaldean folk-traditions. Here the folk-lore of numbers has a germ of scientific truth in that there is a certain periodicity in some of the phenomena of disease. Another superstition which came from Chaldean astrology was the belief that the heavenly bodies had an influence upon disease. The sun, moon, stars, and planets were regarded as sentient, animated beings, exerting a profound influence upon human weal and woe, and, late into the seventeenth century, European mankind resorted to horoscopes (the "judicia astrorum") before attempting any enterprise of moment, and in particular to determine the proper time for blood-letting, emesis, and purgation. Moonshine was supposed to be potent alike in causing lunacy, conferring beauty, or curing warts and asthma; and the lunar influence is further seen in the common superstition that death occurs, as in the case of Shakespeare's Falstaff or of Barkis in "David Copperfield," at the turning of the tide. Comparable with the influence attributed to the stars is the idea, already mentioned, that disease is a scourge or punishment inflicted by gods or demons alike and remediable only through divine or diabolic intervention. The mischievous powers, whose ideas of good and evil were apparently so interchangeable, could be propitiated or conciliated only by sacrifice, which, as Jakob Grimm pointed out, had the double purpose (like the graft given to politicians) of keeping the powers in a good humor or of restoring good humor when necessary. The Greek myth of the arrows of far-darting Apollo, Bhowani, the cholera goddess of the Hindus, the many medical divinities of the Romans, the Indian and Samoyed lore of "magic bullets" (a *motif* in "Der Freischütz"), the passage in the Book of Job in which the patriarch attributes his sufferings to "the arrows of the Almighty," Martin Luther's conviction that "pestilence, fever and other severe diseases are naught else than the devil's work," Cotton Mather's definition of sickness as "Flagellum Dei pro peccatis mundi," the medieval figurations of death as a reaper (the "Schnitter Tod" of German folk-song), the folk-superstition that erysipelas (or "wild fire") originates from fairy malice, all illustrate the strength of this deep-rooted belief, which survived in the many sermons and prayers delivered in time of pestilence throughout the seventeenth and eighteenth centuries and even crops up in our day under various guises. Of a piece with this theory of disease was the malignant or benignant power which was supposed to attach to certain personalities. A child born on Easter Eve could cure tertian or quartan fever. Persons born "with a caul" were supposed to be clairvoyant. The power to heal scrofula by royal touch was part and parcel of the divine right of kings. In the West of Ireland, the blood of the Walshes, Keoghs, and Cahills is held to be an infallible remedy for erysipelas or toothache.[1] The medical lore of holy men, their special days, the diseases they presided over and the holy wells and other things blessed by them, form a special field in itself. The saints were supposed, as usual, to have the power of both inflicting and healing diseases, most of which were, however, associated with the names of several saints. Thus the names of St. Guy, St. Vitus, and St. With are eponymic for chorea; St. Avertin, St. John, and St. Valentine stood sponsors for epilepsy, while St. Antony, St. Benedict, St. Martial, and St. Genevieve presided over ergotism. Kerler[2] has compiled a bulky volume made up of indices of these patron saints of medicine alone.

A remarkable example of belief in the malevolence of personality is the superstition of the evil eye which causes Levantines to cross their fingers and Orientals to wear a crescent of horns over the forehead as a safeguard. In the Purana legend, Siva destroys a whole town with one withering glance, as Wotan destroys Hunding in "Die Walküre." There is a strong human prejudice against disconcerting, intensive, or forbidding appearances of the eye, as, indeed, for any abnormity, whether it be the strabismic *regard louche* of the French writers, the *jettatura* of the Corsican, the *mal-occhio* of the Italian, the filmy glance of some gypsies, the "steady, ambiguous look" which Arthur Symons ascribes to Orientals, or the stony stare of the blue-eyed northern races which a line of Tennyson's likens to the effect of the Gorgon's head. We dislike a stare. The phrase, *Sie fixieren mich, mein Herr!* has caused many a duel in Germany. We have a natural aversion for a person having but one eye, because, as Charles Dickens neatly said, "popular prejudice is in favor of two." Parti-colored eyes or eyes each of a different color are nowise re-

---

[1] Black: "Folk-Lore," London, 1883, p. 140.

[2] D. H. Kerler: "Die Patronate der Heiligen," Ulm, 1905.

assuring. The blind are sometimes known to develop dubious tendencies along sexual and other lines. It is easy to see from facts of this kind how the notion of the "evil eye" came to be ingrained in the beliefs of the Eastern and Levantine races, the Celts and the African Negro, and, in some cases, not without reason.

An essential part of the theory of divine or personal influence is the doctrine of amulets and talismans and, of course, the appropriate charms and spells that go with them. The amulet (from the Arabic "hamalet," a pendant) was an object usually hung or worn about the patient's body as a safeguard against disease or other misfortune. Amulets include a motley array of strange and incongruous objects, such as the bits of crania excised in prehistoric trephining, the voodoo fetishes of Hayti and Louisiana, teeth from the mouths of corpses, bones and other parts of the lower animals, the

> Finger of birth-strangled babe,
> Ditch-delivered by a drab

of the Weird Sisters in Macbeth, rings made of coffin-nails, widows' wedding-rings, rings made from pennies collected by beggars at a church porch and changed for a silver coin from the offertory, "sacrament shillings" collected on Easter Sunday, and the ikons and scapularies blessed by the dignitaries of the church. In the interesting exhibit of folk-medicine in the National Museum at Washington[1] a buckeye or horse-chestnut (*Æsculus flavus*), an Irish potato, a rabbit's foot, a leather strap previously worn by a horse, and a carbon from an arc light are shown as sovereign charms against rheumatism, and as Dr. Oliver Wendell Holmes used to point out, in his quizzical way, a belief in the efficacy of some of these anti-rheumatics is by no means confined to the European peasant and the negro. Other amulets in the Washington exhibit are the patella of a sheep and a ring made out of a coffin-nail (dug up out of a graveyard) for cramps and epilepsy, a peony root to be carried in the pocket against insanity, and rare and precious stones for all and sundry diseases.

The folk-lore of stones is of great antiquity, and the oldest prescription in existence,—that discovered in Egypt by W. Max Müller,—on exhibition in the Museum of Natural History in New York, calls for the exhibition of a green stone as a fumigation against hysteria. Dr. Robert Fletcher has shown[2] that "scopelism," the

---

[1] Visitors in Washington who are interested in folk-medicine and the cultural aspects of medical history will do well to see this unique collection, which was prepared by Rear-Admiral James M. Flint, Surgeon, U.S.N. (retired).

[2] American Anthropologist, Washington, 1897, x, pp. 201–213.

ancient Arabic custom of piling up stones in a field, either to prevent its tillage or as a menace of death to the owner, is to be found
everywhere as a symbol of the hatred of Cain for Abel, of the outlaw for the worker, of the barbarian for civilization. The lore
relating to mad-stones, snake-stones, eye-stones, and wart-stones
is considerable. Bezoars (enteroliths or other concretions from
the bodies of animals) were supposed to prevent melancholia and
all kinds of poisoning, including snake-bite. In England and Scotland, holed stones (fairy mill-stones, pixy's grindstones) and elf-
bolts (flint arrow-heads) were sometimes handsomely mounted
and worn about the person for protection. Precious stones came
to be esteemed, in the first instance, no doubt, for their rarity,
but equally for their supposed potency against disease. From the
engraved stones in the High-Priest's breast-plate, representing the
Twelve Tribes of Israel, to the birth-stones and month-stones of
our own day, there is a continuity of belief in the power of these
precious objects. Many women dread to wear an opal; there is
a supposed fatality about pearls, and the diamond now, as of
yore, will "preserve peace" and "prevent storms" in a household.
M. Josse, in Molière's "L'Amour Médecin," archly opines that
nothing is so well calculated to restore a drooping young lady to
health as "a handsome set of diamonds, rubies or emeralds."

Talismans (from the Arabic "talasim") were amulets or other
charms that were carefully guarded but not necessarily worn about
the person. These often consisted of written charms or "char-
acts," such as the Hebrew phylacteries or verses from the Bible,
Talmud, Koran, or Iliad. When the Indians saw Catlin, the ex-
plorer, reading the New York Commercial Advertiser, they thought
it was "a medicine cloth for sore eyes."[1] In the category of spoken
charms we must include all prayers, incantations, conjurations
and exorcisms used to drive away disease, as well as mystic words
like ABRACADABRA, SICYCUMA, Erra Pater, Hax Pax Max,
and the like.[2] Cato the Censor, who hated Greek medicine, endeavored to treat dislocations by repeating the following bit of
gibberish: "Huat hanat ista pista sista domiabo damnaustra
et luxato." The charms of the Byzantine period imposed a very
heavy onus of responsibility upon the several saints.

In surveying these different superstitions, one point becomes of
especial moment. It is highly improbable that any of the remedies mentioned actually cured disease, but there is abundant evidence of the most trustworthy kind that there have been sick
people who got well with the aid of nothing else. How did they
get well? Short of accepting the existence of supernatural forces,

---

[1] Black: Op. cit., p. 49.
3

[2] Ibid., pp. 167, 168.

we can only fall back upon such vague explanations as "the healing power of nature," the tendency of nature to throw off the
materies morbi or to bring unstable chemical states to equilibrium,
the latter being the most plausible. But, in many cases of a
nervous nature or in neurotic individuals, there is indubitable
evidence of the effect of the mind upon the body, and in such cases
it is possible that a sensory impression may so influence the vasomotor centers or the internal secretions of the ductless glands as to
bring about definite chemical changes in the blood, glands, or other
tissues, which, in some cases, might constitute a "cure." We know
that the reverse is possible, for example, in such occurrences as the
whitening of the hair from intense grief or fear, or the production
of convulsions in a suckling infant whose mother has been exposed
to anger, fright or other violent emotions before nursing it. As
Loeb strongly puts it, "Since Pawlow and his pupils have succeeded
in causing the secretion of saliva in the dog by means of optic and
acoustic signals, it no longer seems strange to us that what the
philosopher terms an "idea" is a process which can cause chemical
changes in the body."[1] Billings compares the sensation obtained
by placing the hand on a cold object in a dark room with the way
in which the blood "runs cold" when one realizes that this object
is a corpse.[2] Crile's important studies of surgical shock show the
strong analogy existing between the phenomena produced by
shock, the extreme passion of fear, and the symptom-complex of
Graves' disease, particularly in regard to the pouring out of the
thyroid secretions and the destruction of the Purkinje cells in the
brain. W. B. Cannon has shown that the adrenal veins in frightened animals are so full of adrenalin that this blood will inhibit
peristalsis when applied to the intestines. Extreme mental irritation or depression can produce dyspepsia, jaundice, chlorosis, or
general decline; the outward manifestations of hysteria are innumerable; and it is well known that it is bad for any person to go
under a surgical operation with the idea that he or she will not recover. A number of cases are on record of persons mentally depressed but not otherwise unwell who have realized the imminence
of their own death and predicted it with certainty. An impressive
instance was given from personal recollection by Dr. John S. Billings,
in his Lowell Institute lectures on the history of medicine in 1887.[3]
An officer of unusually strong and active physique and in the best
of health had sustained a slight flesh wound at the battle of Gettys-
burg. Becoming depressed in mind at the start, he declared he

[1] J. Loeb: "The Mechanistic Conception of Life," Chicago, 1912, p. 62.
[2] J. S. Billings: Boston Med. & Surg. Jour., 1888, cxviii, p. 59.
[3] J. S. Billings: Boston Med. & Surg. Jour., 1888, cxviii, p. 57.

would die, which he did on the fourth day. The postmortem showed that every organ was healthy and normal and the wound itself so trivial as to be a negligible factor. Crile's whole philosophy of "anoci-association" in surgery turns upon these mysterious mental influences, the combating of which constitutes the essence of psychotherapy. People who have become dyspeptic, bilious, or melancholy from worry or hope deferred, green-sick girls and women grown hysteric from disappointment in love, usually brighten up on receipt of good news. Babinski's dismemberment of hysteria identifies its phenomena solely with those capable of being produced in the hypnotic state. In treating the different neuroses, Charcot was guided almost entirely by his favorite maxim (from Coleridge): "The best inspirer of hope is the best physician," an aphorism which contains the germ of the Freudian theory of psychoanalysis—to "minister to the mind diseased" by removing the splinter of worry or misery from the brain, in order to restore the patient to a cheerful state of mental equilibrium. This fact has been utilized by all "nature healers" and faith-curists with varying degrees of success, and it is the secret of all charlatans, from Apollonius of Tyana, Valentine Greatrakes, Cagliostro, "Spot" Ward, Joanna Stevens, Mesmer, James Graham, John St. John Long, and the Zouave Jacob down to the days of Dowieism and Eddyism. It is also the secret of the influence of religion upon mankind, and here the priest or pastor becomes, in the truest sense, *ein Arzt der Seele.* In practical medicine, the principle now has a definite footing as psychotherapy. Psychotherapy cannot knit a fractured bone, antagonize the action of poisons, or heal a specific infection, but in many bodily ills, especially of the nervous system, its use is far more efficient and respectable than that of many a drug which is claimed to be a specific in an unimaginable number of disorders.

In fine, the lesson of the unity of primitive medicine, which is only a corollary to the general proposition of the unity of folk-lore, is that certain beliefs and superstitions have become ingrained in humanity through space and time, and can be eradicated only through the kind of public enlightenment which teaches that prevention is better than cure. The tendency of humanity to seek medical assistance in time of sickness or injury has been compared with the emotional element in religion, both being based upon "a deep-lying instinct in human nature that relief from suffering is an obtainable goal."[1] As the supernatural element in religion appeals to humanity in its moments of dependence and weakness, so for the weary and heavy-laden, the down-trodden of the earth in the

---

[1] B. M. Randolph: Washington Med. Ann., 1912, xi, p. 152.

past, medical superstitions were simply a phase of what Stevenson calls "ancestral feelings."

Thus the history of medicine is also the history of human fallibility and error. The history of the advancement of medical science, however, is the history of the discovery of a number of important fundamental principles leading to new views of disease, to the invention of new instruments, procedures, and devices, and to the formulation of public hygienic laws, all converging to the great ideal of preventive or social medicine; and this was accomplished by the arduous labor of a few devoted workers in science. The development of science has never been continuous, nor even progressive, but rather like that tangled, tortuous line which Laurence Sterne drew to represent the course of his whimsical narrative of Tristram Shandy. Ideas of the greatest scientific moment have been throttled at birth or veered into a blind alley through some current theologic prepossessions or deprived of their chance of fruition through human indifference, narrow-mindedness, or other accidental circumstances. It is no exaggeration to say that science owes most to the shining individualism of a few chosen spirits. Apart from this, "the success of a discovery depends upon the time of its appearance."

Buckle maintained that ignorance and low-grade minds are the cause of fanaticism and superstition, and, although his equation is reversible, we may consider this proposition true if we apply it to certain fanatical leaders of mankind, savage or civilized, who, as "moulders of public opinion," have retarded human progress. Chamfort said that there are centuries in which public opinion is the most imbecile of all opinions, but this reproach cannot be entirely saddled upon "the complaining millions of men." History teaches everywhere that permanent ignorance and superstition are the results of the oppression of mankind by fanatical overmen. In medicine, this is sometimes ludicrously true. "There is nothing men will not do," says Holmes, "there is nothing they have not done to recover their health and save their lives. They have submitted to be half-drowned in water, and half-choked with gases, to be buried up to their chins in earth, to be seared with hot irons like galley-slaves, to be crimped with knives like codfish, to have needles thrust into their flesh, and bonfires kindled on their skin, to swallow all sorts of abominations, and to pay for all this, as if to be singed and scalded were a costly privilege, as if blisters were a blessing, and leeches a luxury. What more can be asked to prove their honesty and sincerity?"[1] Yet while the lack of public enlightenment in certain periods produced the stationary or dis-

---

[1] O. W. Holmes: "Medical Essays," Boston, 1883, pp. 378, 379.

continuous mind, there are signs that the modern organized advancement of science may bring forth rich fruit for the medicine of the future through the social coöperation of the mass of mankind with the medical profession. As the ancient Greeks hung upon the teachings of Empedocles and Hippocrates, as modern humanity responded beautifully to the ideas of Jenner, Pasteur, and Lister, so there has been at no time a greater interest in the advancement of medicine and public health, as manifested in periodicals and newspapers, than in our own. The awakening of the people to looking after their own interests in regard to the organization and administration of public hygiene is, no doubt, the hope of the preventive medicine of the distant future. Yet, ever under the best conditions, it is still possible and probable that many highly intelligent and highly educated persons will continue to hug their whims and superstitions, consult quacks, and be otherwise amenable to psychotherapy.

EGYPTIAN MEDICINE

WHETHER the human race is descended from several distinct species or from a single common ancestor, "probably arboreal in his habits," is lost in the dim and unattainable past. The discoveries of the skeletal remains at Neanderthal (1856), Spy (1886), Krapina (1899), Heidelberg (1907), Le Moustier (1908), La Chapelle-aux-Saints (1909), and the recent Sussex find (Eoanthropus Dawsoni, 1912) indicate that, even in the paleolithic or chipped-flint period, there was already considerable diversity in the cranial characters of mankind and that, in prehistoric times, the human brain was developed at the expense of a simian body, increasing in volume as we go backward, which would seem slightly in favor of the contention of Virchow and other German anthropologists that humanity is diverse in origin. But whether the Pithecanthropus found in Java in 1891 be simian or human or, as its discoverer Dubois claimed, a mixture of both, all craniologic evidence seems to prove that prehistoric man was more closely akin to the higher (anthropoid) apes in structure than they are to the lower, a kinship which is also borne out by the medico-legal or "precipitin" test of blood-relationship. At the same time the gap between paleolithic and neolithic man is much greater than that between the people of the Later Stone Age and the civilizations of Egypt and Mesopotamia. There is no evidence of the existence of man before the Ice Age, and whether flint implements were actually chipped in the Eolithic period is not positively known; but the fact that all subsequent remains are found embedded in successive layers of strata points to a gradual and inevitable cultural development. In the Mousterian period[1] (the age of the Neanderthal skull), man was probably more ape-like than the Australian savage; in the Solutrian period, he was like the Bushmen and was already skilful in chipping flints; in the Magdalenian, he resembled the Mongolians and the Esquimaux. The Solutrians and Magdalenians were already mighty big-brained warriors and skilled artists, who knew how to bridle horses, make specialized weapons, devise clothing,

---

[1] The terms Acheulean, Mousterian, Solutrian, Magdalenian were introduced by the French anthropologist Gabriel de Mortillet to indicate the successive stages in the specialization of flint and other prehistoric implements found at St. Acheul, Le Moustier, Solutré and La Madeleine. They are now used in a purely arbitrary way to indicate cranial and skeletal remains found in sites corresponding, in order of geologic time, with these localities.

and execute most striking and life-like mural paintings and line engravings on stone, bone and ivory. That the Egyptian and Sumerian civilizations were nearer to these people than had formerly been conceived is indicated by the results of modern cave explorations and excavations. One of the most interesting facts of recent development is that arthritis deformans or rheumatic gout, a disease found in so many Egyptian mummies, is identical with the "cave-gout" (Höhlengicht) which Virchow found in bones of prehistoric men and bears and which is also common in the skeletons of the inhabitants of the early German forests. The fact that the neolithic chipped-flint knife was continually used by the Egyptians in embalming the dead connects their already complex civilization with prehistoric man.

Our principal sources of knowledge of the earliest known phases of Egyptian medicine are the Brugsch, Ebers and Hearst papyri; but even antedating these are certain pictures engraved on the door-posts of a tomb in the burial ground near Memphis and described by their discoverer, Mr. W. Max Müller, as being the earliest known pictures of surgical operations (2500 B. C.). Although we have reasons for believing that the Egyptians never carried surgery to the extent of opening the body, yet here[1] are clear and unmistakable representations of circumcision and possibly of surgery of the extremities and neck, the attitudes and the hieroglyphic inscriptions affixed indicating that the patients are undergoing great pain. The medicine chest of an Egyptian queen of the eleventh dynasty (2500 B. C.)[2] containing vases, spoons, dried drugs and roots is another important find. There is also an inscription on a tomb near the pyramids of Sakarah which shows it to be the resting place of a highly esteemed practitioner who served the fifth dynasty of Pharaohs about 2700 B. C. I-em-hetep ("He who cometh in peace") was a celebrated physician of the third dynasty (4500 B. C.) who was afterward worshiped at Memphis and had a temple erected in his honor upon the island of Philæ. He was the earliest known physician.

Besides the hieroglyphics, which were usually engraved or painted on stone, like the picture-writing of American or Australian savages, the Egyptian employed certain cursive scripts (hieratic and demotic), usually inscribed upon thin sheets of the papyrus plant. The most important of the medical papyri is that discovered by Georg Ebers at Thebes in 1872, which dates back to about 1550 B. C. It consists of 110 pages of hieratic or cursive

---

[1] W. Max Müller: Egyptological Researches, Washington, Carnegie Institution, 1906. See also J. J. Walsh: Jour. Am. Med. Assoc., Chicago, 1907, xlix, pp. 1593–1595.

[2] For a picture of the same, see Jour. Am. Med. Assoc., Dec. 23, 1905, 1392.

script, the text in black letter, the rubrics in red. Ebers himself supposed it to be one of the lost sacred or Hermetic Books of Thoth (Hermes Trismegistus), the moon god, who, like Apollo in Greece, was the special deity of medicine. This assumption has not stood the test of time, and the Ebers Papyrus, with its marginal notes and comments, is now regarded as a simple compilation.[1] It begins with a number of incantations against disease and then proceeds to list a large number of diseases in detail, with about 700 different remedies for the same. The most interesting parts are the extensive sections on the eye and ear and the descriptions of the ĀAĀ disease, the UHA disease and the Uhedu (painful swelling), all three of which have been thought by Joachim to be identical with different stages of the hookworm infection (chlorosis Ægyptiaca).[2] The large number of remedies and prescriptions cited in the Papyrus points to a highly specialized therapeusis, even in the sixteenth century B. C., but it cannot be claimed, as many seem to contend, that these 700 odd remedies indicate any special scientific advancement of the art of healing. We do not find a few well-selected drugs, as opium, hellebore, hyoscyamus, used, as the later Greek physicians employed them, with skill and discrimination, but Egyptian therapy must have been, of necessity, haphazard because, as we shall see, each Egyptian physician was a narrow specialist, confining himself to one disease or to diseases affecting one part of the body only. Many minerals and vegetable simples are mentioned, from the salts of lead and copper to squills, colchicum, gentian, castor oil and opium, and, as in some pharmacopeias of even the seventeenth and eighteenth centuries, these were compounded with such filthy ingredients as the blood, excreta, fats and visceral parts of birds, mammals and reptiles. A favorite Egyptian pomade for baldness consisted of equal parts of the fats of the lion, hippopotamus, crocodile, goose, serpent and ibex. Another consisted simply of equal parts of writing ink and cerebrospinal fluid. An ointment for the eye consisted of a trituration of antimony in goose-fat. Another for conjunctivitis employs a copper salt. A poultice for suppuration consisted of equal parts of a meal of dates and wheat chaff, bicarbonate of soda and seeds of endives.

---

[1] The hieratic writing of the Ebers Papyrus had first to be rendered into hieroglyphics, by a method devised at the Orientalists' Congress in 1874, and these were finally translated into German by Dr. H. Joachim of Berlin in 1890. One of the first to attempt to decipher the hieroglyphics on the Rosetta Stone (1799) was the English physician and physicist, Thomas Young. The difficult task was finally accomplished by Champollion.

[2] Joachim, Papyros Ebers, Berlin, 1890. Edwin Pfister, however, thinks that the āaā disease of the Ebers and Brugsch papyri was bilharziosis. See, Sudhoff's Arch., 1912–13, vi, pp. 12–20.

The most interesting part of the Ebers Papyrus is the last section of all, which treats of tumors. Here, as in the description of the ẮẮẮ disease, we find some approach to the accurate clinical pictures of Hippocrates, and many have supposed, on this slender evidence, that the Father of Medicine was indebted to Egypt for much of his knowledge. Some ethical precepts of the ancient Egyptian physicians are very much like the Hippocratic Oath in sentiment and expression, and this alone would point to the fact that pre-Hippocratic medicine in Greece had an origin closely connected with Egyptian medicine. There is, however, one marked point of divergence, namely, that later Egyptian medicine was entirely in the hands of priests, while Greek medicine, even at the time of the Trojan War, would seem to be entirely free from priestly domination, surgery in particular being often practised by Homer's warrior kings. Our principal authorities for the state of Egyptian medicine during the fifth century B. C. are Herodotus and Diodorus Siculus. From Herodotus we learn of the hygienic customs of the Egyptians, the gods of their worship, their ideas about medicine and their methods of embalming dead bodies. "The art of medicine," says Herodotus, "is thus divided among them: Each physician applies himself to one disease only, and not more. All places abound in physicians; some physicians are for the eyes, others for the head, others for the teeth, others for the intestines, and others for internal disorders."[1] Medical practice was rigidly prescribed by the Hermetic Books of Thoth, and if a patient's death resulted from any deviation from this set line of treatment, it was regarded as a capital crime. Aristotle, writing one century later, says, in his Politics, that physicians were allowed to alter the treatment after the fourth day if the patient did not improve.[2] The simple dress and frequent baths of the Egyptians were what is suitable in a subtropical climate and not unlike those of the Greeks. "They purge themselves every month, three days in succession," says Herodotus, "seeking to preserve health by emetics and clysters; for they suppose that all diseases to which men are subject proceed from the food they use. And, indeed, in other respects, the Egyptians, next to the Libyans, are the most healthy people in the world, as I think, on account of the seasons, because they are not liable to change."[3] This view of the old historian does not harmonize with the great frequency of rheumatoid arthritis in the Egyptian mummies, which was probably due to exposure to a moist climate during the inundations of the Nile. The account of Egyptian embalming in Herodotus is, in the

[1] Herodotus: ii, 84.   [2] Aristotle: Politics, iii, 15.
[3] Herodotus: ii, 77.

light of all recent investigations, authentic and accurate[1] and it shows that the Egyptians already knew the antiseptic virtues of extreme dryness and of certain chemicals, like nitre and common salt. The brain was first drawn out through the nostrils by an iron hook and the skull cleared of the rest by rinsing with drugs; the abdomen was then incised with a sharp flint knife, eviscerated, cleansed with wine and aromatics, filled with myrrh, cassia and spices and the wound sewed up. The body was then steeped for seventy days in sodium chloride or bicarbonate (natron) and afterward washed and enveloped completely in linen bandages smeared together with gum. The relatives put it in a wooden coffin, shaped like a man, which was deposited in the burial chamber along with four Canopic jars containing the viscera. As with our North American Indians, the departed spirit was furnished with food, drink and other appointments and conveniences, and there was a special ritual or Book of the Dead, which every Egyptian learned by heart, as a sort of Baedeker to the other world. According to Diodorus Siculus, the "parachistes," who made the initial incision with the flint knife, was held in such aversion that he was driven away with curses, pelted with stones, and otherwise roughly handled, if caught. On the other hand, the "taricheutes," who eviscerated the body and prepared it for the tomb, was revered as belonging to the priestly class. But this was probably only a perfunctory piece of ritualism. Sudhoff has recently published some interesting plates[2] representing the characteristic stone knives and iron hooks used by the Egyptian embalmers, and Comrie, in an interesting paper in Sudhoff's Archiv,[3] describes what are probably the earliest known surgical instruments of the ancient Egyptians (about 1500 B. C.), consisting of three saber-shaped copper knives with hooked or incurvated handles, found in a tomb near Thebes. They are characteristic specimens of the Bronze Age. Elliot Smith and Wood Jones have described the splints of palm fiber employed to mend fractures, and the mummies show that many fractures so healed did not escape shortening. Elliot Smith and Ruffer, in a most interesting monograph, have described a genuine case of Pott's disease in a mummy of the twenty-first dynasty (circa 1000 B. C.[4]).

The main interest of Egyptian medicine lies in its proximity and relationship to Greek medicine. The references in Homer to the skill of the Egyptian physicians in compounding drugs bring to

[1] Herodotus: ii, 86.

[2] Sudhoff: Arch. f. Gesch. d. Med., Leipz., 1911, v, pp. 161–171, 2 pl.

[3] Arch. f. Gesch. d. Med., Leipz., 1909, iii, pp. 269–272, 1 pl.

[4] G. Elliot Smith and M. A. Ruffer: "Pott'sche Krankheit an einer ägyptischen Mumie," Giessen, 1910.

mind the fact that the word "chemistry" itself is derived from *chemi* (the "Black Land"), the ancient name of Egypt, whence the science was called the "Black Art." Doubtless the ancient Greeks learned as much of medicine as of chemistry from these wise elders across the sea, who told Solon that his people were "mere children, talkative and vain, knowing nothing of the past"; who were so skilled in metallurgy, dyeing, distillation, preparing leather, making glass, soap, alloys and amalgams, and who, in Homer's time, probably knew more anatomy and therapeutics than the Hellenes. Yet, long before the Alexandrian period, Egyptian civilization had become absolutely stationary in character, and, in medicine, Egypt was going to school to Greece.[1] As the Egyptian gods—the dog or ibis-headed Thoth (the Egyptian Hermes), the cat-headed Pacht, their deity of parturition, the beak-nosed Horus, the horned Chnum, the veiled Neith at Sais, remained forever the same, while the Greek mythology was a continuous and consistent evolution of deific figures of permanent beauty and human interest, so Greek medicine was destined to go beyond Egyptian or Oriental medicine as surely as Greek poetry, sculpture and architecture surpassed the efforts of these peoples in the same kind.

---

[1] See, for example, Sudhoff's studies of the Greek papyri of the Alexandrian period (Studien z. Gesch. d. Med., Puschmann-Stiftung, Nos. 5, 6, Leipzig, 1909).

SUMERIAN AND ORIENTAL MEDICINE

In the book of Genesis we read that Nimrod was "a mighty hunter before the Lord" and that "the beginning of his kingdom was Babel and Erech, and Accad and Calneh in the land of Shinar." The land of Shinar (Shumer or "Sumer") was the southern part of Babylonia, comprising the strip of country between the Euphrates and the Tigris down to the Persian Gulf, and northern Babylonia was called Accad. The Babylonian sovereigns and their Assyrian conquerors always styled themselves "kings of Sumer and Accad." Before the advent of the Babylonians, it is supposed that an original non-Semitic or Sumerian race existed, about 4000–3000 B. C., who laid the foundations of modern civilization by the invention of pictorial writing and the development of astronomy. Others assume that the cursive script of the Sumerians, which, like Chinese writing, runs from right to left, was in the first instance only a sort of cipher-code used by the dominant Semitic race. In any case Mesopotamia was the starting-point of Oriental civilization, of which the Babylonians were undoubtedly the principal founders. They were skilled in mathematics and astronomy, originated the decimal system of notation, weights and measures, made the divisions of time into twelve months in the year, seven days in the week, sixty minutes and seconds in the hour and minute respectively, and divided the circle, as we do, into 360 degrees. They invented the cuneiform inscriptions, reading from left to right, they knew much about military tactics and the art of war and were variously skilled in music, architecture, pottery, glassblowing, weaving and carpet-making. Layard found a plano-convex lens of rock-crystal in his explorations at Nineveh.

It is said that astronomy is the oldest of the sciences and, in all early civilizations we find it applied to the practical affairs of life as astrology. This trait is the essence of Sumerian or Accadian medicine. Wars, epidemics, famines, successions of monarchs and other affairs of public or private life were closely studied in relation to the precession of the equinoxes, eclipses, comets, changes of the moon, and stars, and other meteorologic and astronomic events, and from these fatalistic coincidences arose the idea that certain numerals are lucky or unlucky. Thus astrology and the interpretation of omens merged into prognosis and, as with all early civilizations, the first Babylonian physician was a

44

priest or the first priest a physician. Inspection of the viscera, an essential part of augury, led to inspection of the urine, and, among the Babylonians, soothsaying was concentrated upon the liver, terra-cotta models of which, about 3000 years old, have been found, divided into squares and studded with prophetic inscriptions. Neuburger points out how the priestly interest in omens might have led to the collection and collocation of clinical observations, such as facial expression, the appearances of the urine, the saliva, the blood drawn in blood-letting, and other signs which were used as indices or tokens of recovery or death; and he goes on to say that the next step in the direction of scientific advancement would be the elimination of the supernatural from the matter. This step, unfortunately, is and has been the hardest one to take in medical reasoning. So we find the Babylonian physicians regarding disease as the work of demons, which swarmed in the earth, air and water, and against which long litanies or incantations were recited. The real beginnings of the practice of medicine among them have been described by Herodotus as follows: "They bring out their sick to the market place, for they have no physicians; then those who pass by the sick person confer with him about the disease, to discover whether they have themselves been afflicted with the same disease as the sick person, or have seen others so afflicted; thus the passers-by confer with him, and advise him to have recourse to the same treatment as that by which they escaped a similar disease, or as they have known to cure others. And they are not allowed to pass by a sick person in silence, without inquiring into the nature of his distemper."[1] With the Babylonians, as Montaigne quaintly observes, "the whole people was the physician," and they eventually reached the stage at which, like the Egyptians, they had a special physician for every disease. Whether they ever got beyond this stage we do not know, but we learn from the Code Hammurabi (2250 B. C.) that the medical profession in Babylon advanced far enough in public esteem to be rewarded with adequate fees, carefully prescribed and regulated by law. Thus ten shekels in silver was the statutory fee for treating a wound or opening an abscess of the eye with a bronze lancet, if the patient happened to be a "gentleman"; if he were a poor man or a servant, the fee was five or two shekels respectively. If the doctor caused the patient to lose his life or his organ of vision, he had his hands cut off in the case of the gentleman or had to render value for value in the case of a slave. It is clear from all this that the Babylonian physicians owned slaves and sometimes operated for cataract. Here as everywhere, it was surgery that made the first

---

[1] Herodotus: i, 80.

step in the right direction. Internal medicine, among both the Persians and the Babylonians, was occupied mainly in endeavoring to cast out the demons of disease. Some advance in hygiene was made, however, for the excavations of the huge Babylonian drains, of which models were recently exhibited at the Dresden Exposition, show that they understood the proper disposal of sewage.

Closely connected with Sumerian medicine in point of time is the medicine of the Jewish people, in relation to the Assyrian captivity (B. C. 722) and the Babylonian captivity (B. C. 604). The principal sources of our knowledge of Jewish medicine are the Bible and the Talmud, the first throwing only such light upon the subject as we should expect to find in the details of a legendary historic narrative. In the Old Testament, disease is an expression of the wrath of God, to be removed only by moral reform, prayers and sacrifice; and it is God who confers both health and disease: "I will put none of these diseases upon thee, which I have brought upon the Egyptians: for I am the Lord that healeth thee" (Exodus xv, 26). The priests acted as hygienic police in relation to contagious diseases, but there is not a single reference in the Bible to priests acting as physicians. The latter were a class apart, of whom we read, for example, that Joseph "commanded his servants the physicians to embalm his father" (Gen. l, 2), that King Asa consulted physicians instead of the Lord and "slept with his fathers" for his pains (II. Chron. xvi, 12, 13), or that if two men fight and one of them be injured to the extent of having to keep his bed, the other "shall pay for the loss of his time, and shall cause him to be thoroughly healed" (Exodus xxi, 19). The Prophets, on the other hand, frequently performed miracles, as where both Elijah and Elisha raised children from the dead. A striking example of relation between the Divine wrath and the efficacy of prayer is to be found in the case of Hezekiah, who, "sick unto death," and told by the Lord to set his house in order, turned his face to the wall; his prayers were answered by the Prophet Isaiah who, at the Divine instance, ordered that a lump of figs be applied to the afflicted part, with the result that Hezekiah recovered (II Kings xx, 1–8). Besides the physicians and the high priests, who acted as public health officers, there were professional midwives, who are mentioned in the cases of Rachel, of Tamar, and particularly in the striking reference to the ancient Oriental usage of the obstetric chair, in the first chapter of the second book of Exodus, where Pharaoh commands the midwives to slay all Jewish infants of the male sex, "when ye do the office of a midwife to the Hebrew women, and see them upon the stools." Maternal impressions form the subject of the second half of the thirtieth chapter of Genesis, in which Jacob retaliates upon Laban for the deception which the latter practised upon him about Leah and Rachel by outwitting him in a method of raising speckled and spotted live-stock hardly explicable by Mendel's law. The use of the primitive chipped flint in ritual circumcision is referred to in the second book of Exodus (IV, 25) where Zipporah, the wife of Moses, "took a sharp stone and cut off the foreskin of her son." This is the only surgical procedure mentioned in the Bible, but the use of the roller-bandage in fractures is referred to in Ezekiel (XXX, 22) as follows: "Son of man, I have broken the arm of Pharaoh king of Egypt; and, lo, it shall not be bound up to be healed, to put a roller to bind it, to make it strong to hold the sword." Wounds were dressed, as among all ancient peoples, with oil, wine and balsams. Of the different diseases referred to in the Bible, the most important are leprosy, the "issue," and the several plagues visited upon Israel, notably the plague of Baal-peor, in which twenty-four thousand perished (Numbers XXV, 9). Yet these diseases are so vaguely alluded to that it is impossible to identify them with any latter-day equivalents. Modern dermatologists contend, for instance, that Biblical leprosy (zaraath), of which Naaman was healed by dipping himself "seven times in Jordan," and which was transferred (in the folk-lore sense) to Gehazi, so that "he went out from his presence a leper as white as snow," was, in reality, psoriasis. On the other hand, Iwan Bloch and others maintain that the venereal plagues mentioned in the Bible (Baal-peor and the rest) are not the same as present-day lues or gonorrhea.[1] The fiery serpents mentioned in Numbers (XXI, 7) may have been the dracunculus, and Castellani holds that the disease with "emerods" in I. Samuel (V, 6) was bubonic plague, because the "mice died and marred the land."

The principal interest in these Biblical diseases lies in the remarkable efforts made to prevent them. The ancient Hebrews were, in fact, the founders of public hygiene and the high priests were true medical police. The book of Leviticus contains the sternest mandates in regard to touching unclean objects, the proper food to be eaten, the purifying of women after child-birth, the hygiene of the menstrual periods, the abomination of sexual perversions and the prevention of contagious diseases. In the remark-

---

[1] Medical scholars, who speculate about these uncertain details in such dogmatic fashion, fail to consider the point, well known to mathematicians and physicists, that the inherent probability of any occurrence tends the closer to zero the further we get away from it, and that the effect of any event tends to "die out asymptotically" in indefinite or infinite time. Æsculapius was very much of a reality to Homer, Hippocrates and Celsus. To us he is well-nigh a myth. Bloch forgets that the logical opposite of the "morbus Americanus" theory of syphilis, which he advances with such fanatical zeal, is just as likely to be true as the theory itself.

able chapters on the diagnosis and prevention of leprosy, gonorrhea and leukorrhea (Leviticus XIII–XV), the most definite common-sense directions are given in regard to segregation, disinfection (even to the point of scraping the walls of the house or destroying it completely), and the old Mosaic rite of incineration of the patient's garments and other fomites. In the Middle Ages, these precepts from Leviticus were still in force against leprosy. Who but does not admire the rigorous Hebrew regulation of sexual hygiene which, however severe, enforced exogamy, put a ban upon perversions, and invested the figure of a good and virtuous woman with that peculiar halo of respect which has been preserved by all highly civilized nations down to the present time.[1] The institution of the Sabbath day gave tired workaday humanity a sort of permanent splint to rest upon. In short the chief glory of Biblical medicine lies, as Neuburger rightly says, in the institution of social hygiene as a science. How highly the physician was esteemed by the Hebrews of a later time may be gathered from the impressive language of Jesus, son of Sirach (180 B. C.):

1. Honour a physician according to thy need of him with the honours
   due unto him:
   For verily the Lord hath created him.
2. For from the Most High cometh healing:
   And from the King he shall receive a gift.
3. The skill of the physician shall lift up his head:
   And in the sight of great men he shall be admired.

The Talmud is essentially a law book, dating from the second century A. D., and the information about Jewish medicine conveyed in it is, in consequence, of a more definite and detailed character than we should expect to find in the half-legendary narrative of the Bible. Its most interesting feature is the light it throws upon later Jewish anatomy and surgery and upon the knowledge of post-mortem appearances which the Hebrews gained through the inspection of meat for food. Anatomy of any kind before the time of Vesalius was a thing of shreds and patches and Jewish anatomy was no exception to the rule. Only a very few of the parts of the body are mentioned in the Bible and these references are as vague and general as those in the Iliad. In the Talmud, the number of bones in the skeleton is variously estimated at 248 or 252, and, of these, one, the bone Luz, which was supposed to lie somewhere between the base of the skull and the coccyx, was regarded as the indestructible nucleus from which the body is to be raised from the dead at the Resurrection. This myth, which modern

---

[1] It is worthy of note that the Mosaic mandates against bestiality, sexual inversion, etc., in Exodus (xxi, xxii) and Leviticus (xviii) are the beginnings of medical jurisprudence.

rabbinical authority holds to have originated from the ancient Egyptian rite of "burying the spinal column of Osiris," was exploded by Vesalius in a striking passage in the "Fabrica."[1] The Talmud displays considerable knowledge of the œsophagus, larynx, trachea, the membranes of the brain and the generative organs. The pancreas is called the "finger of the liver" and structures like the spleen, kidneys and spinal cord are frequently mentioned but not described. The blood is held to be the vital principle, identical with the soul, and the heart is essential to life. Respiration is likened to burning. The effect of the saliva upon food and the churning movements of the stomach are noted, and the liver is believed to elaborate the blood. Among the Hebrews, the flesh of diseased or injured animals was always considered unfit for food, and the autopsies, made upon slaughtered animals to determine what was "kosher" and "trepha," threw a light upon pathologic appearances which the ancient Greeks never gained. Hyperemia, caseous degeneration and tumors of the lungs were noted, as also atrophy and abscess of the kidneys and cirrhosis and necrosis of the liver. Talmudic surgery included the usual "wound-surgery," with treatment by sutures and bandages, applications of wine and oil and the device of freshening the edges of old wounds to secure more perfect union. Venesection, leeching and cupping were common and, before attempting the major operations, a sleeping draught ("samme de-shinta") was administered. Cesarean section, excision of the spleen, amputations, trephining, and the operation for imperforate anus in infants were known, as also the use of the speculum and the uterine sound. Fractures and dislocations were discussed and crutches, artificial limbs and artificial teeth employed.[2] There is no evidence of specialized medical education among the Jews until the Alexandrian period, and individual Hebrew physicians did not attain any particular prominence until the Middle Ages and, more especially, in the Modern Period.

As the Hebrews attained the highest eminence among Oriental peoples in hygiene, so the ancient Hindus excelled all other nations of their time in operative surgery. In the earliest Sanskrit documents, the Rig Veda (1500 B. C.) and the Atharva Veda, medicine is entirely theurgic, and treatment consists of the usual spells and incantations against the demons of disease or their human agents, the witches and wizards. In the Brahminical period (800 B. C.–1000 A. D.), medicine was entirely in the hands of the

---

[1] See F. H. Garrison, "The Bone called 'Luz,'" New York Med. Jour., 1911, xcii, pp. 149–151.

[2] For further information about Biblical and Talmudic medicine, see Julius Preuss, Biblisch-Talmudische Medizin, Berlin, 1911, and the article by Dr. Charles D. Spivak in the Jewish Encyclopedia, N. Y., 1904, viii, pp. 409–414.

Brahmin priests and scholars, and the center of medical education
was at Benares. The three leading figures of Brahminical medicine were Charaka, who lived about the beginning of the Christian
era, Susruta (fifth century A. D.) and Vagbhata (seventh century
A. D.). Of these the most remarkable is Susruta, whose work,
bearing the same name, is the great storehouse of Aryan surgery.
Indian medicine was particularly weak in its anatomy, which consisted of purely fanciful numerations of unimaginable parts of the
body, as 360 bones, 800 ligaments, 500 muscles, 300 veins and so
on. Hindu physiology presupposes that the vital processes are
actuated by means of the air (below the navel), the bile (between
the navel and the heart) and the phlegm (above the heart), from
which are derived the seven proximal principles, chyle, blood,
flesh, fat, bone, marrow, and semen. Health consists in a normal
quantitative relationship of these primary constituents, disease in a
derangement of their proper proportions. Diseases are again
minutely subdivided, the Susruta enumerating as many as 1120,
which are classed in the two grand divisions of natural and supernatural diseases. Diagnosis was carefully made and included
inspection, palpation, auscultation and the use of the special senses.
Semeiology and prognosis combined acute observation with the
usual folk superstitions. As examples, witness the Susruta's very
recognizable description of malarial fever, which is attributed to
mosquitos, or the passage in the Bhâgatava Purana which warns
people to desert their houses "when rats fall from the roofs above,
jump about and die," presumably from plague. In therapeutics,
a proper diet and regimen were carefully detailed, and baths, enemata, emetics, inhalations, gargles, blood-letting and urethral
and vaginal injections employed. The materia medica of India
was particularly rich. Susruta mentions 760 medicinal plants, of
which nard, cinnamon, pepper, cardamoms, spices and sugar were
native. Especial attention was paid to aphrodisiacs and poisons,
particularly antidotes for the bites of venomous snakes and other
animals. The soporific effects of hyoscyamus and *Cannabis indica* were known, and their employment in surgical anesthesia was,
according to Burton, of great antiquity. The surgical arm of
treatment reached, as we have said, the highest point of development attained in antiquity. The Susruta describes about 121
different surgical instruments, including scalpels, lancets, saws,
scissors, needles, hooks, probes, directors, sounds, forceps, tro-
cars, catheters, syringes, bougies and a rectal speculum.[1] These
were properly handled and jointed, the blade instruments sharp

---

[1] See, "A Short History of Aryan Medical Science," by Sir Bhagvat Sinh
Jee, London, 1896, 176–186, with pictures of surgical instruments and other
apparatus, on plates 1–10.

enough to cut a hair and kept clean by wrapping in flannel in a box. The Hindus apparently knew every important operative procedure except the use of the ligature. They amputated limbs, checking hemorrhage by cauterization, boiling oil or pressure. They treated fractures and dislocations by a special splint made of withes of bamboo which was subsequently adopted in the British Army as the "patent rattan cane splint." They performed lithotomy (without the staff), Cesarean section, excision of tumors and the removal of omental hernia through the scrotum. Their mode of extracting cataract has survived to the present day and they were especially strong in skin-grafting and other phases of plastic surgery. Their method of rhinoplasty was probably learned from them in the first instance by the itinerant Arabian surgeons and so transmitted through private families, like the Norsini, from generation to generation up to the time of Tagliacozzi. The Hindus were especially clever in their method of teaching surgery. Realizing the importance of rapid, dexterous incision in operations without anesthesia, they had the student practise at first upon plants. The hollow stocks of water lilies or the veins of large leaves were punctured and lanced as well as the blood-vessels of dead animals. Gourds, cucumbers and other soft fruits, or leather bags filled with water were tapped or incised in lieu of hydrocele or any other disorder of a hollow cavity. Flexible models were used for bandaging, and amputations and the plastic operations were practised upon dead animals. In so teaching the student to acquire ease and surety in operating by "going through the motions," the Hindus were pioneers of many recent wrinkles on the didactic side of experimental surgery.[1]

Whether the Hindus influenced Greek medicine before the time of Alexander the Great or were themselves influenced by it is not known; but it is certain that, at the time of Alexander's Indian expedition (327 B. C.), their physicians and surgeons enjoyed a well-deserved reputation for superior knowledge and skill. Some writers even maintain that Aristotle, who lived about this time, got many of his ideas from the East.

With the Mohammedan conquest, Indian medicine passed under the sway of the Arabic domination and virtually ceased to be. Its only survival in our own time consists apparently in the Vedantic practices of the various Swamis and Mahatmas who oc-

---

[1] Readers of Captain Marryat's novels may recall how the apothecary, Mr. Cophagus, taught venesection to the fatherless Japhet by making him, "in the first instance, puncture very scientifically all the larger veins of a cabbage leaf, until, well satisfied with the delicacy of my hand and the precision of my hand, he wound up his instructions by permitting me to breathe a vein in his own arm." Marryat, Japhet in Search of a Father, ch. iv.

casionally visit this country and whose strange cult has driven many of its American adherents insane. It is interesting to note, however, that the three Englishmen who did most to put hypnotism upon a permanent basis in practical therapeutics—Braid, Esdaile and Elliotson—undoubtedly got their ideas and some of their experience from contact with India.

Chinese medicine is what our own medicine might be, had we been guided by medieval ideas down to the present time, that is, absolutely stationary. Its literature consists of a large number of works none of which are of the slightest scientific importance. Their characteristics are reverence for authority, petrified formalism and a pedantic excess of detail. Chinese anatomy accounts for 365 bones in the human body, of which the cranium in some systems consists of only one bone, in others of eight in the male sex, six in the female. The larynx opens into the heart, the spinal cord into the testicles, the lung has eight lobes, the liver seven. The spleen and the heart are the organs of reason. With such inadequate knowledge of human structure there could be very little surgery, particularly among a people whose religious convictions were against the drawing of blood or the mutilation of the body. Castration is in fact the only operation they perform, and, while they use dry cupping and massage, they do not resort to venesection, but substitute the moxa and acupuncture. The moxa consists of little combustible cones which are applied all over the body and ignited. Acupuncture is the insertion into the stretched skin, of fine gold or silver needles, which are twisted about. Both procedures are employed for purposes of counter-irritation in gouty and rheumatic disorders. The Chinese were wonderfully clever at massage and were the first to employ the blind as masseurs. Chinese pathology is characterized by an excessive amount of detail; for example, 10,000 varieties of fevers or 14 kinds of dysentery. In diagnosis they attach great importance to the pulse, the varieties of which are minutely subdivided and investigated by touching different parts of the radial artery of either hand with the fingers, after the fashion of striking the keys of a piano. In this way, six sets of pulse-data are elicited, which are connected with the different organs and their diseases. The Chinese materia medica is unusually extensive and includes such well-known drugs as ginseng, rhubarb, pomegranate root, aconite, opium, arsenic, sulphur and mercury (for inunction and fumigation in syphilis), and many disgusting remedies, such as the parts or excreta of animals. The ancient Chinese knew of preventive inoculation against smallpox, which they probably got from India.

The Japanese are noted for their remarkable power of assimilating the culture of other nations, and, before they came in contact

with European civilization, their medicine was simply an extension of Chinese medicine.   Up till 96 B. C., the healing art in Japan
was passing through the mythical phases common to all forms of
early medicine.[1] Disease was supposed to be caused by divine
influence (Kamino-no-ke), by devils and evil spirits or by spirits
of the dead.   Two deities, with particularly long names, presided
over healing, which was further helped out by prayers and incantations, and at a later period, by internal remedies, venesection, and
mineral baths.   The period 96 B. C.–709 A. D. marks the ascendancy of Chinese medicine, which was introduced by way of Corea.
The practitioners and teachers were priests.   Pupils were sent to
China at government expense, and by 702 A. D. there were native
medical schools, with seven-year courses in internal medicine and
shorter periods for the other branches.   The students were made
ishi or doctors after passing a final examination in the presence of
the Minister, and women were occasionally trained as midwives.
During the succeeding periods (710–1333), called the "Nara,"
"Heian," and so on, after the names of the different capitals of
Japan, the influence of the Chinese priest-healers was still dominant, with some advances in surgical procedure, such as suturing
intestinal wounds with mulberry fiber or couching a cataract with
needles.   The oldest Japanese book is the Ishinho, written by
Yasuhori Tambu in 892, which describes these surgical novelties.
During the medieval period, personal observations of clinical cases
were recorded.   The moxa, acupuncture, and many of the Chinese
herbal or mineral remedies were in vogue and massage was delegated to the blind as a suitable occupation.   A striking contribution of the ancient Japanese to therapeutics was their use of
red hangings in the treatment of smallpox, the remedy afterward
employed by John of Gaddesden and Finsen.   The first Portuguese
ship touched Japan in 1542, and with the arrival of St. Francis
Xavier in 1549 begins the rise of European influences.   The
physicians who came with him and with the later missionaries—
there was a Catholic church at Kyoto in 1568—treated the sick
gratuitously, did surgical work, founded hospitals, and planted
botanic gardens.   After the expulsion of the missionaries, two of
their Japanese pupils settled at Sakai and founded a school.   The
Dutch traders came in 1597 and their ship's surgeons also exerted
some influence.   A translation of Ambroïse Paré's works was made
in the seventeenth century, but the importation of European books
was forbidden until the year 1700, after which time translations of
Boerhaave, Van Swieten, Heister, and other writers began to ap-

---

[1] Most of these details are taken from Y. Fujikawa's "Geschichte der
Medizin in Japan," Tokyo, 1911.

pear. Vaccination was introduced by Mohmike in 1848. The medical school founded by the Dutch physicians at Yedo in 1857 passed into the hands of the government in 1860 and became in time the present University of Tokyo. The modern or Meiji period of Japanese medicine begins with the year of revolution, 1868, and its distinctive feature is the rise of German influences. The universities and medical academies, the state examinations, the medical societies and medical journals, are all copied after German models, and the ablest Japanese medical men of today have received their education and training in Germany. Under such influences as these, the modern Japanese physician aspires not so much to be classed among the two-sworded Samurai as to have the thorough scientific training of a Shiga or a Kitasato, a Noguchi or a Hata.

To sum up what we owe to Oriental medicine, the Babylonians specialized in the matter of medical fees, the Jews originated medical jurisprudence and public hygiene and ordained a weekly day of rest, and the Hindus demonstrated that skill in operative surgery which has been a permanent possession of the Aryan race ever since.

GREEK MEDICINE

I. Before Hippocrates

The Greeks were a *Sammelvolk*, a composite people, and their diverse elements—Ionian, Thessalian, Arcadian, Achaian, Æolian, Dorian—gave them the self-willed independence, the restless individuality, of a mountaineer and sea-faring race, traits which were at once the secret of their greatness and their downfall. The physical geography of insular and peninsular Greece, with its deep coastwise indentations and abrupt mountain walls, isolated the whole country and its separate states in a way that made at once for intense local patriotism, and at the same time gave the cultural advantages of abundant maritime intercourse with other nations, while such grandeur in external nature could only inspire the loftiest freedom of mind and spirit. Yet this very freedom of thought prevented Greece from becoming a nation in the end, for her people were too diverse in racial strain, pulled too many different ways, to become permanently united. "Her city states were too wilful to combine."[1]

Of the Pelasgians, the prehistoric inhabitants of Greece, we know little beyond the evidence of such massive remains as the Lion's Gate at Mycenæ, and of the early achievements of their successors, the Hellenes, Thucydides himself says, at the beginning of his history, that "they were no great things." He points out that ancient Hellas had no settled population, wars and factions keeping the people in a state of constant migration, so that "the richest soils were always the most subject to change of masters." Under conditions like these, a restless, athletic, warlike and sea-faring people were developed whose chief interest were the active lives they led and the influence exerted upon their affairs by the gods of their worship.

As Walter Pater has so charmingly set forth, in his studies of Dionysus and "Hippolytus Veiled,"[2] it is a common error to suppose that the ancient Greeks everywhere worshiped the same Pantheon of gods. In point of fact, as being a divided people, the Hellenes of the mountains, the coast, the valleys, farms and river-

---

[1] Sir T. Clifford Allbutt: "Science and Mediæval Thought," London, 1901, p. 21.

[2] Walter Pater: Greek Studies, London, 1895, pp. 1–48 and 158–194.

sides had each a separate religion of their own, the whole forming, of course, an essential polytheism, in that every little clan or village community worshiped its special god, at the same time paying a vague general reverence to the greater gods. Thus, Demeter was the special divinity of those who lived on farms and among corn-fields, Dionysus of those who cultivated vineyards, Poseidon of those who dwelt by the sea, Pallas Athene of the Athenians, while the lesser gods had each a particular locality where their worship was a cult. "Like a network over the land of gracious poetic tradition," says Pater, "the local religions had been never wholly superseded by the worship of the great national temples."[1] Thus we find, at the start, that there were many tutelary divini-ties of medicine among the Greeks. Artemis (Diana), Demeter (Ceres), Hermes (Mercury), Hera (Juno), Poseidon (Neptune), Dionysus (Bacchus) were, all of them, patron gods and goddesses of the healing art, and were able, at need, to produce disease themselves.[2]

The chief god of healing in the Greek Pantheon was Apollo, commonly called Alexikakos (the averter of ills), whose far-darting arrows visited plagues and epidemics upon mankind and who could, at need, avert them. He was also the god of purity and well-being in youth, and, as Homer relates, the physician to the Olym-pian gods, whose wounds or diseases he cured by means of the root of the peony. Hence his name "Pæan," and the epithet "sons of Pæan," as applied to physicians. Legend relates that a knowledge of medicine was communicated by Apollo and his sister Artemis to the Centaur Chiron, the son of Saturn. As one skilled in music and surgery and especially versed in ancient lore, Chiron was entrusted with the rearing and education of the heroes Jason, Hercules, Achil-les, and, in particular, Æsculapius, the son of Apollo by the nymph Coronis. As Pindar sings, in his fourth Isthmian ode, Æsculapius became so proficient in the healing art that Pluto accused him of diminishing the number of shades in Hades, and he was destroyed by a thunderbolt of Zeus. After his death he became an object of worship, and the temples of his cult were the famous Asclepieia, of which the most celebrated were those at Cos, Epidaurus, Cnidus and Pergamus. These temples, commonly situated on wooded hills or mountain sides, near mineral springs, became popular sanitaria,

---

[1] Pater: "Hippolytus Veiled," op. cit., p. 162.

[2] In the Hippocratic treatise "On the Sacred Disease," it is said of epi-leptics that "if they imitate a goat, or grind their teeth, or if their right side be convulsed, they say that the mother of the gods (Cybele) is the cause. If they speak in a sharper, shriller tone, they liken this state to a horse and say that Poseidon is the cause. . . . but if foam be emitted by the mouth and the patient kick with his feet, Ares (Mars) gets the blame."

managed by trained priests and, in intention, not unlike the health-resorts of modern times. The patients were received by the physician-priests, who stirred their imaginations by recounting the deeds of Æsculapius, the success of the temple treatment and the remedies employed. After appropriate prayers and sacrifice, the patient was further purified by a bath from the mineral spring, with massage, inunction and other methods, and, after offering up a cock or ram before the image of the god, was inducted into the special rite of "incubation" or the temple-sleep. This consisted in lying down to sleep in the sanctuary, and during the night, the priest, in the guise of the god, presented himself before the patient to administer medical advice, if he happened to be awake. If he slept, as was usually the case, the advice came in a dream, which was interpreted afterward by the priests, who then prescribed catharsis, emesis, blood-letting or whatever remedies seemed appropriate. If the treatment was successful and the patient cured, he then presented a thank-offering to the god, usually a model of the diseased part in wax, silver or gold, while a votive tablet giving the history of his case and its treatment was suspended in the temple. The whole rite of incubation has been facetiously described in the "Plutus" of Aristophanes, and in more elevated and dignified style in the third chapter of Walter Pater's romance of Roman antiquity, "Marius the Epicurean." The votive tablets in the Asclepieia at Cos and Cnidus became the permanent clinical records of the Coan and Cnidian Schools of Medicine, of the first of which Hippocrates was himself a pupil. The Greek traveler Pausanias noticed six of these votive columns when he visited the temple at Epidaurus about 150 A. D., and two of them were excavated in recent times by Cavvadias. Engraved upon these last were about thirty clinical cases, giving the names of the patients, their bodily ills and what was done for them. The details of symptoms and treatment are very meager. In most cases it sufficed if the god anointed the patient in his sleep or if one of the sacred dogs or snakes in the temple licked the diseased part. One patient came with four fingers of his hand paralyzed, another was blind of one eye, another had carried a spear-point in his jaw for six years, another had an ulcer of the stomach, another empyema, another was infested with vermin. All were reported as cured.[1] These fragmentary case-histories, none of them conveying any medical information of positive value, are sometimes supposed to have been the starting-point of the Hippocratic descriptions of disease.

---

[1] For further details, see E. T. Withington, "Medical History," London, 1894, Appendix ii (pp. 370–397).

Among the legendary children of Æsculapius were his daughters
Hygieia and Panacea, who assisted in the temple rites and fed the
sacred snakes. Of the sons of Æsculapius, two, Machaon and
Podalirius, are mentioned in Homer's Catalogue of the Ships as
leaders, commanding thirty vessels and "good physicians both."
Æsculapius is himself referred to in the Iliad as a real chieftain of
Thessaly who learned medicine from the centaur Chiron, from
whose teaching, again, Achilles was able to impart his knowledge
of the healing art to his friend Patroclus. Machaon and Podalirius
are often referred to in Homer's narrative as men skilled in extracting weapons, binding up wounds and applying soothing drugs.
In the fourth Iliad, Machaon is summoned to remove an arrow
which was driven through the belt of Menelaus, King of Sparta.
He arrives to find a circle of warriors gathered about the hero, and
"instantly thereupon he extracted the arrow from the well-fitted
belt. But while it was being extracted the sharp barbs were
broken. Then he loosed the variegated belt and the girdle beneath, and the plated belt which brass-workers had forged. But
when he perceived the wound, where the bitter shaft had fallen,
having sucked out the blood, he skilfully sprinkled on it soothing
remedies, which benevolent Chiron had formerly given to his
father." In the eleventh Iliad, Idomeneus refers to Machaon as
follows: "O Neleian Nestor, great glory of the Greeks, come, as-
cend thy chariot and let Machaon mount beside thee; and direct
thy solid-hoofed horses with all speed towards the ships, for a
medical man is the equal of many others, both to cut out arrows,
and to apply mild remedies." At the end of the same book, Eury-
pylus, wounded with an arrow in the thigh, calls upon Patroclus
to remove it. He is borne to a tent, and there, Patroclus, "laying
him at length, cut out with a knife the bitter, sharp arrow from
his thigh, and washed the black blood from it with warm water.
Then he applied a bitter, pain-assuaging root, rubbing it between
his hands, which checked all his pains; the wound indeed dried up,
and the bleeding ceased." In the thirteenth Iliad, Helenus, son
of Priam, is smitten through the hand by the brass spear of Menelaus and we have a glimpse of the "great-hearted Agenor" extracting it and binding the wounded hand "sling-wise in well-
twisted sheep's wool, which his attendant carried for the shepherd
of the people." In the eighth Iliad (lines 81–86) there is a striking picture of the rotatory movements made by a horse which had
been wounded in the brain by an arrow. That women sometimes
rendered medical aid we gather from both Iliad and Odyssey, as
in the references in the former to "yellow-haired Agamede, who
well understood as many drugs as the wide earth nourishes,"
or, in the latter, to the soporific which Helen casts into the wine, a

drug "which Polydamna, the wife of Thon, had given her, a woman of Egypt." In the Odyssey, a healer of diseases is said to be as welcome at a feast as a prophet, a builder of ships, or even a god-like minstrel. From these specimens of the war-surgery of the Iliad it is plain that the surgeon's art was held in high esteem by the ancient Greeks, and that chieftains of high rank did not disdain to follow it. It is said that over forty different wounds are described by Homer, but no details are given as to febrile or other symptoms. The anatomic terms used are, according to Malgaigne and Daremberg, more or less identical with those employed by Hippocrates.

There is no mention of the Asclepieia in the Homeric poems, which date back to at least 1000 B. C., but we may assume that, even then, physicians and surgeons were a distinct class from priests, although perhaps associated with the latter in time of peace. Apart from such "priests" and the medical men proper, the healing art was studied by the philosophers, and practised in some details by the "gymnasts," who bathed and anointed the body and tried to treat wounds and injuries and even internal diseases. Greek medicine, as Osler has said, "had a triple relationship with science, with gymnastics, and with theology," and before the time of Hippocrates, it was regarded simply as a branch of philosophy.

Greek philosophy before the age of Pericles was of Ionian origin and was derived from Egypt and the East. The founder of the Ionic School was Thales of Miletus (639–544 B. C.), who had studied under the Egyptian priests, and taught that water is the primary element from which all else is derived. He was followed by Anaximander of Miletus (611), Anaximenes of Miletus ((570–500 B. C.) and Heraclitus of Ephesus (circa 556–460 B. C.), who, in succession, assumed that indivisible matter (earth?), air, or fire respectively are the primordial elements. These four elements, earth, air, fire, water, were assumed by Anaxagoras of Clazomenæ (500–428 B. C.) to be made up of as many parts or "seed" as there are varieties of sensible or perceptible matter. These categories were thrown into striking relief in the teaching of Empedocles of Agrigentum in Sicily (504–443 B. C.), the picturesque hero of Matthew Arnold's poem, who as philosopher, physician, poet, traveled through the Greek cities, clad in a purple robe, gold-cinctured, laurel-crowned, long haired, severe of mien, and on account of his medical skill, was held by the people to be endowed with supernatural powers. One of his poetic fragments shows the unusual reverence in which the Greek physician was held at this time:

> Ye friends, who in the mighty city dwell
> Along the yellow Acragas hard by
> The Acropolis, ye stewards of good works,
> The stranger's refuge venerable and kind,
> All hail, O friends! But unto ye I walk
> As god immortal now, no more as man,
> On all sides honored fittingly and well,
> Crowned both with fillets, and with flowering wreaths.
> When with my throngs of men and women I come
> To thriving cities I am sought by prayers,
> And thousands follow me that they may ask
> The path to weal and vantage, craving some
> For oracles, whilst others seek to hear
> A healing word 'gainst many a foul disease
> That all too long hath pierced with grievous pains.[1]

Empedocles introduced into philosophy the doctrine of the elements, earth, air, fire, water, as "the four-fold root of all things." The human body is supposed to be made up of these primordial substances, health resulting from their balance, disease from imbalance. He holds that nothing can be created or destroyed, and that there is only transformation, which is the modern theory of conservation of energy. Everything originates from the attraction of the four elements and is destroyed by their repulsion, and he applies the same idea, under the forms of love and hate, to the moral world. Development is due to the union of dissimilar elements, decay to the return of like to like, air to air, fire to fire, earth to earth. Empedocles is said to have raised Pantheia from a trance, to have checked an epidemic by draining swampy lands and to have improved the climatic condition of his native town by blocking a cleft in a mountain side. Legend relates that he ended his life by throwing himself into the crater of Mount Etna. His pupil Pausanias is said by Plutarch to have used fire in checking an epidemic.

The Italian School of Philosophers was founded by Pythagoras of Samos (580–489 B. C.) at Crotona. Pythagoras had also studied in Egypt, from which he probably acquired his doctrine of the mystic power of numbers. He held that unity being perfection and representing God, the number twelve represents the whole material universe, of which the factors three and four represent the worlds, the spheres and the primordial elements. As the monad (1) denotes the active or vital principle in nature, so the duad (2) represents the passive principle or matter, the triad (3), the world, formed by the union of the two former, and the tetrad (4), the perfection of eternally flowing nature. Heaven is made up of ten celestial spheres (nine of which are visible), the fixed stars, the seven planets and the earth. The distances of the celestial spheres

---

[1] From the interesting translations of the poetic fragments of Empedocles, by William Ellery Leonard in the Monist, Chicago, 1907, xvii, p. 468.

from the earth correspond with the proportion of sounds in the musical scale. Pythagoras was the first to investigate the mathematical
physics of sound, and in the following way: In passing a blacksmith's shop, one day, he noticed that, when the smith's hammers
were struck in rapid succession upon the anvil, the chords elicited
(the octave, thirds and fifths) were all harmonious; the chord of
the fourth was not. Going into the shop, he found that this was
due, not to the shapes of the hammers or the force with which they
were struck, but to the differences in their individual weights.
Upon this hint, he went home and stretched four strings of the same
material, length and thickness, suspending weights at the lower
end of each, equal to the weights of the four hammers respectively.
Upon striking these strings, he got the chords which he had heard
in the smithy, and by subdividing the strings with other weights,
he was able to construct the musical scale. This was the earliest
recorded experiment in physics, and the scale was, after his death,
engraved on brass, and set up in the temple of Juno at Samos.
Pythagoras reasoned that the celestial spheres might produce
sounds by striking upon the surrounding ether, and these sounds
would vary with the velocity of impact and the relative distance.
The distances of the spheres from the earth correspond, as we have
seen, to the proportion of sounds in the scale, and as the heavenly
bodies move according to fixed laws, the sounds produced by them
must be harmonious. This is the doctrine of the "harmony of the
spheres." The number-lore of Pythagoras is thought to have
exerted a profound influence upon the Hippocratic doctrine of
crises and critical days, which assigned fixed periods to the resolution of different diseases. More than to anything else, the Greek
physicians aspired to the scientific power of prediction. In pathology, the plastic significance of the number four was combined, in
the teaching of Plato and Aristotle, with the doctrine of the four
elements, as follows: Corresponding with the elements of earth,
air, fire and water were the qualities dry, cold, hot and moist, according to the scheme:

$$\text{hot}+\text{dry}=\text{fire}; \quad \text{cold}+\text{dry}=\text{earth}.$$
$$\text{hot}+\text{moist}=\text{air}; \quad \text{cold}+\text{moist}=\text{water}.$$

By reversing these equations, the four elements could be resolved
into their qualitative components, and, long before Aristotle,
probably before Hippocrates, it was held that, corresponding to
these four elements, fire, air, water, earth, and the four qualities,
hot, cold, moist, dry, are the four humors of the body, viz., blood,
phlegm, yellow bile, and black bile. These three sets of elements,
qualities and humors could then be brought, by permutation and

combination, into a complex system of arrangements, based upon
the following scheme:

hot + moist = blood;   cold + moist = phlegm.
hot + dry   = yellow bile;   cold + dry   = black bile,

the different combinations giving the qualitative aspects of disease,
and, by the same token, of the physiologic action of drugs. The
whole arrangement made up the "humoral pathology" which
regarded health and disease as the proper adjustment or imbalance
respectively of the different components mentioned, and the
scheme was further elaborated by Galen and the Arabian physicians, in that remedies and their compounds were classified in nu-
merical scales according to the "degrees" or relative proportions
of their several qualities. Thus the Arabian pharmacists held that
sugar is cold in the first degree, warm in the second degree, dry in
the second degree, and moist in the first degree; cardamoms are
warm in the first degree, cold by one-half a degree, dry in the first
degree, and so on. In Galen's system, the Pythagorean doctrine
of numbers was applied to every aspect of medicine. For example,
there are three faculties, natural, spiritual, animal. There are
three spirits: the natural, arising from the liver; the vital, from
the heart; the animal, from the brain, the three being distributed
and diffused through the body by the veins, arteries and nerves.
There are four ages of man, adolescence (hot and moist); manhood
(hot and dry); advanced age (cold and dry); old age (cold and
moist). The eye has seven coats and three humors. There are
three kinds of drinks, pure, as water; containing food, as wine;
or a mixture of both, as syrups and medicinal drafts. There are
three kinds of fevers, the ephemeral, in the spirit; the ethic (hec-
tic?), in the solids; and the putrid, in the humors; and the putrid
are of four varieties, the continued (synochal), in the blood; the
quotidian, in the phlegm; the tertian, in the yellow bile; the
quartan, in the black bile.[1] In short, everything in Galenic and
Arabic medicine was mathematically subdivided, usually by the
sacred numerals of Pythagoras.

In Egypt, Pythagoras learned the doctrine of transmigration of
souls or metempsychosis, and he is credited with being the first to
establish the fact that the brain is the central organ of the higher
activities, a proposition which was long afterward put to experimental proof by Flourens and Goltz.

After Pythagoras, the most important of the Greek philosophers, with the exception of Plato and Aristotle, was Democritus

---

[1] For further illustrations, see the very thoroughgoing account of Galen's
system by Johannitius in the "Medical History" of E. T. Withington
(London, 1894), pp. 386–396.

of Abdera (460–360 B. C.), who first stated the theory that every-thing in nature, including the body and the soul, is made up of atoms of different shapes and sizes, the movements of which are the cause of life and mental activity.

During the Heroic Age, and at the time of the Trojan war, the dominant people in the Peloponnesus were the athletic, simple-minded Achaians, whose high regard for surgery and the surgeon was in striking contrast with the attitude of the ancient Romans. In later times, Greek civilization was made up of two main elements, the Ionian or Attic, and the Doric or Spartan. The composite, imaginative, artistic peoples of Ionia and the islands were inter-ested in everything, and at once brave and warlike, keen and busi-ness-like, serious and high-minded, or, at need, flippant and ironi-cal. As we see them in the comedies of Aristophanes, Lucian's dialogues and the idyls of Theocritus, the city-bred Greeks were a gay, quick-minded, supremely talkative people, adoring intelli-gence for itself, fonder of speculation than of material facts, keen at taking an advantage, and cheerfully complaisant as to their neighbors' morals. Yet they were the same people who could listen with reverent attention to the dramas of Æschylus and Sophocles. In striking contrast were the Dorians or Spartans, who were essentially robust, unimaginative warriors, severe in such morals as they had, and like the Homeric Greeks and the ancient Romans, cultivating the body rather than the mind, as an essential part of their scheme of military government. As with all military peoples, they were narrowly jealous, suspicious or contemptuous of achievement or prosperity in other nations. Both Ionians and Spartans were extremely curious about the fu-ture, and, like all people of early civilizations, attached enormous importance to oracles, presages and omens, so that prognosis was still the essential feature of Greek medicine before Hippocrates. Among the Spartans, the surgeon was held in the same high regard as among the Homeric heroes, and Lycurgus classed them as non-combatant officials. Among the Attic or Ionian Greeks, the medi-cal profession, as we approach the Age of Pericles, is found to be more highly specialized. In the first place, general practitioners began, toward the later period, to receive stipulated fees for their services instead of the usual thank-offerings of the temples, and, further, city and district physicians came to be appointed at an annual salary which, for the times, was quite high—in the case of Democedes at Athens, in the second half of the sixth century B. C., about $2000. There were also military and naval surgeons among the Athenians, as among the Spartans. Xenophon records that there were eight army surgeons with the expedition of the Ten Thousand, at the end of the fifth century. There were again midwives, professional lithotomists, druggists and veterinarians, and finally a special class, the "rhizotomi," or root gatherers, who wandered through the fields and forests collecting vegetable simples. The physician's office was called the Iatreion, and was used indifferently as a dispensary, consulting room and operating theater. In the larger cities there were public Iatreia, supported by special taxes.

Medical instruction was not organized and was, in effect, private, either under some renowned physician or received from the adherents of the different schools. On finishing his course, the graduate simply took the physician's oath of the particular medical clan or sect to which he belonged.

Such human anatomy as the Greek physicians and surgeons learned was identical with the sculptor's knowledge of the subject, which the latter acquired through constant familiarity with the appearance of the nude body in action, either during the athletic contests celebrated by Pindar or in the palæstra. "It was here," says Waldstein, "with hundreds of nude youths, not only wrestling, jumping and running, but endeavoring by systematic practice to remedy any defect or abnormality in any one limb or organ, that the artist, day by day, studied his anatomy of the human figure without the need of entering the dissecting room."[1] What Pater calls "the age of athletic prizemen" was also the great age of Greek sculpture, and in nothing is the discriminating power of Greek intelligence more beautifully and nobly shown than in the masterpieces of the great artists of this period. In reference to their remarkable capacity for close observation, Waldstein notes that the pectineus muscle, hidden at the base of Scarpa's triangle, but highly developed in the stress of Greek athletics, appears in some of their statues, although it has escaped the attention of modern artistic anatomists.[2]

In regard to education and personal hygiene, the Greeks cultivated that ideal of a harmonious development of all the individual faculties which was set aside or lost sight of during the Middle Ages, but has been steadily coming more and more to the front in later times. With such training, it is not strange that the Hellenes of the fifth century attained a degree of civilization and a supremacy in philosophy, lyrical and dramatic poetry, sculpture and architecture, which has not been equaled by any people who came after them. And this culminating period was also the Age of Hippocrates.

---

[1] See Charles Waldstein: "The Argive Heræum," Boston, 1902, pp. 400, 401.

[2] See Waldstein: Op. cit., 186, pl. xxx and xxxiv; also editorial in Jour. Am. Med. Assoc., Chicago, July 15, 1911, p. 222.

II. The Classic Period (460–146 B. C.)

European medicine begins properly in the Age of Pericles and its scientific advancement centers in the figure of **Hippocrates** (460–370 B. C.), who gave to Greek medicine its scientific spirit and its ethical ideals. A contemporary of Sophocles and Euripides, Aristophanes and Pindar, Socrates and Plato, Herodotus and Thucydides, Phidias and Polygnotus, he lived at a time when the Athenian democracy had attained its highest point of development. Never, before or since, had so many men of genius appeared in the same narrow limits of space and time. Hippocrates was born, according to Soranus, in the island of Cos, at the beginning of the eightieth Olympiad, of an Asclepiad family. He received his first medical instruction from his father, studied at Athens, and acquired extensive experience in travel and practice among the cities of Thrace, Thessaly, and Macedonia. The date of his death is unknown, his age being variously given as anywhere from 85 to 109 years. The eminence of Hippocrates is three-fold: he dissociated medicine from theurgy and philosophy,[1] crystallized the loose knowledge of the Coan and Cnidian Schools into systematic science, and gave physicians the highest moral inspiration they have. No future facts that may be dug up about cuneiform or papyric medicine will quite impair the value of the great advance he made in synthetic science. Before the Age of Pericles, the Greek physician was either an associate of priests in times of peace or a surgeon in time of war. As the Greek mind was essentially plastic, so, in anatomy, his knowledge was mainly the sculptor's knowledge of visible or palpable parts, and, for this reason, his clinical knowledge of internal diseases was confined to externalities also. Even as

> The Grecian gods were like the Greeks,
> As keen-eyed, cold and fair,

so the early Hellenic physician remained essentially a surgeon rather than a clinician in his attitude toward his patients, considering only the surface indications. In cold, dry enumeration of symptoms, the Coan and Cnidian tablets and sentences, like the Egyptian papyri, might have been scientific, if the physicians of the time had known how to group and coördinate symptoms and consequently to interpret them. All this was changed with the advent of Hippocrates. All that a man of genius could do for internal medicine, with no other instrument of precision than his own open mind and keen senses, he accomplished, and, with these

---

[1] "Primus quidem ex omnibus memoria dignus, ab studio sapientiæ disciplinam hanc separavit." Celsus, De re medica, Proœmium.

5

reservations, his best descriptions of disease are models of their kind today.   To him medicine owes the art of clinical inspection and observation, and he is, above all, the exemplar of that flexible, critical, well-poised attitude of mind, ever on the lookout for sources of error, which is the very essence of the scientific spirit.   As Allbutt points out,[1] Hippocrates taught the Coan physicians that, in relation to an internal malady like empyema or malarial fever, the basis of all real knowledge lies in the application of the inductive method, that "grinding or rubbing in," which, better than the mere haphazard notation of symptoms, consists in going over them again and again, until the real values in the clinical picture begin to stand out of themselves.   Thus, instead of attributing disease to the gods or other fantastic imaginations, like his predecessors, Hippocrates virtually founded that bedside method which was afterward employed with such signal ability by Sydenham, Heberden, Laënnec, Bright and Addison, the Dublin clinicians of the fifties, Frerichs, Duchenne of Boulogne, and Charcot.   Huchard says that the revival of the Hippocratic methods in the seventeenth century and their triumphant vindication by the concerted scientific movement of the nineteenth, is the whole history of internal medicine.   The central Hippocratic doctrine, the humoral pathology, which, as we have seen, attributes all disease to disorders of the fluids of the body, has, in its original form, long since been discarded, although some phases of it still survive in the modern theory of serodiagnosis and serotherapy.   It is the method of Hippocrates, the use of the mind and senses as diagnostic instruments, together with his transparent honesty and his elevated conception of the dignity of the physician's calling, his high seriousness and deep respect for his patients, that make him, by common consent, the "Father of Medicine" and the greatest of all physicians.

Claude Bernard said that observation is a passive science, experimentation an active science.   Hippocrates was not acquainted with experiment, but no physician ever profited more by experience. Although Asclepiades called this observational method "a meditation upon death," the work of Hippocrates must be judged by its results.   He described the "bilious, malarial, hemoglobinuric" fevers of Thessaly and Thrace very much as the modern Greek writers, Cardamatis, Kanellis, and the rest, have found them today. and it has often been remarked that his clinical pictures of phthisis, puerperal convulsions, epilepsy, epidemic parotitis, and some other diseases might, with a few changes and additions, take their place in any modern text-book.   Of the forty-two clinical cases he has

---

[1] Sir T. C. Allbutt: "The Historical Relations of Medicine and Surgery," London, 1905, pp. 6–13.

left us—almost the only records of the kind for the next 1700 years —twenty-five are reported with characteristic sincerity as fatal, while, unlike Galen, the author has nothing whatever to say about clever diagnoses, remarkable cures, or blunders on the part of his fellow practitioners. "He seems," says Billings, "to have written mainly for the purpose of telling what he himself knew, and this motive—rare among all writers—is especially rare among writers on medicine."[1] Through Hippocrates, it was the chief glory of Greek medicine to have introduced that spontaneous, first-hand study of nature, with a definitely honest intention, which is the motor power of modern science. After the Hippocratic period, the practice of taking clinical case-histories died out, for Galen's cases were written only to puff his own reputation, and there was nothing of value until the time of Benivieni's postmortems.

The works attributed to Hippocrates are usually divided into four groups—the genuine, the spurious, the works of his predecessors, and those of his contemporaries and followers. Written in Ionic Greek, the genuine writings include, at least, those remarkable clinical jottings, the aphorisms (Books I–III), the treatises on prognosis, on epidemic diseases (Books I and III), wounds, dislocations, fractures and ulcers, and the excursus, "On Airs, Waters and Places," which is at once the first book ever written on medical geography, climatology and anthropology, if we except the contemporary narrative of Herodotus, with whom Hippocrates is often in such striking accord. The ὅρκος, or physician's oath, the earliest and most impressive document in medical ethics, is not usually regarded as a genuine Hippocratic writing, but is thought to be an ancient temple oath of the Asclepiads. Yet both the Oath and the Law are so much in keeping with what we know of the ethical spirit of the great Coan that they are usually included in the Hippocratic Canon. To a modern reader, the best of the Aphorisms seem like the short-hand notes of a keen mind at the bedside, intent on establishing a true relation between generals and particulars, accidentals and essentials. While many of them go straight to the mark, others are strongly suggestive of the kind of inadequate information that was probably conveyed in the Coan and Cnidian sentences. The "Prognostics," the finished net result of the "Coan Prenotions" and "Prorrhetics" of his predecessors, show that the dignity of the Greek physician was based more upon his ability to predict clinical happenings than his power to control them. To this end Hippocrates instituted, for the first time, a careful, systematic, and thoroughgoing examination of the patient's condition, including the facial appearance,

---

[1] J. S. Billings: "History of Surgery," New York, 1895, p. 24.

pulse, temperature, respiration, excreta, sputum, localized pains, and movements of the body. He even notes the ominous symptom of picking at the coverlid in fevers. The books on epidemic diseases contain the remarkable case histories and clinical pictures to which we have referred. Not the least among these is the famous "facies Hippocratica," that wonderful thumb-nail sketch of the signs of approaching dissolution,[1] some touches of which are given in Shakespeare's account of Falstaff's death. While there is much in the surgical writings of Hippocrates that is faulty, incomplete or not in accordance with modern practice, they are the only thing of value on the subject before the time of Celsus. The treatises on fractures, dislocations and wounds may be thought of as modern works in the same sense in which Matthew Arnold regarded Thucydides as a modern writer, illustrating the wonderful capacity of Greek intelligence for separating essentials from accidentals, "the tendency to observe facts with a critical spirit; to search for their law, not to wander among them at random; to judge by the rule of reason, not by the impulse of prejudice or caprice."[2] Some of the greatest medical scholars, Malgaigne, Littré, Allbutt, and the rest, have pronounced the Hippocratic books on fractures, dislocations and wounds, given the limitations under which they were written, to be the equal of any similar work of a more recent day. Dislocations of the shoulder, Hippocrates says, are "rarely inwards or outwards, but frequently and chiefly downwards," and his methods of reduction are practically those of modern times. He was particularly strong in his account of congenital dislocations, and in reducing and bandaging fractures. He was the first to notice that deformity of the spine often coexists with tubercle of the lungs. He was acquainted with fracture of the clavicle and dislocation of its acromial end, and knew how to treat both conditions. In the treatment of wounds, he says that they should never be irrigated except with clean water or wine, the dry state being nearest to the healthy, the wet to the diseased, and the antiseptic advantages of extreme dryness were utilized in the avoidance of greasy dressings and the effort to bring the fresh edges of the wound into close apposition, sometimes by the use of astringents. Hippocrates recognizes that "rest and immobilization are of capital importance," and to keep still is even a better splint than bandaging. He describes the symptoms of suppuration, and says that, in such cases, medicated dressings, if applied at all, should be "not upon the wound itself, but around it." If water was used for irrigation, it had either to be very pure or else boiled, and the hands and nails

---

[1] Prognosis, § 2.

[2] Matthew Arnold: "Essays in Criticism," third series, Boston, 1910, p. 48.

of the operator were to be cleansed. Hippocrates gives the first description of healing by first and second intention. In his description of the operating-room, he lays stress upon good illumination, posture of the patient and the presence of capable assistants. He refers to trephining and paracentesis, but apparently knew nothing of amputation. In his directions for trephining in head injuries he notes that a wound of the left temporal region will cause convulsions on the right side and *vice versâ*. The Hippocratic aphorism that diseases not curable by iron are curable by fire, which caused no end of surgical bungling and malpractice down to the time of Paré, is really pre-Hippocratic, being already

mentioned in the Agamemnon of Æschylus. It has been traced by Baas to the ancient Hindus. In clinical diagnosis, Hippocrates was the first to note the "succussion sound," obtained by shaking the patient on a rigid seat, the ear being applied to the chest. Littré also comments on a "boiling sound," and a sound like that made by new leather. Cheyne-Stokes respiration ("like that of a person recollecting himself") is noted in the case of Philiscus.[1]

In therapeutics, Hippocrates believed simply in assisting nature, and although he knew the use of many drugs, his scheme of treatment was usually confined to such plain expedients as fresh air, good diet, purgation, tisans of barley water, wine, massage, and hydrotherapy.

In literary style Hippocrates is like the best Greek writers of the classic period, clear, precise and simple. The

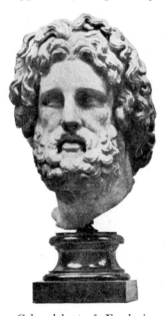

Colossal bust of Æsculapius in the British Museum.

Law, the Oath and the discourse "On the Sacred Disease" are the loftiest utterances of Greek medicine, and, whether due to Hippocrates or not, they represent the essence of his teaching. The argument of the latter treatise, which deals with the supposed divine origin of epilepsy, was the highest reach of free thought for centuries, and had it been heeded, would have done away forever with the foolish idea that human ills are caused by gods or demons.

The usual portraits of Hippocrates represent a tall, bearded

---

[1] Epid. Dis., Bk. i, Sect. 3, § 13, Case 1. Cited by Finlayson.

man of venerable aspect. They are in no sense "counterfeit presentments," but only traditional. In the "Clouds" of Aristophanes, there is a satirical reference to physicians as lazy, long-haired foppish individuals with rings and carefully polished nails, which is supposed to have been, incidentally, a slap at the Father of Medicine. It is highly probable that physicians of the Periclean age wore their hair and beards as much like the figures of Jove or Æsculapius as possible, and were otherwise not lacking in the self-sufficiency which characterized the Greeks of the period. We may therefore infer that the supposed portraits of Hippocrates are only variants of the bust of Æsculapius, as rendered into marble by Praxiteles (in the British Museum), or as seen in statuettes from the shrine of Epidaurus or on the Greek coins of Cos, Pergamus, and Epidaurus, representing him enthroned.

The most important editions of Hippocrates are:

1. The folio Latin text of the *Opera Omnia*, translated and edited by Fabius Calvus, the friend and patron of Raphael, and published at Rome under the auspices of Pope Clement VII in 1525. This was the first complete edition of Hippocrates to be printed.

2. The folio *editio princeps* of the Greek text, published in the following year (1526) by Aldus at Venice.

3. The Basel *Opera Omnia*, edited by Janus Cornarius and printed by Froben (1538), highly prized on account of its textual and critical accuracy.

4. The Greek text and Latin translation of Hieronymus Mercurialis, printed by the house of Giunta at Venice in 1538.

5. The Frankfurt edition of 1595, containing the valuable translation and commentary of Anutius Foesius, the most learned, industrious and able of the Hippocratic commentators before the time of Littré.

6. The magnificent ten-volume edition of Littré himself (Paris, 1839–61), containing the Greek text, a French translation (all the readings known having been carefully collated with critical notes), a biographic introduction and special introductions to each separate treatise. It was the work of a lifetime and is one of the triumphs of modern scholarship.

The first Greek text of the Aphorisms was edited by François Rabelais, and published at Lyons in 1532. Of English translations, the most valuable is that of the Scotch scholar, Francis Adams (London, 1849), which is limited to the genuine works of Hippocrates. Next to this, the handiest for practical use is the "Œuvres choisies" of Charles Daremberg (Paris, 1834).

Hippocrates voiced the spirit of an entire epoch, and after his time there was a great gap in the continuity of Greek medicine. In succeeding centuries, the open-minded, receptive spirit of his teaching became merged into the case-hardened formalism of dogmatists like Praxagoras, who cared more for rigid doctrine than for investigation.

The greatest scientific name after Hippocrates is that of "the master of those who know," the Asclepiad **Aristotle** (384–322 B. C.) of Stagira, who gave to medicine the beginnings of zoölogy, comparative anatomy and embryology, and the use of formal logic as an instrument of precision. Aristotle was a pupil of Plato, whose "Timæus" imposed some very fantastic theories upon medical teaching for centuries, but he improved upon his master to the extent, at least, of describing about 500 species of animals (some of them fictitious), and studying their bodily structure. He noted a number of facts in embryology, such as the punctum saliens, the movements of the fetal heart, and the possibility of superfetation. He was the first to use the term "anthropologist," but in the sense of a vain, self-important person, the logical opposite of the "high-minded man" of his "Ethics." His "entelechies," which he regarded as intermediaries between the soul and the body, have been revived, as a substitute for "vital principles," by the morphologist Driesch.

A worthy successor of Aristotle was his friend and pupil, **Theophrastus** of Eresos (370–286 B. C.), who was also a physician, and was called the "protobotanist" because he did for the vegetable kingdom what Hippocrates had previously done for surgery and clinical medicine, in that he collated the loose plant-lore of the woodmen and rhizotomists into a systematic treatise. The "De Historia Plantarum" of Theophrastus contains descriptions of some 500 different plants, and is a good example of the power of the Greek mind to select what is important and reject the superfluous. As Greene has shown,[1] he first divided plants into flowering and flowerless, seed-plants into angiospermous and gymnospermous, describing their external organs in sequence from root to fruit. Before Goethe and Linnæus, he recognized the flower as "a metamorphosed leafy branch." He differentiated aërial roots from tendrils, and regarded fruit as "every form and phase of seed encasement, seed included." He understood how the annual rings on the stems and trunks of trees are formed, and "without having seen a vegetable cell, yet distinguished clearly between parenchymatous and prosenchymatous tissues." The most important editions of Theophrastus are the two Aldines of 1497 (Greek) and 1504 (Latin), and Stapel's Greek and Latin text of 1644.

The colonization of Greek medicine in Egypt led to brilliant developments in anatomy and surgery, but our knowledge of the two great Alexandrian anatomists, **Herophilus** and **Erasistratus,** the originators of dissecting, is not based upon any textual record of their writings, but was pieced together by the scholarship of Marx and Hieronymus. Both Herophilus and Erasistratus made important investigations of the nervous system, showing the relations of the larger nerves to the brain and spinal cord, and distinguishing sensory and motor nerves, with which they sometimes confused the tendons. Both are credited with a vague reference to the lacteal vessels. Herophilus in particular described the

[1] E. L. Greene: "Landmarks of Botanical History," Washington, Smithsonian Inst., 1909, pp. 52–142.

torcular Herophili and the fourth ventricle of the brain, including the calamus scriptorius. He also described the hyoid bone, the duodenum, and the prostate gland, and, in the eye, the retina, vitreous and ciliary body. Erasistratus described the trachea, the auricles and chordæ tendineæ of the heart, but claimed that the heart contains no blood. The Egyptians of the Alexandrian period were almost entirely under the sway of Greek medicine.

Considerable light is thrown upon the Hellenic medical culture grafted upon Egypt in the Alexandrian period—the, dietetics, materia medica, pathology, wet-nursing, public baths, the surviving "etiquette" of circumcision and embalming, the temples of Serapis and Isis (Serapieia, Isieia, corresponding to the Greek Asclepieia)—in Karl Sudhoff's splendid monograph, "Aerztliches aus griechischen Papyrus-Urkunden. Baustein zu einer medicinischen Kulturgeschichte des Hellenismus," in Studien z. Gesch. d. Med. (Puschmann-Stiftung), Nos. 5, 6, Leipzig, 1909.

The tendencies of the school of Empirics who flourished in the second century before Christ culminated in an actual development of quasi-experimental pharmacology and toxicology at the hands of physicians and wary dilettante rulers, of whom Mithridates, King of Pontus, achieved a reputation in the art of giving and taking poisons. He is said to have immunized himself against poisoning by means of the blood of ducks fed upon toxic principles, and he aspired to make a universal antidote (alexipharmacy). These "mithridates" and "theriacs," as they were called, engaged the talents of pharmacists up to the beginning of the eighteenth century, and, in a manner, Mithridates may be regarded as the originator of the idea of polyvalent drugs and sera. The principal relics of this empirical poison-lore are the two hexameter poems of Nikander on poisonous animals (Theriaca), and antidotes for poisons (Alexipharmaca), which have been preserved in the two Aldine editions of 1499 and 1523, and in the French versification of these poems of Jacques Grevin (Plantin imprint, Antwerp, 1568).

III. The Græco-Roman Period (146 B. C.–476 A. D.)

After the destruction of Corinth (146 B. C.), Greek medicine may be said to have migrated to Rome. Before the Greek invasion, the Romans, as the younger Pliny tells us, "got on for 600 years without doctors," relying mainly on medicinal herbs and domestic simples, superstitious rites and religious observances. To the Romans of the Empire, the Greek of any description was the *Græculus esuriens* of Juvenal. The proud Roman citizen, who had a household god for nearly every disease or physiologic function known to him,[1] looked askance upon the itinerant Greek physi-

---

[1] These Roman gods were worshiped under fanciful but appropriate names, as Febris, Scabies, Angeronia, Fluonia, Uterina, Cloacina, Mephites, Dea Salus, and the like.

cian, despising him as a mercenary for accepting compensation for his services, and otherwise distrusting him as a possible poisoner or assassin. Apart from the writings of a private littérateur like Celsus, the principal Roman contribution to medicine was the splendid sanitary engineering of the architect Vitruvius. Greek medicine was finally established on a respectable footing in Rome through the personality, tact, and superior ability of **Asclepiades** of Bithyna (124 B. C.), whose fragments are presented in Gumpert's Greek text (Weimar, 1794). Asclepiades was a formal opponent of the Hippocratic idea that morbid conditions are due to a disturbance of the humors of the body (Humoralism), and attributed disease to constricted or relaxed conditions of its solid particles (Solidism). This is the so-called doctrine of the "strictum et laxum," which was derived from the atomic theory of Democritus and has been revived at different times under such various guises as the Brunonian theory of sthenic and asthenic states, Friedrich Hoffmann's idea of tonic and atonic conditions, Broussais' theory of irritation as a cause of disease, and Rasori's doctrine of stimulus and contra-stimulus. As a logical consequence of his antagonism to Hippocrates, Asclepiades founded his therapeutic scheme on the efficiency of systematic interference as opposed to the healing power of nature; but in practice he was a real Asclepiad, wisely falling back upon the Coan régime of fresh air, light, appropriate diet, hydrotherapy, massage, clysters, local applications, and sparing internal medication. He was the first to mention tracheotomy. His influence for good was that of a superior personality and died with him. His pupils and adherents, Themison and others, exaggerated his doctrines into a formal "Methodism,"[1] while the followers of the Stoic philosophers endeavored to found a system of medicine based upon the physical action and status of the vital air, or *pneuma*. The Hellenic Renaissance in Rome was thus characterized by three different ways of looking at disease as disturbances of the liquid, solid or gaseous constituents of the body, viz., Humoralism, Solidism, and Pneumatism. In all this welter of theorizing, six names stand out above the rest—Celsus, Dioscorides, Rufus, Soranus, Galen, and Antyllus, and most of these were free-lances, that is, "Eclectics."

Although Roman medicine was almost entirely in Greek hands, the best account of it we have was the work of Aurelius Cornelius

---

[1] Allbutt says that the Methodists and the Empirics were, in some sort, a continuation of the Coan and Cnidian schools, the former considering the whole patient and his environment, the latter the locality of the disease and its local treatment. The Cnidians and the Empirics merely listed symptoms without coördinating them and were, in consequence, only haphazard therapeutists. See Allbutt's lectures on Greek medicine in Rome, Brit. Med. Jour., London, 1909, ii; 1449; 1515; 1598.

Celsus, who lived during the reign of Augustus Cæsar. Celsus was, inferentially, not a physician, but a private gentleman of the noble family of the Cornelii, who wrote encyclopedic treatises on medicine, agriculture, and other subjects for the benefit of the Admirable Crichtons of his own station in life. Celsus wrote on medicine in the same spirit in which Virgil treated of veterinary matters in the third book of the Georgics, and we are led to suppose that, in accordance with Roman usage, he rendered medical assistance gratis, very much as the mistress of an old English estate or Southern plantation played Lady Bountiful among her friends and dependents. Classed by Pliny among the men of letters (*auctores*) rather than the *medici*, Celsus was ignored by the Roman practitioners of his day, and his name is mentioned only four times by the medieval commentators; but with the Revival of Learning, he had his revenge, in that his work ("De Re Medicina") was one of the first medical books to be printed (1478), afterward passing through more separate editions than almost any other scientific treatise. This was due largely to the purity and precision of his literary style, his elegant Latinity assuring him the title of "Cicero medicorum." Celsus is the oldest medical document after the Hippocratic writings, and, of the seventy-two medical authors mentioned by him, only the work of Hippocrates himself has come down to us. The "De Re Medicina" consists of eight books, the first four of which deal with diseases treated by diet and regimen, the last four describing those amenable to drugs and surgery. He begins his fifth book with a classified list of drugs, followed by a chapter on weights and measures, pharmaceutic methods and prescriptions, very much like a modern hand-book of therapeutics. He was the first to recommend nutritive enemata. The sixth book treats of skin[1] and venereal diseases as well as those of the eye, ear, nose, throat and mouth. The seventh book is surgical, and contains one of the first accounts of the use of the ligature, and his classic description of lateral lithotomy. Under the Romans, surgery (including obstetrics and ophthalmology) attained to a degree of perfection which it was not to reach again before the time of Ambroise Paré. Surgical instrumentation, in particular, was highly specialized. Over two hundred different surgical instruments were found at Pompeii. Herniotomy and plastic surgery were known, as well as the operations for cataract, version, and Cesarean section. Sufficient reason for all this may be found in the constant contact of the Romans with gladiatorial and military surgery, and the fact that the dissection of executed criminals was

---

[1] Of the forty skin diseases described by Celsus, alopecia areata is still remembered as "area Celsi."

sometimes allowed. Hippocrates said that "war is the only proper school for the surgeon." Celsus is also very full on the different malarial fevers of Italy and their treatment, on gout, and on the treatment of different kinds of insanity. He was the first important writer on medical history,[1] and, in his Prooemium, establishes the status of Hippocrates, Herophilus, Erasistratus, and other great names of the past in the spirit of one who might himself have said

> I write as others wrote
> On Sunium's height.

Of the 105 different editions of Celsus extant, the most interesting are the Florentine *editio princeps*, the Milan imprint of 1481, the Venetian imprint of 1524 (the rarest and costliest of all), the Aldine of 1525, and the handsome Elzevir of 1657. The standard modern edition is that of Daremberg. The best account of Celsus in any language is unquestionably the lucid and scholarly essay of Paul Broca.[2]

The three leading Greek surgeons of the period contemporary with Celsus were Heliodorus, Archigenes (both mentioned in Juvenal's Satires), and Antyllus, all of whom have come down to us in the compilations of the Byzantine writers. **Heliodorus,** who antedated Celsus, gave the first account of ligation and torsion of blood-vessels, and was one of the first to treat stricture by internal urethrotomy. He also described head injuries, the operative treatment of hernia, circular and flap amputation. The latter procedure was fully described by **Archigenes,** and both surgeons employed ligatures, which, in Galen's time, were to be bought at a special shop in the Via Sacra. **Antyllus,** long before Daviel, mentions the removal of cataract by extraction and suction, but his name and fame are permanently associated with his well-known method of treating aneurysms by applying two ligatures and cutting down between them, which held the field until the time of John Hunter.

Pedacius **Dioscorides,** the originator of the materia medica, was a Greek army surgeon in the service of Nero (54–68 A. D.), and utilized his opportunities of travel in the study of plants. His work is the authoritative source on the materia medica of antiquity, of which he describes about 600 plants and plant-principles, over a hundred more than Theophrastus. As Theophrastus was the first scientific botanist, so Dioscorides was the first to write on medical botany as an applied science. His first book deals with

---

[1] The others are Hippocrates (On Ancient Medicine), and, as Professor Sudhoff informs me, Oseibia and Menon (Iatrike).

[2] "Conférences historiques de la Faculté de médecine," Paris, 1865, pp. 445–497.

aromatic, oily, gummy or resinous plant products; the second with
animal products of dietetic and medicinal value and with cereals
and garden herbs; the third and fourth, with the other medicinal
plants. His classification was qualitative, as in a materia medica,
rather than botanical, but, like Theophrastus, he recognized natural
families of plants before Linnæus, Adanson, and Jussieu. His
descriptions were followed, "word by word," for sixteen centuries,
and his book, says Greene,[1] has been more attentively studied by
learned men than any other botanical work, with the possible exception of Bauhin's "Pinax" (1623). Up to the beginning of the
seventeenth century the best books on medical botany were still
simple commentaries on the treatise of Dioscorides, the most interesting editions of which are the Aldine of 1499 (Greek text), the
Stephanus of 1516 (Latin translation of Ruellius), the rare bilingual text of Cologne (1529), and the Italian commentary of Mattioli (Venice, 1544), also extremely rare.

Aretæus the Cappadocian, who also lived in the reign of Nero,
comes nearer than any other Greek to the spirit and method of
Hippocrates, and is on this account more readily appreciated by
modern readers. As a clinician, he ranks next to the Father of Medicine for the graphic accuracy and fidelity of his pictures of disease,
of which he has given the classic first-hand accounts of pneumonia, diabetes, tetanus, elephantiasis, diphtheria (ulcera Syriaca),
the first clear differentiation between cerebral and spinal paralysis,
indicating the decussation of the pyramids, and a very full account
of the different kinds of insanity. Aretæus is easily the most attractive medical author of his time. His work is preserved in the
faulty Greek text of 1554 and in Wigan's valued Clarendon Press
edition (Oxford, 1723).

Another great eclectic was **Rufus of Ephesus,** who lived in the
reign of Trajan (98–117 A. D.), and whose literary remains and
fragments have been preserved in the Paris text of 1554. He
wrote a little work on anatomy in which he described the capsule
of the crystalline lens, the membranes of the eye, the optic chiasm,
and the oviduct in the sheep. He also gave the first descriptions of
traumatic erysipelas, epithelioma, and bubonic plague. He added
many new compounds to the materia medica, of which his "hiera,"
a purgative containing colocynth, became celebrated.

Soranus of Ephesus, of the second century A. D., a follower of
the Methodist school of Asclepiades, is our leading authority on
the gynecology, obstetrics, and pediatrics of antiquity. His
treatise on midwifery and diseases of women, preserved in Dietz's
Greek text (Königsberg, 1838), was the original of such famous

---

[1] E. L. Greene: "Landmarks of Botanical History," Washington, 1909,
pp. 151–155.

works as Röslin's Rosegarten (1513), and Raynalde's "Byrthe of Mankynde" (1545); and most of the supposed innovations in these books, such as the obstetric chair or podalic version, have been traced back to Soranus. After Soranus, there were no real additions to obstetrics before the time of Paré, some fifteen hundred years later.

The "Natural History" of **Pliny** the Elder (23–79 A. D.) is a vast compilation of all that was known in his time of geography, meteorology, anthropology, botany, zoölogy, and mineralogy and is interesting for its many curious facts about plants and drugs, its sidelights on Roman medicine, and its author's many slaps at physicians. After the invention of printing it passed through more than eighty editions. It contains the original references to many unique things, such as Mithridates' experiments with poisons, or Nero's use of the monocle or lorgnette ("Nero princeps gladiatorum pugnas spectabat in smaragdo"), which, some writers think, may have been an actual eyeglass. The botanical errors of Pliny remained unchallenged until the time of Nicholas Leonicenus (1492).

The ancient period closes with the name of the greatest Greek physician after Hippocrates, **Galen** (131–201 A. D.), the founder of experimental medicine. Born an architect's son at Pergamus, Galen's youth and old age were those of a peripatetic. His life was one long *Wanderjahr*. At Rome, where he commenced practice in 164 A. D., he soon attained the leadership of his profession, but retired early to devote himself to study, travel, and teaching. Compared with Hippocrates, Galen seems like the versatile many-sided man of talent as contrasted with the man of true genius. He was the most skilled practitioner of his time, but left no good accounts of clinical cases, only miraculous cures. He usually got his patients well, and to this end instituted an elaborated system of polypharmacy, the memory of which survives in our language in the term "galenicals," as applied to vegetable simples. Galen was fond of botanizing in his travels, and his roving disposition undoubtedly did much to develop that cocksure attitude of mind which made his writings the fountain-head of ready-made theory, or what the Germans call "polypragmatism."[1] He had an answer ready for every problem, a reason to assign for every phenomenon. He elaborated a system of pathology which combined the humoral ideas of Hippocrates with the Pythagorean theory of the four elements and his own conception of a spirit or "pneuma" penetrating all the parts. Referring all pathologic phenomena back to

[1] Asclepiades, Allbutt says, tended to dissipate the specific in the universal (physiologic therapeutics); Galen, proceeding from a theoretic monotheism, tended to lose the universal in the particular (polypharmacy).

these postulates, Galen, with fatal facility and ingenuity, proceeded to explain everything in the light of pure theory, thus substituting a pragmatical system of medical philosophy for the plain notation and interpretation of facts as taught by Hippocrates. The effect of this dogmatism and infallibility upon after-time was appalling; for while Galen's monotheism and piety appealed to the Moslems, his assumption of omniscience was specially adapted to appease the mental indolence and flatter the complacency of those who were swayed entirely by reverence for authority. Up to the time of Vesalius, European medicine was one vast *argumentum ad hominem* in which everything relating to anatomy and physiology, as well as disease, was referred back to Galen as a final authority, from whom there could be no appeal. After his death, European medicine remained at a dead level for nearly fourteen centuries.

Galen was the most voluminous of all the ancient writers and the greatest of the theorists and systematists. His works are a gigantic encyclopedia of the knowledge of his time, including nine books on anatomy, seventeen on physiology, six on pathology, sixteen essays on the pulse, the Megatechne (Ars magna) or therapeutics (fourteen books), the Microtechne (Ars parva) or "practice," and thirty books on pharmacy. He gave us the four classic symptoms of inflammation, differentiated pneumonia from pleurisy, was the first to mention aneurysm,[1] differentiating the traumatic from the dilated form, described the different forms of phthisis, mentioning its infectious nature and proposing a full milk diet and climatotherapy (sea voyages and dry elevated places) for the disease; he understood the diathetic relation between calculus and gout, and his prescriptions indicate a most intelligent use of opium, hyoscyamus, hellebore and colocynth, hartshorn, turpentine, alcohol (wine), sugar diet (honey), grape-juice, barley-water, and cold compresses. He set the pace for a fantastic pulse-lore or "ars sphygmica," which was still in vogue in the eighteenth century. As an anatomist, he gave many excellent descriptions, especially of the motor and locomotor systems, but his work was faulty and inaccurate, as being based largely on the dissection of apes and swine. His contributions to the science were accepted as finalities up to the time of Vesalius. But if Galen was little of an anatomist, he was the first and only experimental physiologist before Harvey. He was the first to describe the cranial nerves and the sympathetic system, made the first experimental sections of the spinal cord, producing hemiplegia; produced aphonia by cutting the recurrent laryngeal; and gave the first valid explanation of the mechanism of respiration. In these matters Galen gave to

---

[1] "Methodus Medendi," lib. v, f. 63 (Linacre's translation of 1519).

medicine that method of putting questions to nature and of arranging matters so that nature may answer them, which we call experiment. His contributions to the physiology of the nervous, respiratory, and circulatory systems, however faulty, were the only real knowledge for seventeen centuries.[1]

There are three Galenic superstitions which, through their plausible character, have had a great deal to do with preventing the advancement of medical science. First, the doctrine of Vitalism, which maintained that the blood is endued with "natural spirits" in the liver, with "vital spirits" in the left ventricle of the heart, and that the vital spirits are converted into "animal spirits" in the brain, the whole organism being animated by a "pneuma." Modifications of this theory, however attractive, have driven physiology into many a delusive blind alley, even up to the time of Driesch. Second, the notion that the blood, in its transit through the body, passes from the right to the left ventricle by means of certain imaginary invisible pores in the interventricular septum, prevented theorists from having real insight into the circulation until the time of Harvey.[2] Third, the idea that "coction" or suppuration is an essential part of the healing of wounds led to those Arabist notions of "healing by second intention," setons and laudable pus, which, although combated by Mondeville, Paracelsus and Paré, were not entirely overthrown before the advent of Lister.

Of the many editions of Galen's works, the most important are the Aldine Greek text of 1525 (five volumes), the Basel edition of 1538, with the initial letter by Holbein, and the nine different editions of the Latin text published by the house of Giunta at Venice between the years 1541 and 1625. Of Latin translations, Conrad Gesner's (Basel, 1562), with the biographic illustrations on the title page, is perhaps the most famous. Among the modern editions, the best are the twenty-volume Greek and Latin text of Kühn (Leipzig, 1821–33) and Daremberg's anthology in two volumes (Paris, 1854–6). The most famous single treatise of Galen is his monograph on the physiologic and teleologic aspects of the different parts of the human body ("De Usu Partium"), the prototype of all subsequent "Bridgewater treatises."

---

[1] A possible exception to this statement would be the few physiologic experiments made by Vesalius which, however, passed unnoticed in his time.

[2] Galen regarded the arterial blood (charged with "vital spirits) and the venous blood (charged with "natural" spirits) as ebbing and flowing, back and forth, through their respective channels, but having no connection with each other except through the interventricular pores. In like manner the "animal spirits" were supposed to course back and forth through the hollow nerves, which became solid after death. For a good account of this phase of Galenic physiology, see Sir Michael Foster, "Lectures on the History of Physiology," Cambridge, 1901, pp. 12, 13.

Of the condition of medicine under the Romans, considerable is known but little need be said. Before the second century A. D., they employed medical slaves (*servi medici*), or relied upon their special medical gods (Febris, Scabies, Uterina, and the rest), with an occasional dilettante interest in healing on their own account. How the early Roman citizens looked upon the Greek physicians has been seen. But even after Asclepiades, Galen, and Soranus had made the status of medicine respectable, the Roman Quirites continued to regard the profession as beneath them. Some Romans, early and late, practised or wrote upon medicine, such as Scribonius Largus, the compiler of drugs and prescriptions (47 A. D.), who left an important expectorant mixture for phthisis and first suggested the use of the electric ray in headaches; Cælius Aurelianus, the neurologist, who translated Soranus of Ephesus; Quintus Serenus Samonicus, who wrote a didactic poem on popular medicine in the third century A. D., and Theodorus Priscianus, court physician to Gratian. Besides the "medici" proper, there were the herb gatherers (*rhizotomi*), the drug-peddlers (*pharmacopolæ*), the salve-dealers (*unguentarii*), the army surgeons, and the *archiatri* or body physicians to the emperors, some of whom were also public or communal (*archiatri populares*). There were also the less reputable *iatroliptæ*, or bath attendants, *obstetrices*, or midwives, the professional poisoners (*pharmacopœi*), and the depraved characters who sold philters and abortifacients. A very dubious and much satirized class were the eye specialists or oculists (*medici ocularii*) who, each of them, sold a special eye salve stamped with his own private seal and compounded of zinc and calamine. Nearly two hundred of these seals have been found.

A special feature of Roman medicine was the cultivation of warm public baths (*thermæ*) and of mineral springs. General hydrotherapy was introduced by Asclepiades, and no less than 1800 public baths had been founded during the period 334 B. C.–180 A. D. (Haeser). The baths of Caracalla and Diocletian had marble accommodations for 1600 and 3000 persons respectively, the water being supplied from the great aqueducts. The establishments for cold bathing (*frigidaria*) often had a swimming-pool (*piscina*) attached, but it is not known whether the warm baths (*tepidaria, calidaria*) were heated as to the water or the air of the room. The principal natural springs were the thermæ at Baiæ near Naples, Thermopylæ in Greece (especially patronized by the Emperor Hadrian), and, in the Roman Colonies, Aix les Bains (*Aquæ Gratianæ Allobrogum*), Aix in Provence (*Aquæ Sextiæ*), Bagnères de Bigorre (*Vicus Aquensis*), Baden in Switzerland (*Thermopolis*), Baden near Vienna (*Aquæ Pannonicæ*), Baden Baden (*Civitas Aquensis*), Aix la Chapelle (*Aquisgranum*), and Wiesbaden (*Aquæ Mattiacenses*).[1]

The Etruscans were wonderfully skilled in dentistry. Some remarkable specimens of Etruscan bridgework are preserved in the museum of Corneto and have been described by Guerini and Walsh.[2]

---

[1] Haeser: "Lehrb. d. Gesch. d. Med." 3. Aufl., Leipz., 1875, i, 494.

[2] Guerini: "History of Dentistry," New York, 1909, 67–76, and J. J. Walsh, "Modern Progress and History," New York, 1912, 79–103.

The special talent of the Romans was for military science and the making and administration of laws. Their hygienic achievements, such as cremation, the sensible, well-ventilated houses, the great aqueducts, sewers, drains and public baths, were of far greater consequence than their native literary contributions to medicine. Yet even here, as Sudhoff says, they often produced hygienic results without intention, things of hygienic value but of non-medical origin.[1] Roman medicine, at best, can only be regarded as an offshoot or subvariety of Greek medicine.

[1] Karl Sudhoff: "Hygienische Gedanken und ihre Manifestationen in der Weltgeschichte," Deutsche Revue, Stuttgart, Oct., 1911, p. 43.

6

THE BYZANTINE PERIOD (476-732 A. D.)

THE downfall of the Western Roman Empire was mainly due to the degeneration of the Roman stock through mixture with weaker and inferior races, and the soldiers who had never known defeat became an easy prey to the invading barbarians of the North, informed with the rugged and primitive virtues which they themselves had once possessed. In the days of the Republic, the Roman had matched the Spartan as a virile soldier and law giver, essentially simple in mind and morals. In a state of society "where wealth accumulates and men decay," he could not hold his own with the flexible, wily Greek of later times, nor with the subtle, fatalistic Oriental, both of them more agile in mind and more dexterous in action than he. Like the Normans in Sicily, or those English colonists in Ireland, who became proverbially "Hibernis ipsis Hiberniores," he fell under that strange law by which the conqueror, in the end, assimilates himself to the conquered people. By process of race-inmixture the Romans of the fifth century A.D. had acquired the "serene impartiality" of spirit which Professor Huxley attributes to the mongrel races, and some think that the malarial fevers which had begun to devastate the Italian peninsula had as much to do with weakening their fiber as the luxuries and dissipations to which they were continually exposed. Degeneration of mind and body, with consequent relaxation of morals, led to mysticism and that respect for the authority of magic and the supernatural which was to pave the way for the bigotry, dogmatism and mental inertia of the Middle Ages. Under these conditions, the physician became more and more of a mercenary, parasite and vendor of quack medicines. Long before the downfall of Rome the magician, the thaumaturgist, the professional poisoner, and the courtezan who peddled drugs—

> Ambubaiarum collegia, pharmacopolæ,
> Mendici, mimæ, balatrones, hoc genus omne,

were familiar figures. In the Eastern Empire, the decomposition of intelligence was even more pronounced, and today the adjective "Byzantine" connotes little more than luxury, effemination and sloth. Through the conflict of Pagan and Christian modes of thought, almost all of the intellectual energy of the period was dissipated in religious controversy, while medicine had become an affair of salves and poultices, talismans and pentagrams, with a mumbling of incantations and spells very like the backwoods pranks of Tom Sawyer and Huckleberry Finn, or some of the vagaries of Christian Science. There were doubtless good people, then as now, but they did not come to the front, and there is pith in Gibbon's sarcasm about two pious characters of the period: "We know his vices and are ignorant of her virtues." This supine cast of mind and morals is well reflected in the Byzantine mysticism of Wagner's Parsifal, and the figure of Kundry, the sorcerer's minion, who brings nostrums from the far East to alleviate the sufferings of Anfortas, may serve as a sort of type and symbol of Byzantine medicine. The solitary thing the Eastern Empire did for European medicine was to preserve something of the language, culture and literary texts of Greece. Although the Byzantine power lasted over a thousand years (395–1453 A. D.), medical history is concerned chiefly with the names of four industrious compilers who were prominent physicians in the first three centuries of its existence. Of these, the courtier **Oribasius** (326–403 A. D.), a friend and physician-in-ordinary to Julian the Apostate and sometime quæstor of Constantinople, is chiefly remarkable as a torch-bearer of knowledge rather than as an original writer, but his compilations are highly valued by scholars in that he always gives his authorities, and so far as is known, quotes them exactly. Medicine is indebted to him for a remarkable anthology of the works of his predecessors, many of whom (the surgeons Archigenes, Heliodorus, Antyllus, for instance) might otherwise have been lost to posterity. Galen in particular he expounded with loving care and did much to establish him in his central position of authority during the Dark Ages. Like Galen, Oribasius took all knowledge for his province. His great encyclopedia of medicine comprised indeed over seventy volumes, dealing with all aspects of the subject. Much of this has been lost, but its author epitomized his knowledge in the little "Synopsis" which he made for the use of his son. His "Euporista," or popular treatise on medicine, had the rare merit of avoiding any current superstitions and inculcating sound therapeutic doctrine. The student of medical history will read Oribasius to best advantage in Daremberg's splendid six-volume edition, with the parallel French translation (Paris, 1851–76).

Ætius of Amida, who lived in the sixth century, A. D., was also a royal physician (to Justinian I, 527–65) and *comes obsequii* (lord high chamberlain) at the court of Byzantium. He left an extensive compilation, usually called the "Tetrabiblion," which is a principal authority for what we know of the work of Rufus of Ephesus and Leonides in surgery, Soranus and Philumenus in gynecology and obstetrics. Ætius gives a description of epidemic

diphtheria not unlike that of Aretæus, and his work contains the
best account of diseases of the eye, ear, nose, throat and teeth in
the literature of antiquity. He has also interesting chapters on
goitre and hydrophobia. In surgery he supplies many of the lost
passages in Oribasius, and describes modes of procedure (tonsillotomy, urethrotomy, treatment of hemorrhoids) not found elsewhere. He recommended many salves and plasters, and is supposed to have been a Christian by reason of the charms and spells
he proposes for their preparation.[1] Thus, in preparing a plaster,
he says, one should intone repeatedly, "The God of Abraham, the
God of Isaac, the God of Jacob, give virtue to this medicament."
To remove a bone stuck in the throat, one should cry out in a loud
voice: "As Jesus Christ drew Lazarus from the grave, and Jonah
out of the whale, thus Blasius, the martyr and servant of God,
commands 'Bone come up or go down.'"

Alexander of Tralles (525–605), a much traveled practitioner
who finally settled in Rome, was the only one of the Byzantine
compilers who displayed any special originality. Although a
follower of Galen, his "Practica" (first printed at Lyons in 1504)
contains some descriptions of disease and some prescriptions which
seem to be his own. His accounts of insanity, gout and the dysenteric and choleraic disorders are above the average. He has a highly
original chapter on intestinal worms and vermifuges and he is said
to have been the first to mention rhubarb. Like Galen, he recommends a full milk diet, change of air and sea voyages for phthisis,
but his other prescriptions are often disfigured by the obtrusion
of the usual Byzantine spells and charms.

Paul of Ægina (625–690), the last of the Greek eclectics and
compilers, was the author of an "Epitome" of medicine in seven
books, first printed by the Aldine press at Venice in 1528. Although he was a physician of high repute, we may judge how low
medicine had sunk in the seventh century by his apologetic statements in regard to any lack of originality on his part. He frankly
admits that the ancients have said all that could be said on the
subject and that he is only a humble scribe. Paul was, however, a
very capable surgeon, and the sixth book of his Epitome was the
standard work on the subject up to the time of Albucasis, who indeed drew upon it for most of his information. Paul gives original
descriptions of lithotomy, trephining, tonsillotomy, paracentesis
and amputation of the breast, but stopped short of opening the
chest for empyema. In describing herniotomy, he recommends
removal of the testicles, a mutilation which was perpetuated by

---

[1] A definitive and complete edition of the Greek text of Ætius still remains
to be published.

the Arabians and continued to be the vogue with the outcast medieval surgeons until far into the sixteenth century. Paul gives the fullest account we have of the eye surgery and military surgery of antiquity. He omits all reference to podalic version, and as his authority was upheld by the Arabians, the procedure disappears from literature until the time of Röslin and Paré.

Among the minor writers of the Byzantine period, we may mention Publius Vegetius Renatus, a horse trader and farrier of the fifth century, A. D., whose "Ars Veterinaria," published at Basel in 1528, contains the first authentic account of glanders; and Theophilus Protospatharius, physician and captain of the guard to the Emperor Heraclius (603–641), and a contemporary of Paul of Ægina, who left an original description of the palmaris brevis muscle and the olfactory nerve, and wrote a treatise on the urine which for centuries upheld the Galenic doctrine that the latter is a filtrate of the blood, secreted in the portal vein and vena cava. The same doctrine was maintained unchanged in the thirteenth century by Johannes Actuarius, the last of the Byzantine writers, whose elaborate treatise on the urine made the notion authoritative with the absurd "water-casters" of a later time. He is memorable as the first to use a graduated glass for examining the urine, although the markings upon it were not quantitative but qualitative, indicating the possible position of the different scums, precipitates and sediments.

During the Byzantine period, an interesting contribution to clinical medicine was made by the Fathers of the Christian Church, namely, the description of the earlier epidemics of smallpox. Eusebius described a Syrian epidemic in 302 A. D., another was described by Gregory of Tours in 581, and the term "variola" was first employed by Marius, Bishop of Avenche, in 570. It is said that the disease was also described in the Irish monastery records of 675 A. D. as "Bolgagh" and "Galar Breac."

THE MOHAMMEDAN AND JEWISH PERIODS
(732–1096 A. D.)

By the swords of Mohammed and his emirs, the wild outlaw clans of the Asian and African deserts were converted into nations capable of acting as military and social units, but it was not until long after his death, when the mighty empire which he founded was subdivided into caliphates, that the sciences and arts were permitted to develop. During the period of conquest and conversion, the fanatical, fatalistic zeal of the Moslems tended naturally toward the destruction and persecution of the things of the mind. While the principal service of Islam to medicine was the preservation of Greek culture, yet the Saracens themselves were the originators not only of algebra, chemistry and geology, but of many of the so-called improvements or refinements of civilization, such as street-lamps, window-panes, fireworks, stringed instruments, cultivated fruits, perfumes, spices, and that "often-changed and often-washed undergarment of linen or cotton which still passes among ladies under its old Arabic name."[1] In the intellectual sphere, the monotheism and the dialectic tendencies of Galen and Aristotle appealed strongly to the Mohammedans. Galen's polypharmacy in particular appealed to these natural chemists, and his haphazard "polypragmatism" was molded by them into iron-clad dogma. The Oriental idea that it is sinful to touch the human body with the hands did little to advance anatomy or surgery. The general trend of Oriental religious fatalism was toward contemplative brooding and resigned submission to authority and such eagerness or free-play of the mind as the Moslems possessed was expended in hair-splitting subtleties. Thus the intellectual tendencies of the Middle Ages were determined for them in advance. We call the medical authors of the Mohammedan period "Arabic" on account of the language in which they wrote, but, in reality, most of them were Persian or Spanish-born, and many of them were Jewish.

The Mohammedan physicians themselves owed their medical knowledge, in the first instance, to a persecuted sect of Christians. Nestorius, a priest who had been made patriarch of Constantinople in 428, taught the heretical doctrine that Mary should not be

---

[1] Draper: "History of the Intellectual Development of Europe," New York, 1876, ii, pp. 33, 34.

styled the "Mother of God" but the "Mother of Christ." In consequence, he and his followers were driven into the desert and, like the Jews after them, took up the study of medicine because of religious and social ostracism. The Nestorian heretics gained control of the school at Edessa in Mesopotamia, with its two large hospitals, and made it a remarkable institution for teaching medicine, but were driven out by the orthodox Bishop Cyrus in 489. Fleeing to Persia, where their theologic doctrines were welcome, they established the famous school at Gondisapor, which was the true starting-point of Mohammedan medicine.

The Eastern (or Bagdad) Caliphate (750–1258) was under the sway of the Abbasides, who were friends of learning and science and included such liberal-minded rulers as the caliphs Al-Mansur (754–775), Harun al-Rashid (786–802) and Al-Meiamun (813–833). These monarchs encouraged the collection and copying of Greek manuscripts, and the earlier centuries of the Mohammedan period were occupied in translating the works of Hippocrates, Galen, Dioscorides and other Greek classics into Arabic. The principal Arabic translators in the eighth and ninth centuries were the Syrian family of Mesuë and the Nestorian teacher Honain (or Johannitius) (809–873), whom Withington calls "the Erasmus of the Arabic Renaissance." Johannitius had an adventurous career, translated Hippocrates, Galen, Oribasius, and Paul of Ægina, and was in his day the leading medical spirit of Bagdad. The greatest physicians of the Eastern Caliphate were the three Persians, Rhazes, Haly Abbas, and Avicenna.

Rhazes (860–932), a great clinician, ranks with Hippocrates, Aretæus, and Sydenham as one of the original portrayers of disease. His description of smallpox and measles is the first authentic account in literature, a classic text, preserved in the original Arabic, with parallel Latin translation, in Channing's edition (London, 1766). Although smallpox had been vaguely described as early as the sixth century by some of the church fathers and by the Arabic chronicler Aaron, the account of Rhazes is so vivid and complete that it is almost modern. His great encyclopedia of medicine, the *El Hawi*, or "Continens," which Haller preferred to any other Arabic treatise, is preserved in the Latin translation of Feragus (Brescia, 1486). Made up of an enormous mass of extracts from many sources, together with original clinical histories and experiments in therapeutics, it reveals Rhazes as a Galenist in theory, although he was a true follower of Hippocrates in the simplicity of his practice.

Haly ben Abbas, a Persian mage, who died in 994, was the author of the "Almaleki" ("Liber regius" or "Royal Book"), a work which was the canonical treatise on medicine for a hundred years, when it was superseded by the "Canon" of Avicenna. It has never been printed in the original Arabic, but was translated into Latin in 1080 by Constantinus Africanus, who published it as his own work.[1]

Avicenna (980–1036), called "the Prince of Physicians," a convivial Omarian spirit, eminently successful in practice as court physician and vizier to different caliphs, was one who trod the primrose path at ease and died in the prime of life from the effect of its pleasures. He was physician in chief to the celebrated hospital at Bagdad, and is said to have written over one hundred works on different subjects, only a few of which have been preserved. His wonderful description of the origin of mountains (cited by Draper and Withington) fully entitles him to be called the "Father of Geology," and it is interesting to note that two physicians, widely separated in space and time—Avicenna and Fracastorius—are the only writers who contributed anything of value to this science for centuries. Avicenna is said to have been the first to describe the preparation and properties of sulphuric acid and alcohol. His "Canon,"[2] which Haller styled a "methodic inanity," is a huge, unwieldy storehouse of learning, in which the author attempts to codify the whole medical knowledge of his time and to square its facts with the systems of Galen and Aristotle. Written in clear and attractive style, this gigantic tome became a fountain-head of authority in the Middle Ages, for Avicenna's elaborated train of reasoning, a miracle of syllogism in its way, appealed particularly to the medieval mind, and indeed set the pace for its movement in many directions. In fairness to Avicenna, it is proper to say that his clinical records, which he intended as an appendix to the "Canon," were irrecoverably lost, and only the Arabic text of the latter, published at Rome in 1593, survives. That Avicenna must have been a clever practitioner we should naturally infer from his great reputation. For example, the striking plates in the Giunta edition of 1595 show that he must have known and practised the method of treating spinal deformities by forcible reduction which was reintroduced by Calot in 1896. Avicenna also described the guinea-worm (Vena Medinensis).[3] Yet upon the whole, the influence of the "Canon" upon medieval medicine was bad in that it confirmed physicians in the pernicious

---

[1] The two principal Latin editions are the Venetian of 1492 and the Lyons of 1523.

[2] The principal Latin editions of the Canon are the Milan imprint of 1473, the Paduan of 1476 and 1497, the Venetian of 1482, 1486, 1490, 1491, 1494 and 1500, the Giuntas of 1527, 1544, 1555, 1582, 1595, and 1608. The Arabic text was printed at Rome in 1593.

[3] Avicenna, Canon, sect. III, tract. II, cap. XXI.

idea that ratiocination is better than first-hand investigation. It also set back the progress of surgery by inculcating the novel doctrine that the latter art is an inferior and separate branch of medicine and by substituting the use of the cautery for the knife.

Other prominent medical figures of the Eastern Caliphate were the Hebrew physician Isaac ben Solomon, called Isaac Judæus (850–950), who wrote a treatise upon dietetics ("De Diæta," Padua, 1487), which became deservedly popular in Europe; and the Arabian traveler Abdollatif (1161–1231), who visited Egypt at Saladin's instance, and while there had opportunities for studying human skeletons which convinced him that Galen's osteology must be wrong in many important respects.

The Western or Cordovan Caliphate (755–1236) attained highest prosperity under the Spanish or Ommiade dynasty (755–1036), and its leading medical authors were the surgeon Albucasis, the philosopher Averroes, and the Jewish physicians Avenzoar and Moses Maimonides.

Abulkasim, called **Albucasis,** a native of Cordova, flourished in the eleventh century, and was the author of a great medico-chirurgical treatise called the "Altasrif" (or "Collection"), of which the surgical part survives in Channing's Arabic text (Oxford, Clarendon Press, 1778). It is remarkable as containing the first pictorial representations of surgical (including dental) instruments, and was the leading text-book on surgery in the Middle Ages up to the time of Saliceto. It consists of three books, founded upon the work of Paul of Ægina. The first of these deals with the use of the actual cautery, the special feature of Arabian surgery, and gives descriptions and figurations of the peculiar instruments used; the second book contains full descriptions of lithotomy, lithotrity, amputations for gangrene and the treatment of wounds; the third book deals with fractures and dislocations, including fracture of the pelvis and a mention of paralysis in fracture of the spine. Albucasis was apparently the first to write on the treatment of deformities of the mouth and dental arches, and he mentions the obstetric posture which is now known as the "Walcher position."[1]

Averroës, also Cordovan-born (1126–1198), was more noted as a philosopher and free thinker than as a physician. His *Ketab* or "Colliget"[2] ("Book of Universals"), an attempt to found a system of medicine upon Aristotle's philosophy, advanced the Pantheistic doctrine that the soul or nature of man is absorbed into universal nature at death. This denial of personal immortality

---

[1] "Tum decumbat mulier in collum suum, pendeantque deorsum pedes, ejus, illa vero in lectum decumbat, etc.," cited by Dr. Herbert Spencer in Lancet, London, 1912, i, p. 1568. Mercurio, in La Comare (1596), also described the hanging position of Walcher.

[2] Published at Venice in 1482.

caused Averroës to be persecuted in his own lifetime, and his followers to be anathematized during the Middle Ages. His work is of interest only as a relic of Arabic modes of thought.

The greatest of the Jewish physicians of the Western Caliphate was the Cordovan **Avenzoar,** who died in 1162. He was one of the few men of his time who had courage enough to tilt against Galenism, and by his description of the itch-mite (*Acarus scabiei*) he may be accounted the first parasitologist after Alexander of Tralles. He also described serous pericarditis, mediastinal abscess, pharyngeal paralysis, and inflammation of the middle ear, and he recommended the use of goat's milk in phthisis and tracheotomy. His "Teisir" or "Rectification of Health" is preserved in the Latin translation published at Venice in 1490.

The Rabbi Moses ben Maimon, called **Moses Maimonides** (1135–1204), was court-physician to Saladin, and his treatise on personal hygiene ("Tractatus de Regimine Sanitatis") was written for that sultan's private use. It contains some admirable precepts of diet and regimen, including a rhubarb and tamarind pill, and its first edition, the Florentine imprint of 1478, is esteemed as one of the rarest of books.

Such able chemists as the Arabians could not fail of being good pharmacologists, and their descriptions of the materia medica and of the preparation of drugs became standard authority throughout the Middle Ages. Even to this day what Osler calls "the heavy hand of the Arabian" is sensed in the enormous bulk of our own pharmacopeias. The principal storehouse of the Arabian materia medica is the "Jami" of Ibn Baitar, a huge thirteenth century compilation, describing some fourteen hundred drugs of which about 300 are said to be new. **Mesue** junior, a mysterious personage of the tenth or eleventh century, who used this name as an eponym or pseudonym, was the most popular Arabic writer on drugs in medieval Europe, and his "Grabadin," or apothecary's manual ("Antidotarium"), was used everywhere in their preparation. His treatise on purgatives divides the latter into mild (wormwood, tamarind, rhubarb) and drastic (scammony, colocynth). The esteem in which these works were held is shown by the fact that a Latin translation of both was one of the first medical books to be printed (Venice, 1471). An important work in the Persian language was the materia medica of **Abu Mansur,**[1] containing descriptions of 585 drugs, of which 466 are vegetable, 75 mineral and 44 animal. A Persian manuscript of the eleventh century by Ismail of Jurjani contains probably the most complete directions of the period for examining the urine.

---

[1] Epitomized in Latin by R. Seligmann, Vienna, 1830–33.

Cultural Aspects of Mohammedan Medicine.—In Sir Richard Burton's translation of the Arabian Nights,[1] there is a tale of a spendthrift heir who has squandered all his substance except a beautiful slave girl of extraordinary talents, who, realizing her master's plight, urges him to bring her before the Caliph Harun al-Rashid to be sold for a sum large enough to cover his loses. On seeing her, the Caliph decides to test the extent of her knowledge, and has specialists put her through a lengthy cross-examination which, incidentally, furnishes us a good documentation of the social aspects of Arabian medicine. As the fair slave exploits her extensive knowledge of Mohammedan theology, law, philosophy, medicine, astronomy, astrology, music, chess-playing and other arts and sciences, we perceive that these accomplishments were also an essential part of the Arabian physician's training and, at the same time, that a certain acquaintance with the Galenical system of medicine was a feature of the cultural equipment of any well-educated Mohammedan of the time. The Arabians derived their knowledge of Greek medicine from the Nestorian monks, many practical details from the Jews, and their astrologic lore from Egypt and the far East. So the slave girl follows the Talmud in regard to the number of the bones (249), gives an exact account of the four humors, and details at length the effects of different conjunctions of the planets. Diagnosis of internal disease is founded upon six canons: (1) The patient's actions; (2) his excreta; (3) the nature of the pain; (4) its site; (5) swelling; (6) the effluvia of the body; and further information is elicited by "the feel of the hands," whether firm or flabby, hot or cool, moist or dry, or by such indications as "yellowness of the whites of the eye" (jaundice) or "bending of the back" (lung disease). The symptoms of yellow bile are a sallow complexion, dryness of the throat, a bitter taste, loss of appetite and rapid pulse; those of black bile, "false appetite and great mental disquiet and cark and care," terminating in melancholia.[2] Medicinal draughts are best taken "when the sap runs in the wood and the grape thickens in the cluster and the two auspicious planets, Jupiter and Venus, are in the ascendant." Cupping is most effective at the wane of the moon, with the weather at set-fair, preferably the seventeenth of the month and on a Tuesday. This, or something like it, was about the character of Mohammedan practice toward the end of the fourteenth century, the period assigned for the composition of the Arabian Nights, and we may reasonably infer that is also fairly representa-

[1] Denver edition, 1899, vol. v, pp. 189–245 ("Abu al-Husn and his Slave-girl Tawaddud"), the medical portion being on pp. 218–226.

[2] Maurice Girardeau, in his Paris Dissertation (No. 107, 1910), points out that the cholemic diathesis was perhaps the most prominent feature of Arabic pathology.

tive of the best period of Moslem medicine as handed down by tradition. The Arabian physician, whose professional importance was gauged by the height of his turban and the richness and length of his sleeves, was usually an astrologer and a magician, who regarded the heart as "the prince of the body," the lungs as the fan of the heart, the liver as the guard of the heart and the seat of the soul, the pit of the stomach as the seat of pleasure and the gallbladder as the seat of courage. From the Arabic medical texts, we know that their authors upheld the Galenic pulse-lore, affected to arrive at inaccessible data, such as the sex of the child in pregnancy, by inspection of the urine (uroscopy), wrote charms in cups with "purgative ink" to mystify their patients, indeed, resorted to all manner of sensational trade-tricks and surprises in order to impose their authority. They abstained from dissecting out of religious conviction, left operative surgery and venesection to the wandering specialists, and the care of women's diseases and obstetric cases to midwives; were constantly squabbling among themselves, stipulated their fees in advance and tried to collect at least half, if the case took an unfavorable turn or did not improve. Some of the fees they received were phenomenal. Gabriel Batischua, a favorite of Harun al-Rashid, got about $1500 per annum "for bleeding and purging the Commander of the Faithful," besides a regular monthly salary of about $2500 and a New Year's purse of $6250. He estimated his total fortune in fees at $10,000,000, and on being recalled from banishment to heal Al-Meiamun, he received $125,000, which Withington regards as the largest fee on record. Abu Nasr, according to the same authority, received more than $60,000 for curing one of the Caliphs of stone. Most all the prominent physicians of the period aimed to curry favor with the reigning potentates or to supplant rival colleagues in their good graces. The Caliphs themselves, after the Mohammedan passion for conquest had been sated, became loyal supporters of science and were instrumental in founding hospitals, libraries and schools. Even private collections of books were sometimes of extraordinary extent, and all Greek, Egyptian, Indian and Jewish culture that did not conflict with the creed of Islam was rapidly assimilated. As early as 707 A. D., the Caliph El Welid had founded a hospital at Damascus. Another was established at Misr in Egypt in 597, another at Cairo in 874, two at Bagdad in 918, two others in the same city in 925 and 977. In course of time dispensaries and infirmaries existed in all the important cities of the Eastern Caliphate and about 1160 a Jewish traveler found as many as sixty of these institutions in Bagdad alone. The largest and best appointed of the Mohammedan hospitals were those founded at Damascus (1160) and Cairo (1276). In the former of these, treatment was given and drugs dispensed free of charge for three centuries. As late as 1427, it was said its fires had never been put out since its opening. The great Al-Mansur hospital of Cairo was a huge quadrangular structure with fountains playing in the four court-yards, separate wards for important diseases, wards for women and convalescents, lecture rooms, an extensive library, out-patient clinics, diet kitchens, an orphan asylum and a chapel. It employed male and female nurses, had an income of about $100,000, and disbursed a suitable sum to each convalescent on his departure, so that he might not have to go to work at once. The patients were nourished upon a rich and attractive diet, and the sleepless were provided with soft music or, as in the Arabian Nights, with accomplished tellers of tales. The Cordovan Caliphate was equally well off in the number, if not the extent, of its hospitals, while the Bagdad Caliphate was especially noted for its ophthalmic dispensaries and lunatic asylums. The Arabians were far ahead of their European contemporaries in their kindly treatment of the insane. Medical instruction was given either at the great hospitals at Bagdad, Damascus and Cairo, or as a special course at the academies which existed in all the cities. Of these, the Hall of Wisdom at Cairo was the most famous. The principal courses were clinical medicine, pharmacology and therapeutics. Anatomy and surgery were neglected but chemistry was held in special esteem. Arabian medicine was, in fact, the parent of alchemy, the founder of which was Geber (702–765), the discoverer of nitric acid and aqua regia and the describer of distillation, filtration, sublimation, water-baths and other essentials of chemical procedure. Alchemy was combined with astrology in this wise. The ancient Chaldaic Pantheism, the doctrine of an *anima mundi*, or "soul of the world," with indwelling spirits in all things, was applied to whatever could be extracted from substances by fire, as "spirit" of wine, "spirit" of nitre, or the various essences and quintessences; while to the seven planets (the sun, the moon, Mars, Mercury, Jupiter, Saturn, Venus) corresponded the seven days of the week and the seven known metals (gold, silver, iron, quicksilver, tin, lead and copper). As these metals were supposed to be "generated" in the bowels of the earth, the special aim of alchemy was to find the fecundating or germinal substance, under appropriate planetary influences. Thus Geber's parable of a medicine which could heal any of six lepers was regarded by Boerhaave as nothing more than allegory of the philosopher's stone for transmuting the six baser planetary metals into gold. Hand in hand with this idea of transmutation of metals went the notion of a polyvalent "elixir of life," which could cure all diseases and confer immortal youth and which was supposed to be of the nature of a "potable gold" (*aurum potabile*).

The search for potable gold led to the discovery of aqua regia and the strong acids by Geber and Rhazes, and the quest of the elixir became the foundation of chemical pharmaceutics. Even as late as the sixteenth century, we find Paracelsus still upholding Geber's idea that everything is made of mercury, sulphur and salt, and that as "the sun rules the heart, the moon the brain, Jupiter the liver, Saturn the spleen, Mercury the lungs, Mars the bile, Venus the kidneys," so the seven planetary metals and their compounds were specifics for the diseases of these organs under the will of the stars. Arabian chemistry probably survived beyond the decadence of Arabian medicine, for Leo Africanus, a traveler of the fifteenth century, mentions a chemical society which existed at Fez at that time. From their constant contact with strange lands and peoples, the Arabian pharmacists or "sandalani" were the exploiters if not the introducers of a vast number of new drugs; in particular, senna, camphor, sandalwood, rhubarb, musk, myrrh, cassia, tamarind, nutmeg, cloves, cubebs, aconite, ambergris and mercury; besides being the originators of syrups, juleps, alcohol, aldehydes (all Arabic terms), and the inventors of flavoring extracts made of rose-water, orange and lemon peel, tragacanth, and other attractive ingredients. The effect of Arabian chemistry and pharmacy upon European medicine lasted long after the Mohammedan power itself had waned and, with the simples of Dioscorides and Pliny, their additions to the materia medica made up the better part of the European pharmacopeias for centuries.

Closely connected with Mohammedan medical culture is the influence of the Jews upon European medicine. Under the Arabian domination, Jewish physicians were prominent figures at the courts of the caliphs and a common belief in a stern monotheism created a strong bond of sympathy between Moslem and Hebrew. Another point of contact was the fact that the Hebrew and Mohammedan physicians, with their peculiar analytic cast of mind, their intensive modes of thought and their appreciation of "values," soon acquired a right materialistic way of looking at concrete things. Thus while medical men under Christianity were still trifling with charms, amulets, saintly relics, the Cabala, and other superstitions, many of the Jewish and Mohammedan physicians were beginning to look upon these things with a certain secret contempt.

During the Middle Ages and long after, the lot of the Hebrew physician in Europe was to be used and abused. In the tenth and eleventh centuries, he was, as Billings says, "a sort of contraband luxury,"[1] resorted to by and protected by prince and prelate alike,

---

[1] J. S. Billings: "The History and Literature of Surgery" (Dennis's System of Surgery, New York, 1895, vol. i, p. 38).

on account of his superior scientific knowledge, but hardly coun-
tenanced for any other reason. The Council of Vienna in 1267
forbade the Jews to practise among Christians. Under the Western Caliphate, Jewish physicians were prominent figures in Spain
until they were banished the country in 1412, and the School of
Salerno utilized them as teachers until it had developed enough
home-grown talent to get along without them. The same thing
was true of Montpellier, which was closed to the Jews in 1301.
Although the different emperors continued to retain Jews as their
body physicians, yet, up to the time of the French Revolution,
they were not allowed to study at the European universities and,
being moreover excluded from the liberal professions, played little
part in medicine during this period. At the outset of the modern
industrial movement, they were admitted to the rights of citizenship all over Europe and given the freedom of the universities.
The effect of this liberal policy was to bring forth a great array of
brilliant talent which contributed very materially to the development of medicine in all its branches, as witness the work of Henle,
Cohnheim, Weigert, Traube and Pick in pathology, Senator,
Hayem and Boas in internal medicine, Romberg, Moll and Freud
in neurology, von Hebra, Kaposi, Neumann, von Zeissl and Unna
in dermatology, Caspar, Lesser, Ottolenghi and Lombroso in forensic medicine, Hirsch, Marx, Pagel, Magnus and Neuburger in
medical history, and, in the science of infection, Metchnikoff,
Fränkel, Friedländer, Marmorek, Haffkine, Neisser, and Paul
Ehrlich,[1] to mention only a few well-known names.

---

[1] For a more complete list of modern Jewish physicians, see F. T. Haneman's paper in the Jewish Encyclopædia, New York, 1904, viii, 421, 422.

THE MEDIEVAL PERIOD (1096-1438)

THE Middle Ages, the period of feudalism and ecclesiasticism, are commonly decried for servile obeisance to authority, with its attending evils of bigotry, pedantry and cruelty. We regard any one who seeks to suppress the truth by overbearing or underhanded methods as "medieval-minded," and we think of special privileges, vested interests, unearned increments, *Faustrecht*, and other phases of Rob Roy's "simple plan," as smacking of feudalism. Yet, in the Middle Ages, there was true "consent of the governed." The people aspired toward nationhood and solidarity rather than toward personal independence and, under these conditions, preferred rather to be led and directed than to think for themselves. In the welter of race-inmixture and race-absorption that followed the downfall of the Roman Empire, it was found that Greek philosophy (neo-Platonism) was a total failure as a moral force, and the greatest need of European humanity was for a spiritual uplift, for regeneration and renewal of character rather than for intellectual development. Mental and moral activities were simply paralyzed by that great cataclysm. To understand the impulses which drove the hermits to the desert and founded the monasteries, one can read Gibbon, Lecky, Montalembert, Gregorovius, Froude on the break-up of Roman society, Turgenieff's wonderful evocation of a Cæsarean triumph or Flaubert's miracle-play of The Temptation of St. Anthony. Matthew Arnold, with his fine historic sense, summed all this up in stirring verses:

> On that hard Pagan world disgust
> And secret loathing fell.
> Deep weariness and sated lust
> Made human life a hell.

> She veiled her eagles, snapp'd her sword,
> And laid her sceptre down;
> Her stately purple she abhorr'd,
> And her imperial crown.

> She broke her flutes, she stopp'd her sports,
> Her artists could not please;
> She tore her books, she shut her courts,
> She fled her palaces.

Thus, the Christian Church, with its spiritual appeal, its attractive symbolism, its splendid organization and its consolidation with Feudalism in protecting Europe from Moslem invasion, could not

96

but triumph. In the great struggle between collectivism and individualism which began from that hour, intellectual independence was bound to go to the wall if it came into conflict with Church or State. In the Middle Ages there was immense concern lest "the centrifugal forces of society overcome the centripetal."[1] The growth of the Christian virtue of compassion toward weakness and suffering, and the more elevated and enlarged conception of the position and mission of women that grew out of it, led to new departures in medicine along untried paths, particularly in nursing the sick and in erecting hospitals everywhere for their care. Only idle bigotry could affirm that Pope and Emperor did not do a great deal for medicine in the advancement of good medical legislation, in the chartering and upbuilding of the medieval universities, in the great hospital movement of the Middle Ages and in the encouragement of individual medical talent in many cases. Yet, as Allbutt has shown, the strife of intellects during the Ages of Faith was manifested in a way that tended to the absolute suppression of experimental science or even of the actual verification of premises. The Greek philosophers, as we have seen, held opinions the most disparate without any special strife among themselves, and above all with a certain definite immunity from persecution. To those who can appreciate the fine individualism of the Greeks, the sentiment of the English poet will not seem exaggerated:

Greece, where only man whose manhood was as godhead ever trod,
  Bears the blind world witness yet of light where with her feet are shod:
Freedom, armed of Greece, was always very man and very God.

The medieval thinkers were all under the ban of authority, and this for the strangest, yet most potent, of reasons. From the earliest times, human ideas as to the meaning of life and the forces behind the material world have usually progressed along two distinct, often parallel, lines, viz., a tendency to deify and worship the objects or forces of external nature, culminating logically in either Pantheism or Buddhistic Pessimism; and the rude fetishism of the savage, which passed through the successive stages of idolatry, hero-worship, ancestor-worship, polytheism, shamanism, finally merging into the pure monotheism of Israel, Christianity and Islam. Christian Theism assumes that God is a spirit, omnipresent and immanent in nature, yet different from it, accessible to prayer, and capable, at need, of divine intervention in human affairs. Pantheism simply identifies God with nature and natural forces. Now, in medieval times, the opposition between Theism and Pantheism took the form of a dispute between "Realists"

---

[1] The phrase is used as a criterion of good and bad government in Roosevelt's Romanes lecture on "Biological Analogies in History," Oxford, 1910, p. 23.

7

and "Nominalists," which, says Allbutt (paraphrasing the language of John of Salisbury), "engaged more of the time and passions of men than for the house of Cæsar to conquer and govern the world."[1] To the medieval logician, "Realism" was just the opposite of our modern concept of a knowledge of material things. The Realist assumed, with Plato, that the idea is as actual as the thing itself and creative of it, the form as real as the matter or substance and anterior to it, whence it follows that all things proceed from the will of God. The Nominalist, on the other hand, affirmed that the form or idea is only a name or abstract conception, existing in the mind of the observer alone, and that God, therefore, exists impersonally in each and every object of the material world. To medieval theologians, such Pantheism as this could be no less than infidelity and unbelief, since it tended to dissolve the dogmas of faith and was subversive of the ideas of divine revelation and of personal immortality, the hope held out to the Christian. To medieval physicians, such a manifesto of free-thought as the Hippocratic treatise "On the sacred disease" would have been abhorrent, while Galen, with his devout monotheism and his careful Bridgewater teleology, became an object of almost veneration. Aristotle, in his Logic and Metaphysics, never made an absolutely clear distinction between the supposed reality of idea and substance, and although proscribed under excommunication by the Synod of Paris in 1209, was restored to favor by Gregory IX in 1231, and later regarded as an almost infallible authority. His more scientific writings were never studied in the critical, inquiring way in which the Greeks would have regarded these things. The natural histories of Pliny and Aristotle were accepted by medieval authorities as beyond cavil, and imitated in the queer "Herbals" and "Bestiaries" (or Beast-Books) of the time. All reasoning was formal and deductive. Until the Renaissance, there was neither induction nor experiment. Grown-up men accepted such a tissue of solemn nonsense as the "Timæus" of Plato for sound physiologic doctrine. Nature herself was never questioned for her secrets, and, as Allbutt puts it, "Logic, which for us is but a drill, and, like all drills, a little out of fashion, was for the Middle Ages a means of discovery, nay, the very source of truth. . . . The dialectically irresistible was the true."[2] In the "Golden Legend" of Longfellow, medieval physicians and medical students are represented as frittering away their time in endless discussions about the nature of universals, the relation between the idea and

---

[1] For a full account of the subject, see Sir Clifford Allbutt's splendid Harveian oration, "Science and Mediæval Thought" (1901), to which the writer is very deeply indebted.

[2] Allbutt: op. cit., pp. 50, 51.

matter, and other dialectic subtleties. The Nominalist of advanced and dogmatic type was even liable to persecution. Without going further into the lengthy disputes between Nominalists and Realists, it may be said that their adjustments of cause and effect have been traced through the ages in the "pneuma" of Galen, the "archæus" of Paracelsus, the "animism" of Van Helmont and Stahl, the "thought and extension" of Descartes and Spinoza, the "noumenon" and "phenomenon" of Kant, the "being and becoming" of Hegel, the "will and idea" of Schopenhauer, and in such modern concepts as natural law and natural phenomenon, type and individual, force and matter, statics and dynamics, vital principles and "the fortuitous concurrence of physico-chemical forces." In our own day, the controversy has become merged into the opposition between Vitalism and Materialism. In the Middle Ages, the enormous expenditure of mental energy over this sterile, insoluble problem led the top-heavy feudalized scholastic to entertain an ill-concealed contempt for all manual arts and crafts, especially for anatomy and surgery. Hence the surprising ignorance of Hippocrates in medieval times. "Had Galen's works been lost," says Withington, "there can be little doubt that the dark age of medicine would have been darker and more prolonged than it was, for the medieval practitioner could no more have appreciated the higher and freer teaching of the physician of Cos than he could have understood those grand words, 'It seemed good to the Demos,' which Hippocrates saw inscribed at the head of every decree, and heard proclaimed in every assembly."[1]

The fundamental error of medieval medical science, as Guy de Chauliac originally pointed out, and as Sir Clifford Allbutt, in a masterly survey,[2] has demonstrated, was in the divorce of medicine from surgery. Greek intelligence, as personified in Hippocrates, saw internal medicine in terms of surgery and saw surgery not only as a mode of therapy, but as "the very right arm of internal medicine," since, in diagnosis, the outward and visible signs of internal malady (the only indices the Greek surgeon had) were also the mainstay of the clinician. Beginning with Avicenna, medieval medical authority pushed Galen's dictum that surgery is only a mode of treatment to the extreme limit of treating the surgeon himself as a lackey and an inferior. The Arabian commentators of Galen and the medieval Arabists who copied them were much obsessed with the idea, peculiar to Oriental religions, that it is unclean or unholy to touch the human body with the hands under certain conditions. As this tenet gained ground,

---

[1] Withington: Medical History, London, 1894, 104.

[2] Sir Clifford Allbutt: " The Historical Relations of Medicine and Surgery," London and New York, 1905.

scholastic and monastic minds became, as we have said, gradually penetrated with the conviction that redecraft is superior to hand-craft, culminating in the famous edict of the Council of Tours, "Ecclesia abhorret a sanguine" (1163). The general practice of surgery, including most of the major operations, was, in the end, relegated to barbers, bath-keepers, sowgelders and wayfaring mountebanks, and the surgeon came to be regarded in such a menial light that, even in Prussia, up to the time of Frederick the Great, it was still one of the duties of the army surgeon to shave the officers of the line. Then the heresy imposed by the Arabist com-mentators of Galen, that "coction" (suppuration) and "laudable pus" are essential to the healing of wounds, made operative sur-gery a perilous and meddlesome undertaking, all the more danger-ous, indeed, in that the surgeon, whether scholar or mountebank, stood in jeopardy of life or limb if he operated unsuccessfully on any of the feudal lords of earth. The greatest surgeons of the time shrewdly advised their professional brethren to avoid the operative treatment of difficult or incurable cases, and, when they attempted the major operations, their custom was to require a guarantee that no harm should come to them in the event of a fatal termination. To lift the surgical art to its modern scientific (aseptic) status required the genius and personal influence of the three greatest surgeons of all time—Ambroise Paré, John Hunter and Lord Lister. The principal interest of the medieval period, therefore, lies not in its internal medicine, for there was precious little of it, but in the gradual development of surgery from the ground up by faithful, sometimes obscure, followers of the craft, who (in France at least) were kept ostracized and short-coated by the edicts of the clerical bigots of St. Côme—the "chirurgiens de longue robe."

Nicaise divides the medical history of the Middle Ages into four periods—the Arabian, covering the period between the fifth and eleventh centuries, the Salernitan (eleventh and twelfth cen-turies), the pre-Renaissance period of the Crusades (twelfth to fourteenth centuries) and the Monastic and Scholastic periods (fifteenth and sixteenth centuries); but medieval medicine, in the sense of medicine under the Christian church, began in the **School of Salerno,** the origin of which is obscure. We only know that it came into existence in "a most mysterious way." Some hold that it was founded by clerics connected with the Benedictine monastery at Monte Cassino, eighty miles away, and twice destroyed in the sixth and ninth centuries; others regard this theory as an agree-able *fable convenue*. The little seaside town of Salerno, near Naples, was known even to the ancient Romans as an ideal health resort, and here for nearly three centuries we find monastic medicine thriving under conditions most favorable to its development, namely, ecclesiastical organization of hospitals and sick-nursing, especially at the hands of women. Here, too, were those beginnings of organized medical education which were to attain such remarkable developments in the great universities of the thirteenth century. The Salernitan instructors, some of them Jewish, included such compilers and commentators as Copho, Gariopontus, Constantinus, Africanus, Nicolaus Salernitanus and Ægidius Corboliensis, while among the "Ladies of Salerno," Trotula and Abella are especially remembered. The leading productions of the School of Salerno were the "Breslau Codex," most of which has been reproduced in the collections of De Renzi (1853–6) and Giacosa (1901), the "Compendium Salernitanum," the first example of an encyclopedic textbook of medicine written by many authors; and the "*Regimen* (or *Flos*) *Sanitatis*," a poem in double rhymed hexameter (leonine) verse, written about 1101 and first printed in German (1472), later in Latin (1480). The latter consists of a string of very sensible dietetic and hygienic precepts composed for the benefit of Robert, son of William of Normandy, who was cured of a wound in the arm at Salerno about 1101. It passed through more than 240 separate editions and has been translated into nearly every language, including Irish, Bohemian, Provençal and Hebrew. The "Antidotarium" of Nicholas the Salernitan[1] was the first formulary and one of the first medical books to be printed (Venice, 1471), containing many new Eastern drugs and a table of weights and measures. Copho, one of the Jewish instructors at Salerno in the twelfth century, wrote a little primer on the dissection of the pig (Anatomia porci), which was reprinted in the little anatomic manual of Dryander (1537). Gilles de Corbeil (Ægidius Corboliensis), canon of Paris and physician to Philip Augustus of France (1165–1213), wrote two poems on the pulse and the urine,[2] based upon the Byzantine treatises of Theophilus Protospatharius, and an elegy in verse lamenting the decline of Salerno, after it had been sacked by Henry VI in 1194. After this terrible event, according to Ægidius, the Salernitan professors degenerated into beardless striplings who cared only for books of prescriptions. In the thirteenth century, the medical authority of Salerno was gradually impinged upon by the great rival schools at Naples, Palermo and Montpellier and its fame and influence became more and more of a vanishing fraction, until the famous university itself was finally abolished by Napoleon in 1811.

---

[1] As Wickersheimer has shown (Bull. Soc. franç. d'hist. de méd., Par., 1911, x, 388–397), Nicolaus Præpositi (Nicole Prevost), a French physician, and the Salernitan Nicolaus Præpositus were two entirely different persons. The "Præpositus" in the latter case was probably synonymous with "Præses."

[2] Printed at Padua (1484) and Venice (1494).

The principal outcome of the school of Salerno was the work of two surgeons, **Roger** (Ruggiero) of Palermo and **Roland** of Parma, who, as Allbutt says, "stand like Twin Brethren in the dawn of modern Medicine, bearing the very names of romance." Roger's *Practica*, written about 1180, re-edited by his pupil Roland about 1250,[1] and commented upon by the "Four Masters" a little later, was never separately printed but exists apart in manuscript, although Daremberg published a unique edition of the famous commentary (*Glossulæ quatuor magistrorum*) in 1854. Roger's work became a standard text-book at Salerno, where he himself had been a student and teacher. He knew of cancer and (possibly) syphilis, described a case of hernia of the lungs, prescribed ashes of sponge and sea-weed (iodides) for goiter or scrofula, introduced the seton, and taught the use of styptics, sutures and ligatures in hemorrhage and the healing of wounds by second intention. Roger, Roland and the Four Masters were succeeded by Hugh of Lucca (Ugo Borgognoni), who left no record of his work behind him, and his son or disciple, **Teodorico Borgognoni** (1205–1296), Bishop of Cervia, whose treatise (completed in 1266) is preserved in the surgical anthology ("Cyrurgia") of 1498 and 1499. Theodoric was reviled by Guy de Chauliac as a copyist and plagiarist, probably because, like Hugh before him, he contradicted the pseudo-Galenist dogma of "coction" or "laudable pus" and stood out in his day as a sturdy pioneer of a rational asepsis: "For it is not necessary, as Roger and Roland have written, as many of their disciples teach, and as all modern surgeons profess," he says, "that pus should be generated in wounds. No error can be greater than this. Such a practice is indeed to hinder nature, to prolong the disease, and to prevent the conglutination and consolidation of the wound." (Book II, ch. 27.) This simple statement, as Allbutt points out, makes Theodoric one of the most original surgeons of all time, for only Mondeville, Paracelsus and Lister upheld these principles after him. In the long interregnum between Mondeville and Lister, "the advocates of suppuration won all along the line." Hugh and Theodoric are also memorable for their use of a soporific sponge (*spongia somnifera*) steeped in a mixture of opium, hyoscyamus, hemlock, lettuce and mulberry juice ("oleum de lateribus") which, inhaled by the patient, produced the equivalent of surgical anesthesia.

The ablest Italian surgeon of the thirteenth century was Guglielmo Salicetti, called **Saliceto** or Salicet (1201–1277), a man well educated in hospital and on the battlefield, as also in respect of university training. He was city physician at Bologna, later at

---

[1] Printed in the Venetian encyclopedic collections (entitled "Cyrurgia"), of date 1498 and 1499.

Verona, and wrote his "Cyrurgia" (first printed at Piacenza in 1476) for the benefit of his son, whom he brought up to the profession of medicine. Although far shorter than his treatise on internal medicine, his Surgery stands out as a great landmark or seamark in the history of the craft, and for the following reasons:[1] Saliceto did not separate surgical diagnosis from internal medicine; and kept a good record of case histories, which he held to be the foundation of his subject. He restored the use of the knife, which Arabian practice had set aside in favor of the cautery; he showed how to suture divided nerves and to diagnose bleeding from an artery by the spurt of blood. He was the first to assign venereal contagion as the real cause of chancre and phagedenic ulcers, and has left a classic description of dropsy due to contracted kidney ("durities in renibus").[2] The sound surgical principles of Saliceto were very ably upheld by his pupil, **Lanfranchi** of Milan, who became involved in the squabbles of the Guelphs and Ghibellines and was driven out of his native town by the Visconti. Arriving in Paris in 1295, he found himself, as a married man, shut out of teaching at the university, where the professors were celibate clerics; and he therefore became associated with the College de Saint Côme, organized by Jean Pitard. Here, by his straightforward style of lecturing and his use of bedside instruction, he became the virtual founder of French surgery, and died in 1315. In his "Chirurgia magna," published at Venice in 1490,[3] Lanfranc made a resolute and valiant stand against the medieval schism between surgery and medicine which had existed since Avicenna's time. He was the first to describe concussion of the brain, and his chapter on the symptoms of fracture of the skull is accounted a classic. He also differentiated between venous and arterial hemorrhage and between cancer and hypertrophy of the female breast; and such procedures as intubation of the esophagus, reunion of divided nerves, and neurotomy for tetanus are among his innovations. Unlike Saliceto, Lanfranc was a cauterist and averse to the knife. He therefore avoided trephining, cataract extraction, or lithotomy, but did not hesitate to operate for empyema and wounds of the intestines, treating hemorrhage by styptics, compression, torsion, or even the ligature. His ethical advice to the surgeon is quaint and characteristic, and although he looked upon

---

[1] See Allbutt: "The Historical Relations of Medicine and Surgery," London, 1905, pp. 32, 33.

[2] Saliceto: "Liber . . . in scientia medicinali," Placentiæ, 1476, ch. 140. See also Haeser, "Zur Geschichte der Bright'schen Krankheit," Janus, Breslau, 1848, iii, 371, which gives interesting references to nephritis by the Arabic writers, Serapion and Rhazes.

[3] Also printed in the surgical anthologies of 1498–9. A superb black-letter translation of Lanfranc into Spanish was printed at Seville in 1495 by "tres alemanes compañeros."

Paris as an earthly paradise he held the French surgery of his day in sovereign contempt. The work of Saliceto and Lanfranc, coincident with the development of the great medieval universities— Paris (1110), Bologna (1113), Oxford (1167), Montpellier (1181), Padua (1222)—and the brilliant false dawn of culture and liberalism in the thirteenth century,[1] did much to further the growth of surgical talent in France, England and Flanders.

Contemporary with Lanfranc was his loyal follower, **Henri de Mondeville** (1260–1320), a hardy and original thinker, endowed with great powers of wit and sarcasm, who made a valiant last stand for the principle of avoiding suppuration by simple cleanliness, as originally taught by Hippocrates and as reintroduced by Hugh and Theodoric. The surgical treatise of Mondeville was first edited and printed from the several manuscripts by Professor Pagel of Berlin in 1892, and later translated into French by Professor Nicaise (Paris, 1893). It abounds in directions of the rarest common sense for the aseptic treatment of wounds and in shrewd practical advice to the surgeon as to the conduct of his professional life. In opposition to the salve surgery of the Galenists, Mondeville advises simply to wash the wound clean and put nothing whatever into it, since "wounds dry much better before suppuration than after it." For hemorrhage he recommends styptics, digital compression, acupressure and torsion of the isolated vessel by means of a sliding-noose ligature. His biting wit is shown in such utterances as these: "God did not exhaust all His creative power in making Galen." "Many more surgeons know how to cause suppuration than to heal a wound." "Keep up your patient's spirits by music of viols and ten-stringed psaltery, or by forged letters describing the death of his enemies, or by telling him that he has been elected to a bishopric, if a churchman." "Never dine with a patient who is in your debt, but get your dinner at an inn, otherwise he will deduct his hospitality from your fee." Henri's rapacity in the matter of fees shows how hard they were to get in the Middle Ages, and what he says about the subject suggests the type of surgeon who had to succeed by dint of hard knocks. Like the heroes of Smollett, as described by Sir Walter Scott, his cynical spirit seemed to delight in things "attended with disgrace, mental pain, and bodily mischief to others," yet it is hard to say offhand whether this was the fruit of harsh experience or the expression of supreme irony.

A man of far different type was **Guy de Chauliac** (1300–70), the most distinguished authority on surgery in the fourteenth and fifteenth centuries. A country boy from Auvergne, Guy managed,

---

[1] For an interesting account of this *Aufklärung*, which unfortunately did not last long, see J. J. Walsh, "The Thirteenth Greatest of Centuries," New York, 1912.

through friends, to take holy orders and to get an excellent medical
education at Toulouse, Montpellier and Paris, with a special course
in anatomy at Bologna. He was thus the most highly educated
surgeon of his time, and, in due course, settled down at Avignon
as physician and "commensal chaplain" to Pope Clement VI and
to his successors, Innocent VI and Urban V (1352–78). He was
a writer of rare learning, endowed with a fine critical and historic sense, and, indeed, the only medical historian of consequence
between Celsus and Haller. As an operator, he set great store by

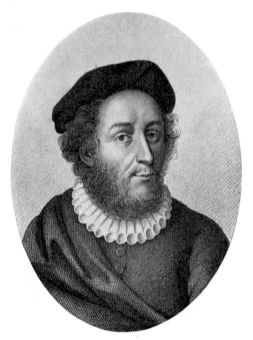

Guy de Chauliac (1300–1370).

the study of human anatomy and was one of the first to take the
operations for hernia and cataract out of the hands of the strolling
mountebanks, although he hesitated to cut for stone. He believed
in cutting out cancer at an early stage with the knife, but employed
the actual cautery in the fungous variety as well as in caries, anthrax and similar lesions. Ulcers he treated by means of an investing collar or guard of sheet lead, and he suspended fractures in
a sling bandage or (when in the thigh) by means of weight and pulley. He also gives an interesting summary of the dentistry of the

period.[1] He throws a great light upon the operative procedure of
his time by his description of the narcotic or soporific inhalation,
originally attributed to Theodoric. This, the medieval substitute
for anesthesia, as above described, was in vogue up to the seventeenth century, and is frequently referred to by the Elizabethan
poets and dramatists, for instance, in the well-worn citation from
Thomas Middleton's tragedy of "Women Beware Women" (Act
IV, sc. 1):

> I'll imitate the pities of old surgeons
> To this lost limb, who, ere they show their art,
> Cast one asleep, then cut the diseased part.

Yet, in spite of his wide experience, Guy de Chauliac was on the
whole a reactionary in the important matter of the treatment of
wounds and, by his great authority, threw back the progress of
surgery for some six centuries, giving his personal weight to the
doctrine that the healing of a wound must be accomplished by the
surgeon's interference—salves, plasters and other meddling—
rather than by the healing power of nature. As an ethical teacher,
Guy holds up a far nobler ideal to the surgeon than Henri, and his
mode of expression reveals the gentleman as well as the scholar.
During the epidemics of plague at Avignon in 1348 and 1360, he
stuck manfully to his post as a healer of the sick, while other
physicians fled the locality. His most important work is the
"Chirurgia magna," written in 1363, and first published in French
translation at Lyons in 1478.[2] Guy's most distinguished pupil was
Pietro **d'Argelata** (died 1423), a professor at Bologna, whose
"Cirurgia" was printed at Venice in 1480. Argelata taught the
dry treatment of wounds, but powdered them; he also used sutures
and drainage-tubes in wounds, trephined the skull and sometimes operated for hernia, stone, and fistula in ano. The
latter operation attained a high degree of perfection in the
hands of **John of Arderne** (1306–90 [?]), the earliest of the
English surgeons. Arderne was a well-educated man who got
his training by an adventurous career as army surgeon in the
Hundred Years War. He wrote treatises on intestinal obstruction (*Passio iliaca*) and gout; and an essay on clysters (1370),
advocating an instrument of his own invention. His treatise on
fistula in ano (1376), in the opinion of its editor, D'Arcy Power,
introduced a well-described surgical operation for a condition which
most of his predecessors had abandoned as incurable. Getting his

---

[1] For which see V. Guerini's "History of Dentistry," Phila., 1909, pp. 142–
149, and J. J. Walsh's "Old-Time Makers of Medicine," New York, 1912, pp.
319–323.

[2] La pratique en chirurgie du maistre Guidon de Chauliac, Lyon, Barth-
elemy Buyer, 1478. The Latin text (Chirurgia) was first printed at Venice
in 1490.

patient into the lithotomy position, Arderne boldly incised the outer wall of the fistula in all its branches instead of fretting it by probes and ligatures; checking any hemorrhage with sponges, and avoiding all corrosive or irritating after-treatment of the wound. This asepsis, akin to Mondeville's, is a reflex of Arderne's training as a Norman surgeon. The Saxon leech crops out in his leaning towards astrology, charms and wort-cunning. "Nothing pleased him more than a charm."

Giovanni **Arcolani** (died 1484), or **Arculanus,** a professor of medicine and surgery at Bologna (1422–1427) and Padua, whose treatise on surgery ("Practica") was published at Venice in 1483, is memorable as one of the leading pioneers of dentistry and the surgery of the mouth, his work giving figurations of the instruments used.[1]

The Flemish surgeon, Jean **Yperman** (1295–1351), whose "Chirurgie" was printed from the manuscript by Carolus (Ghent, 1854) and again by Broeckx (Antwerp, 1863),[2] was a pupil of Lanfranc's who worthily upheld his master's teaching, especially in regard to ligation and torsion of arteries. In the fourteenth century, he was the great authority on surgery in the Low Countries.

Hand in hand with the medieval development of surgery, there necessarily went some effort to improve the status of human anatomy. Dissecting, at first rigorously prescribed by law and sentiment, became more and more a matter of course, following the decree of Emperor Frederick II in 1240. Payne has divided medieval anatomic teaching into three periods: First, the Salernitan (800–1200), in which instruction was based upon the dissection of animals as set forth in the "Anatomia Porci" of Copho, one of the Jewish instructors at Salerno; second, the Arabist period (thirteenth century), in which such dissections were superseded by books and lectures. The leading authorities of this time were Richard, Canon of Wendover, called Ricardus Anglicus (1252), whose work is preserved in the text of Robert Töply (Vienna, 1902); and Henri de Mondeville, who, long before Ambroise Paré, prefixed an anatomic treatise to his surgery, and who improved upon Wendover's teaching by the use of pictures, diagrams and a model of the skeleton. The interest of the third period centers in the revival of human dissecting by Mondino de'Luzzi, called **Mundinus,** whose Anathomia was completed in 1316 and first published at Padua in 1478, and later at Leipzig in 1493 by Martin Pollich von Mellerstadt. In intention, this work was really a little horn-book of dissecting,

[1] For an account of his work, see the interesting essays by J. J. Walsh in "Old-Time Makers of Medicine," New York, 1911, and in "Modern Progress and History," by the same author, New York, 1912, pp. 116–118.

[2] A "Traité de médecine pratique du maître Jehan Yperman" was also edited and published by Broeckx (Antwerp, 1867).

rather than a formal treatise on gross anatomy. Although full of Galenical errors in regard to the structure of the human frame, it was yet the sole text-book on anatomy for over a hundred years. After this time, dissecting gained a firmer foothold as a mode of instruction, and public dissections were decreed at the universities of Montpellier in 1366, at Venice in 1368, at Florence in 1388, at Lerida in 1391, at Vienna in 1404, at Bologna in 1405, at Padua in 1429, at Prague in 1460, at Paris in 1478, and at Tübingen in

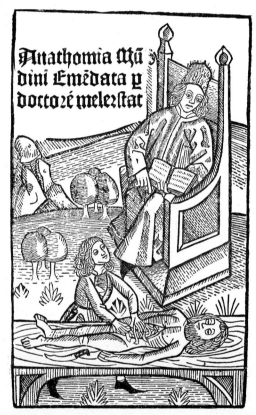

Title-page of Mundinus: "Anathomia," Leipzig, 1493.

1485.[1]   An anatomic theater was erected at Padua in 1446, and, at the Paris Faculty, four dissections annually had been required from the latter half of the fifteenth century on.   Even before the advent of Vesalius we find the great artists of the Renaissance making dissections, even in the hospital of Santo Spirito at Florence.

---

[1] See F. Baker: Johns Hopkins Hosp. Bull., Balt., 1909, xx, footnote to p. 331.

In regard to the bull *De sepulturis*, issued by Pope Boniface in 1300, which many suppose to have put a damper upon anatomical research, Walsh shows that it was, in intention at least, a simple mandate to prevent the bodies of dead Crusaders from being boiled and dismembered before returning them to their relatives.

Internal medicine during the Middle Ages was essentially scholastic and monastic, that is, its votaries were either monks or schoolmen of the type of the foremost intellectual leaders of the thirteenth century—Roger Bacon, Thomas Aquinas, Duns Scotus and Albertus Magnus. The medieval logicians did good service in sharpening men's minds and teaching them how to use dialectics as an instrument or weapon, but science itself could not advance so long as the pitfalls of syllogism were preferred to inductive demonstration of fact. The medieval writers on practice of medicine are commonly described as Arabists on account of their unswerving fidelity to Galenic dogma as transmuted through Mohammedan sources. Characteristic Arabist texts are the "Conciliator differentiarum" (Venice, 1471) of the heretic Peter of Abano (1250–1320), who, as the title of his work implies, tried to reconcile the views of the Arabists and Grecians; the "Liber Pandectæ Medicinæ" of Matthæus Sylvaticus (died–1342), of Mantua, one of the first incunabula to be printed (Strassburg, 1470[?]), which also attempts a conciliation between Greeks and Arabists; and the "Practica" (Venice, 1483) of Giovanni d'Arcoli. The most prominent of the Arabists, however, were associated with the rise of the medical school at Montpellier. Founded about 738, this famous school, like that of Salerno, was charmingly situated near the sea and not far from mineral baths. As early as 1137, Bishop Adelbert of Mainz visited the school to listen to its medical lecturers, and its influence in France has survived to this day. A prominent early representative of the Arabist teachings of Montpellier was the alchemist Raymond Lully (1235–1315), a native of Majorca, who, in addition to the philosopher's stone, sought the "aurum potabile" or liquid gold as a sovereign elixir against disease. Having entered the order of the Minorites, he learned Arabic through his desire to convert the Moslems of North Africa and, in this way, became acquainted with Arabian chemistry and brought some of its ideas into Europe. A man of similar type was **Arnold of Villanova** (1235–1312), also a Spaniard, who was a doctor of theology, law, philosophy and medicine, and physician to Peter III of Aragon. A follower of the Arabian chemists, he also sought an universal elixir of life, and his alchemistic tendencies, taken together with his theological heresies, caused him to be anathematized after his death. He is credited with the introduction of tinctures and of brandy into the pharmacopeia, and his

"Breviary of Practice" (Pavia, 1488) combines the Salernitan régime of dietetics and hygiene with the contemporary belief in astrology, charms and spells. Other prominent pupils of Montpellier were the surgeons Guy de Chauliac, Arderne and Mondeville; Valescus de Taranta (1382–1417), physician to Charles VI of France, whose "Tractatus de peste" was one of the earliest incunabula (1470[?]); Johannes de Tornamira, physician to Popes Gregory IX and Clement VII, for many years chancellor of Montpellier and remembered by his "Introductorium" (Lyons, 1490), a popular text-book on practice in the fourteenth and fifteenth centuries; Peter of Spain (1277), called Petrus Hispanus, physician to Pope Gregory X and afterward himself Pope John XXI, whose "Thesaurus Pauperum" was the most popular of the medieval formularies; and the leading representatives of Anglo-Norman medicine, Bernard de Gordon, Richard of Wendover (the anatomist), Gilbertus Anglicus and John of Gaddesden. Before the advent of the Norman conquerors, English medicine was entirely in the hands of the Saxon leeches, whose practice was made up of charms, spells and herb-doctoring, and whose folk-medicine is preserved in the "Leech-Book" of Bald and other Anglo-Saxon "leechdoms." [1] The Normans raised the social and intellectual status of their physicians by having them educated abroad as clerics. **Bernard de Gordon,** presumably a Scotchman, did not practise in England, but was a teacher at Montpellier from 1285 to 1307. His *Lilium Medicinæ,* which exists in several rare manuscripts and was first published at Venice in 1496, is a characteristic Arabist text-book of the practice of medicine, nowise classical, and typical of the Middle Ages in scholastic subtlety and rigid adherence to dogma. The subject matter is well arranged; acute fevers, anthrax, phthisis, leprosy, scabies and St. Anthony's fire are described as contagious, and the book is notable as containing the first description of a modern truss and the first mention of spectacles as "oculus berellinus." The "Compendium medicinæ" (London, 1510) of **Gilbertus Anglicus** (died 1230), the leading exponent of Anglo-Norman medicine, is very much like Gordon's Lily in style, arrangement of contents and modes of thought. Its most important feature is an original account of leprosy which became the basis of medieval information upon the subject. Gilbert was the first to refer to smallpox as a contagious disease, a view afterward contradicted, even by Sydenham. **John of Gaddesden** (1280 [?]–1361), a prebendary of St. Paul's, whom some think the original of Chaucer's Doctor of Physic, was physician to King Edward II of England and a fellow and professor of Merton Col-

---

[1] See, Oswald Cockayne, Leechdoms, wortcunning and starcraft of early England. 3 vols. London, 1864–6.

lege, Oxford. His *Rosa Anglica*, compiled in 1314, and printed at Pavia in 1492, contains an early reference to the red-light[1] or Finsen treatment of smallpox, but is otherwise mainly a farrago of Arabist quackeries and countryside superstitions. Guy de Chauliac called it "a vapid rose, devoid of fragrance," and Haller referred to its author as "an empiric, full of superstition, obviously untrained, a lover and eulogist of quack medicines, greedy of gain, an expert in kitchen-lore."

The most eminent naturalist of the thirteenth century was the Dominican monk, Albert von Bollstädt (1193–1280), called *Albertus Magnus*, who was successively a teacher at Paris and Cologne, Bishop of Ratisbon (1260–1263), ending his days in Cologne. His descriptions of plants (*De vegetabilibus*) were based upon his own observations and, according to Haller, contain the beginnings of plant geography. His work on animals is of the same character, and he assisted Frederick II in his work on falconry. The often reprinted work on cosmetics (*De secretis mulierum*), which usually goes by his name, was in reality a huge compilation made by his pupil, Henry of Saxony. Albertus Magnus did not write on medical practice, a subject forbidden to the Dominicans.

The *Physica* of St. Hildegarde (1099–1179), Abbess of Rupertsberg, near Bingen, contains descriptions of the healing properties of the known plants, minerals and animals, emphasizing the most reliable of these, and giving the German names by preference. It is held to be of especial value for its sidelights upon the medicine, botany, gardening and other social phases of the twelfth century.

Two other medieval writers on medical plants and simples deserve mention, viz., Giacomo de Dondis (1298–1359), whose "Aggregator de medicinis simplicibus," printed at Strassburg, *circa* 1470, by Adolf Rusch (the "R." printer[2]), is one of the earliest known of medical incunabula;[3] and Simone de Cordo (died 1330),

---

[1] H. P. Cholmeley: John of Gaddesden and the Rosa Medicinæ, Oxford, 1912, 41, points out that Gaddesden probably got the notion of the red-light treatment from Gilbertus Anglicus. "Compendium Medicinæ," Lyons, 1510, fol. 348, *verso*, col. I: "Vetulæ provinciales dant purpuram combustam in potu, habet enim occultam naturam curandi variolas. Similiter pannus tinctus de grano." Gaddesden (fol. 51 recto, col. II) reads: "Deinde capiatur scarletum rubeum, et involvatur variolosus totaliter, vel in panno alio rubeo, sic ego feci de filio nobilissimi Regis Angliae quando patiebatur istos morbos, et feci omnia circa lectum esse rubea, et est bono cura, et curair cum in sequente sine vestigiis variolarum."

[2] The fact that the "R" printer was Adolf Rusch, and not his employer Mentelin, was settled by the distinguished Göttingen philologist Karl Dziatzko, in his essay "Der Drucker mit dem bizarren R" (Samml. bibliothekswissensch. Arbeiten, Halle, 1904, Heft 17, 13–24). Rusch, it seems, married Mentelin's daughter, Salome, and eventually took over his business. The much disputed "R" is in reality a monogram of the initial letters of Rusch's name, which he was in the habit of inserting here and there in the books printed by him, as a sign of his handiwork during the days of his apprenticeship.

[3] The question, "What is the earliest printed medical book of size?" is still unsettled. The Guttenberg "Laxierkalender" of 1457 of course antedates everything else, but it is only a sheet of paper. The date "1468" has been claimed for Roland of Parma's pest-tract and 1469 for Giamatteo Ferrari's *Practica* (Pt. 1). The question cannot be finally decided until all the known medical incunabula have been catalogued, collated and compared as to fonts of type, filigrams (water-marks), "majuscules" (initial letters) and the internal evidence of biographical and other data.

whose "Synonyma medicinæ" (1471) was the first dictionary of drugs and simples.

A striking feature of clinical medicine in the fourteenth and fifteenth centuries was the writing of "Consilia" or medical case-books, consisting of clinical records from the practice of well-known physicians and letters of advice written by them to imaginary patients or else to real pupils or country doctors, who appealed to their superior knowledge as consultants. The most important Consilia were those written by the Paduan professors Gentile da Foligno, who was a victim of the Black Death in 1348 and was the first to observe gallstones; and Bartolommeo Montagnana (1470) a descendant of a long line of physicians, an anatomist who had dissected as many as fourteen bodies, and a surgeon who described strangulated hernia, operated for lacrimal fistula and extracted decayed teeth. These Consilia, of which Montagnana gives some 305, usually run over the patient's physical condition and disease, winding up with seasonable advice as to what to eat, what drugs to take and what things to avoid. Being personal histories, they have not the classical flavor of the cases described by Hippocrates and Aretæus, and are of interest chiefly as showing that physicians had already begun to keep careful records of their daily practice.

Cultural and Social Aspects of Medieval Medicine.—During the Dark Ages (476–1000), Western European civilization was in a chaotic, formless state, the turbulent fermentation of barbaric or decadent peoples resolving themselves into new nations. Feudalism put nationhood on its feet, while the Church was the only foster-mother that science could find. In the Dark Ages, the clergy were the only class who had any pretence to education and, before the time of the School of Salerno, medicine was entirely in the hands of Jewish and Arabian physicians. The rest were simply vagrant quacks or stationary humbugs whose practice was discountenanced by the Church on the ground that faith, prayers and fasting were better than pagan amulets, while the sick were advised to emulate the saints in their capacity for endurance of suffering. With the rise of the School of Salerno, European medicine began to look up a little, but, as soon as monks and clerics began to practise medicine, it was found that the acceptance of medical fees, the sight of many aspects of the sick that might offend modesty, the possibility of being the cause of a patient's death and other happenings were somewhat inconsistent with the original intention of holy orders, and so we find the Church instituting that long series of edicts which, in the first instance, were aimed not so much at medicine as at its malpractice by monks. These were the decrees of the councils of Rheims (1131), the Lateran (1139), Montpellier (1162),

Tours (1163), Paris (1212), the second Lateran (1215), and Le Mans (1247), and their general effect was, unfortunately, not only to stop the monks from practising but to extend the special odium of these decrees to the whole medical profession.[1] The famous maxim of the Council of Tours ("Ecclesia abhorret a sanguine"), for example, went wide of its supposed intention, since, in casting discredit upon the sometimes murderous vagabond surgeon, the weight of its authority made the surgeon of best type still an inferior to the average practitioner, even in Protestant Germany to the end of the eighteenth century. Worse still, the bigots of the Paris Faculty went much further than the Papal See in widening the gap between surgery and medicine. The Roman Pontiffs themselves were, some of them, liberal-minded men of the world, who did not hesitate to employ talented Jewish physicians at need and, in later times, did much to foster the arts and sciences, in Italy at least. John XXI and Paul II were physicians. While great harm was done to medicine by the Papal decrees which degraded the surgeon's status, we should not forget that, up to the time of the crusades, all Europe outside of Italy was in a state of barbarism and that the status of surgery in these countries was lower than it was among the Greeks at the time of the Trojan War. A few shreds of technical knowledge may have drifted over from far Byzantium, but the evidence of the Niebelungenlied, the Anglo-Saxon Leech-Books, and the Norse Sagas all point to the same conclusion, viz., that the care of the sick and wounded was first in the hands of women and later entrusted to a class of men who, in war-time, were in great request but, in times of peace, ranked on a level with menials. In Russia, for instance, medicine was originally in the hands of the volkhava or wolf-men, who, like the Druids and weise Frauen, culled medicinal herbs and resorted to charms and spells. The earliest relic of Russian medicine is a vase of Greek pattern excavated at Koul-Oba, representing a Scythian chieftain in consultation with a volkhava, a Scythian warrior examining another's teeth and a surgeon bandaging an injured leg. This unique vase epitomizes medieval medicine and surgery up to the time of the School of Salerno.[2] After the introduction of Christianity in the tenth century, Russian medicine passed into the hands of the priesthood, the wolf-men gave place to the monks of Mount Athos, and the Russian Church, like the Roman, put severe interdictions upon sorcery and magic. Thus religion at the start tended to improve the status of medicine, but

---

[1] As Allbutt says, "If Papal bulls conferred privileges, they usually implied or imposed restrictions."

[2] For a photograph of the Koul-Oba vase, see "Nouvelle Iconographie de la Salpêtrière," Paris, 1901, xiv, plate no. 72, opposite page 528.

speedily, if unintentionally, degraded it, as soon as it found its own medical ministrants falling into evil ways. Even the special nurses or "parabolani,"[1] whom the Church employed to seek out the sick and convey them to places of shelter and safety, were soon shorn of their powers as they became uppish, quarrelsome and overbearing. Even before this time, however, the Visigothic Code of the seventh century put the same severe **restrictions upon medical practice** that we find in the Code Hammurabi. Before taking up a case, the physician, under the Visigothic Code, had to make a contract and give pledges, and, if his patient died, he got no fee. If he injured a nobleman in venesection he had to pay 100 solidi (about $225); if the nobleman died, the physician was turned over to the relatives of the deceased to be dealt with as they pleased. If he killed or injured a slave, he had to replace him by one of equal value. He was forbidden to bleed a married woman in the absence of her relatives, for fear of the commission of adultery, and he could not visit a prisoner lest he defeat the ends of justice by furnishing him with poison. On the other hand, it is stated that no one might cast a physician into prison without a hearing, except in case of murder, and that the statutory fee for instructing medical students should be twelve solidi ($27) each. From these regulations, made by the secular arm of authority, and designed to protect the public as well as the physician, it may be gathered that, with medicine in such an unorganized condition, something more than the guardianship of Church and State was necessary to elevate the status of the healing art, and this was accomplished by improved medical legislation, by the foundation of the great medieval universities and the subsequent formation of "guilds" by the physicians themselves. Under the legal restrictions of medieval times, the surgeon worked daily and hourly in jeopardy of life or limb.[2] In the seventh century, Guntram, King of Burgundy, had two physicians executed upon his wife's tomb because the latter died of plague in spite of their treatment. In 1337, a strolling eye surgeon was thrown into the Oder because he failed to cure John of Bohemia of his blindness, and in 1464, Matthias, King of Hungary, issued a proclamation that whoever cured him of an arrow wound should be richly rewarded, but, failing that, should be put to death. These barbarities point their own moral, for the strolling medieval mountebanks, in couching a cataract, sometimes put out an eye, mangled the viscera in "cutting" for stone and, in attempting to effect a "radical cure" for hernia, as Baas says, not infrequently excised

---

[1] First mentioned, A. D. 416.

[2] For a careful study of this subject, see Sir John Tweedy on "The Deterrent Influence of Social and Legal Restrictions on Medical Thought and Practice," Tr. Med. Leg. Soc., London, 1911, viii, pp. 1–8.

"the radix of humanity itself."[1] Allbutt gives a striking picture
of a medieval incisor who, in ligating an artery, paralyzed his
patient's arm by crushing the musculo-spiral nerve and was afterward pursued with curses by his miserable victim whenever he
dared show himself in the street. If the Church "abhorred the
shedding of blood," therefore, it is fair to suppose that, in the first
instance, its aversion had the same human significance as the well-
founded horror of hospitals and surgical operations which existed
in the minds of the laity up to the end of the nineteenth century.
As the physicians looked down upon the surgeons, so the surgeons
of higher education, who in the Middle Ages could be counted on
the fingers, looked down upon the barbers. The latter were, in the
first instance, trained for the purpose of bleeding and shaving the
monks. In the thirteenth century, the Collège de Saint Côme
was organized at Paris (circa 1210), constituting a guild the members of which were divided into the clerical barber-surgeons or
surgeons of the long robe and the lay barbers or surgeons of the
short robe, and, in 1311, 1352 and 1364, royal decrees were issued
forbidding the latter to practise surgery without being duly examined by the former. In 1372, Charles V decreed that the barbers should be allowed to treat wounds and not be interfered with
by their long-robed confrères. The same thing happened in England, where the surgeons formed a separate guild in 1368, combined
with the physicians about 1421, while the barbers obtained a separate charter from Edward IV in 1462. In this way, barber-
surgery (the surgery of the common people) became "wound-surgery," that is, was restricted to blood-letting and the healing of
wounds. The barbers (tonsores) themselves owed their business
largely to the fact that, after the monks were forbidden to wear
beards in 1092, smooth chins and shaving became the fashion.
In Germany the barber was often a bath keeper, who, in addition
to bleeding, cupping and leeching, gave enemas, picked lint and
extracted teeth, and his examination or "Meisterstück" consisted
in sharpening a knife or in preparing certain salves and plasters.

Throughout the Middle Ages, there were some vague attempts to formulate the principles of medical jurisprudence, the earliest of these being, as
Cumston points out, in the laws of the Germanic and Slavic tribes, the Salic
law, the Capitularies of Charlemagne (ninth century) the Assizes of the Crusaders, and, in the thirteenth century and after, the Decretals of the Popes
and general canon laws. The procedure in such cases was often of the crudest
kind, the tests being by ordeal, torture, de facto verification of impotence, and
"cruentation," or the spontaneous bleeding of a corpse in the presence of the
true murderer. The expert opinions given were usually in the nature of hair-

---

[1] The strolling herniotomists believed castration to be necessary because
they thought the intestines and testicles were inclosed in the same sac, which
must be removed in its entirety to obviate relapses and faulty healing of the
peritoneum.

splitting casuistry, but Cousin and Cumston[1] give a number of cases from French legal procedure of the fourteenth century in which surgeons were commonly consulted in cases of wounds, homicide, rape, and the like.

In the year 1140, Roger II of Sicily issued an edict forbidding any one to practise medicine without proper examination, under pain of imprisonment and the sale of his belongings at auction. This important law was followed by an ordinance of larger scope issued by Roger's grandson, the generous and liberal-minded Hohenstauffen Emperor, **Frederick II,** in 1224. Frederick's edict required that a candidate for license to practise must be properly examined in public by the masters at Salerno, the license being issued by the Emperor himself or his representative; failure to comply with the statute being again punishable by a year's imprisonment and forfeiture of property. The examination was based upon the genuine books of Hippocrates, Galen and Avicenna, and before taking it the candidate must have studied logic for three years, medicine and surgery for five years and have practised for one year under some experienced physician. The candidate in surgery had to give evidence that he had studied the art for at least a year, in particular human anatomy, "without which no incision can be safely made nor any fracture treated." The physician was required to treat the poor for nothing; to visit his patients twice a day and once a night, if necessary; to avoid collusion with apothecaries and to inform upon them, if they adulterated or substituted drugs. The medical fee was fixed at half a tarenus (about 35 cents) for office practice or for patients residing in the city; four tareni ($3.00) for out-of-town visits, the physician paying his expenses, or three tareni ($2.25), if the patient paid them. The purchasing power of money in this period is said to have been fifteen or twenty times what it is now. The sale of poisons, magic potions and aphrodisiac philters was punishable by death if any person lost his life thereby; drugs and apothecaries' mixtures were examined at stated intervals by inspectors; and timely regulations were made in municipal hygiene and rural hygiene, such as for the proper depth of graves or the suitable disposal of refuse. Given the time at which it was issued, it would be hard to improve upon the plain scope and intention of this law, which was followed by similar ordinances for Spain in 1283 and Germany in 1347, and was again confirmed by Joanna of Naples in 1365.[2] Frederick's edict

---

[1] André Cousin: "Essai sur les origines de la médecine légale," Paris diss. No. 252, 1905. C. G. Cumston: Jour. Am. Inst. Crim. Law, Chicago, 1913, iii, 855–865.

[2] Sudhoff states that the alleged ordinance for city physicians of 1426, attributed to Kaiser Sigmund (1410–37), is probably mythical, although he has discovered a city ordinance of 1439, which he reproduces in Mitt. z. Gesch. d. Med., Leipzig, 1912, xi, 126, 127.

did much to elevate the status of the respectable physician and to correspondingly diminish the number of quacks; and this end was further approached by the introduction of a new element—the rise and growth of the great **medieval universities,** which usually began as a *"studium generale,"* *i. e.,* migration or assemblage of students in some locality. The earliest of these were at Paris (1110), Bologna (1113), Oxford (1167) and Montpellier (1181), and the Italian universities at Padua (1222), Messina (1224), and Naples (1225) were founded by Frederick II himself. Those at Cambridge (1209), Siena (1241), Salamanca (1243), Piacenza (1248), Seville (1254), Lerida (1300), Perugia (1308), Coimbra (1309), Palermo (1312), Florence (1320), Grenoble (1339), Pisa (1343), Valladolid (1346) and Pavia (1361) followed, while the fourteenth and fifteenth centuries witnessed also the rise of the principal German and Slavic universities, in particular, Prague (1347), Cracow (1364), Vienna (1364), Erfurt (1379), Heidelberg (1385), Würzburg (1402), Leipzig (1409), Rostock (1419), Greifswald (1448), Freiburg in Breisgau (1455), Basel (1460), Budapest (1465), Ingolstadt (1472) and Tübingen (1477); of the Scandinavian, Copenhagen (1475) and Upsala (1477); and, in Scotland, St. Andrew's (1411), Glasgow (1453) and Aberdeen (1494). All these were soon thronged with great concourses of students and it was through the influence of the medieval universities that the physician came to be regarded in the end as a member of a "learned profession." At first, philosophy was the chief end of study, with law and theology as the main objects of interest, and medicine was taught as a mere branch of philosophy as set forth in Aristotle, Averroes and other Arabic writers. Before the Revival of Learning and the Invention of Printing, the Greek writers were seldom read in the original or even in a straight translation, but "doubly disguised and half buried in glosses which not only overlaid the text but often supplanted it."[1] Thus the curriculum at Tübingen in the fourteenth century, as given by Haeser, comprised, in the first year, the first canon of Avicenna and the ninth book of Rhazes, as expounded by Jacob of Forli and Arculanus; in the second year, the Ars parva of Galen with the commentary of Torrigiani, and the fourth canon of Avicenna; in the third year, the Aphorisms of Hippocrates and (again) Avicenna, with suitable commentaries. The courses and text-books were usually determined by papal bulls and the libraries of the medieval universities were small in extent, seldom exceeding a hundred or two volumes. The professors' salaries usually ranged from $35 to $50 per annum. The term "doctor of medicine" was first applied to the Salernitan graduates by Gilles de Corbeil, in the twelfth century, and the

---

[1] Allbutt: Science and Medieval Thought, London, 1901, 69.

graduation ceremonies were commonly modeled after the Salernitan pattern. The candidate was first required to defend
four theses from Aristotle, Hippocrates, Galen and a modern
writer and to take an oath, the conditions of which corresponded,
in the main, with the decree of Emperor Frederick. He then
received "a ring, a wreath of laurel and ivy, a book first closed
and then opened, the kiss of peace" and the rank of "Doctor in
Philosophy and Medicine." John Locke describes very much the
same thing at Montpellier in 1675, and the custom of the modern
German universities is along similar lines.

The chief glory of medieval medicine was undoubtedly in the
organization of **hospitals and sick nursing,**[1] which had its origin in
the teachings of Christ. For while the germ of the hospital idea
may have existed in the ancient Babylonian custom of bringing the
sick into the market-place for consultation, as it were, and while
the Iatreia and Asclepeia of the Greeks and the Romans may have
served this purpose to some extent, the spirit of antiquity toward
sickness and misfortune was not one of compassion, and the credit
of ministering to human suffering on an extended scale belongs to
Christianity. The Arabian hospitals, large and liberal as were
their endowments and capacity, came long after the beginning of
the Christian era, and the Mohammedans probably got the idea
from the Christians. The Asclepeia and other pagan temples were
closed by the decree of Constantine, A. D. 335, and, very soon after,
the movement of founding and building the Christian hospitals
went forward, in which Helena, the mother of Constantine, is said
to have played an active part. These were, in all probability,
small at first, the wealthier Christians taking care of the sick in
Valetudinaria, but by the accession of Julian the Apostate in 361,
the movement was in full swing. In 369, the celebrated Basilias at
Cæsarea in Cappadocia was founded by St. Basil, consisting of a
large number of buildings, with houses for physicians and nurses,
workshops and industrial schools. It was followed by a charity
hospital of 300 beds for the plague-stricken at Edessa, which was
founded by St. Ephraim in 375. A hospital was founded at Alexandria by St. John the Almsgiver in 610, and, during the Byzantine
period, other large hospitals arose at Ephesus, Constantinople and
elsewhere. These eventually became specialized, according to
Christian ideas of the obligation of charity and hospitality, as
Nosocomia, or claustral hospitals for the reception and care of the
sick alone; Brephotrophia, for foundlings; Orphanotrophia, for
orphans; Ptochia, for the helpless poor; Gerontochia, for the

---

[1] In the preparation of this section, I have been much indebted to the
interesting article by Dr. James J. Walsh in the Catholic Encyclopædia, *sub
voce* "Hospitals," and to the references given by him.

aged; and Xenodochia, for poor and infirm pilgrims. At the beginning of the fifth century, hospitals began to spring up in the Western Empire. The first nosocomium in Western Europe was founded by Fabiola about 400, "to gather in the sick from the streets and to nurse the wretched sufferers, wasted with poverty and disease" (St. Jerome). Others were founded in Rome by Belisarius, in the Via Lata, and by Pelagius; and, further west, by Cæsarius at Arles in 542, by Childebert at Lyons in 542 and by Bishop Masona at Merida in 580. The Hôtel Dieu is said to have been founded between 641 and 660 by St. Landry, Bishop of Paris, and was first mentioned in 829. St. Albans Hospital in England dates from the year 794. The mountain xenodochia or hospices at Mont Cenis (825) and the Great St. Bernard (962) are still in existence. After the death of Charlemagne, the larger hospitals began to decline through subdivision or loss of revenue and, at this period, we find the monasteries, such as those of the Benedictine order at Cluny, Fulda and elsewhere, provided with private infirmaries and "eleemosynary hospitals." About this time, also, arose the various Catholic hospital orders and fraternities for looking after the sick, of which the earliest were the Parabolani who, according to Gibbon, were first organized at Alexandria during the plague of Gallienus, A. D. 253–268. Parabolani sought out the sick, not unlike the monks of St. Bernard today, but soon exceeded their authority and were gradually suppressed. The term "sorority" probably comes from Soror, who founded the hospital Santa Maria della Scala at Siena in 898. Other religious orders which sprang up about the time of the Crusades were the Alexians, the Antonines, the Beguins and the Hospitallers, the latter comprising the followers of St. Elizabeth of Hungary, who founded two hospitals at Eisenach with a third on the Wartburg, the Sisters of St. Catherine, the order of St. John of Jerusalem, which was founded when the Crusaders reached the Holy City in 1099 and the Teutonic Order, which was started in a field hospital outside the walls of Acre and was approved by Clement III in 1191. The members of the latter order vowed themselves to care for the sick and to build a hospital wherever their order was introduced, and played a great part in Germany in medieval times, eventually dying out from lack of funds in the fifteenth century. Similarly, the Order of St. John of Jerusalem became merged into a purely military order and declined in the thirteenth century. Parallel with the specialization of nursing orders during the Crusades, however, there went the great medieval hospital movement initiated by Pope Innocent III in 1198, which has received the just encomium of Virchow. In 1145, Guy of Montpellier opened a hospital in honor of the Holy Ghost, which was approved by the Pope in 1198, he himself building the hospital in Rome called Santo Spirito in Sassia in 1204. The example of the Pontiff was soon followed all over Europe, with the result that nearly every city had its Hospital of the Holy Ghost, and it became the ambition of many a prince or landgrave to found a "xenodochium pauperum, debilium et infirmorum." Virchow, in his essay on the hospitals of the Middle Ages,[1] gives a remarkable catalogue of these institutions in 155 German cities. Many of these were, of course, merely first aid and nursing stations of the charitable order of Teutonic knights, but Virchow's list shows the definite social character of the movement. In Rome, says Walsh, there were four city hospitals in the eleventh century, six in the twelfth, ten in the thirteenth. Another circumstance which vastly aided the city hospital movement was the immense growth of leprosy in the Middle Ages. Already known to the ancient Hebrews, Greeks and Romans, this disease began to appear in Northern Europe in the sixth and seventh centuries A. D., and its spread in connection with the Crusades was appalling, reaching its full height in the thirteenth century. The leper, wandering abroad, an outcast from human society, living apart in huts in the open field, became a common figure, and the subject of frequent reference in the chronicles and romances of the period, such as "Der arme Heinrich" of Hartmann von Aue,[2] the "Frauendienst" of Ulrich von Lichtenstein,[3] the Grandes Chroniques de France[4] or the unforgetable passage in the Lüneburger Chronik, which Heine paraphrased:

Living corpses, they wandered to and fro, muffled from head to foot; a hood drawn over the face, and carrying in the hand a bell, the Lazarus-bell, as it was called, through which they were to give timely warning of their approach, so that every one could get out of the way in time.[5]

Leper hospitals were already mentioned by Gregory of Tours (*circa* 560) and, as leprosy spread far and wide, the advantage of these retreats for purposes of segregation became apparent and they turned out to be a potent factor in the eventual stamping out of the disease. The number of these lazar-houses (leprodochia or leprosoria), as they were then called, was extraordinary. Baas estimates that there were some 19,000 of them in Europe during

[1] R. Virchow: "Krankenhäuser und Hospitalwesen," in his Ges. Abhandl. a. d. Gebiete d. öffentlichen Medicin u. d. Seuchenlehre, Berlin, 1879, ii, 1–130.

[2] In this poetical romance of the thirteenth century, "poor Henry," the hero, journeys to Montpellier and Salerno to be cured of leprosy.

[3] The "Frauendienst" gives a ludicrous sidelight on the excesses of chivalry, the leper episode representing the henpecked hero as consorting with lepers to gratify the caprices of his exacting "lady."

[4] Swinburne's poem of "The Leper," filled with the fantastic "Frauendienst" spirit of the Middle Ages, is based upon an episode in this chronicle.

[5] Heinrich Heine: "Geständnisse" (Sämmtl. Werke, Cotta ed., x, 241, 242).

the thirteenth century, 2000 of which were in France alone. Virchow, in his wonderful study of leprosy in the Middle Ages, has listed and described, with his usual patient fidelity, an amazing number of these leper hospitals in all the Germanic cities of the thirteenth and fourteenth centuries,[1] and it is clear, from his thoroughgoing narrative, that the building of the leprosoria represented a great social and hygienic movement, a wave of genuine prophylaxis as well as of human charity. Billings characterizes the true spirit of the hospital movement of the Middle Ages in the following language:

> When the medieval priest established in each great city of France a Hôtel Dieu, a place for God's hospitality, it was in the interests of charity as he understood it, including both the helping of the sick poor and the affording to those who were neither sick nor poor an opportunity and a stimulus to help their fellow men; and doubtless the cause of humanity and religion was advanced more by the effect on the givers than on the receivers.[2]

About the beginning of the thirteenth century, the hospitals began to pass, without friction and by mutual agreement, from the hands of the ecclesiastical authorities into those of the municipality. By this time, there were many splendid city hospitals, like the Hôtel Dieu or the Santo Spirito, and hospital construction attained its height in the fifteenth century. Prominent English hospitals of the medieval period were the Hospital St. Gregory, founded by Archbishop Lanfranc in 1084; St. Bartholomew's, founded in 1137 by Rahere, a jester, who joined a religious order and obtained a grant of land from Henry I about 1123; the Holy Cross Hospital at Winchester, founded 1132, St. Mary's Hospital, founded in London in 1197; and St. Thomas's Hospital, founded by Peter, Bishop of Winchester, in 1215 and rebuilt in 1693.

In studying the cultural phases of medicine, there is no documentation so effective or instructive as the graphic, and for a period so remote and well-nigh inaccessible to modern comprehension as the Middle Ages, the great cathedrals, with their stained glass windows, the liturgies, Books of Hours and illuminated missals, the chansons and epics, the miracle plays and moralities furnish us the shortest path to such comprehension. Perhaps the best sidelights upon earlier medieval medicine that we have are afforded in the **miniature paintings** which illuminate certain manuscript codices of the Salernitan masters, compiled and edited by Piero Giacosa in 1901.[3] One of these, an illustration to the Turin Codex of Pliny's

---

[1] R. Virchow: "Zur Geschichte des Aussatzes und der Spitäler," Arch. f. path. Anat. (etc.), Berlin, 1860, xviii, 138; 273; xix, 43; 1861, xx, 166.

[2] J. S. Billings: "Description of the Johns Hopkins Hospital," Baltimore, 1890, p. 48.

[3] Piero Giacosa: "Magistri Salernitani nondum editi," one vol. and atlas, Turin, fratelli Bocca, 1901.

Natural History, represents an imposing interior, showing three physicians with features of unmistakeably Jewish cast, clad in flowing Oriental robes and turbans, in professional attendance upon some great personage. One of them is feeling the patient's pulse, the other two stand in grave consultation while their horses champ outside; and within, long-haired pages in doublet and hose remain in waiting or converse among themselves. Another miniature on the same page shows a number of monks in a magic circle, exorcising the devil. A cut from the Bolognese Codex of the Canon of Avicenna shows the medieval physician, in gown and biretta, lecturing to his students, as on the title page of the Mellerstadt Mundinus. A superb miniature from the Turin Codex of the El Hawi of Rhazes shows a Salernitan master inspecting urine in a glass, while a humble looking patient of rustic mien, stands uncovered before him, holding the urine basket in his hand. The contrast between the professional gravity of the doctor's face and the pathetic solemnity of his mute, enduring patient is one of the cleverest things in medieval art. Uroscopy or water-casting was, in fact, a favorite theme of the painter and wood-engraver down to the beginning of the eighteenth century, and the accessaries in these representations are nearly always the same. The urine was always contained in a characteristic flask of Erlenmeyer shape, sometimes graduated, and this flask was carried in an osier basket with lid and handle, looking very like a modern champagne bucket. The physician, of whatever period, is always represented as inspecting the urine in a most judicial way, often holding it up to the light in such wise that there will be no reflection or refraction from the sun's rays. Some medieval pictures represent the physician as disdaining to touch the Erlenmeyer urinal with his hands. In the frontispiece of Montagnana's treatise (1487), for instance, two Venetian pages hold up the urine in glasses while the doctors, in gowns and skull-caps, inspect it and comment upon it. An effective miniature from Avicenna, in Giacosa's collection, shows a physician in office consultation with a number of patients, each of whom stands with his osier basket in his hands while the practitioner descants upon the properties of each individual specimen of urine. As may be imagined, offhand diagnoses of this kind were a favorite imposture of the strolling quacks, who reaped a rich harvest from the deception. Another miniature, in the Bolognese Codex of Avicenna, shows us the front of an apothecary's shop, with the apprentices braying drugs in mortars, a physician riding by on horseback, the medicine jars upon the shelves being labeled with Arabic inscriptions. The cuts around the border represent a cold bath in a running torrent of water, another bath of a quasi-social character taken by several persons together in one of the piscines or circular bathing pools, with further representations of cupping, blood-letting and the exploration of a chest wound. The most striking cuts in Giacosa's collection, however, are the rude pen drawings from the Codex of Roland's Surgery in the Biblioteca Casanatense, representing different episodes in the surgeon's experience, such as the diagnosis of a fracture, the reduction of a dislocation, the inspection, widening, or suturing of a wound, the withdrawal of an arrow, the setting of a fracture of the jaw and so on. These pictures, crude as they are, will decidedly enhance anyone's opinion of the Salernitan surgeons and must be seen to be appreciated. Of the costume and personal appearance of the fourteenth century surgeon we get a faint, far-away impression from the illuminated picture of John of Arderne in the Sloane MS., representing the blond-bearded Saxon surgeon in gown, cloak and cap, seated in a throne-like chair, in the act of demonstrating his mode of procedure in fistula; and from the miniature frontispiece in Nicaise's edition of Mondeville (1314), representing that sharp-featured, gray-haired master, tall and slim, in a purple gown of clerical cut, black skull-cap, red stockings and slippered feet, reading lectures with uplifted forefinger. The faces in all these medieval pictures have the curious wall-eyed expression which is found even in the paintings of such masters as Giotto, Cimabue and Lucas Cranach, and which seem to suggest that there was no self-revelation in the workings of the medieval mind. The methods of the medieval artists were unmistakeably objective, as in Holbein's portraits, or the life-like representations of the nude by Jan van Eyck and Pollaiuolo. In this connection, we may mention Ghirlandajo's picture of rhinophyma in the Louvre and another representation of the same disease by the younger Holbein in the Prado.

In the fifteenth century, there were numbers of pictures painted representing scenes in the lying-in chamber. These, contrary to modern custom and sentiment, are usually thronged with figures plying various avocations about the sick-room and some of them frankly represent the act and moment of delivery. In the foreground of each, there is the inevitable nursemaid in the act of washing the newborn infant, and, from some of these pictures, we gather the curious fact that, in the Middle Ages, the sensitive naked foot was used as a sort of clinical thermometer. In a fresco of Luini's, in the Brera Gallery at Milan, the nursemaid is dipping her hand into the basin to ascertain if the water is too hot or too cold for the infant. In most of the pictures, however, a wooden tub is used, and in quite a number, notably in those representing the "Birth of the Virgin," by the elder Holbein (Augsburg Gallery), Bernhard Strigel (Berlin Gallery), and Bartholomäus Zeit-

blom (Augsburg and Sigmaringen Galleries), particularly in a
"Wochenstube" of an unknown Tyrolese artist in the Ferdinandeum at Innsbruck, the nursemaid is represented, like the Highland
laundresses in "Waverley," with "kilted kirtle," her bare feet
testing the temperature of the water in the tub. The different
methods of investing an infant in its swaddling clothes are strikingly shown in the bas-relief figures in glazed clay by Andrea della
Robbia in the loggia of the Spedale degli Innocenti at Florence. [1]

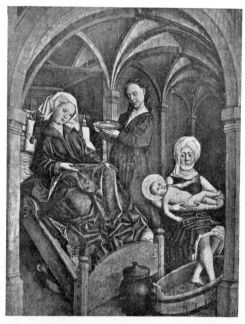

The Human Foot as a Thermometer. (Painting by a Tyrolese artist in
the Ferdinandeum at Innsbruck.) From Dr. Robert Müllerheim's "Die
Wochenstube in der Kunst" (Stuttgart, 1904).

Another important fact which is brought out in the fifteenth century
pictures is that the use of *spectacles* had by this time become quite common.
The discovery of spectacle-lenses has been variously attributed to the Chinese,
to the Romans and to Roger Bacon. The only authentic reference is Pliny's
statement that Nero looked at the gladiators through an emerald (smaragd),
which Lessing discussed at great length in his "Antiquarian Letters," and
which, at best, can be construed only as a sort of lorgnette. It has been inferred that spectacles were invented about 1285 from the following data:
An inscription on a tomb in the chapel adjoining the church of Santa Maria
Maggiore (Florence) reads: "Here lies Salvino de'Armato degli Armati, of
Florence, the inventor of spectacles. May God forgive his sins. He died

[1] Those who wish to study the relation of the fine arts to early obstetrics
will find all the pictures in Witkowski's 'Histoire des accouchements," Paris,
1887, and in Robert Müllerheim's "Die Wochenstube in der Kunst," Stuttgart,
1904.

A. D. 1317."[1] In the dictionary of the Florentine Academy (1729) we read, *sub voce* "occhiali" (spectacles), that Giordano da Rivalto (1311), a monk of Pisa, stated, in a sermon of February 23, 1305, that spectacles had been invented less than twenty years before and that he himself had seen and conversed with the inventor, who was either Salvino de'Armati or the Dominican monk, Alessandro della Spina, who died in 1313. A manuscript of 1289, by Sandro di Pifozzo, published by Redi in 1648, mentions spectacles as of recent invention. Bernard de Gordon first referred to them, about 1305, as "oculus berellinus," because they were originally made from a smoky stone (berillus), whence the German "Brillen" (Parillen) and the French *besicles* (bericles). Arnold of Villanova terms them "vitrea vocata conspicilia," and Guy de Chauliac, in his Chirurgia Magna (1363), recommends them, if collyria fail. During the

fourteenth and fifteenth centuries, spectacles consisted of convex lenses in heavy unsightly frames which were sold at an uncommonly high price. They figure as a detail in Jan van Eyck's Madonna at Bruges in the hand of the donor, Georg van der Pale; in Ghirlandajo's Saint Jerome in the church of Ognissanti at Florence, in a woodcut of the book-worm in Sebastian Brand's "Narrenschiff" (1494) ; in Martin Schöngauer's engraving of the Death of Mary; in the decorations of the altar of St. Jacob's Church at Rothenburg an der Tauber; and in a colored picture in a manuscript in the University Library at Prague, representing the investiture of the Elector of Brandenburg (1417). In the last, they give the wearer the appearance of a Chinese mandarin. The earliest known pair of spectacles, consisting of two large circular lenses connected by a nosebridge of pince nez pattern, and once the property of the Renaissance humanist, Willibald Pirkheimer (1470–1530), are now on exhibition in the Wartburg.[2]

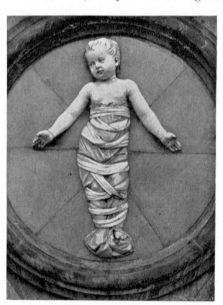

Bas-relief of Bambino in glazed clay in the Foundling Asylum at Florence, by Andrea della Robbia (1437–1525), showing method of swaddling infants. From Dr. Robert Müllerheim's "Die Wochenstube in der Kunst" (Stuttgart, 1904).

---

[1] Through the courtesy of Hon. Leo J. Keena, U. S. Consul at Florence, I am informed that the tombstone of Salvino degli Armati, which was originally over his remains in the cloister adjoining the church of Santa Maria Maggiore in Florence, was removed, with a portrait-monument, from his grave, and placed in the chapel of the Virgin Mary, on the right side of the church, for preservation. The inscription, as verified, reads:

QUI DIACE SALVINO D'ARMATO DEGLI ARMATI
DI FIRENZE, INVENTOR DEGLI OCCHIALI
DIO GLI PERDONI LE PECCATA
ANNO D. MCCCXVII.

[2] See R. Greeff: "Die ältesten uns erhaltenen Brillen," in Arch. f. Ophth., Wiesbaden, 1912, lxxii, 44–51.

During the Middle Ages, European humanity was plagued with **epidemic diseases** as never before or since, and these were variously attributed to comets and other astral influences, to storms, the failure of crops, famines, the sinking of mountains, the effects of drought or inundation, swarms of insects, poisoning of wells by the Jews and other absurd causes. The real predisposing factors were the crowded condition and bad sanitation of the walled medieval towns, the squalor, misrule and gross immorality occasioned by the many wars, by the fact that Europe was overrun with wandering soldiers, students and other vagabond characters, and by the general superstition, ignorance and uncleanliness of the masses, who, even in their bath-houses, were crowded together in one common compartment, sometimes with the sexes commingled. The earliest of the great medieval pandemics were the leprosy, Saint Anthony's fire or ergotism (857),[1] scurvy (1250),[2] influenza, the "Dancing Mania" (epidemic chorea), sweating sickness and plica Polonica (1287); the most formidable were the Black Death and syphilis. Of the former, leprosy, scurvy and influenza were either introduced or spread by the Crusades. Chorea, or Saint Vitus's dance (dancing mania), was probably the result of physical degeneracy plus fanatical religious enthusiasm, and acquired the latter name from the processions of dancing patients in the Strassburg epidemic of 1418, who proceeded in this wise to the chapel of St. Vitus in Zabern for treatment. Plica Polonica, the unsightly disease of matted hair, was introduced into Poland by the Mongol invasion (1287). Ergotism, variously known as *ignis sacer, ignis infernalis,* or St. Anthony's fire,[3] was a characteristic disease of the Middle Ages, due to the formation of the fungus *Claviceps purpurea* in spur-shaped masses upon rye, the common bread-staple of the poorer classes. The first allusion to it occurs in the Annals of the Convent at Xanten, near the Rhine, of date about 857, and, even in this brief paragraph, reference is already made to its gangrenous character and the eventual dropping off of the limbs from mortification. Later French epidemics occurred in 944, 957, 1039, 1089, 1096 and 1129, which were described, in the chronicles of the

---

[1] Mezeray, in his history of France, describes the epidemic of 944 and 1090, to the latter of which he gave the name St. Anthony's fire.

[2] First described by Joinville in his Histoire de St.-Loys, Paris, 1617, 121.

[3] The name St. Anthony's fire was first used by the French historian Mezeray, in speaking of the epidemic of 1090. The Order of St. Anthony for the care of the sufferers was founded in 1093. The patron saint was usually represented as a venerable figure, bearing a tau cross with bells, and attended by a hog, the ear of which was also belled. St. Martial, St. Genevieve and St. Benedict were also regarded as patron saints of ergotism, a fuller account of which may be found in the valuable historical monograph of Edvard Ehlers. See, also, the paper of Dr. Robert Fletcher in Bristol Med.-Chir. Journal, Dec., 1912, 295–315.

time, by Frodoard, Felibien and Siegebert. The disease usually began with sensations of extreme coldness in the affected part, followed by intense burning pains; or else a crop of blisters broke out, the limb becoming livid, foul and putrescent, and eventually dropping off: in either case, after causing great suffering in the unfortunate victim. Recovery commonly followed the loss of a limb and, by some cruel sport of fate, patients sometimes survived after losing all four limbs. When the gangrene attacked the viscera, however, it was speedily fatal. In the different chronicles, true ergotism was undoubtedly confused with erysipelas, gangrene, and bubonic plague, and the so-called *mal des ardents* was probably the latter disease. The convulsive form of ergotism did not appear until a later period.

The Black Death, which caused the unprecedented mortality of one-fourth of the population of the earth (over sixty millions of human beings), appeared in Europe about 1348, after devastating Asia and Africa. From a focus in the Crimea, it spread, *viâ* Turkey, Greece and Italy, northward and westward over the whole of Europe, again attacking it from a second focus by way of lower Austria. It broke out anew, at intervals, up to the end of the seventeenth century. Sweeping everything before it, this terrible plague brought panic and confusion in its train and broke down all restrictions of morality, decency and humanity. Parents, children and lifelong friends forsook one another, everyone striving to save only himself and to come off with a whole skin. Some took to vessels in the open sea only to find that the pestilence was hot upon them; some prayed and fasted in sanctuaries, others gave themselves up to unbridled indulgence or, as in the Decameron of Boccaccio, one of the most graphic accounts of the plague of 1348, fled the country to idle away their time in some safe retreat; others lapsed into sullen indifference and despair. The dead were hurled pell-mell into huge pits, hastily dug for the purpose, and putrefying bodies lay about everywhere in the houses and streets. "Shrift there was none; churches and chapels were open, but neither priests nor penitents entered—all went to the charnel-house. The sexton and the physician were cast into the same deep and wide grave; the testator, and his heirs and executors were hurled from the same cart into the same hole together."[1] In short, the Black Death, with its dark stains upon the skin, its hemorrhages and gangrenous destruction of the lungs, its paralyzing effect upon mind and body, was, in the grim phrase of the Italians, the *mortalega grande*, a veritable sign and symbol of the

---

[1] Cited from an old writer of the period by Dr. Robert Fletcher, in his "Tragedy of the Great Plague of Milan," Johns Hopkins Hosp. Bull., 1898, ix, 176.

King of Terrors.   The axillary and inguinal, with the pulmonary, lesions would make it identical with modern bubonic plague.   It was ably described by Guy de Chauliac, Boccaccio and Simon de Covino.   The epidemic had at least this good effect, that it led the Venetian Republic to appoint three guardians of public health and to make the first *quarantine* of infected areas, so called because it lasted forty days (*quaranta giorni*); while, in other cities, there were plague ordinances and private personal directions (*Pests-schriften*), pesthouses and other hygienic improvements.

The other great scourge of the Middle Ages was syphilis, which broke out in epidemic form at the siege of Naples in 1495, and was supposed to have been communicated to the French invaders by the Spanish occupants, who got it (modern authorities conjecture) from Columbus's sailors, a visitation from the New World.   That sporadic syphilis existed in antiquity and even in prehistoric times is quite within the range of probability, but never before had it taken on such a virulent aspect as about the time of the supposed Neapolitan epidemic of 1495–96, and, if Columbian in origin, its malignancy was perhaps the usual result of the contact of civilized and primitive races, as in the "Black Lion" of the Peninsular Wars, or the syphilis of Mexico, Japan, and the South Seas. Syphilis is first mentioned in the following works, recently printed in facsimile by Professor Karl Sudhoff:[1]

   1. The Edict against Blasphemers (*Gottesläster-Edikt*) of Emperor Maximilian I, issued August 7, 1495.
   2. The Vaticinium or "astrological vision" of the Frisian poet-physician Theodoricus Ulsenius (Dietrich Uelzen), printed at Nuremberg August 1, 1496, with a colored print of a syphilitic by Albrecht Dürer.   (Reprinted at Augsburg by Johann Froschauer, 1496.)
   3. The "Eulogium," a poem by Sebastian Brant, printed in September, 1496, by Joh. Bergmann von Olpe at Basel.
   4. The "Tractatus de pestilentiali Scorra" (Augsburg, Hans Schauer, October 18, 1496), and "Ein hübscher Tractat von dem Ursprung des Bösen Franzos" (Augsburg, Hans Schauer, December 17, 1496), the first of these reprinted three times at Nuremberg, Cologne, and Leipzig (1496), and the latter once at Nuremberg early in 1497.
   5. The "Enarratio Satyrica," a poem of the Veronese patrician, Giorgio Sommariva, printed at Venice in December, 1496.
   6. The "Concilium breve contra malas pustulas" of Konrad Schellig (Schelling), physician to the Elector Palatine (printed at Heidelberg in 1496).
   7. Four prayers, one to St. Minus (Nuremberg, 1496), one to St. Dionysius (Nuremberg, 1496), one printed at Vienna, 1497, and one in low German of uncertain date.
   8. A letter from Barcelona (1495) by Nicolò Scillacio of Messina, printed in his "Opuscula," March 9, 1496, at Pavia showing that, in June, 1495, syph-

---

[1] Karl Sudhoff: Graphische und typographische Erstlinge der Syphilis-literatur, Leipzig, 1912.   This work should be read by every one who wishes to know the most recent views of the subject as controlled by first-hand investigation (with typographic and photographic reproduction) of the original texts and documents.   Sudhoff has continued these investigations in "Aus der Frühgeschichte der Syphilis" (Stud. z. Gesch. d. Med., Hft. 9), Leipzig, 1912.

ilis had broken out at Barcelona, simultaneously with the Naples epidemic, and was thought to have come from France (qui nuper ex Gallia defluxit in alias nationes).

All these tracts tend to show, Sudhoff thinks, that syphilis was known in Europe before the siege of Naples, since the name of the disease had already so many different synonyms and its general semeiology seems to have been definitely outlined as early as 1495.

It is also mentioned before the year 1501 in various tracts by Niccolò Leoniceno (1497), Johannes Widmann (1497), Bartolommeo Montagnana (1498), Bartholomæus Steber (1498), Cino da Pistoia (1500), and Gasparo Torella (1500).

The first reference to the supposed West Indian origin of syphilis is contained in a work of Diaz de Isla, written about 1510, and published in 1539 and 1542, in which the disease is said to be described as an absolutely new and unheard-of affection in Barcelona, brought from Hayti by Columbus' sailors in April, 1493. Isla is one of the rarest of books, and, if we may trust current accounts, its author had treated sailors in Columbus' fleet for syphilis before they landed at Palos, and it is said that both Monardes and Montejo speak of the disease as then prevalent in near-by Seville, where a special hospital was built for syphilitics. The "Lucubratiuncula" of Leonhard Schmaus (1518) also refers to the West Indian origin of the disease on the authority of sea-captains of the period. In favor of the West Indian hypothesis, Hutchinson contended that, if transmissible syphilis existed in Europe before 1492, it would have been mentioned in Chaucer and Boccaccio, while it was found in Hayti and San Domingo after Columbus' second voyage. Virchow maintained that the *caries sicca* of prehistoric and pre-Columbian skulls was not true syphilis but either identical with the arthritis deformans (*Höhlengicht*) of old cave-bears, or else caused by plants and insects, which would eliminate the question of prehistoric syphilis in Europe. Medieval syphilis was first known as *mal franzoso, morbus Gallicus, mala napoletana*, after the supposititious siege of Naples (1495), where it is supposed to have been communicated to the French soldiers under Charles VIII by the Spanish inhabitants. After it became epidemic, it was called the Spanish, Polish, German, or Turkish "pocks," from the anxiety of the different nations to shift the blame upon one another. Iwan Bloch has attempted to prove that the evidences of *mal franzoso* in the cases of King Wenzel, the chorister of Mainz (1473), and Peter Martyr's letter (1488) were either fabrications or forgeries. On the other hand, the exhaustive studies recently made by Karl Sudhoff show that, in the "Gottes-lästereredikt" of Emperor Maximilian (August 7, 1495), mention is made of "malum francicum," but nothing is said about syphilis in relation to the siege of Naples. According to Guicciardini, there was no actual siege at Naples, since Charles VIII passed through the city without opposition on February 21, 1495. Furthermore, in moving homeward through Tuscany, the troops were besieged at Novara early in July, and did not get away until October 10th, two months after the date of Maximilian's Edict (August 7th); yet the latter shows that the disease was well known in Germany in July, while the actual march of events makes it clear that it could not have been spread about by wandering soldiery until long after, as Sudhoff shows. Sudhoff also gives a large number of recipes for syphilis, indicating that, far from being helpless in the treatment of the disease, physicians at the end of the fourteenth century were already prescribing the mercurial inunctions which had been used as far back as the twelfth century for leprosy, chronic eczema, and various skin eruptions. A special group of the latter, as yielding to mercury, were, Sudhoff thinks, an endemic spirochetosis, in all probability syphilis.[1] The most interesting of these recipes are two which Sudhoff found in an old Italian manuscript at Copenhagen, dated 1465, the handwriting of which has been assigned by the directors of the State Archives in the Uffizi at Florence to the first quarter of

---

[1] It is interesting to note that Sydenham thought that syphilis was identical with West African yaws; that Castellani's *Treponema pertenue* is hardly distinguishable from Schaudinn's parasite, and that, for the former, "606" is a true *therapia sterilisans*.

9

the fifteenth century.[1]   These recipes read (*16*) *Electuario optimo al mal franzoso* and (*77*) *Per fare siropi da male franzoso*, and contain ingredients identical with those employed in the vegetable electuaries (*Kräuterlatwergen*) of the early German and Italian writers on syphilis.   Thus, from the internal evidence of handwriting in some of the Uffizi manuscripts, syphilis may have been endemic in Italy as early as 1429.   Sudhoff also shows that the alleged 90 per cent. mortality of French troops at Naples is a nursery tale (*Ammenmärchen*), and that the Nuremberg prohibition of public bathing in a common chamber or tank (November 16, 1496) was similar to those already issued years before against leprosy and plague.   At the end of his interesting studies,[2] he quotes a prognostication made by Paul von Middelburg on the occasion of the conjunction of Jupiter, Mars and Saturn in the sign of the scorpion (November 25, 1484), which announces the approach of a fearful venereal disease, to reach its height about 1492–1500, and gives, along with a lurid purview of sexual debauchery, a series of resulting symptoms which are strikingly like those of syphilis.

Aside from the astrologic view of its causation, lues was latterly attributed to the rains and inundations of the same period (Leonicenus, intercourse of a leper with a prostitute (Monardi and Paracelsus), poisoning of the wells by the Spanish viceroys of Naples (Fallopius), or to disguised human flesh eaten by the French for ordinary meat (Fioravanti).   It is evident that the disease was not clearly understood at first, but, after it became pandemic, its sexual origin was recognized, and, as it spread northward and southward from Italy, its different stages were more or less accurately described between the years 1494 and 1550.   Meanwhile humanity of high and low degree had to learn the hard lesson that syphilis is "no respecter of persons."   Like the omnipresent grim skeleton in Holbein's "Dance of Death," it laid hold of lords and commons, just or unjust, in the same impartial spirit, and the illustrated books of a later time, Blancard's, for instance, teem with pictures representing the miseries wrought by lues and the inconveniences of the clumsy, if heroic, modes of treatment in vogue.   Apart from wars and famine, and even up to Ehrlich's time, syphilis has held its own, with tuberculosis and alcoholism, as a prime factor in bringing about the degeneration of the human stock.

---

[1] Sudhoff: Mal franzoso in Italien, Giessen, 1912.
[2] Sudhoff: Aus der Frühgeschichte der Syphilis, Leipzig, 1912, pp. 159–168.

THE PERIOD OF THE RENAISSANCE, THE REVIVAL OF LEARNING, AND THE REFORMATION (1438-1600)

In the transition of civilized mankind from medieval to modern conditions, many forces were operative, but undoubtedly the most potent were the invention of gunpowder, which gave the *coup de grace* to feudalism, and the discovery of printing, the greatest agent in uplifting mankind by self-education. The effect of the revival of Greek culture by the Byzantine scholars who poured into the Italian peninsula after the fall of Constantinople (1453) was to substitute the spontaneous receptive attitude of Plato and Hippocrates for the dialectics and logic-chopping of Aristotle and the Galenists. Prime movers in this change for medicine were the great printers of the Renaissance and the so-called "medical humanists." The sack of Mainz, by Adolph of Nassau, in 1462, scattered the German printers over Europe, and the first book to be printed in Italy was the Lactantius of 1465. The Florentine press was set up in 1471, and later the printing-houses of the Aldi and Giunti in Venice, Stephanus and Colinæus in Paris, Herbst (Oporinus) and Froben in Basel, Wynkyn de Worde and Wyer in London, Plantin at Antwerp, Elzevir in Leyden, vied with one another in the issue of stately folios and beautiful texts, while such editors and translators as Niccolò Leoniceno at Ferrara, Rabelais at Meudon, Günther of Andernach at Strassburg, Hagenbut (Cornarus) at Marburg, and Anutius Foesius at Metz, did for Hippocrates what Linacre and Caius in England did for Galen. These Renaissance imprints and editions are not only remarkable for unapproachable typography (those of Oporinus, Colinæus, and the early German printers in Spain bearing away the palm in this respect), but are usually furnished with good tables of contents and oftentimes with subject and author indices at the end, giving accurate paginations.

Of the **medical humanists,** Niccolò Leoniceno (**Leonicenus**) (1428–1524), professor of medicine at Padua, Bologna, and Ferrara, a friend of Politian and Linacre, and, like them, an elegant Latinist, made a famous translation of the aphorisms of Hippocrates, and, toward the close of his life, had even begun, by request, an accurate Latin translation of the works of Galen. He also wrote one of the earliest of the Renaissance tracts on syphilis (1497),[1] but his chief service to science lay in the difficult task of correcting the botanical errors in the Natural History of Pliny. In Leonicenus' day, this was a feat of the rarest intellectual courage. Hermolaus Barbarus, an earlier commentator, had already corrected some 500 orthographic and grammatic blunders perpetrated by the copyists of Pliny's manuscripts, but to assert that Pliny himself could be fallible in his statements of fact savored of rankest heresy, for his writings, like those of Galen and Aristotle, were regarded as sacrosanct and unimpeachable. Accordingly, when Leonicenus, who was a good botanist, published his little tract on the errors of Pliny[2] (1492), a violent storm of controversy broke loose over his head. His friend Poliziano, Colinuccio, and other non-botanists, who cared more for the letter than for the import of the old Roman's text, blazed away at the luckless commentator in truly medieval style for daring to challenge the accuracy of "our Pliny." Leonicenus stuck to his guns, however, with this important sequel, that all true botanists of later times— Ruellius, Matthiolus, Cesalpinus, Cordus—accepted his emendations without cavil. In this respect Leonicenus may be said to have cleared the ground for the German "Fathers of Botany." Without the careful work of these botanist-commentators there could have been no scientific description of the materia medica.

Thomas **Linacre** (1460–1524), physician to Henry VII and Henry VIII, was educated in Italy and graduated at Padua. On account of his services to humanism he was called by Fuller the "restorer of learning" in England. He is remembered especially for his grammatic works (Payne thought him the original of Robert Browning's "Grammarian"), for his foundations of lectures on medicine at Oxford and Cambridge (1524), and for his Latin versions of Galen's treatises on hygiene (1517),[3] therapeutics (1519),[4] temperaments (1521),[5] natural faculties (1523),[6] the pulse (1523),[7] and semeiology (1524).[8] These faithful and accurate translations had a wide circulation on the continent and made it clear to physicians of the day that for centuries they had relied upon garbled and second-hand versions of their favorite author.

---

[1] "Libellus de epidemia, quam Itali morbum gallicum vocant vulgo brossulas," Venice, 1497 (Hain, 10019); another edition was published at Milan in 1497 (Hain, 10020), and a third, printed in Gothic type, without place or date (Hain, 10018), is the earliest and rarest of all.

[2] "Plinii et aliorum auctorum, qui de simplicibus medicaminibus scripserunt, errores notati," Ferrara, 1492.

[3] De sanitate tuenda, Paris, 1517.

[4] Methodus medendi, Paris, 1519.

[5] De temperamentis, Cambridge, Siberch, 1519.

[6] De naturalibus facultatibus, London, Pynson, 1523.

[7] De pulsuum usu, London, Pynson, 1523.

[8] De symptomatum differentiis, London, Pynson, 1524.

François **Rabelais** (1490–1553), who, like Linacre, was a priest as well as a physician, made one of the first Latin translations of the aphorisms of Hippocrates (Lyons, 1532), the original edition of which is much prized by bibliophiles.[1] Rabelais is best known, of course, by his immortal humorous works "Gargantua" and "Pantagruel," which are not only filled with the strangest kind of medical erudition, but are exponents of Renaissance humanism in the broadest sense.[2]

Anutius **Foesius,** or Foes (1528–95), devoted forty years of a laborious and useful life, as city physician in his native town of

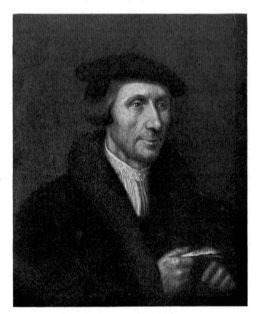

Thomas Linacre, M.D. (1460?–1524).

Metz, to the completion of a critical edition of the Greek text of Hippocrates (1595), which is recognized by scholars everywhere as unquestionably the best of its kind before the time of Littré.

Some time after the invention of printing Germany entered the field of medicine with a remarkable array of semi-popular treatises, most of them written, contrary to custom, in the vernacular—the language of the people. According to Sudhoff, the

[1] Earlier Latin versions were published at Venice in 1495 (Hain, 8674) and at Nuremberg in 1496 (Hain, 8675).

[2] The old medieval custom of stuffing the youthful mind with book-learning is keenly ridiculed, and the Greek ideal of education as a drawing out of all the faculties, including the physical and social, is upheld by Rabelais.

earliest printed document relating to medicine is the unique
"Purgation-Calendar" (*Laxierkalender*) of 1457, printed in the
type of Guttenberg's 36-line Bible,[1] and contained (a sheet of paper
only) in the Bibliothèque nationale at Paris. A unique copy of
a "Calendar for Blood-Letting" (*Aderlasskalender*), printed at
Mainz in 1462,[1] is one of the treasures of the Fürstenberg Library
at Donaueschingen (Baden). These popular almanacs, consisting

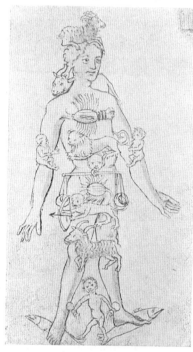

of loose leaves or broadsides,
printed on one side only, show
the hold which judicial astrology (the *Lasstafelkunst*) had
taken upon the people. In
some of them, a special figure,
the "zodiac-man" (*Tierkreiszeichenmann*), indicates, as in
drug-store almanacs of more
recent date, the parts of the
body influenced by the different planetary conjunctions the
proper times and places for
bleeding and purgation under
each sign of the zodiac, with
gloomy prognostications of the
terrible diseases, wars, famines,
and other pests which were
to befall humanity under dif-
 erent ascendancies and conjunctions of the planets. More
scientific interest attaches to
the *Regiment der jungen Kinder*
of Bartholomæus Metlinger
(Augsburg, 1473), a little book
on infant hygiene, which would
be the first Renaissance contribution to pediatrics had it
not been preceded by Paolo

Zodiac-man. Miniature, from a
blood-letting calendar by Johann Nider
von Gmünd (Vienna), painted at Brau-
nau in 1470. Courtesy of Professor
Karl Sudhoff, Leipzig, Germany.

Bagellardo's *De ægritudinibus infantum* (Padua, 1472).

The *Arztneibuch* of **Ortollf of Bavaria** (Nuremberg, 1477) was an
important German text of popular medicine in its day, followed,
about 1500, by Ortollf's quaint little *Frauenbüchlein*, or popular
handbook for lying-in women. A few years later (in 1513) there
appeared, at Worms, the *Rosegarten* of Eucharius **Röslin,** a work

---

[1] For a facsimile of either, see Sudhoff's interesting "Lasstafelkunst in
Drucken des 15. Jahrhunderts," in his Arch. f. Gesch. d. Med., Leipzig, 1907,
8, i, pp. 223 and 227 and p. 135 (opposite).

Coniuctioes z oppoſicoes ſolis et lune ac miucoes electie nec no dies p medicis
laxatiuis ſumendis In anno dni M cccc lviii Cui b lra dnicalis xiii aure nis
Intecuallu ix ebdomde Concurrentes una dies ⁖

Jannarius ⟨ Oppoſicie feria ſcda p echardi hora ix p meridie Intcentio in die couctionis
pauli hora v poſt meridie Minutioes fcia ſcda et tercia poſt circucifiois dni
laxatiua ſumenta ix x xi xviii xix xx xxviii die bui menſis

Februarius ⟨ Oppoſie die applonie hora xi an meridie Intctio die machie apli hora v an
meridie Minutoes fabbo z dnica p applonie v x vi p valctini z iii p machie
laxatiua ſumenda v v vi vii xiii xx xxi xxiii xxiiii ac xxv die huius menſis

Marcius ⟨ Oppoſie fecia quita an gregorii hora xi p meridie Intctio annuciacois marie hora ſecta poſt meridiem Minutoes pdie z die gettcudis et dnica p gettcud
laxatiua ſumenta iiii v vi xiii xiiii xx xxiii xxiiii die huius menſis

Aprilis ⟨ Oppoſie fabbo poſt ambroſij in meridie Intctio craftino georgii hod fecta
an meidiem Minutoes fecta p ambroſij pdie z die tyburcii dnica z fcia ſcda p
tyburcii laxatiua ſumenta i ii iii x xi xii xix xx xxi xxviii xxix ac xxx die h menſis

Maius ⟨ Oppo ſcda p gotchardi in media nocte Intctio ſcda an urbani hod vi p meid
Minutoes die gotchardi z die ſecti die gordiani z die ſecti pdie ſophie z die
eusdem laxatiua ſumeta vii viii ix xii xiii xviii xx xxvi z xxvii die h menſis

Junius ⟨ Oppoſicio tercia poſt bonifacii hod pma p meidie Intctio qrta poſt albani
hod vii an meid Minutoes qrta z v an bonifacii vi z fabbo p bonifacii v z vi
ante albani laxatiua ſumeta iii iiii v xiii xxiii xxv xxvi ac xxiiii die h menſis
Oppo qrta p utalrici hod xi p meidie Intctio pdie marie magtal hod v p

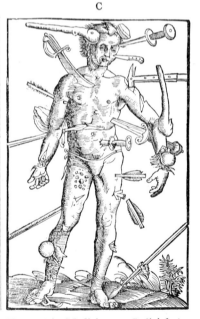

Specimens of the *Lasstafelkunst* (Horoscopic Medicine or Judicial Astrology). (By kind permission of Professor Karl Sudhoff, University of
Leipzig.) A: Fragment of Purgation Calendar (*Laxierkalender*), printed with
the types of Guttenberg's 36-line Bible (1457), and discovered by Professor
Sudhoff in the Bibliothèque nationale, Paris. B: Blood-letting man (*Aderlassmann*), from the Calendar of Regiomontanus (1475), showing the points
of election for blood-letting under the signs of the Zodiac. C: Wound-man
(*Wundenmann*), from Gersdorff's *Feldtbuch* (1517), showing the sites for
ligation of the different arteries or for blood-letting. C is a later evolutionary
form of the old zodiacal diagrams, which combined an exposition of planetary
influences with schemata of the viscera (B).

which bears about the same relation to Renaissance obstetrics that the "Anathomia" of Mundinus does to medieval anatomy. Although mainly a compilation from Soranus of Ephesus, as filtered through the manuscript codices of Moschion, it was still the only text-book in the field after a lapse of fourteen centuries. Three first editions were issued simultaneously, both extremely interesting for their quaint cuts (already faintly outlined in the Moschion codices), for the revival of podalic version as originally described by Soranus, and for the fact that Röslin's text was miserably plagiarized by Walther Reiff in 1545,[1] and also translated and reissued by William Raynalde as "The Byrthe of Mankynde," London, 1545. The ordinance issued by the city of Ratisbon in 1555 for the direction of midwives (*Regensburger Hebammenbuch*) has been proved by Mr. Felix Neumann[2] to be the earliest public document of this kind in the vernacular.

Perhaps the earliest European text of medical jurisprudence of consequence is the "Constitutio Criminalis Carolina" (*Peinliche Gerichtsordnung*) issued by Emperor Charles V in 1533, as an extension of a similar ordinance issued by the Bishop of Bamberg in 1507. Interesting relics of the great medieval pandemics of syphilis and bubonic plague are preserved in the curious tracts of Widman (1497), Steber (1498), Pollich (1501), Konrad Schelling (1502), Grünpeck (1503), Ulrich von Hutten (1514), and Schmaus (1518), and sweating sickness is the subject of the little treatise of John Kaye or Caius (1552). Early German botany had its beginnings in the queer wood engravings of the *Hortus sanitatis* attributed to Johan von Cube (1491), which was rendered into German as the "Gart der Gesundheit." This work contained some 500 engravings, which, as Greene says, are "most wretched caricatures of plants," but it became so popular as to be the principal incentive for the work of the "German Fathers," Brunfels, Fuchs, Bock, and Valerius Cordus.

Early German surgery begins with the *Bündth-Ertznei* of Heinrich von **Pfolspeundt**, a Bavarian army surgeon, whose work, written in 1460, remained long in manuscript, until it was discovered at Breslau and edited by Haeser and Middeldorpf in 1868. Pfolspeundt was only a wound surgeon, had no skill in the major operations, which he left to the cutters or "incisors," and did not know how to treat fractures and dislocations; but he learned how to make artificial noses (by the Hindu method) from the wandering Italians. His military experience gave him a large practice in arrow wounds, and his book contains the first faint allusion to

---

[1] The plagiarist Reiff should not be confused with the Swiss obstetrician Jacob Rueff (1500–58), author of the "Trostbüchle" (Zürich, 1554), a midwifery of sterling character.

[2] Arch. f. Gesch. d. Med., Leipzig, 1911–12, v, 132–141.

"powder-burns" and to the extraction of bullets by means of the sound.[1] He treated wounds by second intention, used the narcotic recommended by Theodoric, and, like Mondeville and other surgeons of earlier times, gave his patients strengthening "wound-drinks." After Pfolspeundt came two Alsatian army surgeons, Hieronymus Brunschwig (*circa* 1450–1533) and Hans von Gersdorff, called Schyllhans, both natives of Strassburg. The *Buch der Wund-Artzeny* (Strassburg, 1497) of **Brunschwig** contains the first detailed account of gunshot wounds in medical literature. He regarded such wounds as poisoned, and thought the poison could be best removed by promoting suppuration, usually by means of the seton. As an army surgeon, Brunschwig did no major operations, confining himself to wounds, bone-setting, and amputation. In performing the latter, he applied the actual cautery or boiling oil to check hemorrhage from the stump. This book contains some of the earliest specimens of medical illustration by wood-cuts, rare and curious in their kind, and the same thing is true of Gersdorff's Field-Book of Wound Surgery (*Feldtbuch der Wundtartzney*), which was published at Strassburg in 1517. **Gersdorff** goes even more fully into gunshot wounds than Jerome of Brunswick. He did not regard them as poisonous, but probed for the bullet with special instruments and, like most surgeons of his time, poured hot oil into the wound. In amputating, he "Esmarched" the limb by means of a constricting band, and, discarding the cautery, checked hemorrhage by a styptic of his own devising (containing lime, vitriol, alum, aloes, and nut-galls), inclosing the stump in "the bladder of a bull, ox, or hog," which may, in some cases, have been a good Listerian protective. Gersdorff's book contains some of the most instructive pictures of early surgical procedure in existence; in particular, the first picture ever made of an amputation, and unique plates of diseases like leprosy and St. Anthony's fire. The wood-cut of the latter condition ("ignis sacer" or ergotism) represents the victim of the disease as hobbling upon a crutch and holding up a shriveled, gangrenous hand, bursting into flame, to excite the pity of Anthony, the patron-saint of the disease, who stands leaning upon his tau-cross, attended by his faithful swine. Another interesting picture book in the vernacular is the *Augendienst* (Dresden, 1583) of the court oculist, George **Bartisch** (1535–

---

[1] Haeser and Middeldorpf at first asserted, in their commentary on Pfolspeundt (pp. xxii, xxvii), that there is no mention of gunshot wounds in the Bündth-Ertznei. This was afterward shown to be incorrect by H. Frœlich (Deutsche mil.-ärztl. Ztschr., Berlin, 1874, vol. iii, pp. 592–594), who points out the "Item vor das büchsenpülüer auss den wünden" (Pfolspeundt, p. 10), and the following (p. 60): "Auch machstu solchs suchel [Sonde] wol von eissen machenn . . . mith dem hebstu die kleine gelödt oder *kugel* hiraus, die von buchsenn hinein geschossenn sein, unnd auch was sunst in den wunden ist."

1606), the striking illustrations of which give us a complete purview of Renaissance eye-surgery. Among these may be mentioned the cuts showing the patient tied in a chair and ready for
operation, the modes of procedure in cataract, and the perforated
spectacles or visors (originally recommended by Paul of Ægina[1])
for strabismus. As Bartisch, originally an unlettered barber-
surgeon, makes a great parade of learning and Latinity in his text,
aside from its pompous title,[2] he is supposed to have employed

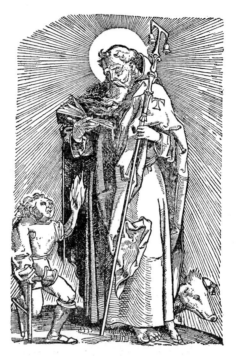

St. Anthony with a victim of ergotism. (From Hans von Gersdorff's
Feldtbuch der Wundtartzney, Strassburg, 1540.)

a famulus or hired scribe to polish his book for him. None the
less, this work did much to lift ophthalmology above what its
author calls the "couchers and eye-destroyers" of his time. The
earliest printed book on the eye was the "De oculis, eorumque
egritudinibus et curis" of Benvenuto Grassi of Salerno (printed
at Ferrara in 1475), which follows the ancients.

---

[1] Paul's visor-mask is described in the Basel (Oporinus) edition of 1546,
lib. iii, cap. 22, p. 182.

[2] 'Οφαλμώδουλεῖα, das ist, Augendienst, Dresden, 1583.

In the vernacular group may be mentioned the little eye-books of G. Vogtherr (Strassburg, 1538) and Walter Bailey (London, 1586), and the "Traité des maladies de l'œil" by Jacques Guillemeau (Paris, 1585), decidedly the best of the Renaissance books on ophthalmology. Even the English treatise of Richard Banister (1622) is only a translation of this work.

The first medical book to be printed in England was called "A Passing Gode Lityll Boke Necessarye and Behovefull Agenst the Pestilence," being a small quarto of twelve leaves, attributed to the press of William de Machlinia (London, circa 1485), translated from the "Tractatus contra pestilentiam" (1485), ascribed to Kanutus (Bengt Knutsson), Bishop of Västerås, Sweden, but which, as Sudhoff has shown, by parallel comparison of texts, was really written by the Papal physician Johannes Jacobi of Montpellier in 1373.[1] The English version was afterward reprinted by Wynkyn de Worde in 1510.

Next came "The Governayle of Helthe" printed at Caxton's press about 1491, followed, in 1510, by "The Judycyal of Urins," sometimes attributed to John of Arderne, and probably printed by Wynkyn de Worde. In 1516, Peter Treverus, a printer in Southwark, published "The Grete Herball," and, in 1521, Siberch of Cambridge printed Linacre's translation of Galen's "De temperamentis," after which Pynson of London published other versions of Galen by the same scholar. The first work on anatomy to be printed in England was David Egar's little tract of 15 pages entitled, "In anatomicen introductio luculenta et brevis," and the first English work in the vernacular on the same subject was "The Englishman's Treasure" by Thomas Vicary (London, 1548).[2]

The effect of these vernacular writings was to get men's minds away from scholasticism and turn them toward realities. This Renaissance tendency reached its highest development in the most prominent of the medical leaders of the sixteenth century, Paracelsus, Vesalius, and Paré—three strong men of aggressive temperament, who, by shouldering past other men, literally "blazed the way," not only for the general advance of medicine, but for keen and liberal thinking in all its branches.

Aureolus Theophrastus Bombastus von Hohenheim, or **Paracelsus** (1493–1541), the founder of chemical pharmacology and therapeutics, was, in spite of his bombastic claims to rank and lineage,[3] a striking example of the very raw materials from which such aspirations are sometimes fashioned. His coarseness of fiber, though a better possession to him than vulgarity of spirit, often impeded his power to "think straight and see clear." A native of Einsiedeln, near Zürich, Switzerland, he had the truculent, independent spirit commonly ascribed to the man of mountaineer race, and was one of the few writers who ever advanced medicine by quarreling about it. Like the "roarers" in Elizabethan comedy, or the Zankbauer in German farce, he tried to bully and browbeat his auditors and readers into accepting his views, and the writings which he dictated to his pupils are often a curious

---

[1] Sudhoff: Arch. f. Gesch. d. Med., Leipzig, 1911–12, v, 56–58.

[2] These data are given in a paper by the late Dr. J. F. Payne in the Brit. Med. Jour., London, 1889, i, 1085.

[3] The name "Paracelsus" is supposed to be either a free translation of "Hohenheim" or else an indication of his superiority to Celsus. He usually calls himself "Theophrastus ex Hohenheim eremita," i. e., of Einsiedeln.

mixture of credulous fustian and swagger, set off by many successful guesses at truth, the work of a noisy declaimer who sometimes hits the nail on the head. His humorous sallies, if he intended them as such, are usually of the lumpish kind that drift
"from the obscene into the incomprehensible." Paracelsus was
the son of a physician, from whom he learned medicine while
picking up an unusual knowledge of alchemy, astrology, and
other occult sciences from the learned abbots and bishops of the
country round, as also in the laboratory and mines owned by the

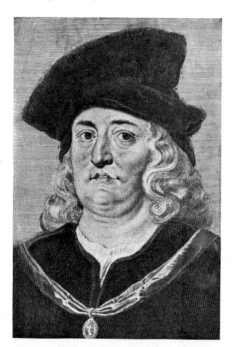

Paracelsus (1493–1541).

Tyrolese alchemist, Sigis-
mund Fugger. Having
the Swiss *Wanderlust*, he
traveled far and wide,
collecting information
from every source, and by
his relations with barbers,
executioners, bathkeepers,
gypsies, midwives, and
fortune-tellers, he learned
a great deal about medical
practice, and incidentally
acquired an unusual
knowledge of folk-medicine
and a permanent taste for
low company. Appointed
professor of medicine and
city physician at Basel in
1527, he began his cam-
paign of reform by publicly
burning the works of Galen
and Avicenna in his lec-
ture room, but, a year later
(1528), he was already in
violent conflict with the
authorities about fees, and
forced to leave the city. Resuming his wandering habits, he
practised all over Germany with varying success, finally dying
from the consequences of an injury in a tavern brawl at Salzburg. As a pioneer in chemistry, Paracelsus was preceded by
the alchemists Albertus Magnus (Albrecht von Bollstädt) and
Cornelius Agrippa, and by the (probably mythical) fifteenth-
century Benedictine monk, Basil Valentine, who is supposed
to have given to chemistry hydrochloric acid, sugar of lead,
the means of preparing ammonia and sulphuric acid, and, in
his "Triumphant Chariot of Antimony" (1604), fastened the

latter metal upon medical practice for centuries.[1] Paracelsus took Valentine's three chemical elements—combustible sulphur, volatile mercury, residual salt—and mixed them up with a species of theosophic lore not unlike that of the far East, in which he is supposed to have traveled. Baas has compared reading Paracelsus to delving in a mine. We are in a strange world of mystic principles, archæi and arcana, enlivened by gnomes, sylvans, sprites, and salamanders. Existence proceeds from God, all material things from the Yliaster, or primordial substance, while the force in nature which sets things going (the vital principle) is the Archæus. The Archæus is the essence of life, contained in an invisible vehicle, the Mumia, and in diseased conditions this Mumia must be magnetically extracted from the patient's body and inoculated into a plant bearing the signature of the disease, so that it may attract the specific influence from the stars, diseases being caused by astral influences acting upon the "astral body" of man. Yet the author of all this high-flown verbiage, the actual Paracelsus, was a capable physician and surgeon, generous to the poor, and however despised and rejected for coarseness, charlatanry, and possible drunkenness, a man deserving of better human remembrance. For Paracelsus was neither the refined, supersubtle mystic of Browning's poem, nor yet the roistering, lying, tippling blackguard and quacksalver of tradition. His influence was far reaching, and his real services were great. Far in advance of his time, he discarded Galenism and taught physicians to accept chemical therapeutics; he attacked witchcraft and the strolling mountebanks who butchered the body in lieu of surgical procedure, and he opposed the silly uromancy and uroscopy; he was the first to write on miner's (occupation) diseases, and the first to establish a correlation between cretinism and endemic goiter; almost the only asepsist between Mondeville and Lister, he taught that nature (the "natural balsam") heals wounds, and not officious meddling; he introduced mineral baths, and was one of the first to analyze them; he made

---

[1] In the opinion of Kopp (Die Alchemie, 1886), John Ferguson (Bibliotheca Chimica, 1906), and Professor Karl Sudhoff, the pseudonymous writings of Basil Valentine were written by their "editor," the chemist, Johann Thölde, owner of the salt-works at Franckenhausen in Thuringia, and unquestionably belong to the early seventeenth century literature. See, on this head, Sudhoff's Bibliographia Paracelsica (Berlin, 1894), C. S. Pierce, in Science, N. Y., 1898, N. S. viii, 169–176, and "Basil Valentine, a seventeenth century hoax," by J. M. Stillmann, in Pop. Sci. Monthly, New York, 1912, lxxxi, 591–600. The picture of Basil Valentine in the Royal Cabinet of Etchings at Munich represents a monk, with retort and pentagram, looking very like the usual pictures of Paracelsus. The "Currus triumphalis antimonii" led all practitioners to prescribe antimony at the start in fevers. The vogue died out, but the drug was revived in 1657, when its exhibition cured Louis XIV of typhoid fever. Valentine refers to syphilis as the "Neue Krankheit der Kriegsleut," recommending a mixture of antimony, lead, and mercury against it.

opium (laudanum),[1] mercury, lead, sulphur, iron, arsenic, copper
sulphate, and potassium sulphate (called the "specificum purgans
Paracelsi"), a part of the pharmacopeia, and regarded zinc as an
elementary substance; he distinguished alum from ferrous sulphate, and demonstrated the iron content of water by means of
gallic acid; his "doctrine of signatures" was revived by Rade-
macher and Hahnemann, and, in comparing the action of the
"arcana," or intrinsic principles of drugs, to a spark, he grasped
the idea of catalytic action. As a theorist, he believed in the
descent of living organisms from the *Urschleim*, or primordial
ooze, and Baas credits him with anticipating Darwin in his observation that the strong war down and prey upon the weak—a
fact, unfortunately, within the range of any beggar or footman.
But none of these things can outweigh the influence which Paracelsus exerted on his time through his personality. In an age
when heresy often meant death, he wasted no time in breaking
butterflies upon wheels, but drove full tilt at many a superstition,
risking his neck with all the recklessness of a border reiver. The
importance attached to his name may be gathered from the line
in Shakespeare's comedy which brackets it with that of Galen.[2]
Paracelsus was great in respect of his own time. He does not
seem particularly great in relation to our time.

The most exhaustive study yet made of Paracelsus and his
writings is that of Professor Karl Sudhoff (1894–9).

The principal works of Paracelsus are the treatise on open
wounds (1528), his *Chirurgia magna*, 1536), his manual introducing
the use of mercurials in syphilis (Frankfurt, 1553), the treatise
"De gradibus" (Basel, 1568), which contains most of his innovations in chemical therapeutics, his monograph on miner's diseases
(*Von der Bergsucht*, Dilingen, 1567), and his booklet on mineral
baths (Basel, 1576), recommending Gastein ("Castyn"), Töpp-
litz, Göppingen, and Plombières ("Blumbers"). The treatise on
miner's diseases, the result of his observations in Fugger's mines
in Tyrol, giving descriptions of miner's phthisis and the effects of
choke-damp, was one of the few original contributions of the time
to clinical medicine. In his chapter, "De generatione stultorum,"[3]
Paracelsus first notes the coincidence of cretinism and endemic

---

[1] "Ich hab ein Arcanum, heiss ich Laudanum, ist über das alles, wo es
zum Tod reichen will," Grosse Wundarznei, i, Tr. 3, cited by Haeser.

[2] In "All's Well That Ends Well," Act. II, sc. 3, where Lafeu refers to the
King's case as incurable, "to be relinquished of the artists," and Parolles replies: "So I say, both of Galen and Paracelsus"—meaning, of course, that
neither the Galenical nor the alchemical school of physicians could help him
in any way.

[3] Printed in his posthumous "Opera Omnia," Strassburg, 1603, ii, pp.
174–182.

goiter, a discovery also based upon original observations in the Salzburg region.

Apart from the huge output of the syphilographers,—Leonicenus (1497), Fracastorius (1530), Niccolò Massa (1532), Fernelius (1538), Fallopius (1564), and Luisinus (1566),—the Renaissance literature dealing with the actual portrayal of disease is meager. In this group we may include the original descriptions of typhus fever by Fracastorius (1546), of sweating sickness by Caius (1552), of varicella by Ingrassias (1553), of "tabardillo" (Spanish or Mexican typhus) by Francesco Bravo (1570), of whooping-cough ("*quinta*") by Guillaume Baillou or Ballonius (1578), of chlorosis (*morbus virgineus*) by Johann Lange (1554), and of the syndrome "mountain sickness" by the Jesuit traveler José d'Acosta (1590). Geronimo Mercuriali (1530–1606) wrote the first systematic treatise on skin diseases (1572) and one of the earlier works on diseases of children (1583). The pediatric treatise of Sebastianus Austrius (1540) deserves mention, as also the work of Prospero Alpino on Egyptian medicine (1591).

Dr. Chas. Singer points out[1] that some beginnings of tropical medicine were made in Oviedo's description of yaws as "bubas," afterward identified by André Thevet, in 1558, as "no other thing than the pocks which rageth and hath power over all Europe, specially among the Frenchmen." Oviedo and Thevet also mention the sandflea (Pulex penetrans). Singer draws attention to the first book on tropical medicine, an anonymous tract, entitled *The Cures of The Diseased In Remote Regions* (London, 1598), the scope of the work being indicated by the versified table of contents:

"The burning fever, calde the Calenture,
The aking Tabardilla pestilent,
The Espintas prickings which men do endure,
Cameras de sangre, Fluxes violent,
Th' *Erizipila*, swelling the Pacient,
Th' *Tiñoso*, which we the Scurvey call,
Are truly here described and cured all."

For a long time after Paracelsus, **chemistry** still remained alchemy, and, in the following century, became merged into the fantastic pseudo-science of the Rosicrucians. The arch-patron of alchemy in the sixteenth century was the Emperor Rudolph II of Germany (1576–1612), who devoted much of his fortune and the whole of his life to the quest of potable gold, the philosopher's stone, and the elixir of life. In the spacious and gloomy chambers of his palace, the Hradschin at Prague, he held high court with alchemists, spiritualists, judicial astrologers, clairvoyants, and other followers of psychic "science," and no reward was considered too great for any adventurer, however disreputable, who might manage to wheedle this fantastic monarch "of dark corners." The credulous Rudolph was continually the prey of all sorts of impudent knaves and sharp practitioners, upon whom he speedily revenged himself by imprisonment or execution if they failed to perform their promises.[2] Hither came the learned Cambridge scholar, John Dee, a solemn humbug, and his assistant, Edward

---

[1] Ann. Trop. Med. and Parasitol., Liverpool, 1912, vi, 87–101.

[2] For a full account of all this, see Henry Carrington Bolton's delightful book, "The Follies of Science at the Court of Rudolph II," Milwaukee, 1904.

Kelley, a sharp-witted impostor, to make "projections" of the baser metals into gold, and, by crystal gazing in a shew-stone (now in the British Museum), to indulge the kind of self-hypnotism familiar to-day as "automatic writing," Kelley acting as "skryer," or clairvoyant, in the maneuver. Both were richly rewarded, Dee escaping to England in the nick of time, Kelley remaining to become a landed proprietor and *eques auratus* of the Bohemian Kingdom, but subsequently losing his life as a punishment for his brawls and impostures. To "Gold Alley," the charlatan street of Prague, came also Michael Sendivogius, "Count" Marco Bragadino, Gossenhauer, and Cornelius Drebbel, the perpetual motion man; and it was for the sake of alchemy that Rudolph brought Tyco Brahe and Kepler together, to the material advantage of future astronomy. The foregatherings of Rudolph's physicians, Crato von Kraftheim, Oswald Croll, Guarinonius, Michael Maier, and the rest, made up the Rudolphine Academy of Medicine, of which an extraordinary session was once convened to hear Andreas Libau (Libavius) read an essay on the "aurum potabile." This Libavius (1546–1616), a physician and teacher of Coburg, made a real start in chemistry, and his "Alchymia" (Frankfurt, 1595) is usually regarded as the first systematic treatise on the science. He had, says Bolton, "a sumptuous laboratory, provided not only with every requisite for chemical experimentation, but also with means of entertaining visiting guests, including such luxuries as baths, inclosed corridors for exercise in inclement weather, and a well-stocked wine-cellar." He discovered stannic chloride, analyzed mineral waters with the balance (1597), wrote a city pharmacopeia (1606), and was one of the first to recommend the transfusion of blood (1615). His "Alchymia" is divided into two parts, the first dealing with the laboratory operations of chemistry, including instruments and furnaces; the latter half containing accurate and systematic descriptions of chemical substances. Of this, no less than 80 pages are still devoted to the philosopher's stone.

A typical follower of Paracelsus was the adventurous alchemist and swindler, Leonhard Thurnheysser zum Thurn (1531–95), of Basel, who started out as a goldsmith's apprentice, married at sixteen, and was soon embarked in a "gold-brick" imposture (selling tin coated with gold), for which he had to flee the city and take up a roving life. He traveled far and wide, became inspector of mines in Tyrol in 1558, and, after healing the wife of the Elector of Brandenburg of a desperate illness, became his body physician in 1578. In Berlin, he made so much money by pawn-broking, usury, and the sale of calendars, horoscopes, and secret remedies, that he was able to set up a private laboratory and printing office, with type-foundry attached. A scandalous lawsuit with his third wife reduced him to beggary, and he died obscurely in a cloister at Cologne. His writings, full of mystical humbuggery, are without value, although much has been made of his discovery that mineral waters yield a certain residue upon evaporation.

After the time of Mundinus, a number of anatomic treatises appeared containing the first rude attempts at pictorial representation of dissected parts. These include the so-called **"graphic incunabula"** of anatomy and may conveniently take in all published illustrations of the pre-Vesalian period. They are:

1. The 25 editions of Mundinus, printed between 1478 and 1580, including those in Ketham.

2. The "Fasciculus medicinæ" (Venice, 1491) of Johannes de Ketham, a series of writings on uroscopy, venesection, surgery, etc., which passed through six later (Venetian) editions, viz., 1493, 1495, 1500, 1513, 1522, 1522 (Italian translation), all containing the anatomy of Mundinus at the end.

3. The skeleton of Richard Helain, printed at Nuremberg in 1493.

4. An illustration of the abdominal muscles in the 1496 edition of the "Conciliator differentiarum" of Peter of Abano.

5. The Philosophiæ naturalis compendium (Leipzig, 1499) of the Leipzig jurist, Johannes Peyligk (1474–1592?).

6. The "Antropologium" (Leipzig, 1501) of the Leipzig professor Magnus Hundt (1449–1519).

7. Gregor Reisch's Margarita philosophica (1503, 1504), containing a view of the thoracic and abdominal viscera and the oldest schematic representation of the eye, which Sudhoff has traced to a pen drawing in a Leipzig codex of the preceding century.

8. The fugitive anatomic plates (Fliegende Blätter) of Johann Schott of Mainz (1517), Christian Wechel of Paris (1536), Heinrich Vogtherr of Strassburg (1539), and others.

9. The "Spiegl der Artzny" of Laurentius Phryesen (Fries, Friesen) (1519).

10. Giacomo Berengario da Carpi's commentary on Mundinus (1521); and his "Isagogæ breves" (Bonn, 1514).

11. The "Anatomiæ pars prior" (Marburg, 1537) of Johann Eichmann or Dryander (1560).

It has been shown, in the highly original researches of Karl Sudhoff,[1] that none of these earlier anatomic illustrations were based upon original observation or dissection, but that, for the most part, they are purely traditional, servile copies from manuscript sketches of the past, with some little superadded touches here and there. The wood-cuts in Ketham's "Fasciculus" represent a circle of 21 urine glasses which Sudhoff has traced to a manuscript of 1400; sick-room and dissecting scenes, with groups of Venetian gentry in the costumes of the period; and a remarkable series of characteristic figures indicating the sites of injury or disease and the most favorable localities for applying treatment, viz., the "zodiac-man" (*Tierkreiszeichenmann*), in which schemata of the viscera are often overlaid by the zodiacal figures; the "blood-letting man" (*Aderlassmann*), whose body is tattooed with marks indicating the best sites for venesection under the signs

---

[1] Karl Sudhoff: Tradition und Naturbeobachtung in den Illustrationen medizinischer Handschriften und Frühdrucke, vornehmlich des 15. Jahrhunderts, Leipzig, 1907; and Ein Beitrag zur Geschichte der Anatomie im Mittelalter, Leipzig, 1908. For a good account of pre-Vesalian illustration in English, with reproductions of most of the figures, see Prof. William A. Locy's interesting essay in Jour. Morphol., Chicago, 1911, xxii, 945–987.

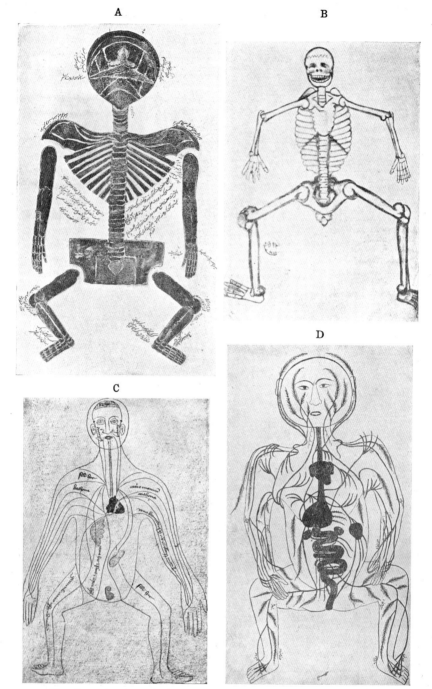

Drawings showing influence of tradition upon early anatomic illustration. (By kind permission of Professor Karl Sudhoff, University of Leipzig.) A: Skeleton from Persian MS. No. 2296, India Office, London. B: Skeleton in aquatint from Dresden MS. Codex 310 (A. D. 1323). C: Arterial system, from a fourteenth century MS. in the Library of Prince von Lobkowicz (Raudnitz, Bohemia). D: Venous system, from Persian MS. No. 2296, India Office, London. Roth called attention to the traditional character of anatomic illustration in the pre-Vesalian period, but the development of the subject is almost entirely the work of Professor Sudhoff.

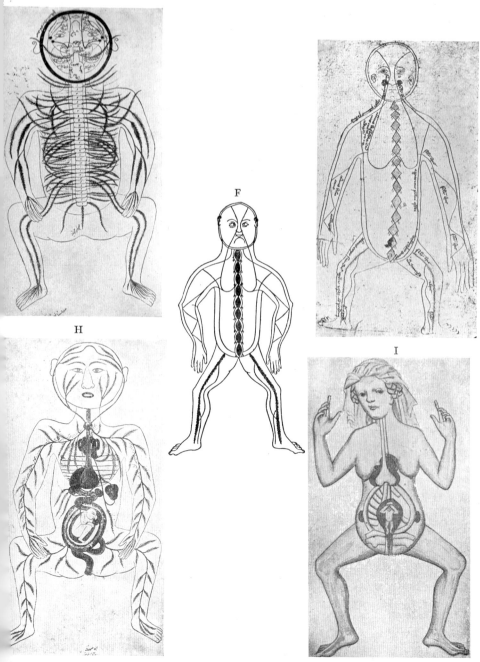

Drawings showing influence of tradition upon early anatomic illustration. (By kind permission of Professor Karl Sudhoff, University of Leipzig.) E: Nervous system, from Persian MS. No. 2296, India Office, London. F: Schema of the nervous system, from a MS. of 1152, discovered by Sir Victor Horsley in the Bodleian Library, Oxford. G, Nervous system, from a fourteenth century MS. in the library of Prince von Lobkowicz (Raudnitz, Bohemia). H: Arterial system of a pregnant woman, from Persian MS. No. 2296, India Office, London. I: Gravida, from a miniature painted about 1400 A. D. in Leipzig MS. Codex No. 1122. Compare G with the two-centuries older F, and note the monotonous similarity in all these frog-like figures.

of the zodiac; the "sick-man" (*Krankheitsmann*), ringed about with names of diseases and vague indications· as to their location in the body; the "wound-man" (*Wundenmann*), whose body is mauled and pierced all over by stones, arrows, swords and spears, the points of incision or lesion showing where the arteries are to be sought for in ligation; and the crouching pregnant woman (*Gravida*), giving a crude, diagrammatic view of the fetus in utero. These strange didactic pictures have all been interpreted by Sudhoff as sidelights on the almost stationary character of the medieval mind, standing out as rude indices of its workings in relation to the three great branches of internal medicine, surgery, and obstetrics.[1] They have all been located by him in manuscripts of earlier centuries, for instance, the bloodletting man of 1432 in the Munich library, or the figures in a thirteenth-century Provençal manuscript at Basel. It was customary for the medieval illustrators to make a series of five schematic pictures (*Fünfbilderserie*), representing the osseous, nervous, muscular, venous, and arterial systems, to which the pregnant woman or a view of the generative organs of either sex was sometimes added, and this series has been found by Sudhoff in many German manuscripts, and even in Persian MS. in the India office at London and the Bodleian Library at Oxford. In Ketham's Gravida of 1491, the parts of the body are labeled for the first time, and this is also true of Richard Helain's skeleton of 1493, a good example of the fugitive anatomic plates which used to be exhibited in the German barber-shops and bath-houses of the period. This skeleton was copied by Grüninger in 1497 and by Johann Schott in 1517. The cuts in Peyligk and Hundt look, in some of their details, like a child's scratching on a slate, and, in the former, they have been traced by Sudhoff to a series of 18 manuscript figures in the Royal Library at Berlin and Erfurt, which were used by Henri de Mondeville to illustrate his anatomic lectures at Montpellier about 1304. Phryesen has a much better executed engraving of the viscera, which is, however, strikingly like the cruder picture in Reisch's Margarita philosophica (1504). Peter of Abano's Conciliator of 1496 contains the first example of the "*Muskelmann*," i. e., a full-length figure exhibiting its dissected muscles. In the works of Berengario da Carpi, this figure is represented as holding up the separate muscles for inspection, and the same *motif* becomes the *écorché* or flayed figure in Vesalius. Berengario has a tolerable skeleton, which is suspiciously like those of Helain, Grüninger, and Schott, and his picture of the pregnant woman in a reclining attitude is

---

[1] Sudhoff: Arch. f. Gesch. d. Med., Leipzig, 1907–8, i, 351; 1908–9, ii, 84.

afterward the theme of many variations by Stephanus and others. These tentative efforts at representation, rare and curious as they are, pale almost into obscurity beside the cartoons, écorchés, and chalk drawings of the great artists of the period—Luca Signorelli, Michael Angelo, Raphael, Verocchio, and his pupil, **Leonardo da Vinci** (1452–1519). Of chief interest are the reproductions of Leonardo's red-chalk drawings from the Ambrosian Library at Milan and the Royal Library at Windsor.[1] Startlingly modern in their accuracy and display of physiologic knowledge, these impromptu sketches, made beside the dissected subject, reveal such acquaintance with muscular anatomy as was possible only to the Greek sculptors, and fully justify William Hunter's claim that their author was "the greatest anatomist of his epoch." Leonardo taught painters and sculptors that a scientific knowledge of artistic anatomy— something quite different from the Greek sculptor's instinctive knowledge of the nude figure in action and repose—can be gained only at the dissecting table. He made over 750 separate sketches, including not only delineations of muscles, but drawings of the heart, the lungs, the cervical, thoracic, abdominal and femoral blood-vessels, the bones and nerves, with deep dissections of the viscera and cross-sections of the brain in different planes. Sometimes his notations of the origin and insertion of the muscles are too minute, because, having no accurate nomenclature to guide him, he had to rely upon his own deductions from what he saw, which was, in any case, a great advance upon servile Galenism. The marginal notes, which Leonardo has recorded in mirror-writing, lest others appropriate his ideas on the physiology of locomotion, reveal the cautious, secretive spirit of the time.

Among the anatomic works of the pre-Vesalian period we should, of course, include Albrecht Dürer's treatise on human proportions (*De simmetria*, Nuremberg, 1532), which was the first application of anthropometry to esthetics, and is technically interesting because it contains the first attempts to represent shades and shadows in wood-engraving by means of cross-hatching.

Thoroughly as the great artists of the Renaissance may have studied external anatomy, yet dissecting for teaching purposes was still hampered by the theologic idea of the sanctity of the human body and its resurrection. Moreover, as very little anatomic material could be obtained among a sparse and slowly growing population, people were naturally averse to the possible dissection of friends or relatives. The anatomy of the schools was still the anatomy of Galen. How far such teaching had progressed may be gathered from the quaint cut on the

---

[1] I manoscritti di Leonardo da Vinci, fol. Paris, 1898.

title-page of the Mellerstadt Mundinus (1493), in which the scholastic instructor, in long robe and biretta, wand in hand, gravely expounds Galen by the book from his pulpit-chair, while below the long-haired barber-servant[1] makes a desperate shift at demonstrating the viscera of the subject before him. The Faust who was to release the subject from these trammels and uphold the doctrine of the *visum et repertum* was Andreas **Vesalius**[2] (1514–64), the most commanding figure in European medicine after Galen and before Harvey. There were plenty of dissectors and dissections before Vesalius, but he alone made anatomy what it is today—a living, working science. It was the effect of his strong and engaging personality that made dissecting not only viable, but respectable. His career is one of the most romantic in the history of medicine. Flemish born, but of German extraction, a pupil of the ardent and bigoted Galenist, Jacobus Sylvius, Vesalius, in his graduating thesis, showed at first the conventional tendencies of the scholiast; but his mind was too active, his spirit too keen and independent, to feed long on the dust of ages, and he soon established a reputation for

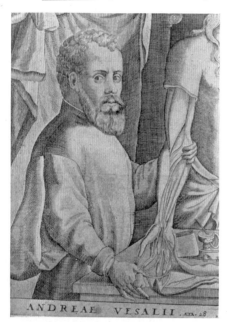

Andreas Vesalius (1514–64).

first-hand knowledge of the dissected human body, even teaching himself the difficult art, so essential to surgeon and gynecologist, of recognizing the palpable structures by an educated sense of touch. Five years' experience as public prosecutor at Padua, where he made students dissect and inspect the parts *in situ*, culminated in the magnificent *De Fabrica Humani Corporis* (1543), a work which marks an epoch in breaking with the past and throwing overboard Galenical tradition. The effect of a publi-

---

[1] It is possible that this may represent Alessandra Giliani, a talented girl of Persiceto, who assisted Mundinus in dissecting.

[2] Vesalius' family name was "Wesel," and Foster thinks his mother (born Isabel Crabbe) may have been an Englishwoman.

cation so radical on a superstitious and forelock-pulling age was immediate and self-evident.   Sylvius, his old teacher, turned against his brilliant pupil with acrimony and coarse abuse, while his own pupil, Columbus, a man of questionable honesty, sought to cast discredit and derision on him by sharp practice. Others were inclined to "damn with faint praise," or joined in a conspiracy of silence, and, as a last straw, he was subjected to subterranean persecution at the instance of authority.   Those things were not without their effect on Vesalius.   His portrait suggests a doughty, swarthy, shaggy, full-blooded nature, like some of Lucas Cranach's worthies—a man ready to give no odds and take none, so long as his opponents confronted him in the open; but nowise intended for the spiritual rôle of a martyr. In a fit of indignation he burned his manuscripts, left Padua, and accepted the lucrative post of court physician to Emperor Charles V.   He married, settled down, became a courtier, and gave up anatomy so completely that, during the long, tedious years in Madrid, "he could not get hold of so much as a dried skull, let alone the chance of making a dissection."   He paid the penalty of "the great refusal" when his favorite pupil, Gabriele Falloppio, came to the front as a worthy successor, and rumor began to make it clear that he himself was fast becoming the shadow of a great name—

> Vesalius, who's Vesalius?   This Fallopius
> It is who dragged the Galen-idol down.

On receiving the Fallopian "Observationes Anatomicæ" in 1561, all the aspirations of his youth revived, if we may trust his own burning, enthusiastic words, language which fully justifies the implications of Edith Wharton's poem:

> At least
> I repossess my past, am once again
> No courtier med'cining the whims of kings
> In muffled palace-chambers, but the free
> Friendless Vesalius, with his back against the wall,
> And all the world against him.

In the year 1563 Vesalius set out on a pilgrimage to Jerusalem, as a penance, some say, for an accidental human vivisection; more probably, the botanist Clusius thought, as a pretext for getting away from his tiresome surroundings.   On his way back, in 1564, he received word of an invitation to resume his old chair at Padua, just vacated by the death of Fallopius.   But his highest wish, to "once more be able to study that true Bible, as we count it, of the human body and of the nature of man," was not to be realized. The sudden access of an obscure malady left Vesalius to die, solitary and unfriended, on the island of Zante.

The principal works of Vesalius include six anatomic plates ("Tabulæ anatomicæ sex"), printed at Venice in 1538, and reprinted in facsimile by Sir William Sterling Maxwell in 1874; the "Epitome" (Basel, 1540), a specimen abstract of the "Fabrica," remarkable for the plates representing two handsome specimens of the human race, usually ascribed to Titian;[1] the epistle on the China root (1546), which contains much acute criticism of Galen, and is especially valuable for the light it throws upon the life of Vesalius; finally the "Fabrica" itself, published in June, 1543, a superb example of the beautiful typography of his friend Oporinus (Herbst) of Basel, sumptuously illustrated by Titian's pupil, Johan von Calcar. The splendid wood-cuts, representing majestic skeletons and flayed figures, dwarfing a background of landscape, set the fashion for over a century, and were copied or imitated by a long line of anatomic illustrators, such as Walther Ryff, Geminus, Tortebat, Valverde di Hamusco, Dulaurens, Casserius, and Bidloo.

While written in Latin, the "Fabrica" is truly vernacular in the sweeping scorn and violence of its language in dealing with Galenical and other superstitions. Although it completely disposes of Galen's osteology for all time, and, indeed, recreates the whole gross anatomy of the human body, it has never been translated. It closes with a chapter on vivisection in which Vesalius verifies Galen's experimental sections of the spinal cord and recurrent laryngeal nerve, proves the general functions of muscle and nerve by section, shows that artificial respiration will keep an animal alive after its chest has been opened, and that a quiescent heart may be resuscitated by the use of the bellows. In his chapter on the brain, he appears, in theory, at least, as a pioneer of experimental and comparative psychology, rejecting the current view that the cerebral action of brutes differs from that of man. He was also a pioneer in ethnic craniology, noting the globular shape of the skull in the Genoese, the Greeks, and the Turks, the flattened occiput and broad head (brachycephaly) in the "Germans" of his time, and the oblong skull of the Belgians. As a clinician, he was the first to diagnose and describe aneurysm of the abdominal and thoracic aorta (1555).[2] However scornful and truculent in his general onslaught against superstition, Vesalius displays the airy skepticism of a man of the world in dealing with these teleologic points so dear to medieval theologians. For instance, touching the Galenical crux that the blood passes through certain, hypothetic pores in the ventricular septum, he says, "We are driven to wonder at the handiwork of the Almighty, by means of which the blood sweats from the right into the left ventricle through passages which escape the human vision."

What fate might have befallen him had he gone further is seen in the case of the heretic Miguel Servede or **Servetus** (1509–53), whom Calvin caused to be burned at the stake for a mere juggling

---

[1] Titian's portrait of Vesalius is in the Pitti Palace at Florence.

[2] See G. H. Velschius, Sylloge, Augsburg, 1667, pt. 4 (Rumler), pp. 46, 47, and Roth's Vesalius, p. 239.

of verbiage, a theological quibble. Servetus was one of the world's martyrs for "the crime of honest thought." The principal discoverer of the truth about the pulmonary circulation, he ranks with Ramon y Cajal as a leader of Spanish medicine. The discovery is recorded in his book, the "Restitutio Christianismi" (1553), of which only the copies at Paris and Vienna are known to exist, the others having been burned with him. The rare Nuremberg reprint was published in 1790.

The surpassing ability of Vesalius is seen not only in his thorough descriptions of such parts as the eye, the ear, the accessory sinuses of the nose, the pituitary body,[1] or the pelvic cavity, but in his clean sweep of the whole subject. His ideas were sustained by his pupil Fallopius, and opposed not only by Sylvius and Columbus, but by an anatomist of equal rank with himself, Bartolommeo Eustachi (1524–74), called **Eustachius**. The latter was professor at the Collegia della Sapienza in Rome, where, in 1552, he completed his "Tabulæ anatomicæ," a set of superb plates, drawn by himself, which remained unprinted in the Papal Library for one hundred and sixty-two years. Finally Pope Clement XI

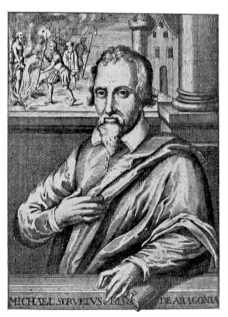

Michael Servetus (1509–53).

presented the engraved plates to his physician, Lancisi, who, by the advice of Morgagni, published them with his own notes in 1714, these being the first anatomic plates on copper. Eustachius discovered the Eustachian tube, the thoracic duct, the suprarenal bodies, and the abducens nerve; described the origin of the optic nerves, the cochlea, the pulmonary veins, the muscles of the throat and neck, gave the first correct picture of the uterus, and wrote an important little treatise on the structure of the teeth (Libellus de dentibus). Although Eustachius professed to

---

[1] Vesalius called it the "glans pituitam excipiens," and thought it secreted the mucous discharges of the nose. (Fabrica, lib. vii, cap. xi.)

follow Galen, he was a natural genius in discovery.   Jacques
Dubois (1478–1555), called **Sylvius,** Vesalius' teacher at Paris,
was, in spite of his large following of pupils, a harsh, avaricious
bigot, whose devotion to Galen was such that he declared
Vesalius to be a madman (*vesanus*), and said, in reference
to Galen's errors in human anatomy, that "Man had changed
but not for the better." Sylvius named the jugular, subclavian,
renal, popliteal, and other blood-vessels, gave equally character-

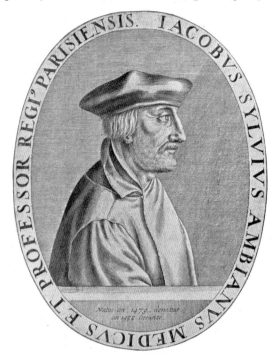

Jacques Dubois (Sylvius) (1478–1555).

istic names to many of the muscles, which we still retain today,
and, in his "Isagoge" (Venice, 1536), was one of the first to mention
the Sylvian aqueduct[1] and the valves in the veins.

The other opponent of Vesalius, Matteo Realdo Colombo
(1516?–1559), called **Columbus,** is sometimes spoken of as the
discoverer of the pulmonary circulation, but the work in which

---

[1] As Dr. Frank Baker has pointed out, the aqueduct between the third and
fourth ventricles of the brain, attributed by various writers indifferently to
Jacobus and Franciscus Sylvius, was described and figured by other anatomists
long before the time of either.   Johns Hopkins Hosp. Bull., Baltimore, 1909,
vol. xx, 329–339.

his undoubtedly excellent account is contained, his "De re anatomica," was published in 1559, at least six years after the burning of Servetus and his book, and there is some internal evidence indicating that Columbus may have plagiarized his facts from Servetus, as he certainly did in the case of Vesalius and Ingrassias (discovery of the stapes in the ear). Columbus begins his work with a title-page engraving, imitated from the frontispiece of the Fabrica, and, like Vesalius, winds up with a chapter on vivisection.[1] In prosecuting the latter, he had the cleverness to substitute dogs for hogs, but while he professed a horror for human vivisections, he seems correspondingly callous in reference to the sufferings of the canine creatures which, as he constantly reminds us, he cut up in such numbers for the amusement of this or that exalted personage.

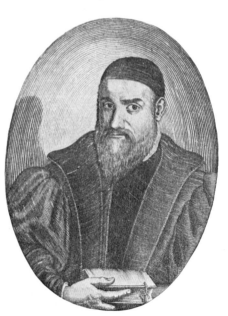

Gabriele Falloppio (1523–62), or **Fallopius,** a loyal pupil of Vesalius, discovered and described the chorda tympani, the semi-circular canals, the sphenoid sinus, the ovaries (Fallopian tubes), the round ligaments, the trigeminal, auditory, and glossopharyngeal nerves, and named the vagina and placenta. He

Gabriele Falloppio (1523–62).

was also a versatile writer on surgery, syphilis, mineral waters, and other subjects. The names of the anatomists Costanzo Varolio (1543–75), or **Varolius,** physician to Pope Gregory XIII, Giulio Cesare Aranzio (1530–89), professor at Bologna, and Guido Guidi (died 1569), called **Vidius,** the organizer of the medical faculty of the Collége de France, have been eponymically preserved in the structures they discovered. Varolius, in particular, made some capital investigations of the nervous system, describing the crura cerebri, the commissure, and the pons.

---

[1] For a very excellent translation of this work see Dr. L. C. Boislinière's paper on Columbus in St. Louis Med. Rev., October 20, 1906.

Apart from the striking woodcuts in Vesalius, France and
Spain furnished two excellent examples of anatomic illustration
in the folios of Stephanus (Paris, 1545)[1] and Juan Valverde di
Hamusco (Rome, 1556).[2] Charles Estienne (–1564), or
Stephanus, a pupil of Sylvius at Paris, and a prominent publisher
of medical books during the Renaissance, was persecuted and
imprisoned for heresy and died in prison.   Estienne was the first
to mention the valves of the veins as "apophyses membranarum,"
and his treatise also contains the first description of syringomyelia[3]
(1545).

The anatomy of Thomas Vicary, published in 1577 and reprinted by Fur-
nivall for the Early English Text Society in 1888,[4] has been proved by the late
Dr. J. F. Payne to be a transcript of a fourteenth century manuscript based
upon the anatomy of Lanfranc, Guy, and Mondeville, and is, therefore, valueless as a representative of Renaissance ideas upon the subject.   The book has
a certain bibliographic interest of a romantic character, in that an edition,
published in 1548, was once seen or heard of by somebody, but has never since
been found.

The effect of Vesalius on **Renaissance surgery** is seen in the
life work of **Ambroïse Paré** (1510–90), who made the "Fabrica"
popular and accessible to surgeons by writing an epitome of it
in the vernacular.   A rustic barber's apprentice when he came
up from the provinces to Paris in 1529, and afterward a dresser
at the Hôtel Dieu, Paré became an army surgeon eight years
later, was incontinently thrown into the wars, where he soon
made himself the greatest surgeon of his time by his courage, ability, and common sense.   Snubbed by the College of St. Côme, and
ridiculed as an upstart because he wrote in his native tongue, he
made his way to the front on the field of battle.   Like Vesalius
and Paracelsus, he did not hesitate to thrust aside ignorance or
superstition if it stood in his way.   Yet this greatest of army
surgeons was so well beloved by his comrades that, one night, when
he slipped into Metz incognito, he was sought out and carried
through the city by them in triumph;   and Brantôme and Sully
record that he was the only Protestant to be spared (by royal
mandate) at St. Bartholomew.   In personality, Paré stands between his surgical peers, the rude, outspoken Hunter, and the

---

[1] Stephanus: De dissectione, Paris, 1545.   As some of the plates in this
work were signed as early as 1530–32, and are not unlike certain plates of
Vesalius, some have charged the latter with plagiarism, but this would
seem to be sufficiently disproved by the appearance of Vesalius' six Venetian
plates in 1538, seven years before Estienne's "De dissectione" was published
(1545).

[2] Juan de Valverde de Hamusco: Historia de la composicion del cuerpo
humano, Roma, 1556.

[3] Stephanus: De dissectione, 1545, iii, ch. 35.

[4] It is thought that there was an edition of Vicary published in 1548.
See Payne: Brit. Med. Jour., London, 1896, i, 200–203.

refined, self-possessed Lister, as a man equally at home in the rigors of camp life and the slippery footing of courts.

Paré's greatest contribution to surgery hinges on the baneful effect which the pseudo-Hippocratic aphorism that "diseases not curable by iron are curable by fire" exerted on the treatment of gunshot wounds, the new feature of Renaissance surgery. Giovanni di Vigo (1460–1520), physician to Pope Julius II, had taught in his "Practica" (1514), like Brunschwig before him, that such wounds were poisoned burns, and, therefore, should be treated with a first dressing of boiling oil. How Paré's supply of boiling oil gave out one night in camp and how he profited by the experience to the extent of letting well enough alone in future is a well-known

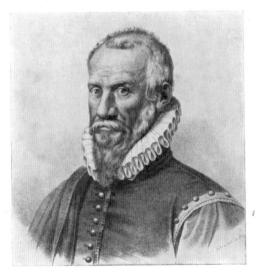

Ambroïse Paré (1510–90).

story. Had it not been for his "fat of puppy-dogs," a lard or salve, which, from some tenacity of superstition, he continued to apply, he would have been a true asepsist. As it is, his relation to the healing power of nature is summed up in the famous inscription on his statue, "Je le pansay, Dieu le guarit." Paré invented many new surgical instruments, made amputation what it is to-day by reintroducing the ligature, which had almost fallen into abeyance since the time of Celsus; was the first to popularize the use of the truss in hernia; did away with the strolling surgeons' trick of castrating the patient in herniotomy; introduced massage, artificial eyes (of gold and silver), and staphyloplasty, and made the first exarticulation of the elbow-joint (1536). He described fracture of the neck of the femur and strangury from hypertrophy of the prostate, and was the first to suggest syphilis as a cause of aneurysm. As Dr. Howard A. Kelly has pointed out,[1] he was probably also the first to see flies as transmitters of infectious disease. In obstetrics, it was his description and use of podalic version that made the procedure viable and practicable, and he had the courage to induce artificial labor in case of uterine hemorrhage. In dentistry, he introduced reimplantation of the teeth, and his little treatise on medical jurisprudence (1575) was the first work of consequence on the subject prior to the "Methodus testificandi" of Codronchi (1597).

Paré is a garrulous, gossipy, sometimes obscure writer, and, like other medical celebrities of his day, by no means free from the "vanity of self-reference which accompanies great and even small reputations."[2] His many references to Hippocrates and the ancients lead us to suppose that, like Bartisch, he employed a secretary or *pion* to embellish his writings for him, since it is most unlikely that he acquired his learning by actual study. His principal works are his treatise on gunshot wounds (1545),[3] his essay on podalic version (1550),[4] his great treatise on surgery (1564), and his discourse on the mummy and the unicorn (1582),[5] which successfully disposed of an ancient therapeutic superstition. A curious book is his treatise on monsters, terrestrial and marine (1573), embellished with pictures of many of the strange, hypothetic creatures which emanated from the brain of Aristotle.

The "Practica Copiosa" of Vigo (1514) had a success out of all proportion to its value, running through some 52 editions and innumerable translations, because it was almost the only book before Paré's time which dealt with the two great problems of Renaissance surgery, epidemic syphilis, and wounds from firearms. Paré's campaign for a soothing treatment of gunshot wounds was very ably seconded by Bartolommeo Maggi (1516–52) of Bologna, who, in 1551, demonstrated experimentally that such wounds could be neither burned nor poisoned. Another book which advanced this view was "An Excellent Treatise of Wounds made by Gonneshot" (London, 1563), by the English surgeon Thomas Gale (1507–86?). The anatomist, Giacomo Berengario da Carpi, was another pioneer in the simple treatment of gunshot wounds. As a gynecologist, he is said to have excised the uterus for prolapse

---

[1] Johns Hopkins Hosp. Bull., Baltimore, 1901, xii, 240–242.

[2] Rodomontades, as they were called, were the fashion of the period, and Brantôme wrote a whole book on the subject.

[3] Paré: La manière de traicter les playes (etc.), Paris, 1545.

[4] Briefve collection de l'administration anatomique (etc.), Paris, 1550.

[5] Discours, à savoir, de la mumie (etc.), Paris, 1582.

on two occasions. Two other Italian surgeons well deserving of mention are Mariano Santo di Barletta (1490–1550), a Neapolitan, who gave the original account of the "Marian operation" or median lithotomy (1535);[1] and Gasparo **Tagliacozzi** (1546–99), of Bologna, who in 1597[2] revived the operation of rhinoplasty, which had been, during the fifteenth century, in the hands of a Sicilian family of plastic surgeons, the Brancas of Catania. For this innovation, Tagliacozzi was roundly abused by both Paré and Fallopius, and satirized during the following century in Butler's "Hudibras," while the ecclesiastics of his own time, we are told, were fain to regard such operations as meddling with the handiwork of God. Tagliacozzi's remains were exhumed from the convent, where they reposed, to be buried in unconsecrated ground, and in 1788 the Paris Faculty interdicted face-repairing altogether. In this way, plastic surgery fell into disrepute and disuse until the time of Dieffenbach. Like the Brancas, were such itinerants as the Norsini, who were skilful in hernia and lithotomy, and the Colots, who cut for stone only. Out of this class was evolved the great Provençal surgeon, **Pierre Franco** (1553–   ), a Huguenot driven by the Waldensian massacres into Switzerland, who did even more than Paré to put the operations for hernia, stone, and cataract upon a definite and dignified basis,[3] and was the first to perform suprapubic cystotomy (1556). Felix **Würtz** (1518–75) was a follower of Paracelsus in the simple treatment of wounds, and a vigorous opponent of the common custom of thrusting "clouts and rags, balsam, oil, or salve" into them. His "Surgical Practice" (*Practica der Wundartzney*) (Basel, 1563) was, like the *Traité des hernies* of Franco (Lyons, 1561), written in the vernacular, and is the fresh, straightforward work of a genuine child of nature. William **Clowes** (1540–1604) was probably the greatest of the English surgeons during the reign of Elizabeth. Experienced both in military and in naval medicine, he became consulting surgeon at St. Bartholomew's Hospital in 1581, served as fleet surgeon against the Armada in 1588, and was afterward made physician to the Queen. His works include a treatise on gunshot wounds (London, 1591),[4] and are pronounced by Dr. Norman Moore to be "the very best surgical writings of the Elizabethan age." As a satirist of the seamy side of medicine in his day, Clowes compares with Gideon Harvey and Butler in

---

[1] Marianus Sanctus Barolitanus: De lapide renum, Venice, 1535.

[2] Tagliacozzi: De curtorum chirurgia per insitionem, Venice, 1597.

[3] Pierre Franco: Petit traité (Lyons, 1556) and Traité des hernies, Lyons, 1561.

[4] "A prooved practise for all young chirurgians concerning burnings with gunpowder and wounds made with gunshot (etc.), London, 1591.

the seventeenth century or Smollett in the eighteenth. The Scotch army surgeon, Peter Lowe, founded the Faculty of Physicians and Surgeons of Glasgow (1599), and made the first English translation of Hippocrates (1597). His "Whole Course of Chirurgerie" (1597) passed through four editions, and contains the first reference in English to ligation of the arteries in amputation. There were a number of Spanish surgeons in the sixteenth century, such as Francisco Arceo (1493–1571), who followed Vigo in the treatment of wounds, or Dionisio Daça Chacon (1510–   ), who opposed him, but their works are only of bibliographic interest.

In the year 1500, Jacob Nufer, a sow-gelder, performed a successful Cesarean section upon his own wife,—she lived to be seventy-seven and bore other children,—and this start in operative **gynecology** was succeeded by other Cesarean operations—those of Bain (1540), Dirlewang (1549), and so on, until we find François **Rousset** enumerating as many as 15 successful cases in his "L'Hysterotomotokie" (1580). Another sow-gelder performed double ovariotomy upon his own daughter, according to Johann Weyer (1515–88), the great Dutch opponent of the persecution of witches, who was himself an able physician and a surgeon enterprising enough to treat amenorrhea from imperforate hymen by incision of the membrane. The growth of interest in diseases of women during the Renaissance period is seen in the huge "Gynæciorum," or encyclopedia of gynecology, issued by Caspar Wolff (1532–1601), of Zürich, in 1566, which was later enlarged by Caspar Bauhin (1550–1624), of Basel, in 1586. These two compilations of the best that had been written upon the subject were afterward reprinted in one volume by Israel Spach, of Strasburg, in 1597. Encyclopedic treatises on medicine by many authors, not unlike the "up-to-date" works written on the coöperative plan in our own time, were a special feature of Renaissance medicine, and of these we may mention, in addition to the Basel encyclopedias of gynecology, the Aldine "Medici Antiqui Omnes" (1547), the "Medicæ Artis Principes" of Stephanus (1567), the Venetian anthology of mineral waters, "De Balneis" (1553), the Gesner collection of surgical treatises (Zürich, 1555),[1] and the medical dictionaries of Lorenz Phryesen (1519), Henri Estienne, or Stephanus (1564) and Jean de Gorris or Gorræus (1564).

The eager, inquiring spirit of Renaissance humanity, greedy as a growing child for new knowledge, is sensed in the immense popularity of such a work as the *Hortus Sanitatis* (1491), with its quaint, colored wood-cuts of real or fanciful animals and plants. This picture book was so much sought after, in fact, that it was

---

[1] De chirurgia scriptores optimi quique veteres et recentiores, 1555.

soon followed by a number of genuinely scientific treatises on botany and by extensive "Bestiaries," or animal-books, which described and figured the actual and mythologic creatures which did or did not exist from the times of Aristotle and Pliny down. Of the latter, we may mention Ambroïse Paré's illustrated treatise on monsters (1573), the "Historia animalium" (Zürich, 1551–87) of the Swiss naturalist Conrad Gesner (1516–65), called the German Pliny, and the many publications of Ulisse Aldrovandi (1522–1605) of Bologna. These rude beginnings of zoölogic science, as Allbutt says, "mostly after Pliny's kind," were far inferior to the works of the **German Fathers of Botany.** The earliest of these, Otho **Brunfels** (1464–1534), of Mainz, originally a Carthusian novice, went over to Luther, graduated in medicine at Basel at the age of sixty-five, and was appointed city physician at Berne in 1533. His "Herbarum Vivæ Icones" (Strassburg, 1530), which marks an epoch in the history of botanic illustration, consists of 135 careful figurations of plants executed by Hans Weydiz, the best wood-engraver of Strassburg in his day. Brunfels prepared the work at his own expense, to offset the wretched engravings of the Hortus Sanitatis. In his text, he makes no attempt at original plant description, but simply follows Theophrastus, Dioscorides, Pliny, and the other authorities up to his time. Next in order came the Bavarian physician, Leonhard **Fuchs** (1501–66), who graduated at Ingolstadt in 1524, and after many vicissitudes (he was also an adherent of Luther), held the chair of medicine at Tübingen for thirty-one years (1535–66), where he occupied his leisure in having artists figure plants which he afterward described. His "De Historia Stirpium" (Basel, 1542), containing over 500 plates, superior to those in Brunfels' book, which had inspired it, created such an interest that it was followed, in 1544, by a new edition, and, after 1545, by many small-sized popular reprints. In purpose, it was entirely utilitarian, the work of a busy practitioner who wished to improve the actual knowledge of the materia medica over and above advancing the science of botany. Plant description, or phytography, took its first fresh start since the days of Theophrastus in the work of Hieronymus **Bock** (1498–1554), called **Tragus**, a poor schoolmaster and gardener, born near Heidelberg, who paid the usual penalties of sympathizing with Luther, and finally died as pastor of a little Protestant church at Hornbach. Tragus loved plants for themselves, and in his "New Kreutterbuch" (1539), and in the "Kreutterbuch" of 1546, wrote down his fresh first-hand descriptions of what he saw in his native tongue. A far greater than Tragus was **Valerius Cordus** (1515–44), the gifted Prussian youth, whose early death robbed science of one of its most promis-

11

ing names. As the son of the physician-botanist, Euricius Cordus, he is known to medicine for his discovery of sulphuric ether (*oleum dulce vitrioli*) in 1540; but botanists revere him as the young Marcellus of their science. Greene styles him "the inventor of phytography," and points out that the field-work and taxonomy of a well-equipped modern botanist were actually done "almost four centuries ago by a German boy in his teens." His posthumous commentary on Dioscorides, edited with pious hand by Conrad Gesner (Strassburg, 1561), not only describes some 500 new species of plants, the ardent search for which eventually cost him his life, but recreates the species listed by Dioscorides in terms of modern botany. The "Dispensatorium" of Cordus (Nuremberg, 1535) is of interest as the first real pharmacopeia to be published.[1]

A remarkable Renaissance figure was Conrad **Gesner** (1516–65), of Zürich, whom Cuvier called "the German Pliny," on account of his equal attainment in botany, zoölogy, bibliography, and general erudition. The son of a poor furrier, and in great want in his early days, he graduated in medicine at Basel in 1541, and after a roving life as a practitioner in many European cities, he was at length appointed professor of natural history at Zürich in 1555, was ennobled in 1564, and sacrificed his life to the plague in the following year. In spite of his struggles with poverty, sickness, and defective eyesight, he was a man of extraordinary industry. His "Bibliotheca universalis," of which 20 volumes were published (1545–49), was the first example of good bibliography before Haller's time, and is, in intention, a catalogue, in Latin, Greek, and Hebrew, of all the writers who have ever lived. The medical part was unfortunately never completed. Gesner's "Historia Plantarum" (Paris, 1541) is a student's handbook of botany, giving the genera in alphabetic order—a sort of pocket dictionary of plants. He edited and published the works of Valerius Cordus in 1561. His "Historia Animalium," published in four folio volumes in 1551–58, with the fifth volume on snakes in 1587, was subsequently translated into German as the "Thierbuch," and became one of the starting-points of modern zoölogy. It contains some 4500 folio pages, comprising a digest of about 250 authors, and illustrated with nearly a thousand wood-cuts, of which Gesner selected some of the best of the period, including Albert Dürer's rhinoceros. Gesner made some curious essays in other directions, such as his "Mithridates," an account of 130 different languages, with the Lord's Prayer translated into 22 of them; and he is known to Alpine enthusiasts through his epistles on mountain climbing and his description of Mount Pilatus (1555). He was also the first to describe the canary-bird.

Caspar **Bauhin** (1550–1624) was professor of anatomy, botany, medicine and Greek at Basel, and afterward city physician and rector of the university. His greatest work is the celebrated "Pinax" (1596), a wonderful index or compend of all the botanic literature up to his time, which, it is said, has been more studied and commented upon by botanists than any other work except that of Dioscorides. Bauhin also wrote a "Theatrum Botanicum" which he left incomplete (1658), and a catalogue of the plants around Basel. His "Theatrum Anatomicum" (1592) is a valuable historic summary. It contains an inter-

---

[1] In this account of the German Fathers of Botany I am much indebted to the "Landmarks of Botanical History," by Dr. Edward Lee Greene (Smithsonian Misc. Collect., v., 54, Washington, 1909, pp. 169–314). Charming in style and irreproachable in scholarship, this work is cordially recommended to physicians as the most interesting history of early botany and materia medica that has yet appeared.

esting account of the ancient Hebrew myth of the bone "Luz," in which the latter term appears for the first time outside the Rabbinical writings.

Pierre **Belon** (1517–64), or Belonius, the author of a valued treatise on coniferous plants (1553), published, in 1555, a monograph on birds, in which he compared the skeletons of birds and man in the same posture and "nearly as possible bone for bone." This was the first of those serial arrangements of homologies which Owen and Haeckel afterward made famous. In 1546–9 Belon traveled in Egypt, Greece, and the Orient, carefully studying the ancient and modern materia medica.

Besides the German Fathers of Botany, all of whom were medical men, we should mention a number of other prominent physician-botanists of the Renaissance period who did much to make the science what it is today. Of these, Jean de la Ruelle (1474–1537), or **Ruellius**, was physician to Francis I, but later became a canon and died in the cloister. Ruellius was an able botanist, who had the courage to accept all of Leonicenus' corrections of Pliny, made the first Latin translation of Dioscorides, with a good commentary, and in his "De Natura Stirpium" (Paris, 1536) was the first to give a full description of each plant, adding many new species and giving to each the popular French names, which he got by questioning the peasants and mountaineers on his excursions. Antonio Musa **Brassavola** (1500–55), of Ferrara, a pupil of Leonicenus, described over 200 different kinds of syphilis, is said to have performed tracheotomy, and wrote a witty imaginary conversation entitled, "An Examination of Medicinal Simples" (Examen omnium simplicium, Rome, 1536), in which new drugs, like Helleborus niger and guaiac, are permanently introduced into the pharmacopœia. This genial idea, so characteristic of the Renaissance, of casting a botanical treatise into the form of a dialogue, had already been utilized by Euricius Cordus (1486–1535), the father of Valerius, in his "Botanologicon" (Cologne, 1534), in which he severely arraigns the German druggists of his time for falsely labeling their jars and receptacles with old Greek names which did not apply. Pietro Andrea **Mattioli** (1501–77), of Siena, called the Brunfels of Italy, wrote a vernacular commentary on Dioscorides (Venice, 1544)—now exceedingly rare—in which, like Brunfels, he illustrated the plants, following Ruellius, in giving a full description of each and adding between 200 and 300 new species from southern Europe.

Andrea **Cesalpino** (1524–1603), professor of medicine at Pisa, and physician to Pope Clement VIII, is regarded by the Italians as a discoverer of the circulation before Harvey (1571–93), and has been honored by them with statues and a medical journal bearing his name. Cesalpinus had indeed grasped, as pure theory, the truth about the systemic and pulmonary circulations, viz., that the heart, in systole, sends blood into the aorta and pulmonary artery, and, in diastole, receives it back from the vena cava and pulmonary vein. But his ideas were not supported by any convincing experiments and were thrown out in a purely controversial spirit, as an additional argument against Galenism. They therefore had no influence upon his contemporaries and are to be entirely dissociated from Harvey's experimental demonstration, as bald theory from actual proof. Cesalpinus was an ardent theologian, and his Pantheism got him into trouble with the Church. He was also an able naturalist, taught botany as well as medicine at Pisa, and was in charge of the Botanic Garden which had been founded there in 1543. Cesalpinus was called by Linnæus the first true systematist (*primus verus systematicus*) in botany. He collected plants from all over Europe, was the first to classify them by their fruits, ranging some 1520 plants into fifteen classes by this plan; and his great work "De Plantis" (Florence, 1583) led to the distinction between systematic and applied (economic) botany.

Giovanni Battista **della Porta** (1536–1615), of Naples, who invented the camera obscura (1588), described the opera glass (1590) and was indeed one of the principal founders of optics, was also an opponent of witchcraft, and, in his "De Humana Physiognomia" (Sorrento, 1586), a forerunner of Lavater in estimating human character by the features. In botany, Porta was the first ecologist, grouping plants, in his "Phytognomonica" (1583), according to their geographic locale and distribution. He went in for magic, and the Accademia de' segrete, which he founded for this purpose in 1560, was suppressed by Pope Paul III.

Pierre Belon (1517–1564), or Bellonius, wrote an important little book on coniferous or resiniferous trees (1553)[1] and the "Semplici" (Venice, 1561) of Luigi Anguillara is a botanical classic. The earliest English contributions to botany were the "Herbals" of Richard Banckes (1525), Peter Treveris (1529), Thomas Petyt (1541), William Middleton (1546), William Turner, called the Father of English Botany (1551), and of the barber-surgeon, John Gerard (1597).[2] The medicinal plants of the New World were described by Oviedo y Valdez, viceroy of Mexico (1525), and by Nicholas Monardes of Seville (1565).

The medical men we have just mentioned are, all of them, examples of the restless Renaissance spirit and, in cast of mind, they were akin to the great pathbreakers of the period, Vesalius, Paracelsus, and Paré. There is yet another group of physicians, each remarkable for achievement along isolated and original lines. Of these, Pierre **Brissot** (1478–1522) stands out as a reformer in the practice of bloodletting. Up to the time of Brissot, physicians had accepted the Arabist teaching that bleeding should be "derivative," that is, on the opposite side from the lesion. In 1514, Brissot, a professor of the Paris Faculty, deeply read in Greek medicine, made a stand for the original Hippocratic method of "revulsive" bloodletting, that is, free venesection on the same side as and near to the lesion, which he believed to be the most effective for the removal of peccant humors. This heresy engendered a storm which resulted in the banishment of Brissot by act of Parliament and a pronouncement of Charles V to the effect that such doctrine was as flagitious as Lutheranism. Clement VII and Vesalius were dragged into the controversy, which was brought to a sudden close by the fact that one of Charles V's relatives died

---

[1] Belon: De arboribus coniferis, Paris, 1553.

[2] Cited by H. M. Barlow: Proc. Roy. Soc. Med., Sect. Hist. Med., London, 1913, 108–149.

11

from venesection by the Arabist method in an attack of pleurisy, and the smug opponents of Hippocrates and Brissot were made ridiculous forever, although blood was still let in quantity until the time of Louis.   Another early disciple of the Father of Medicine was the distinguished Florentine, Antonio **Benivieni** (– 1502), who was an able surgeon and a remarkable pioneer in reporting postmortem sections.   In his posthumous "De Abditis Causis Morborum," published by the house of Giunta in 1507, he appears as a founder of pathology before Morgagni.   "Before

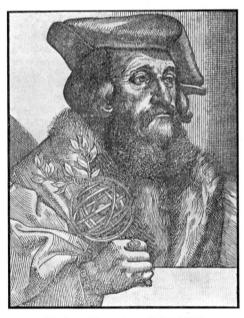

Girolamo Fracastoro (1484–1553).

Vesalius, before Eustachius," says Allbutt, "he opened the bodies of the dead as deliberately and clearsightedly as any pathologist in the spacious times of Baillie, Bright, and Addison," and Malgaigne has described his book as "the only work on pathology which owes nothing to any one."   But with all deference to authority so high, it may be doubted if so slender a performance as Benivieni's (it consists of only 54 pages) can enter into comparison with the vast array of pathologic findings and descriptions of new diseases in Morgagni's majestic treatise.   For such pioneer work as Benivieni's, the time was hardly ripe, and the same thing is true of the theoretic speculations of that most original genius,

Fracastorius. Girolamo Fracastoro (1484–1553), a Veronese of thick-set, hirsute appearance and jovial mien, who practised in the Lago di Gardo region, was at once a physician, poet, physicist, geologist, astronomer, and pathologist, and shares with Leonardo da Vinci the honor of being the first geologist to see fossil remains in the true light (1530). He was also the first scientist to refer to the magnetic poles of the earth (1543). His medical fame rests on that most celebrated of medical poems, *Syphilis sive Morbus Gallicus* (Venice, 1530), which sums up the contemporary dietetic and therapeutic knowledge of the time, recognizes a venereal cause, and gave the disease its present name; and his treatise, "De Contagione" (1546), in which he states, with wonderful clairvoyance, the modern theory of infection by microörganisms (*seminaria contagionum*).[1]

Our account of Renaissance medicine may close with the works of two original characters who were not physicians. The Venetian Luigi **Cornaro** (1467–1566), whose *Trattato della vita sobria* (Padua, 1558) is probably the best treatise on personal hygiene and the "simple life" in existence; and "The Metamorphosis of Ajax" (1596) of Sir John **Harington** (1561–1612), the witty, graceless godson of Queen Elizabeth, who was banished from her court for writing it. The work introduces an important and indispensable improvement in sanitary engineering, but our author's treatment of his theme is entirely in the manner of Aristophanes, Rabelais, or the Zahdärm epitaph in "Sartor Resartus," and the garrulous, whimsical old knight possibly got his invention from Oriental sources.

Carlo Ruini's treatise on the anatomy and diseases of the horse and their treatment (1598) is usually regarded as the foundation of modern veterinary medicine.

It is worth remembering that the first medical books to be printed in the new world, such as the "Opera Medicinalia" of Francesco Bravo (1570) or the "Summa y Recopilacion de Cirugia" of Alphonso Lopez de Hinojoso (1595), were printed in the city of Mexico.

---

[1] It is to be remembered, however, that Fracastorius nowhere refers to the latter as living organisms (*contagia animata*), but describes them (as if in terms of physical chemistry) as something very like our modern "colloidal systems," although he regards them as capable of reproduction in appropriate media. As between Fracastorius and Athanasius Kircher, the decision of priority in regard to the germ theory will depend upon whether the arbiter is a materialist or a vitalist. In the *De Contagione*, Fracastorius also gives the first authentic account of typhus fever (1546), the "tabardillo" of contemporary Spanish and Mexican writers.

CULTURAL AND SOCIAL ASPECTS OF RENAISSANCE MEDICINE

The invention of printing and the Revival of Learning, the discovery of America, and the extension of travel and commerce, the heliocentric astronomy of the physician Copernicus, the beginnings of modern physics and chemistry, the struggle between masses and classes which began with Magna Charta (1215), the reformation (1517) and the growth of vernacular literature, all combined to make the Renaissance a period of incessant intellectual ferment and activity. The Byzantine Greek scholars who poured into Italy after the destruction of Constantinople have been described as "sowers of dragon's teeth," and if we judge them by their effect upon the work of Paracelsus, Vesalius, and Paré, we must regard these Humanists as the true forerunners of modern medicine. The three great leaders of Renaissance medicine were all of them experimenters in the truest sense, but before the common medical mind could be penetrated with the advantages of experimentation over superstitious observances, it was necessary to clear the ground of the accumulated rubbish of the past, and this could be accomplished only by searching, critical study of the medical authorities of antiquity. In the different universities, the courses of **medical instruction** and the text-books used—Avicenna's Canon, Galen's Ars parva, the Aphorisms of Hippocrates—remained about the same, but new and important features were gradually introduced, and the sixteenth century university training had a distinctive character of its own. Bologna, Padua, and Pisa had the most popular medical faculties, and after them Paris, Montpellier, and Basel; but the wide-spread interest in general culture soon led to the foundation of new universities at Valencia (1501), Wittenberg (1502), Santiago (1504), Toledo (1518), Marburg (1527), Granada (1531), Königsberg (1544), Jena (1558), Donai (Lille) (1561), Helmstädt (1575), Leyden (1575), Altdorf (1580), Edinburgh (1582), and Dublin (1593). Each of these Renaissance universities was a little democracy in that the students themselves elected the rector, the professors, and the officers, and had a voice in determining the courses of study. As a rule, the members of the faculty were chosen for only one year, and had to be renominated and reëlected for a further tenure of office. This peculiar arrangement kept the students and professors in continual movement from one university to another; a professor would sometimes give a "Gastspiel" of lectures in order to secure a good position, and even city physicians wandered from place to place after fulfiling their contracts. In Goethe's Faust, Mephistopheles introduces himself for the first time as a "wandering student" (*fahrender Scholastikus*). Characters of this rolling-stone order were a feature of the time. Many of these itinerant scholars were genuine vagabonds, so poor that they had to eke out a livelihood by begging like tramps, singing at doors like Christmas waits, attending to odd jobs, or, their favorite expedient, stealing what they could lay their hands upon.   The fagging and hazing among the different bodies of students were coarse beyond conception, license was unbridled, and many of them went frankly to the devil. Others, in the face of extreme poverty, led lives of noble self-denial for the advancement of learning and science.   The absolute lack of medical periodicals and a slow and expensive postal service made it necessary for even the best to move from pillar to post in order to be in touch with new phases of thought.   The principal innovations in medical teaching were in the branches of anatomy and botany.   There were a few attempts at bedside lecturing, and even postmortem sections for the possible confirmation of diagnoses, but these were soon done away with by popular prejudice.   **Dissections,** however, became more frequent and were regarded, in each case, as a particular and expensive social function, for which a special papal indulgence was necessary.   The cadaver was first made "respectable" by the reading of an official decree, and was then stamped with the seal of the university. Having been taken into the anatomic hall, it was next beheaded in deference to the then universal prejudice against opening the cranial cavity.   The dissection was followed by such festivities as band music or even theatrical performances.   All this led in time to the building of so-called anatomic theaters, notably those at Padua (1549), Montpellier (1551), and Basel (1588).   In England the need for anatomic study led to the passing of the law of 1540 (32 Henry VIII, c. 42), authorizing the barbers and surgeons to use four bodies of executed criminals each year for "anathomyes," a provision which, however enlarged, remained substantially in force until the passing of the Anatomy Act of 1832.   The extreme scarcity of anatomic material everywhere made it a special ambition of each teacher or practitioner to have a skeleton of his own.   This, in due course, became the germinal idea of the splendid anatomic and pathologic museums of later times, from Ruysch to the Hunters and Dupuytren. Botanic teaching in the universities was forwarded by special outdoor excursions in the spring and autumn, to which the apothecaries were invited and which were always followed by banquets and jollifications.   Many universities had separate botanic gardens of their own, notably Padua (1545), Leyden (1577), Leipzig (1579), and Montpellier (1592), and these were again the originals of the great private collections and gardens of the eighteenth century. The salary of a University professor in the sixteenth century was a dependent variable and decidedly low in the northern countries.

In Germany it ranged anywhere from $40 to about four or five times as much. The Linacre foundations at Oxford and Cambridge provided for two professorships at $60 each per annum and one at $30; but Vesalius got $1000 at Pisa. Toward the seventeenth century these sums had a purchasing value equal to about eight times the amount in modern money.[1] The salaries of city physicians and the **fees** charged by physicians in private practice were proportionately low. City physicians in Germany got anywhere from $4.25 to $43, court physicians from $35 to $939. The physicians in ordinary of Henry VII, Henry VIII and Queen Elizabeth all received about $200 annually. In Germany, a simple uroscopy cost about three cents; single visits anywhere from 8 to 50 cents, according to the income of the patient; consultations, $2.50 for each physician, or $1.25 if by letter. The most lucrative phase of practice was in the treatment of syphilis, in which physicians easily made small fortunes, even down to the time of Casanova's Memoirs. Surgeons were fairly well paid, the fee for a fracture, for instance, being about $10.50. John of Arderne is said to have gotten 100 gold sols ($500) for his operation for fistula in ano. The apothecaries fared best of all, if we are to judge by a bill which was sent to Queen Elizabeth amounting to about $216 for one quarter.[2]

Medical practice during the Renaissance period was bound up with superstition, herb-doctoring, and quackery. In the illustrations of the period, the physician, whether in long robe or short fur-edged pelisse, is invariably represented as inspecting a urinal. He usually believed in astrology, and went in for the lore of amulets (*Passauer-Kunst*) and the *Lasstafelkunst*, or the determination of the proper time for purging and blood-letting by the conjunction of the planets. Even a court physician was often an "astronomer royal," that is, a deviser of fortune-tellers' almanacs. The followers of Paracelsus believed in the "doctrine of signatures," in virtue of which a drug is indicated by some fanciful associative resemblance to the disease, as trefoil for heart disease, thistle for a stitch in the side, walnut shells for head injuries, topaz and the yellow celandine for jaundice, and so forth. We may judge of the true greatness of men like Vesalius, Leonicenus, Linacre, Fracastorius, and Benivieni, when we reflect that they alone scorned to credit these things. In like manner only the sur-

---

[1] J. J. Walsh: "Physicians' Fees Down the Ages," Internat. Clinics, Philadelphia, 1910, 20 s., iv, p. 269.

[2] The great center of the London drug trade in the Elizabethan era was Bucklersbury, immortalized in Falstaff's reference to "these lisping hawthorn buds, that come like women in men's apparel, and smell like Bucklersbury in simple time" (Merry Wives of Windsor, Act III, sc. III.).

geons of first rank—Paré, Gersdorff, Franco, Wurtz, Tagliacozzi, Clowes, and Bartisch—were true surgeons.   The unclassed horde of wandering cataract couchers, lithotomists, herniotomists, and booth-surgeons generally were, in the words of William Clowes, "no better than runagates or vagabonds . . . shameless in countenance, lewd in disposition, brutish in judgment and understanding," so disreputable, in fact, that special laws had to be passed to make the status of competent surgeons reputable,— notably the edict of Charles V in 1548, which had to be renewed by Rudolph II in 1577.   The barber surgeon who shaved a criminal condemned to death or dressed the wounds of any one tortured on the rack was regarded as himself a felon.   Quackery was rampant everywhere, and in the vigorous language of the English surgeon just quoted, was practised by "tinkers, tooth-drawers, peddlers, ostlers, carters, porters, horse-gelders and horse-leeches, idiots, apple-squires, broom-men, bawds, witches, conjurers, sooth-sayers and sow-gelders, rogues, rat-catchers, runagates, and proctors of spittle-houses."   Another class of impostors were the tramps of the period, who, in spite of Henry VIII's statute against "sturdy and valiant beggars," tried to impose upon the charity of the hospitals, which in those days gave temporary shelter to all the poor.   Robert Copland (1508–47), the old English printer, who was also a poet, wrote an amusing versified dialogue between himself and the porter of St. Bartholomew's, called "The Hye Way to the Spyttel House," which throws considerable light on the poor-law and free dispensary problems of the sixteenth century.[1]

Perhaps the worst phase of Renaissance medical practice was that of **obstetrics.**   We know little of medieval obstetrics, but we may gauge the extent of its degradation by what happened in the Renaissance period.   In normal labor, a woman had an even chance, if she did not succumb to puerperal fever or eclampsia. In difficult labor she was usually butchered to death, if attended by a Sairey Gamp of the time or one of the vagabond "surgeons." As a rule, only midwives attended women in labor, and in 1580 a law was passed in Germany to prevent shepherds and herdsmen from attending obstetric cases.   The Renaissance pictures show that, as in the Middle Ages, the lying-in room was crowded with people bustling in every direction, giving the general impression, as Baas truly says, of "all sorts of female fussiness."   The obstetric abuses were remedied to some extent by city ordinances governing midwives, notably those of Ratisbon (1555), Frankfurt on the Main (by Adam Lonicerus, 1573), and Passau (1595).

---

[1] See Lancet, London, 1909, ii, 1020.

Certain criminal **laws** issued by the Bishop of Bamberg in 1507, and by the Elector of Brandenburg in 1516, led to the formulation (in 1521 and 1529) of the celebrated C. C. C. (Constitutio Criminalis Carolina), or "Peinliche Gerichtsordnung," published in 1533, which authorized the judge of a court to summon physicians or midwives as expert witnesses in such medicolegal cases as homicide, infanticide, criminal abortion, malpractice, and the like; but, in deference to current superstitions, postmortem examinations were not authorized. The first judicial postmortem was made by Ambroise Paré in 1562, after which time the practice became common. Special laws were passed in regard to the sale of food, the adulteration of alcoholic liquors, street-cleaning, occupations, the plague, and other phases of municipal hygiene, but nothing was done to alleviate the condition of the insane, who were chained, beaten, starved, and otherwise maltreated, and frequently died of cold. In 1547 the monastery of St. Mary of Bethlehem at London (founded in 1246) was converted into a hospital for the insane, popularly known as "Bedlam," and in a few years was amply justifying its reputation as conveyed in this term.

A special feature of Renaissance legislation in France and England was the improvement of the status of the barber surgeons. In 1505, the Paris Faculty took the barber surgeons under its wing, in order to spite the surgeons proper, of whom it was jealous, and a few years later, these "surgeons of the long robe," having failed to become a separate faculty, decided to make the best of a bad bargain by coming under the sway of the physicians. In England, in 1462, the numerous and prosperous Guild of Barbers became the Company of Barbers under Edward IV; the surgeons obtained a special charter in 1492; and in 1540, under Henry VIII, this Barber Company was united with the small and exclusive Guild of Surgeons to form the United Barber-Surgeon Company, with Thomas Vicary as its first Master. A celebrated painting of the younger Holbein represents Henry VIII, huge, bluff, and disdainful, in the act of handing this statute to Vicary, in company with fourteen other surgeons on their knees before the monarch, who does not condescend even to look at them. This picture, one of the best of Holbein's works, not only gives a superb portrait of Henry VIII, but is probably the best representation in existence of the costume and appearance of the sixteenth-century surgeon.

Of the many **epidemic diseases** which had beset Europe in the Middle Ages, three, the sweating sickness, leprosy, and epidemic chorea, had well-nigh disappeared by the middle of the sixteenth century. In France, Italy, Spain, England, Denmark, and Switzerland, leprosy was so well stamped out that the lazar-houses were abolished, but the disease still continued to be epidemic through the seventeenth century in Germany, Scotland, and the Low Countries, and in Sweden and Norway lasted until the eighteenth century. The most formidable epidemics of the sixteenth century were still the plague and syphilis. Between the years 1500–68, the ravages of the plague were particularly severe in Germany, Italy, and France, and, in the sixth decade, spread all over Europe. After this time, it broke out at intervals in different places in 1564, 1568, 1574, and 1591. All through the century a vast number of "Pestschriften" were published, and the most important of these were the public documents recognizing the contagious nature of the plague and proposing various methods of isolation and disinfection. Wittenberg and some of the other cities commemorated the different epidemics by striking off special coins, or pest-dollars (*Wittenberger Pesttaler*). The obverse of these commonly represented Moses' fiery serpent set upon a pole, with the inscription "Who looketh upon the serpent shall live" (Numbers xxi, 8, 9); the reverse represented Christ crucified, with the inscription, "He that believeth on me hath everlasting life" (St. John vi, 47). There were also comet medals (1558), and medals commemorating years of famine. The most remarkable of the latter celebrated the "Annona," or right of the Papacy to limit the price of corn. Famine medals of this kind were struck off in honor of Popes Julius II (1505–8), Pius IV (1560–75), Gregory XIII (1576–91), and Clement VIII (1599). The Wittenberg pest-dollars and the "zenechton," arsenic-paste sewed up in dog-skin, were worn over the heart as amulets against the plague.

Syphilis was less malignant in character than in the former century, and this was perhaps due to a number of really efficient remedies which were a vast improvement upon the mild vegetable concoctions of the earlier period. Mercury had become the great sheet-anchor, whether for internal or external use, although opinion was pretty well divided as to its ultimate value. Leonicenus, Montagnana, and the German writers generally opposed its use; Fracastorius and Benivieni gave it the seal of their approval. A special feature of the antisyphilitic medication of the century was the introduction of new drugs from the Western Hemisphere. As alchemy introduced antimony, mercury, and sugar of lead, so the discovery of America brought in guaiac (introduced in 1508), the root of *China smilax* (1525), exploited by Vesalius, sarsaparilla (1530), and sassafras. Gonorrhea became common about 1520, and one remarkable effect of these venereal diseases was the suppression of common public baths for either sex or both sexes. In the Germanic countries, these bathing establishments were a special feature of city life, and, as depicted by the various Renaissance artists, their status was peculiar. Many of them were frequented indiscriminately by men and women alike, all of whom sat and bathed together in one huge common vat or tank. Dürer's woodcut of 1496 (*Die Badstube*) represents a group of naked men in a common bath vat, some of whom are playing musical instruments, others conversing, while a third is draining a stoup of wine. This *motif* of wine bibbing and general pleasaunce was frequently utilized by the lesser masters, Hans Sebald Beham, Aldegrever, Hans Baldung Grien, Hans Bock, whose pictures show the commingling of nude men and women, with scenes of feasting, cupping, and venesection in the bath. A favorite theme of Lucas Cranach and Beham was the so-called "Jungbrunnen," or "Fountain of Youth," which represent a number of decrepit old women trundled in wheelbarrows to one side of a huge bath tank in which they are supposed to be rejuvenated; on the other side, they are promptly man-handled by a number of amiable youths, who hurry these reinvigorated dames up the bank to appropriate tents. These roguish pictures of the old German masters really point a moral. It was soon found that a general mixing of able-bodied men and women in a state of nature in common bathing pools could lead in the end only to general laxity of morals, and such places could not long be frequented by decent people. Laws were passed segregating the sexes, but the advent of leprosy, plague, and syphilis demonstrated, over and above this that, the idea of a common bath tank was bad in itself, since the latter became a simple medium of infection. In connection with Renaissance art, we should mention Dürer's celebrated wood-cut of a syphilitic (1496);[1] also the picture which he sent to his physician representing himself nude, with the legend, "Where the yellow spot is and my finger points, there am I sick within"; Orcagna's grisly procession of lepers in his "Triumph of Death" (Pisa); the elder Holbein's picture of St. Elizabeth ministering to three lepers (Munich); Matthias Grünewald's representation of bubonic plague (Colmar Gallery, 1515), and Francesco Carotto's St. Roch in the Verona Gallery (1528), showing the typical inguinal bubo. In the Uffizi Gallery at Florence there is a remarkable picture of Ferdinand I of Spain, painted by Lucas van Leyden in 1524, in which the artist has given the characteristic *facies* of adenoid vegetations, without apparently knowing the existence of the condition in his subject.

Of epidemic diseases, smallpox and measles began to appear in the northern countries, notably in Germany (1493) and Sweden (1578). In 1572 there was an epidemic of lead-poisoning (called *colica Pictonum*) in the South of France which resembled the

---

[1] Encircled by 110 Latin lines by Theodoricus Ulsenius and printed at Nuremberg.

"Devonshire colic" of the eighteenth century, in that its probable cause was the use of lead in the cider and wine-presses. Scurvy, which had appeared as early as 1248, and was first described by Joinville (1250), and later, in the narrative of Vasco da Gama's voyage (1497), became quite common along the coast of northern Germany, Holland, and the Scandinavian countries, as described by Euricius Cordus (1534), George Agricola (1539), and other writers. Typhus fever was epidemic in Italy in 1505 and 1524–30, and was described by Fracastorius (1533)[1] and Francesco Bravo (1570).[2] In Spain, after the siege of Granada (1489), where it broke out among the Castilian troops, it was called *el tabardiglo* (the red cloak). The Aztec disease "matlalzuahatl," which Alexander von Humboldt described as already known in Mexico in 1576,[3] was shown to be a tableland disease identical with tabardillo, by Stamm, in 1861.[4] The so-called Hungarian disease (*morbus Hungaricus*), which spread all over Europe in 1501 and, in 1505–87, was frequently epidemic in Italy and France, is now regarded as, in all probability, typhus fever. Another disease of obscure origin and character was a sort of pneumo-typhus or pleurotyphus which was epidemic in Italy, France, Switzerland, Holland, and Germany between the years 1521 and 1598. Diphtheria (garotillo), which had already been described by Gutierrez in the preceding century, was six times epidemic in Spain during the period 1583–1600. Whooping-cough first appeared in the sixteenth century, and was first described by Guillaume Baillou (Ballonius) in 1578. Ergotism in the gangrenous form was prevalent in Spain in 1581 and 1590, while in Germany a convulsive or spasmodic form, preceded by the usual tingling, burning sensations, and known as the *Kriebelkrankheit*, appeared, endemic in the years 1581, 1587, 1592, and 1595–6. In 1597, the Medical Faculty of Marburg issued a pronouncement upon the last epidemic, declaring its cause to be the use of bread made from spurred rye.

Hospital construction approached perfection in the fifteenth century, the greatest technical care being devoted to these structures, as in the hospital at Milan, which was opened in 1445, but not completed until 1456. A painting of Andrea del Sarto's represents the interior of a woman's hospital, probably for lying-in purposes. Before the Reformation, there were 77 hospitals in Scotland alone, but, after that period, hospitals connected with re-

---

[1] Fracastorius: De morbis contagiosis, 1533, cap. vi.

[2] Francesco Bravo: Opera medicinalia, Mexico, 1570.

[3] Humboldt: Reise in die Aequinoctial-Gegenden von Amerika, cited by Haeser.

[4] Stamm: Nosophthorie, Berlin, 1861, cited by Haeser.

ligious institutions began to die out in the northern countries. The lazar-houses also began to diminish in number, as leprosy was gradually stamped out.   Three famous English institutions of the period were the Hospital of St. Mary of Bethlehem, which was converted from a monastery into an insane asylum ("Bedlam") in 1547; Bridewell, anciently a palace, which became a penitentiary and house of correction for vagabonds and loose women in 1553; and Christ's Hospital, formerly the Grey Friars Monastery, which was chartered in 1553 as a charity for fatherless and motherless children, and became the famous school of the "Blue Coat Boys," at which Charles Lamb and Coleridge were educated.

THE SEVENTEENTH CENTURY: THE AGE OF INDIVIDUAL SCIENTIFIC ENDEAVOR

THE seventeenth century, the age of Shakespeare and Milton, Velasquez and Rembrandt, Bach and Purcell, Cervantes and Molière, Newton and Leibnitz, Bacon and Descartes, Spinoza and Locke, was preëminently a period of intense individualism, intellectual and spiritual. What happened to men like Servetus and Sir Thomas More, Bruno and Dolet, Spinoza and Uriel Acosta, Galileo and Copernicus, did but lessen the dominion of the professional theologian, whether Catholic, Protestant, or Jewish. Yet with the decline of collectivism there necessarily went a corresponding decline in the things that had thrived under its régime, in particular, organized nursing, charitable care of the sick, and well-managed hospitals for this purpose.

In the seventeenth century the German people, decimated and torn asunder by the ravages of the Thirty Years War, could do little for medicine, as Baas laments, and the highest distinction in this field was attained by England, Italy, and Holland. The age of the Armada and the Great Rebellion of 1642 was the most glorious period of English history, the age "of her greatest golden-mouthed sons," from Shakespeare, Milton, and the great line of Elizabethan dramatists, to Bacon and Locke, Raleigh and Sidney, Vaughan and More, Herrick and Crashaw, Boyle and Wren. In this age also flourished some of the greatest English mathematicians and astronomers, Newton and Wallis, Halley and Flamsteed, Briggs and Napier. The very beginning of the century (1600) is memorable for the appearance of an epoch-making work in the history of physics—the "De Magnete"[1] of William **Gilbert** (1540–1603), who was physician to Queen Elizabeth and James I,

---

[1] This work ranks beside *Newton's Principia* in that it threw overboard the current Arabian Nights' superstitions attributing the deflection of the compass needle to "magnetic mountains" or magnetic influences from the stars. After a thoroughgoing investigation of the properties of the lodestone, Gilbert establishes the theorem that the earth itself is a gigantic spherical magnet, a proposition which has been the starting-point of all subsequent works on terrestrial magnetic variations, magnetic storms, and of the charting of the earth's magnetic fields by Halley, Gauss, and Sabine. The florid encomium of Dryden—

Gilbert shall live till lodestones cease to draw

is certainly true of human chronology, if not of geological or sidereal time. Gilbert is also memorable for the discovery of frictional electricity, to which he gave its name from the amber (ἤλεκτρων) employed.

176

and left his books and instruments to the Royal College of Physicians, where they were destroyed by the great fire of 1666.

The greatest name in seventeenth century medicine is that of William **Harvey** (1578–1657), of Folkestone in Kent, who studied at Padua (1599–1603) as a pupil of Fabricius and Casserius, and whose work has exerted a profounder influence upon modern medicine than that of any other man save Vesalius. The world has "heard great argument" concerning the merits and status of the "De Motu Cordis," but the following simple facts seem irrefutable and unassailable. The observation that the blood is in motion

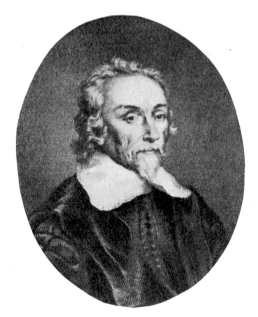

William Harvey (1578–1657).

may have occurred to the first primitive man who ever cut open a live animal or saw a wounded artery. The idea that this motion is along a definite path may well have been entertained by any ancient Egyptian or Greek, as well as by some hypothetical native of Muscovy or Illyria in Harvey's day. Galen's false concept about the pores in the ventricular septum diverted all speculation into the wrong channel for fourteen centuries, and even Servetus, who came nearest the truth, could only admit that some (not all) of the blood takes a circuit through the lungs. In the drawings which Vesalius had made, indicating the close proximity of the terminal twigs of

12

arteries and veins,[1] the truth about the circulation was literally staring in the face of any observer who had eyes to see or wit to discover it. Yet anatomists continued to see everything in the light of Galenical prepossessions. Cesalpinus, at best, made only a clever guess. Columbus, in all likelihood, appropriated the ideas of Servetus. But Harvey, who knew the whole history and literature of the subject, first made a careful review of existing theories, showing their inadequacy, and then proceeded, by experimental vivisection, ligation, and perfusion, to an inductive proof that the heart acts as a muscular force-pump in propelling the blood along, and that the blood's motion is continual, continuous, and in a cycle or circle. The *crux* of Harvey's argument—that the actual quantity and velocity of the blood, as computed by him, make it physically impossible for it to do otherwise than return to the heart by the venous route—was the first application of the idea of measurement in any biologic investigation, and, had he chosen to express this discovery in the language of algebra (by using the symbol of inequality), it would long since have taken its proper place in the application of mathematical physics to medicine. The importance of Harvey's work, then, is not so much the discovery of the circulation of the blood as its quantitative or mathematical demonstration. With this start, physiology became a dynamic science.

In asserting that the heart is a muscular force-pump, Harvey originated the "myogenic" theory of its autonomy, which was a little later confronted by Borelli's idea that the heart-beat has a neurogenic origin, the two views remaining in dispute to this day. In endeavoring to locate the motor power of the muscle itself, Harvey fell into the usual medieval mysticism by assigning, as a final cause for the movements of the heart and the blood, the "innate heat" of the latter, which, he says, is "celestial in nature" and "identical with the essence of the stars." This astrologic theory, which, Allbutt thinks, Harvey got from his reading of Cicero,[2] did much to prevent the development of the true physiology of respiration for a long time. The discovery of the circulation itself was the most momentous event in medical history since Galen's time. While it was opposed by the pedantic Riolanus,[3] Gassendi, Wormius, and others, it was soon supported by some of the ablest spirits of the period, including Rolfink, Sylvius de le Boë, Bartholinus, Ent, and Pecquet. Jan de Wale (1604–49), or **Walæus,** in particular, showed that incisions on either side of a ligature applied to an elevated blood-vessel cause the blood to

---

[1] Vesalius: Fabrica, Basel, 1543, pp. 262, 268, 295, 305, 311, and plate opposite 312.

[2] Sir T. C. Allbutt: Science and Mediæval Thought, London, 1901, 43–48.

[3] Huxley styled Riolanus "a tympanitic Philistine, who would have been none the worse for a few sharp incisions."

ooze or to spurt, according to the direction in which it is flowing, thus affording a convincing proof of Harvey's discovery according to the laws of hydrodynamics (1640).[1]

The status of Harvey's other treatise, "De Generatione Animalium" (1651), is important in the history of embryology and a matter of frequent dispute. Some writers have tended to make Harvey's merits overshadow the just claims of men like Malpighi and von Baer. Of all pronouncements made, that of Huxley still seems the soundest and the best. In his demonstration of the circulation, Harvey was brought to a standstill at one point only, viz., the capillary anastomosis between arteries and veins, which, having no microscope, he could not see. In his investigation of the embryo the minute and patient work of years was driven into an *impasse* for the same reason, while the manuscripts, containing his drawings and other results of experimental investigation of the embryo, were destroyed by the Parliamentary troopers who invaded his chambers in Whitehall in 1642. Long before Wolff and von Baer, he maintained, as pure theory, the doctrine of "epigenesis"—that the organism does not exist encased or preformed in the ovum, but is evolved from it by gradual building up and aggregation of its parts; yet, through his inability to see microscopically, his idea of fecundation was totally wrong, for he believed the fertilization of the ovum to be something "incorporeal"—"as iron touched by the magnet is endowed with its own powers." By such mysticism, the famous dictum, "*Omne vivum ex ovo,*"[2] becomes self-contradictory, since it denies the continuity of the germ-plasm. Its true importance, in Harvey's hands, was that it subverted the ancient concept that life is engendered out of corruption (or putrefaction)—an idea still familiar in the burial service.[3]

Besides the "De Motu Cordis" (1628) and the treatise on generation (1651), we should mention the fac simile reprint of the MS. notes for the "Praelectiones Anatomicæ" of the Lumleian foundation (1616), which shows that Harvey had completed his discovery of the circulation and was lecturing on it at least twelve years before he printed it.

Harvey, as described by Aubrey, was of short stature, with bright black eyes and raven hair, "complexion like the wainscot," quick, alert, choleric, often fingering the handle of his dagger.

---

[1] Walæus: Epistolæ duæ, 1640, [*In:* T. Bartholinus, Anatomia, Leyden, 1541, pp. 539–541 (plate)].

[2] First stated by Francesco Redi in the form, "omne vivum ex vivo."

[3] For a further discussion of this subject, see the admirable essay of the late Professor W. K. Brooks, on "Harvey as Embryologist," in Bull. Johns Hopkins Hosp., Baltimore, 1897, viii, 167–174.

The resemblance of his finely domed head to Shakespeare's is a matter of comment. Like many experimenters, he was but an indifferent practitioner. Yet he was no closet recluse, but highly honored in the worldly affairs of his day, as witness his publicity as Lumleian lecturer, his long association with Charles I, his assistance at the postmortem of "old Parr," or his merciful intervention in the affair of the "late Lancashire witches." Although not a votary of the muse, he was, in the finest sense, a master of Dryden's "other harmony of prose." Read, for instance, his impressionistic account of the Bass Rock in a good English translation. It is a pen-picture which many a modern *prosateur* would be proud to sign. Having survived long enough to live down opposition and see his discovery accepted, Harvey prepared for approaching death with the cool self-possession of his race, meeting the end with a quiet resolution at the age of seventy-nine. While he was not ostentatious in piety, his will, with its liberal legacy to the poor of his native town, reveals the ideal Christian gentleman, tenderly solicitous of all his intimates, from Sir Charles Scarborough down to his humblest body servant.

Although Harvey's publication of his discovery caused an immediate falling off in his practice, its effect upon medical science was as definite and far reaching as that of the Fabrica. The seventeenth century was the great age of specialized anatomic research, and was notable for a long array of individual discoveries and investigations, nearly every one of which had a physiological significance. Earliest among the achievements of the **post-Vesalian anatomists** was the clearing up of the old Galenical error that the veins and lymphatics of the intestines carried chyle to the liver. This was dispelled by the discovery of the lacteal vessels in 1622[1] by Gasparo **Aselli** (1581–1626), who thought they went to the liver, the mistake being corrected by the discovery of the thoracic duct and receptaculum chyli by Jean **Pecquet** (1622–74),[2] and of the intestinal lymphatics and their connection with the thoracic duct by Olof **Rudbeck**[3] (1630–1702), of Sweden, in 1651. The latter discovery was also disputed as to priorty by the Dane, Thomas Bartholinus[4] (1616–80), in 1653, and by Jolyff, an Englishman, who did not publish his claims. Next came the finding of the pancreatic duct in Vesalius' dissecting-room at Padua by his prosector, Georg **Wirsung,** in 1642,[5] to be followed, in order of time, by such im-

---

[1] G. Aselli: De lactibus, Milan, 1627.

[2] J. Pecquet: Experimenta nova anatomica, Paris, 1651.

[3] O. Rudbeck: Nova exercitatio anatomica exhibens ductus hepaticos aquosos et vasa glandularum serosa, Westerås, 1653.

[4] Th. Bartholinus: De lacteis thoracicis, Copenhagen, 1652.

[5] Recorded on a single rare copper plate of 1642.

portant English discoveries as the antrum of **Highmore,** in 1651,[1] **Glisson**'s capsule in 1654,[2] **Wharton**'s duct in 1656,[3] the circle of **Willis** in 1659,[4] Richard **Lower**'s treatise on the heart as a muscle in 1669,[5] Clopton **Havers'** discovery of the Haversian canals in 1691,[6] and **Cowper**'s glands in 1694.[7] Italy won distinction in **Malpighi**'s discovery of the capillary anastomosis in the lungs (1661),[8] which supplied the missing link in Harvey's demonstration; in Lorenzo **Bellini**'s work on the structure of the kidneys (1662),[9] and in Antonis **Pacchioni**'s description of the so-called Pacchionian bodies (1697).[10] Germany is memorable through Conrad Victor **Schneider**'s classic treatise on the membranes of the nose (De catarrhis, 1660), **Meibom**'s demonstration of the conjunctival glands (1666),[11] **Kerckring**'s demonstration of the intestinal valvulæ conniventes (1670),[12] **Brunner**'s discovery of the duodenal glands (1682),[13] and Holland by **Ruysch**'s innovations in anatomic injecting (1665), and his many discoveries, e. g., the valves in the lymphatics (1665),[14] **de Graaf**'s authentic account of the ovary and Graafian follicles (1672),[15] and **Nuck**'s glands and ducts (1685).[16] Bishop Stensen (Nicholaus **Steno**) (1638–86), of Denmark, discovered the parotid duct in 1662,[17] and Johann Conrad **Peyer** (1653–1712), of Switzerland, described the lymphoid follicles in the small intestine (1677),[18] which have such an important rôle in typhoid fever. In France, Joseph Guichard **Duverney** (1648–1730), professor of anatomy in Paris, made some important investigations of the inner structure of the ear which led him to write the first treatise on otology (1683); and Raymond

[1] N. Highmore: Corporis humani disquisitio anatomica, The Hague, 1651.

[2] F. Glisson: De hepate, London, 1654.

[3] T. Wharton: Adenographia, London, 1656.

[4] T. Willis: Cerebri anatome, London, 1659.

[5] R. Lower: Tractatus de corde, London, 1669.

[6] C. Havers: Osteologia nova, London, 1691.

[7] W. Cowper: Glandularum quarundam . . . descriptio, London, 1702.

[8] M. Malpighi: De pulmonibus, Bologna, 1661.

[9] L. Bellini: De structura renum, Florence, 1662.

[10] A. Pacchioni: Diss. epistolaris de glandulis conglobatis duræ meningis humanæ, Rome, 1705.

[11] H. Meibom: De vasis palpebrarum, Helmstadt, 1666.

[12] Th. Kerckring: Spicilegium anatomicum, Amsterdam, 1670.

[13] J. C. Brunner: Glandulæ duodeni, Frankfort, 1687.

[14] F. Ruysch: Dilucidatio valvularum, The Hague, 1665.

[15] R. de Graaf: De mulierum organis generatione inservientibus, Leyden, 1672.

[16] A. Nuck: De ductu salivali novo, Leyden, 1685.

[17] N. Steno: Observationes anatomicæ, Leyden, 1662.

[18] J. C. Peyer: De glandulis intestinorum, Schaffhausen, 1677.

Vieussens (1641–1716), professor at Montpellier, made various studies on the position and structure of the heart and the anatomy of the nervous system.

The seventeenth century was the great age of copper-plate engraving, and **anatomic illustration** reached a high point of perfection in the striking plates in such works as Gottfried Bidloo's "Anatomia" (Amsterdam,1685), Bernardino Genga's "Anatomia" (Rome, 1691), the "Traité de la figure humaine," of the painter Peter Paul Rubens (1577–1640), which was published over a hundred years after his death (1773), or the "Thesauri anatomici decem" (Amsterdam, 1701–16) of Frederik Ruysch (1638–1731). A wonderful union of scientific accuracy with artistic perfection was attained in the "Tabulæ anatomicæ" (1627) of Giulio Casserio (1561–1616), or **Casserius,** one of Harvey's teachers at Padua, whose "eviscerated beauties," as Dr. Holmes has styled them, are as attractive in appearance as their dissected parts were held to be instructive to the student. These Correggio-like plates of Casserius were incorporated in the atlas (1627) of Adrian van Spieghel (1578–1625), or **Spigelius,** who wrote the letter-press around them, and, in this way, is usually credited with the exquisite workmanship of the illustrations. Spieghel's name is associated with the Spigelian lobe of the liver. The 105 plates in Bidloo's Anatomy of 1685 were actually plagiarized by William **Cowper** (1666–1709), whose "Anatomy of Human Bodies" (Oxford, 1698) is only original as to the text, and nine perfunctory plates supplied by Cowper himself. For whimsical originality and exquisite delicacy of detail, the plates drawn by Frederik **Ruysch** (1638–1731) deserve a special mention. Skeletons posed in quaintest attitudes, with appropriate mottoes of the "memento mori" variety attached, surrounded by strange reptiles, stuffed monsters, dried plants and deep-sea creatures, constituted the favorite decorative scheme of the old Dutch anatomist, whose mortuary humors have been sublimated in Leopardi's dialogue.[1]

A very important outcome of Harvey's demonstration of the circulation was the art of **anatomic injection,** which was advanced by Swammerdam, de Graaf, and Ruysch. Berengarius Carpi had filled the blood-vessels with tepid water, Stephanus with air, Eustachius with colored fluids, Malpighi and Glisson with ink, and Willis discovered the circle of Willis by injecting the brain with "*aqua crocata.*" Swammerdam aimed to get a preparation which could be injected warm and solidify afterward. He first tried suet, but, in 1677, hit upon wax. In 1668, de Graaf introduced an improved syringe (*De usu syphonis*), and injected the spermatic vessels with mercury. In 1680, Swammerdam became convinced of the impiety of anatomy, and joined a fanatical religious sect. Before doing so, however, he published his method abroad, sending a preparation to the Royal Society in 1672, and especially training Ruysch

[1] Giacomo Leopardi: "Dialogo di Federico Ruysch e delle sue mummie," in his collective works.

to its use. The latter introduced the new feature of applying the microscope in the injection of the finer vessels. The process was subsequently improved by Monro *primus*, Lieberkühn, Prochaska, Gerlach, and others, up to the time of Hyrtl's wonderful injections in two, three, and four different colors.[1]

The first crude attempt at comparative anatomy was made by Marco Aurelio Severino (1580–1656), whose "Zootomia Democritæ" (1645) antedates Malpighi, Leeuwenhoek, and Swammerdam. The wood-cuts show the viscera of birds, fishes, and mammals, with some phases of their development, and slight as the comparative features are, the book is the only thing of its kind before the eighteenth century.

A remarkable comparative anatomist of the seventeenth century was Edward **Tyson** (1650–1708), of the University of Cambridge, who graduated there in 1678, and lectured on anatomy to the Barber Surgeons up to 1699. Tyson was the first to publish elaborate monographs on the structure of the lower animals, his memoirs on the anatomy of the porpoise (1680), the rattlesnake (1683), and his dissections of such animal parasites as Lumbricus latus, Lumbricus teres (Ascaris lumbricoides), and Lumbricus hydropicus (hydatids), being a great advance on the "Anatomia Porci" of Copho, the first adventure in this kind. The structures in the prepuce known as Tyson's glands are named after him, but his most important contribution to science is his "Orang-Outang, sive Homo Sylvestris" (1699), the first work of consequence in comparative morphology. In this book Tyson compares the anatomy of man with that of monkeys, and between the two he placed what he thought was a typical pygmy—in reality, a chimpanzee, the skeleton of which is now in the South Kensington Museum of Natural History. This was the origin of the "missing-link" idea, which so many confuse with true Darwinism. Tyson's work concludes with a terminal essay setting forth that the satyrs, ægipans, cynocephali, and other mythical creatures of the ancients "are all either apes or monkeys, and not men, as formerly pretended."[2] This hypothesis was accepted by Buffon, and the existence of ape-like or pygmy races of men was doubted until Quatrefages (1887)[3] and Kollmann (1894)[4] proved that they have existed and do exist in space and time.

Another important contribution to anthropology was the idea of "cephalometric lines," conceived by the anatomist Spieghel, and which, says Meigs,[5] "may perhaps be regarded as constituting the earliest scientific attempt at cranial measurements." These "lineæ cephalometricæ," when equal to each other in length, were Spieghel's criterion of a normally proportioned skull, and Meigs observes that "in ascending the zoölogic scale these lines approximate equality just in proportion as the head measured approaches the human form."

The invention of the microscope opened out a new departure for medicine in the direction of the invisible world, as Galileo's telescope had given a glimpse of the infinite vast in astronomy. The earliest of **the microscopists** was the learned Jesuit priest, Athanasius **Kircher** (1602–80), of Fulda, who was at once a mathematician, physicist, optician, Orientalist, musician, and virtuoso, as well as a medical man, and who was probably the first to employ the microscope in investigating the causes of disease.

---

[1] W. W. Keen: Early History of Practical Anatomy, Philadelphia, 1874, *passim.*

[2] See A. C. Haddon: History of Anthropology, New York and London, 1910, pp. 15, 16.

[3] A. Quatrefages: Les Pygmées, Paris, 1887.

[4] J. Kollmann: Pygmäen in Europa, 1894.

[5] J. A. Meigs: N. Am. Med.-Chir. Rev., 1861, v, 840, cited by Haddon.

In his *Scrutinium pestis* (Rome, 1658) he not only details seven experiments upon the nature of putrefaction, showing how maggots and other living creatures are developed in decaying matter, but found that the blood of plague patients was filled with a countless brood of "worms," not perceptible to the naked eye, but to be seen in all putrefying matter through the microscope. While Kircher's "worms," as Friedrich Loeffler[1] claimed, were probably nothing more than pus-cells and rouleaux of red blood-corpuscles, since he could not possibly have seen the Bacillus pestis with a 32-power microscope, yet it is quite within the range of possibility for him to have seen the larger microörganisms, and he was undoubtedly the first to state in explicit terms the doctrine of a

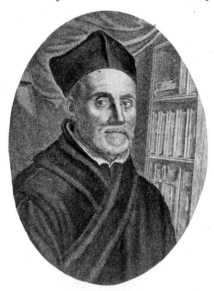

Athanasius Kircher (1602–80).

"contagium animatum" as the cause of infectious disease. In his "Physiologia Kircheriana" he was also the first to record an experiment in hypnotism (1680).[2] Another early worker with the microscope was Robert **Hooke** (1635–1763), a mechanical genius who anticipated many modern discoveries and inventions and who laid claim to all that were thinkable in the period in which he lived. Hooke's "Micrographia" (London, 1665) contains many fine plates of animal and vegetable structures which probably inspired the works of Nehemiah **Grew** (1641–1712) on vegetable histology and physiology (1671, 1682). Grew, whom Haller styled "an industrious observer of nature in every direction," was probably the first to consider the existence of sex in plants.

Jan **Swammerdam** (1637–80), whose interest in natural history was awakened by the fact that his father's apothecary-shop contained the finest collection of exotic fauna in Amsterdam, was an expert in microscopic dissecting long before he began to study

---

[1] Fr. Loeffler: Vorlesungen über die geschichtliche Entwicklung der Lehre von den Bacterien, Leipzig, 1887, pp. 1, 2.

[2] Kircher also treated of the curative powers of magnetism in his "Magnes sive de Arte Magnetica" (1643), which contains a description of "tarantism."

medicine. Having literally grown up among zoölogic specimens, he never practised, but devoted his short life to arduous and splendid labors in minute anatomy and embryology. His career was that of a scientific enthusiast who lived up to the principle *aliis inserviendo consumor*, and his best work is contained in the huge "Bybel der Natuur," which Boerhaave published long after his death (Amsterdam, 1737), comprising some 53 plates with accurate life histories, giving the finer anatomy of the bees, the mayflies, the snail, the clam, the squid, and the frog. The drawings in this collection surpass all other contemporary work in exquisite delicacy and accuracy of detail. Swammerdam was the first to discern and describe the red blood-corpuscles (1658), discovered the valves of the lymphatics (1664), discovered the medicolegal fact that the fetal lungs will float after respiration has taken place (1667), and, in 1677, devised the method of injecting blood-vessels with wax which was afterward claimed by Ruysch. He was also no mean experimental physiologist,[1] studying the movements of the heart, the lungs, and the muscles by plethysmographic methods which are almost modern.

A very great microscopist was Antonj van **Leeuwenhoek,** of Delft (1632–1723), who, as an inheritor of well-to-do brewers, led an easy-going life, the greater part of which was devoted to the study of natural history. He had some 247 microscopes with 419 lenses, most of which were ground by himself, and once sent 26 microscopes to London as a present to the Royal Society, of which he became a Fellow in 1680. The directors of the East India Company sent him specimens, and even Peter the Great visited his collection in 1689. Leeuwenhoek was a strong man of marvelous industry, and during his long life he sent as many as 375 scientific papers to the Royal Society and 27 to the French Academy of Sciences. These *Ontledingen en Ontdekingen* (Leyden, 1696) contain, in addition to a vast amount of work on animalculæ and plant histology, many discoveries of capital importance to medicine. Leeuwenhoek was the first to describe the spermatozoa (originally pointed out to him by the student Hamen in 1674); gave the first complete account of the red blood-corpuscles (1674); discovered the striped character of voluntary muscle and the structure of the crystalline lens; was the first to see protozoa under the microscope (1675); found microörganisms in the teeth, giving,

---

[1] For a good account of Swammerdam's work in experimental physiology see W. Stirling, "Some Apostles of Physiology," London, 1902, pp. 34, 135, with interesting illustrations. The life of Swammerdam has been made the subject of a fascinating "culturhistorischer Roman," by Hermann Klencke, entitled "Swammerdam oder die Offenbarung der Natur" (3 vols., Leipzig, 1860), which is well worth reading for the light it throws upon social life and cultural conditions in the seventeenth century.

for the first time, accurate figurations of bacterial chains and clumps as well as of individual spirilla and bacilli (September 17, 1683); and demonstrated the capillary anastomosis between the arteries and veins, which Malpighi had already seen in 1660 without attaching much importance to it. It was Malpighi's discovery and Leeuwenhoek's thorough work on the capillary circulation which finally completed Harvey's discovery. The portrait of this tremendous worker represents a strong, sturdy figure in whose countenance Richardson discerns "the quiet force of Cromwell and the delicate disdain of Spinoza."

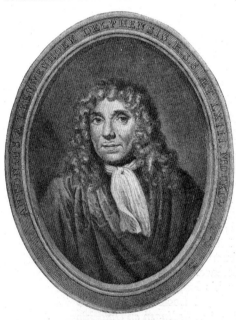

Antonj van Leeuwenhoek (1632–1723).

The greatest of the microscopists, however, was Marcello **Malpighi** (1628–94), the founder of histology, who was professor of anatomy at Bologna, Pisa, and Messina, and physician to Pope Innocent XII (1691–94). Famed in biology for his works on the anatomy of the silkworm and the morphology of plants, he made an epoch in medicine by his investigations of the embryology of the chick and the histology and physiology of the glands and viscera. The 12 plates accompanying his Royal Society memoirs, "De formatione pulli in ovo" (1673) and "De ovo incubato," make him the founder of descriptive or iconographic embryology, surpassing all other contemporary workers on the subject in the accurate notation of such minutiæ as the aortic arches, the head-fold, the neural groove, the cerebral and optic vesicles. Malpighi described the red blood-corpuscles in 1665 (seven years after Swammerdam) as "fat globules looking like a rosary of red coral." He discovered the rete mucosum, or Malpighian layer of the skin, and proved that the papillæ of the tongue are organs of taste. Perhaps his greatest work is the "De Pulmonibus" (1661), which overthrew the current conceptions of the pulmonary tissues as "parenchymatous," demonstrating their true vesicular nature, the capillary anastomosis between arteries and veins, and how the trachea terminates in bronchial filaments. Of his discovery of the capillaries (1660), Fraser Harris has well said that "Harvey made their existence a logical necessity; Malpighi made it a histological certainty."[1] His work on the structure of the liver, spleen, and kidneys[2] (1666) did much to advance the physiological knowledge of these viscera, and his name has been eponymically preserved in the Malpighian bodies of the kidney and spleen. This book also contains the first account of those lymphadeno- matous formations (general enlargement of lymphatics with

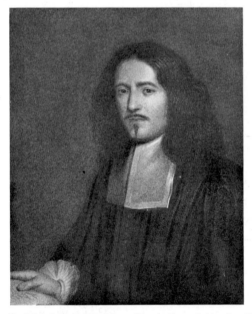

Marcello Malpighi (1628–94). (From the painting by Tabor, Royal Society.)

nodules in spleen)[3] which were fully described by Hodgkin in 1832, and which Wilks, in 1856, called Hodgkin's disease, or pseudoleukæmia. Malpighi's private life was embittered by the coarse personal attacks of his Pisan colleague Borelli, and by an old-time feud (of which he bore the brunt) between his family and a neighboring clan of the ominous and significant name of Sbaraglia. As in the case of Harvey and John Hunter, some of his best work was lost to posterity by the wanton destruction of

[1] Nature, June 29, 1911, 584.   [2] De viscerum structura, Bonn, 1666.
[3] De viscerum structura, Bonn, 1666, 125, 126.

valuable manuscripts. In personality, Malpighi was a gentle, fair-
minded, sympathetic nature, and, among the sick, a patient and
devoted Asclepiad. The memory of Malpighi is one of "sweetness
and light," and, in his capacity for acute observation, he verified
the remark of Thoreau that the laws of the universe are "forever
on the side of the most sensitive." He is not only one of medicine's greatest names, but one of its most attractive personalities.
The first hard blow to the doctrine of spontaneous generation

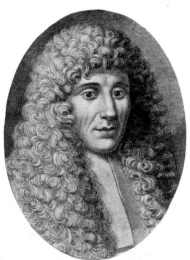

was given by the Italian naturalist, Francesco **Redi** (1626–94),
of Arezzo, who confuted the
idea, then current, that grubs
and maggots develop spontaneously in decaying matter.[1] He
exposed meat in jars, some of
which were uncovered, the
others being covered with
parchment and wire gauze. In
due course maggots appeared in
the first two, but, in the latter,
developed on top of the gauze.
This conclusive object-lesson
settled the matter, so far as
the spontaneous generation of
visible creatures was concerned.
Leeuwenhoek's discovery of bacteria and the yeast plant was to
raise the question in another

Francesco Redi (1626–1694).

form and leave it in dispute until the time of Schwann and Pasteur.

Apart from the productions of the great micrographic or morphologic
botanists of the seventeenth century,—Hooke, Grew, Malpighi,—some good
work was done in systematic or taxonomic botany. The English botanist,
John Ray (1627–1705), separated flowering from flowerless plants in his "Methodus plantarum" (London, 1682), and further divided the former class into
monocotyledonous and dicotyledonous. Ray "stood for the whole plant," as the
botanists say, in his classification. Robert Morison (1620–83), the first professor
of botany at Oxford, made a systematic arrangement of plants in 18 classes,
distinguishing them as woody and herbaceous, flower-bearing and fruit-bearing,
after the fashion of Cesalpinus (1672–80).[2] Rivinus, in 1690, classified plants by
the forms of the flowers. Toward the end of the century the favorite system
of classification was that of Joseph-Pitton **de Tournefort** (1656–1708), the
author of "Élemens de botanique" (1694) and "Institutiones Rei Herbariæ"
(1700), in which he described 8000 species, arranged in 21 classes, according to
the form of the corolla. This system held the field until the time of Linnæus,
who, like Tournefort, exaggerated the importance of the flower as a *fundamentum divisionis.*

---

[1] Experientia circa generationem insectorum, Amsterdam, 1671. Redi
is also said to have been one of the first to analyze food.

[2] Morison: Præludia Botanica, 1672, and Plantarum Historia Universalis,
1680.

The zoölogic investigations of Swammerdam, Leeuwenhoek, Redi, and Malpighi were supplemented by the work of Martin Lister (1638–1711), physician to Queen Anne, Oläus Worm (1588–1654), of the Wormian bones, Antonio Vallisnieri, and others, who, like the great leaders of the time, devoted their attention mainly to entomology.

Theoretical medicine in the seventeenth century naturally followed the trend of physiological doctrine, and this struck into two different paths, the iatromathematical and iatrochemical. Great advances in chemistry were made by Boyle, Willis, Mayow, and others, and the period was preëminently an age of discoveries in astronomy and mathematical physics. Following the publication of Copernicus' treatise on the revolution of the planets around the sun (1543), Galileo had invented the telescope in 1609, Kepler had stated the laws governing planetary motion in 1609–18, and Newton's statement of the law of gravitation (1682) was followed by the publication of his "Principia" in 1687. Logarithms were invented by Napier (1614) and Briggs (1617), Descartes founded analytic geometry in 1637, Pascal published his contributions to the theory of probabilities in 1654, while Newton created the differential calculus in 1665–66, and stated the binomial theorem in 1669. Von

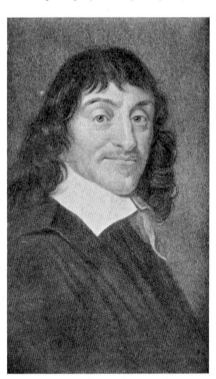

René Descartes (1596–1650).

Guericke, a burgomaster of Magdeburg, invented the air-pump in 1641; Torricelli, the barometer in 1643; and Hooke, a compound microscope in 1665. Such important discoveries and inventions as these were not without their influence upon medicine. The **Iatromathematical School,** by which all physiological happenings were treated as rigid consequences of the laws of physics, was represented by Descartes, Borelli, and Sanctorius. The protagonists of the Iatrochemical School, which regarded all vital phenomena as chemical in essence, were van Helmont, Sylvius, and Willis.

The "De Homine" of René **Descartes** (1622) is usually regarded as the first European text-book on physiology, although it
was only a popular and theoretic exposition of the subject. In
this respect, Sir Michael Foster has likened it to Herbert Spencer's
"Principles of Biology." It treats of the human body as a material machine, directed by a rational soul located in the pineal
gland. Descartes grasped the dynamic importance of Harvey's
discovery, but, like all his contemporaries, was a theoretic Galenist
in ascribing the movements of the heart to its internal fire or
heat. In his treatise, "Des passions de l'âme" (1649), he gives
the first experiment in reflex action—the familiar one of making

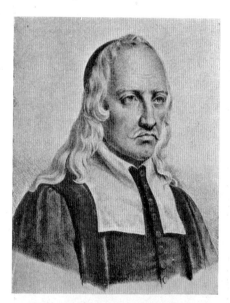

a person bat his eyes by
aiming a mock blow at
them—with the correct
explanation of the phe-
nomenon.

The mechanical view
of the human organism
was pushed to its extreme
limits by the Neapolitan
mathematician, Giovanni
Alfonso **Borelli** (1608–79),
whose *De motu animalium*
(1680–81) at once suggests
a follower of Harvey. A
pupil of Galileo, Borelli
profited much by a long
association with his col-
league Malpighi, and his
r i g o r o u s mathematical
reasoning   swept   away
many current superstitions
about the true functions
of the muscles, the lungs,

Giovanni Alfonso Borelli (1608–79).

and the stomach. He treated locomotion, respiration, and digestion (the grinding and crushing action of the stomach) as purely
mechanical processes. His ultimate theory of muscular action
was dubious, as based upon the erroneous idea that a contracting
muscle actually increases in bulk by reason of a fermentation
started in its substance from a liquid discharged through the
nerves,—the *succus nerveus*,—which was Borelli's substitute for
the Galenic "animal spirits." In this way, Borelli originated
the neurogenic theory of the heart's action, in virtue of which
the heart-beat is attributed to the action of extrinsic or intrinsic
nerves. The men of the Iatromathematical School knew or cared

little about the new science of chemistry, and their efforts finally dwindled away into such sterile eccentricities as Edward Barry's attempts to estimate a man's age from the frequency of his pulse, or Clifford Wintringham's efforts to weigh an individual spermatozoön. The effect of mathematical and experimental physics upon medicine was manifested in more important ways, notably in the first attempt to put pulse counting and clinical thermometry upon a working basis.

In the fifteenth century, as Walsh points out,[1] Cardinal Cusanus (Nikolaus Krebs of Cues) (1401–64), a Roman Catholic churchman who was a good mathematician, made some timely suggestions in his Dialogue on Statics (1450) as to the possible clinical value of weighing the blood and the urine, and of comparing the frequency of the pulse and respiration in disease with that in a normal control, as estimated by the clepsydra, or waterclock. These, however, were not put into effect or carried into practice, and remained unnoticed by succeeding generations. Between 1593 and 1597, as Dr. Weir Mitchell has shown,[2] Galileo had invented a rude thermometer or thermoscope, and as early as 1600 Kepler had used pulse-counting to time his astronomic observations. Later, Galileo conceived the idea of using his own

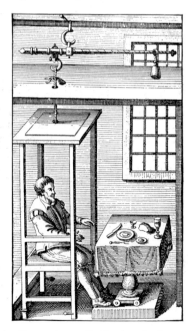

Sanctorius on the Steelyard. (From his Ars de statica medicina, Leyden, 1711.)

pulse to test the synchronous character of a pendulum's vibrations, which led him to the converse proposition of measuring the rate and variation of the pulse by a pendulum, much as a metronome is used to check the tempo of music. These ideas were appropriated and utilized in a remarkable way by the celebrated Paduan professor, Santorio Santorio (1561–1636), usually called **Sanctorius.**

[1] See J. J. Walsh: Old-Time Makers of Medicine, New York, 1912, pp. 336–348.

[2] See S. Weir Mitchell: The Early History of Instrumental Precision in Medicine, New Haven, 1892, p. 10 et seq.

In his commentary on the first book of the canon of Avicenna (Venice, 1625), Sanctorius describes a clinical thermometer[1] and a pulsilogium, or pulse-clock, of his own devising, inventions which soon passed into the limbo of forgotten things for nearly a hundred years. Sanctorius was also the clever inventor of instruments for extracting stones from the bladder and foreign bodies from the ear, as also a trocar, a cannula, and a hygroscope. His medical fame today is best associated with the fact that he founded the physiology of metabolism through his experiments and data upon what he called the "insensible perspiration" of the body. The frontispiece plate in later editions of his "Ars de statica medicina" (1614), representing the famous Paduan seated in his steelyard chair, in act to weigh himself for a metabolism experiment after a meal, is a familiar human document in the annals of medical illustration.

The physical theory of vision, which might be styled the ground-bass of **ophthalmology,** owes its development mainly to the work of great astronomers and physicists. The "Ad Vitellionem, Paralipomena," of the astronomer Kepler (Frankfort, 1604), contains a treatise on vision and the human eye in which is shown for the first time how the retina is essential to sight, the part the lens plays in refraction, and that the convergence of luminous rays before reaching the retina is the cause of myopia. In the "Dioptrica" of René **Descartes** (1637) the eye is compared to a camera obscura, and its accommodation is shown to be due to changes in the form of the lens. It was Edme Mariotte (died 1684) who proved that a luminous eye is due to reflection of light, and discovered the blind spot in the retina (1668). A remarkable pioneer in physiologic optics was the Jesuit astronomer Christoph **Scheiner** (died 1650), of Vienna. In his "Oculus" (Mühldorf, 1619) Scheiner gave an ingenious demonstration of how images fall on the retina, noticed the changes in curvature of the lens during accommodation, and illustrated accommodation and refraction by the pin-hole test which bears his name.

The founder of the **Iatrochemical School** was the Belgian mystic Jean Baptiste **van Helmont** (1577–1644), who, before he studied medicine, was some time a Capuchin friar. Like his master, Paracelsus, van Helmont believed that each material process of the body is presided over by a special archæus, or spirit (which he calls Blas), and that these physiologic processes are in themselves purely chemical, being due in each case to the agency of a special ferment (or Gas). Each Gas is an instrument in the

---

[1] Drebbel is usually regarded as the inventor of the air thermometer, Galileo, of the spirit thermometer, and Roemer, of the mercurial thermometer.

hands of its special Blas, while the latter are presided over by a sensory-motive soul (*anima sensitiva motivaque*), which van Helmont locates in the pit of the stomach, since a blow in that region destroys consciousness. He was the first to recognize the physiological importance of ferments and gases, particularly of carbonic acid, which he described as *gas sylvestre*, and his knowledge of the bile, the gastric juice, and the acids of the stomach was considerable. His claims to the discovery of carbon dioxide (CO_2) are somewhat vitiated by the fact that he regarded this "gas sylvestre," formed in vinous fermentation, as identical with the gas in the Grotto del Cane in Italy, and with the *dunste*, or deadly vapor of burning charcoal, the former of which is CO_2, the latter carbon monoxide (CO). Van Helmont introduced the gravimetric idea in the analysis of urine, and actually weighed a number of twenty-four-hour specimens, but drew no deductions of value from his measurements.

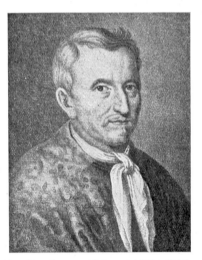

Jean Baptiste van Helmont (1577–1644).

Physiological chemistry was divested of most of the fantastic trappings which van Helmont gave it by the Leyden professor, Franciscus de le Boë, or **Sylvius** (1614–72), and his pupils, Willis, de Graaf, Stensen, and Swammerdam. Sylvius, who did for Harvey's ideas what Paré had done for those of Vesalius, has been described by Sir Michael Foster as an expositor, rather than an investigator of science, but even as a teacher, and there were none greater in his time, he was wonderfully fertile in original ideas about the function of the ductless glands, the thermal and tactile senses, and other things of moment today. He was the first to distinguish between conglomerate and conglobate glands, but his relation to the Sylvian fissure, as described in his "Disputationes medicæ" (1663), is obscure. He regarded digestion as a chemical fermentation, and recognized the importance of the saliva and the pancreatic juice. His real service to medicine was that he took a firm stand upon the ultimate identity of organic and inorganic processes in chemistry, and that, in his little infirmary of twelve beds at Leyden, he was one of the first to introduce ward instruction in medical education.

13

Thomas **Willis** (1621–75), a Wiltshire farmer's son, who graduated from Christ Church College in 1639, was Sedleian Professor of Natural Philosophy at Oxford in 1660, and, moving to London in 1666, acquired the largest fashionable practice of his day. Willis' "Cerebri Anatome" (1664), in the preparation of which he was greatly indebted to Richard Lower and to Sir Christopher Wren (who illustrated it), was the most complete and accurate account of the nervous system which had hitherto appeared. It contains the classification of the cerebral nerves, which held the field up to the time of Soemmerring, the first description of the eleventh cranial (spinal accessory) nerve or

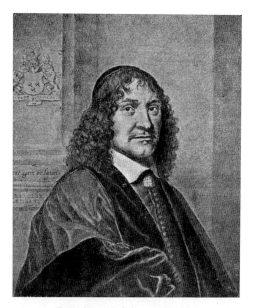

Franciscus Sylvius (1614–72).

"nerve of Willis," and of the hexagonal network of arteries at the base of the brain which is called by his name. His reasoning about the physiology of the nervous system was, in many respects, erroneous and obscure, and this obfuscation has caused some writers, Sir Michael Foster, for instance, to overlook his just merits as a clinician. Willis was, like Sydenham, Heberden, and Bright, a remarkable example of the capacity of the English physicians for close, careful clinical observation. He made the best qualitative examination of the urine that was possible in his time, and was the first to notice the characteristic sweetish taste of diabetic urine, thus establishing the basic principle for the diagnosis between diabetes mellitus and the insipid form. In his "London Practice of Physic" (1685)[1] he described the Erb-Goldflam symptom-complex (myasthenia gravis), and in his "De febribus," he gave the first account of epidemic typhoid fever as it occurred in the troops of the Parliamentary Wars (1643).[2] He was also the first to describe and name puerperal fever. His works on nervous diseases (1667)[3] and on hysteria (1670)[4] are justly esteemed for their many striking clinical pictures, of which his description of dementia paralytica is perhaps the most important. A good example of his talent for locating and

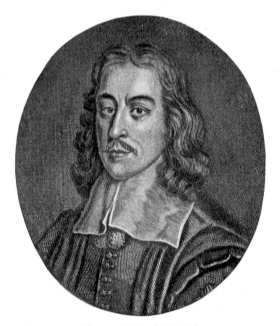

Thomas Willis (1621–75).

isolating important facts is his observation of a deaf woman who could hear only when a drum was beating. This phenomenon is known in modern otology as *paracusis* (or *hyperacusis*) *Willisii*, the test for paracutic hearing being made in the clinics by placing a vibrating tuning-fork on the head of a deaf patient or by means of the "noise machine" recently devised by the

---

[1] Pp. 431, 432.
[2] De febribus, London, 1659, 171 *et seq.*
[3] Pathologiæ cerebri et nervosi generis specimen, Oxford, 1667.
[4] Adfectionum quæ dicuntur hystericæ, etc., Leyden, 1670.

Viennese otologist, Robert Bárány. Willis' "Pharmaceutice rationalis" (1674) gives a valuable epitome of the materia medica of his time.[1]

Regner **de Graaf** (1641–73), of Schoonhaven, Holland, was the first to study the pancreas and its secretions before the time of Claude Bernard. In his disputation on the nature and use of the pancreatic juice (1664),[2] he describes his method of collecting the secretion by means of a temporary pancreatic fistula, noting the small quantity of the juice secreted and its acid character. The monograph is embellished with a picture of the dog employed, showing receptacles depending from a parotid and a pancreatic

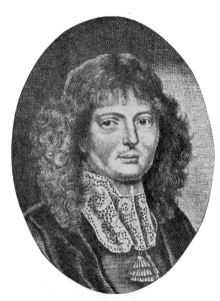

Regner de Graaf (1641–73).

fistula. De Graaf also employed an artificial biliary fistula to collect the bile, in which he was preceded, however, by Malpighi. In 1668,[3] he published a classic account of the testicle, which he described as made up of small tubes folded up into lobules. This work also contains an essay on the use of clysters, which were then coming into fashion. In 1672 appeared his work on the ovary, containing the first account of the structures which Haller called, in honor of his name, the Graafian vesicles (*vesiculæ Graafianæ*).

A prominent German physiologist of this period was Johann **Bohn** (1640–1719), of Leipzig, who experimented upon the decapitated frog (1686)[4] in an entirely modern spirit, declaring the reflex phenomena to be entirely material, as against the current view of "vital spirits" in the nerve-fluid. Baas calls Bohn the founder of state medicine in Germany.

---

[1] The second part has been praised by Osler (Practice of Medicine, 8th ed., 1912, p. 119) for its description of whooping-cough.

[2] De Graaf: Disp. med. de natura et usu succi pancreatici, Leyden, 1664.

[3] De Graaf: De virorum organis generationi inservientibus, Leyden, 1668.

[4] Bohn, Circulus anatomico-physiologicus, Leipzig, 1686, 460. Cited by Neuburger.

Important researches in the physiology of digestion were made by the Swiss anatomists Peyer and Brunner. The name of Johann Conrad **Peyer** (1653–1712), of Schaffhausen, Switzerland, will always be associated with the lesions of Peyer's patches in typhoid fever, although he held that these glands, which he discovered in 1677,[1] were not conglobate or lymphatic, as we now know them, but conglomerate, secreting, as he believed, a digestive juice. He gives an interesting cut of the Peyer glands in the small intestine and the solitary follicles in the large intestine. He also wrote on the physiology of rumination (Merycologia, 1685).

Johann Conrad **Brunner** (1653–1727), of Diessenhofen, Switzerland, discovered Brunner's glands in the duodenum of dogs and man in 1672, publishing his results in 1687.[2] He believed that they secreted a juice similar to that of the pancreas. He also made experimental excisions of the spleen and pancreas in the dog in 1683,[3] keeping the animal alive, with normal digestion, for some time after. In one of these excisions, he found that the dog had extreme thirst and polyuria, which would seem to be a pioneer experiment on the internal secretions of the pancreas.

Niels **Stensen** (1638–86), or Steno, of Copenhagen, was, like Athanasius Kircher, a physician-priest, and, also like him, a man of wonderful versatility. He was at once a great anatomist, physiologist, geologist, and theologian, and became Bishop of Titiopolis some time after his conversion from the Lutheran to the Catholic faith in 1667. In anatomy, his name is permanently associated with the excretory duct of the parotid gland (Steno's duct), which he discovered in the sheep in 1661.[4] In the same year, he investigated the glands of the eye and, in 1664,[5] came his observations on muscles and glands in which he recognizes the muscular nature of the heart. His Paris discourse on the anatomy of the brain (1669)[6] contains much acute criticism of the physiologic errors of his time, particularly those of Willis, who located common sense in the corpora striata, imagination in the corpus callosum, and memory in the cortical substance. Stensen's further studies on the physiology of muscles (1667)[7] treat the subject

---

[1] Peyer: Exercitatio anat. med. de glandulis intestinorum earumque usu et affectionibus, Schaffhausen, 1677.

[2] Brunner: De glandulis in duodeno intestino detectis, Heidelberg, 1687.

[3] Experimenta nova circa pancreas, Amsterdam, 1682.

[4] Steno: Observationes anatomicæ, Leyden, 1662.

[5] De musculis et glandulis observationum specimen, Copenhagen, 1664.

[6] Discours sur l'anatomie du cerveau, Paris, 1669.

[7] Elementorum myologiæ specimen, seu musculi descriptio geometrica, Florence, 1667.

from a purely mechanical and mathematical standpoint, regarding
the individual muscles as parallelepipeds, and opposing the view
entertained by Borelli that the increase in size of a muscle is due
to the influx of hypothetic juices. Stensen was also one of the
leading founders of geology. In 1883, a bust over his tomb, in
the Basilica San Lorenzo in Florence, was erected and unveiled
by geologists of all nations. His treatise, "De solido intra solidum" (1669), contains, after Avicenna and Fracastorius, the
most important work on the production of strata, fossils, and
other geologic formations. He was led to geology by the dissec-

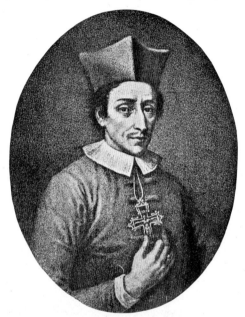

Niels Stensen (1638–1686).

tion of the head of a dog-fish, the teeth of which made it clear to
him that the "glossopetræ" found in Tuscany were in reality
fossil teeth. The story of Stensen's conversion to Catholicism
by a sister of the faith, and of his devotion of the better half of his
short life to the furthering of its cause alone, is one of the romantic
episodes of human history.

Francis **Glisson** (1597–1677), of Rampisham in Dorsetshire,
was a graduate of Cambridge and Regius Professor of Physic in
that University for some forty years. He was also one of the
founders of the Royal Society and president of the Royal College
of Physicians in 1667–69. As anatomist, physiologist, and pathol-

ogist, Glisson was highly praised by Haller and Virchow, and his name is famous for three important things: He gave the original and classical account of infantile rickets (1650),[1] he gave the first accurate description of the capsule of the liver investing the portal vein (Glisson's capsule) and its blood-supply (1654),[2] and, before Haller, he introduced the concept of "irritability" as a specific property of all human tissues (1677).[3] Glisson's view of this property was, however, purely metaphysical, bound up with the current notions about "vital spirits," and, in consequence, it had no effect upon the physiology of his time.

The most brilliant outcome of Harvey's experimental method was in the clearing-up of the obscure matter of the **physiology of respiration,** which, up to the time of Lavoisier, was entirely the work of English scientists. Before Harvey's time, men still believed, with Galen, that the object of respiration was to cool the fiery heart, the purpose of the chest movements being to introduce air for generating vital spirits by the pulmonary vein, and to get rid of the heart's smoky vapors by the same channel. This Galenic notion was not a mere piece of symbolism, as in Richard Crashaw's poem on St. Teresa (The Flaming Heart), but was part and parcel of actual belief about the physics of the circulation. Harvey's demonstration disposed of all this by showing that the blood is changed from venous to arterial in the lungs, but beyond that point, as even Pepys has recorded in his Diary, no one could tell how or why we breathe.[4] The successive steps in what Sir Clifford Allbutt has called "the pathetic quest for oxygen" were as follows: First, the distinguished chemist Robert **Boyle** (1627–91) made experiments with flames and animals *in vacuo* (1660), demonstrating that air is necessary for life as well as for combustion.[5] Next, Robert **Hooke** (1635–1703), in 1667,[6] showed, by blowing a bellows briskly over the open thorax of a dog, that artificial respiration can keep the animal alive without any movement of either chest or lungs. This experiment, which had also been performed by Vesalius, proved that the essential feature of respira-

---

[1] Glisson: De rachitide sive morbo puerili qui vulgo the rickets dicitur, tractatus, London, 1650.

[2] Anatomia hepatis, London, 1654.

[3] De ventriculo et intestinis, London, 1677.

[4] "But what among other fine discourse pleased me most was Sir G. Ent about Respiration; that it is not to this day known or concluded among physicians, nor to be done either, how the action is managed by nature, or for what use it is," Pepys' Diary, Mynors Bright's ed., London, 1900, v, 191.

[5] R. Boyle: Nova experimenta physico-mechanica de vi aëris elastica, Rotterdam, 1669.

[6] R. Hooke: "A supply of fresh air necessary for life," Phil. Tr., 1667, London, 1700, iii, 66.

tion is not in its intrinsic movements, but certain blood changes in the lungs. The next step was made by Richard **Lower,** of Cornwall (1631–91), an able physiologist and successful practitioner, who was the first to perform direct transfusion of blood from one animal to another (February, 1665),[1] and who, with Schneider, overthrew the old Galenic idea (even upheld by Vesalius), that the nasal secretions originate in the pituitary body (1672).[2] About 1669,[3] Lower injected dark venous blood into the insufflated lungs, and concluded that its consequent bright color was due to the fact that it had absorbed some of the air passing

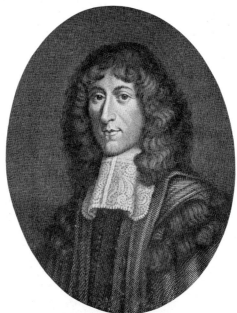

John Mayow (1643–1679).

through the lungs. Finally John **Mayow** (1643–79), another Cornishman, demonstrated, in a series of convincing experiments, that the dark venous blood is changed to bright red by taking up a certain ingredient in this air which, as being a constituent of nitre

[1] R. Lower: "A method of transfusing blood," Phil. Tr., 1666, London, 1700, iii, 226–232.   Denys of Paris was the first to transfuse in man (June 15, 1667), after which Lower performed the operation on Arthur Coga, before the Royal Society (November 23, 1667).

[2] C. V. Schneider, De catarrhis, Wittenberg, 1660–62.   R. Lower: "Dissertatio de origine catarrhi in qua ostenditur illum non provenire a cerebro," in his Tractatus de corde, London, edition of 1680, 163, 175.

[3] R. Lower: Tractatus de corde, London, 1669.

(KNO_3), he termed the igneo-aërial particles or nitro-aërial spirit of air. Mayow was thus, in a sense, very close to the actual discovery of oxygen, and he fully grasped the idea that the object of breathing is simply to cause an interchange of gases between the air and the blood, the former giving up its nitro-aërial spirit (oxygen) and taking away vapors engendered by the blood. He saw that the maternal blood supplies the fetus not only with food, but with oxygen ("nitro-aër"), and was the first to locate the seat of animal heat in the muscles, an idea which fell into abeyance until Helmholtz demonstrated it anew in 1845. He also discovered the double articulation of the ribs with the spine, and discussed the function of the intercostal muscles in an entirely modern spirit. Mayow was a chemist and physiologist of true genius, and his "Tractatus Quinque" (1668) deservedly ranks today with the very best of the English medical classics. Professor Gotch has shown how his ideas were disregarded and discredited through the errors in a garbled English abstract of his Latin text, which some literary hack had made for the Royal Society.[1]

In the latter half of the seventeenth century, **internal medicine** took an entirely new turn in the work of one of its greatest figures, Thomas **Sydenham** (1624–89), the reviver of the Hippocratic methods of observation and experience, who ennobled the practice of physic through those qualities of piety, good humor, and good sense, which Edmund Burke declared to be the genius of the English race. Educated at Oxford and Montpellier, but afterward a Puritan captain of horse in the civil wars, a "trooper turned physician," as he was called, Sydenham's relation to medicine was that of a man of action. A typical Saxon, by no means devoid of *nil admirari*, yet rich in the Saxon's special gift of manly independence and "saving common sense," he stood apart from all the medical theorizing and scientific experimentation of his time, disregarded all his predecessors save Hippocrates, and knew nothing whatever of Vesalius, Harvey, Malpighi, or Mayow. His four favorite books were Hippocrates, Cicero, Bacon, and Don Quixote, and his personal attitude toward his contemporaries was indifferent or scornful. This narrowness and aloofness cost him dear, for he complained bitterly of the neglect and opposition of his own profession, yet it was the very secret of his success as an internist. His theory of medicine was simple. The human mind is limited and fallible, and to it final causes must remain inscrutable. Scientific theories are, therefore, of little value to

---

[1] Francis Gotch: Two Oxford Physiologists, Oxford, 1908, pp. 35–38. See, also, the brilliant chapters on the physiology of respiration in Sir Michael Foster's "Lectures on the History of Physiology," Cambridge, 1901, 174–199; 224–254.

the practitioner since, at the bedside, he must rely upon his powers of observation and his fund of experience. Pathology, for Sydenham, was summed up in the Hippocratic theory of concoction of the humors of the body and the subsequent discharge of the *materies morbi*. Hippocrates was his pattern, and more than any other medical man he resembles the Father of Medicine in his mode of portraying disease and his dignified ethical regard for his patients, holding himself "answerable to God" for their care and, himself a martyr to stone and gout, a fellow-sufferer along with them. This power of imaginative sympathy, a trait not usually found in the self-centered

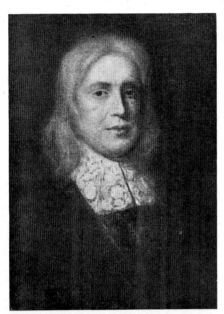

Thomas Sydenham (1624–1689.) (From a painting by Mary Beale.)

Saxon, is prominent in Sydenham's portrait as painted by Mary Beale, representing a Puritan in bearing, like Cromwell or Milton, yet a beautiful face withal, the fine brow, melancholy eye, and sensitive mouth revealing a nature stoical rather than harsh, sad rather than sour, as of a Puritan under protest.

Sydenham's theory of epidemic constitutions, attributing contagion to atmospheric or subterranean conditions, is obsolete, although some features of it were revived in von Pettenkofer's theory of the "soil" (*Boden*) and "soil-water." The fame of Sydenham rests today upon his first-hand accounts of diseases, such as the malarial fevers of his time, gout, scarlatina, measles, bronchopneumonia (*peripneumonia vera*), and pleuropneumonitis (*peripneumonia notha*), dysentery, chorea, and hysteria. His treatise on gout (1683)[1] is esteemed his masterwork. In 1672 he described the articular and muscular pains of dysentery, and, in 1675, gave a full account of scarlatina as it prevailed in London (1661–75), separating the disease from measles and identifying it by its present name. The

---

[1] Tractatus de podagra et hydrope, London, 1683.

"Dissertatio Epistolaris" (1682) contains his classic account of hysteria; and his differentiation of chorea minor is to be found in his "Schedula Monitoria" (1686). In therapeutics, Sydenham popularized the use of Peruvian bark (introduced by the Jesuits in 1632), and was the innovator of fresh air in sick-rooms, horseback riding for consumptives, cooling drafts in small-pox, steel tonics in chlorosis, and the liquid opiate which bears his name. His prescriptions consisted largely of vegetable simples, and he avoided the filthy ingredients recommended, even in the London Pharmacopœia of his time. He was an extensive but not an intensive blood-letter, applying venesection in almost every disease known to him, but with discretion. His "Processus integri" (1692), containing his therapeutic scheme, was the *vade mecum* of the English practitioner for more than a century, and an Oxford enthusiast is said to have committed it to memory.

A group of important monographs which deserve mention in connection with Sydenham's work comprises Daniel Sennert's treatise on fevers (1627),[1] Diemerbroek on the plague (1646),[2] Glisson's original account of rickets (1650),[3] Thuillier's experimental investigation of ergotism (1657),[4] Höfer on cretinism (1657),[5] Wepfer on apoplexy (1658),[6] Solleysel's account of the transmission of glanders from horse to horse (1664),[7] Morton's "Phthisiologia," summing up the knowledge of his time (1689), and Stahl on diseases of the portal system (1698).[8] In 1614 Felix **Platter** (1536–1614) reported the first known case of death from hypertrophy of the thymus gland in an infant. Beriberi was first described, from East Indian cases, by the Dutch physicians, Jacob Bontius (1642)[9] and Nicholas Tulp (1652).[10] Sir John Floyer's "Treatise on Asthma" (1698) gives a postmortem of pulmonary emphysema, and assigns as the cause of spasmodic asthma "a contracture of the muscular fibers of the bronchi." In this group we may also include Felix Platter's "Praxis medicæ" (1602–8), containing the first attempt at a systematic classification of diseases, the "Sepulchretum" of Théophile Bonet (1679), a storehouse of postmortems, Walter Harris's book on diseases of children (1689),[11] and the treatises on medical jurisprudence by Fortunato **Fedeli** (1602),[12] Rodericus à Castro (1614),[13] and Paolo Zacchias (1621–35).[14] Fedeli's little book has an interesting copper-plate frontispiece, in which the attestation of virginity and time of delivery, the jurisprudence of poisoning, lethal wounds, hereditary

[1] Sennert: De febribus, Leyden, 1627.

[2] Diemerbroek: De peste, Arnheim, 1646.

[3] Glisson: De rachitide, London, 1650.

[4] Thuillier: J. d. sçavans, Paris, 1676, iv, 79.

[5] Höfer: Hercules medicus, Vienna, 1657, p. 43.

[6] Wepfer: Observationes anatomicæ ex cadaveribus eorum quos sustulit apoplexia, Schaffhausen, 1658.

[7] De Solleysel: Le parfait mareschal, Paris, 1664.

[8] Stahl: De vena portæ, porta malorum, 1698.

[9] Bontius: De medicina Indorum, Leyden, 1642, pp. 115–120.

[10] Tulp: Observationes medicæ, Amsterdam, 1652, 300–305.

[11] Harris: De morbis acutis infantum, London, 1689.

[12] Fedeli: De relationibus medicorum, Palermo, 1602.

[13] à Castro: Medicus politicus, Hamburg, 1614.

[14] Zacchias: Quaestiones medico-legales, Rome, 1621–35.

disease, torture, monsters, and the formation of the fetus are amusingly "featured," showing the interest which these subjects had acquired; and Paolo **Zacchias** (1584–1659), who was protomedicus of Rome, physician to Popes Innocent X and Alexander VII, is replete with medico-legal information, particularly on wounds of the eye and the jurisprudence of insanity, of which he gives an excellent classification. An important work on the medico-legal relations of surgery was published in 1684[1] by Nicholas de Blegny (1652–1722), who also founded the first medical journal (1679)[2] and made the first city directory (1684). Germany made many contributions to forensic medicine and medical ethics in this period, such as those of Ludwig Hoernigk, on the duties of the profession (1638),[3] Paul Ammann, on lethal wounds (1690),[4] Gottfried Welsch, on lethal wounds (1660) and plural births (1667),[5] Melchior Sebiz, on the signs of virginity (1630).[6] The "Medicus Peccans" of Ahasver Fritsch (Nuremberg, 1684) is an early contribution to medical ethics. The most important medico-legal contribution of the century was undoubtedly Swammerdam's discovery that the fetal lungs will float on water after respiration (1667),[7] which was first put to a practical proof by Johann Schreyer in the case of a fifteen-year-old peasant girl accused of infanticide (1681),[8] the sinking of the infant's lungs securing acquittal.

To English medicine belongs the first book on **vital statistics,** the "Natural and Political Observations upon the Bills of Mortality" (London, 1662) of John **Graunt.** The Hebrews and the Romans had, no doubt, taken the census and counted troops, but Graunt was the first to notice, from the bills of mortality, that more boys are born than girls, and that the population can be estimated from an accurate death-rate, thus making the first step in the application of mathematical methods to the interpretation of statistics. His book was followed, in 1687, by the "Essays in Political Arithmetic" of Sir **William Petty** (1623–87), who took the first census of Ireland.

In 1672 the Welsh physician Charles Clermont published a work with the Hippocratic title, "On the Airs, Waters, and Places of England," in which he plotted off the medical topography of the country as Daniel Drake did long after for the Mississippi Valley. The mineral waters of England were studied by a large number of seventeenth century physicians, notably Edmond Deane (1626), Edward Jorden (1631), Thomas Guidott (1681), Martin Lister (1682), Sir Patrick Dun (1683), Sir John Floyer (An Inquiry into the Right Use of the Hot, Cold and Temperate Baths in England, 1697), and Nehemiah Grew's study of Epsom Wells (1698).[9]

[1] de Blegny: La doctrine des rapports de chirurgie, Lyons, 1684.

[2] Nouvelles découvertes sur toutes les parties de la médecine, Paris,1679–81.

[3] von Hoernigk: Politia medica, Frankfurt, 1638.

[4] Ammann: Praxis vulnerum lethalium, Frankfurt, 1690.

[5] Welsch: Vulnerum lethalium judicium, 1660; and De gemellis et partu numeriori, 1667.

[6] Sebiz: De notis virginitatis, 1630.

[7] Swammerdam: Tractatus phys.-anat.-med. de respiratione usque pulmonum, Leyden, 1667.

[8] Schreyer: Erörterung und Erläuterung der Frage: Ob es ein gewiss Zeichen (etc.), Zeitz, 1690.

[9] These data about mineral baths are given by Handerson in his translation of Baas's History of Medicine, New York, 1889, p. 546.

The first London Pharmacopœia was published in 1618, having been preceded by those of Valerius Cordus (1540), Brice Bauderon (1588), Libavius (1606), Jean de Renou (1615), and other city pharmacopœias of the sixteenth century.[1] It passed through many editions, all of which were disfigured by the retention of the usual vile and unsavory ingredients, which were not thrown out until William Heberden made an onslaught upon these superstitions in 1745. The Pharmacopœia Londinensis was translated into English in 1649 by the famous herbalist and quacksalver, Nicholas Culpeper. Other English Pharmacopœias of the time were Philemon Holland's Latin translation from the French of Bauderon (1639), Salmon's "New London Dispensatory" (1678), and Skipton's "Pharmacopœia Bateana" (1688), compiled from prescriptions of William Bate, physician in ordinary to Charles I, Cromwell, and Charles II.[2] Of continental pharmacopœias, Baas[3] mentions those of Minderer (1621), Poterie (1622), Schröder (1641), Zwelfer of Augsburg (1652), Jüngken (1677), Nicolas Lémery (1697), and C. F. Paulini's "Heilsame Dreckapotheke" (1696), the title of which amply symbolizes the tendency of many seventeenth century prescriptions.

The most important contribution of the seventeenth century to **veterinary medicine** was Jacques de Solleysel's demonstration of the transmission of glanders from horse to horse (1664). Andrew Snape, on "The Anatomy of an Horse," was published in London in 1686, and various French works on farriery appeared, in particular, Francini's translation of Carlo Ruini (1607), Beaugrand (1619, 1646), and de Bouvray (1660). The first German work on veterinary medicine was the "Bellerophon" of Winter von Adlersflügel (1668).[4]

In comparison with the extensive development of anatomy in the seventeenth century, its literature of **surgery** seems meager. Among the Italians, we find no surgeons commensurate in rank with those of the three centuries preceding, and the only names deserving of mention are those of Cesare **Magati** (1579–1647), who followed Paré in holding that gunshot wounds are not poisonous, and taught, in theory at least, the simple expectant treatment of wounds by means of bandages moistened with plain water; and Pietro **de Marchetti** (1589–1673), Professor at Padua, whose "Observationum 'medico-chirurgicarum sylloge" (Padua, 1664) resembles the *Consilia* and the collections of Benivieni, Amatus Lusitanus, and Peter Forest, containing many strange case-histories and valuable surgical observations. The gigantic surgical anthology ("Thesaurus Chirurgiæ") of Peter Uffenbach (1610) deserves mention, although all the authors contained in it are of the sixteenth century.

The leading German surgeons of the period were Fabry of Hilden, Scultetus, and the famous army surgeon Purmann. Wilhelm **Fabry**[5] of Hilden (1560–1624), called Fabricius Hildanus, whose statue was recently unveiled in the city of

---

[1] All mentioned by Baas, *op. cit.*, pp. 436, 437, 546, 547.

[2] Baas: *Op. cit.*, footnote to p. 547.

[3] Baas: *Op. cit.*, p. 547.

[4] *Ibid.*, p. 543.

[5] The name is sometimes given in German as "Fabriz," but Sudhoff regards "Fabry" as the genitive of Faber, or Schmidt (Schmitz), a common family name in the Rhineland (München. med. Wochenschr., 1910, lvii, 1401).

Düsseldorf, is usually regarded as the "Father of German Surgery." Having a good classic education, he was strongly conservative in theory, supporting the views of the ancients, but in practice a bold and skilful operator, inventing many new instruments. In his monograph on gangrene (Cologne, 1593)[1] he was the first to recommend amputation above the diseased part, and is said to have been the first to amputate the thigh. He also wrote a treatise on lithotomy (Basel, 1626), but his most important work is his "Century of Surgical Cases" (1606–46), the best collection of case-records of the time. He showed that head injuries may cause insanity, extracted an iron splinter from the eye with a magnet, explored the auditory canal with a speculum of his invention, and devised the first field-chest of drugs for use in military medicine. In 1657 the Polish army surgeon, Janus Abraham a Gehema (1645–1700), author of a little manual for medical officers in the field (1689),[2] recommended that these chests be supplied, as a matter of course, by the government instead of at the expense of the officers, as formerly. Fabry of Hilden was a reactionary in his use of the cautery, and, like most surgeons of the day, he was a believer in the weapon-salve, which was applied to the weapon instead of the wound.

His contemporary, Johann Schultes (1595–1645), called **Scultetus**, is famous, like Albucasis and Paré before him, as one of the great illustrators of surgery and surgical instruments. His "Armamentarium Chirurgicum" (Ulm, 1653) gives us a good side-light on the operations of the time through its interesting plates, representing such procedures as amputation of the breast, reduction of dislocations, passage of sounds, forceps-delivery, etc.

Matthæus Gottfried **Purmann** (1649–1711) was a surgeon in the Brandenburg army in 1675, and acquired great skill and courage through his pillar-to-post operating in the field. With Fabry of Hilden, he is held in the highest esteem by the German historians of today, because he regarded anatomy as the true basis of the surgeon's knowledge. He seems to have performed most of the operations known or proposed in his time, from trephining (40 cases), transfusion, aneurysm, and bronchotomy, to suturing wounds of the intestines. He left many different works, one of the most interesting of which is "Fifty Strange and Wonderful Cures of Gunshot Wounds" (1693).[3] Needless to say, he was a believer in the weapon-salve and the sympathetic powder for healing wounds at a distance. Another important relic of the Thirty Years' War is the "Medicina

---

[1] De gangræno et sphacelo, Cologne, 1593.

[2] Gehema: Der wohlversuchte Feld-Medicus, Rostock, 1689.

[3] Purmann: Fünfzig sonder- und wunderbare Schusswundkuren, Frankfurt, 1693.

Militaris" of Raimund Minderer (Augsburg, 1620). Among pioneer operations of the German surgeons in the seventeenth century may be mentioned the gastrotomies of Florian Matthis (1602) and Daniel Schwabe (1635), the partial resection of the jaw by Acoluthus of Breslau in 1693, and Schonkoff's "ovariotomy" in 1685. At this time we may judge laparotomy to have been common enough, since plates in Roonhuyze (1663) and Völter's Midwifery (1679) give a very plausible representation of the procedure.

The "Several Chirurgicall Treatises" (1672) of the Royalist surgeon, Richard **Wiseman** (1622–76), is the leading work of a man who played the same part in the English surgery of his day that Sydenham did in the practice of medicine. Wiseman was a skilful operator, amputated above the diseased part, employed primary amputation in gunshot wounds of joints, and was the first to describe tuberculosis of the joints as "tumor albus." He also gave the authentic account of "King's Evil." In his treatise on gonorrhea he mentions the first case of external urethrotomy for stricture, which he performed with Edward Molins in 1652. The first case of amputation by means of a flap is recorded in the "Triumphal Chariot of Turpentine" (1679), by James Yonge (1646–1721).

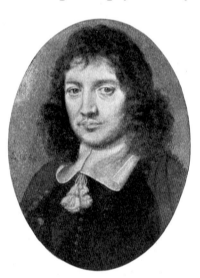

Richard Wiseman (1622–1676).

Seventeenth century **obstetrics** finds expression in the works of Mauriceau, de la Motte, Portal, van Deventer, Roonhuyze, and the midwives Louise Bourgeois, who attended Marie de Medici through her six labors; Justine Siegemundin, "Court Midwife to the Electorate of Brandenburg," whose treatise of 1690 met with great opposition because it was written in the German language, and the perhaps mythical Jane Sharp, whose "Compleat Midwife's Companion" was first published in London in 1671. Of these writers, François **Mauriceau** (1637–1709), of Paris, is in some respects the leading representative of the obstetric knowledge of his time, and his work on the diseases of pregnant and puerperal women (1668),[1] illustrated with exquisite copper plates, was

---

[1] Mauriceau: Traité des maladies des femmes grosses (etc.), Paris, 1668.

a sort of canon of the art in its time, giving a good account of the conduct of normal labor, the employment of version, and the management of placenta prævia. He was the first to correct the ancient view that the pelvic bones are separated in normal labor, and that the amniotic discharge is an accumulation of menstrual blood or milk; he was also the first to refer to tubal pregnancy, difficult labor from involvement of the umbilical cord, and epidemic puerperal fever. His book also gives an account of the author's adventure with the celebrated Hugh Chamberlen, of the Huguenot clan who succeeded in keeping their invention of an

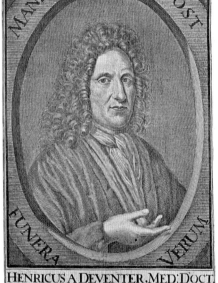

obstetric forceps a family secret for nearly two hundred years.[1]

Paul **Portal**[2] (died 1703), of Montpellier, wrote an obstetric treatise in 1685, in which he taught that version can be done by one foot and that face presentations usually run a normal course.

A far more important work is the *Novum Lumen* of Hendrik **van Deventer** (1651–1724), which, although printed in 1701, properly belongs to the seventeenth century. Van Deventer, a native of Holland, was at first a goldsmith, but turned to medicine at seventeen,

Hendrik van Deventer (1651–1724).

and after studying at Groningen, practised obstetrics and orthopedics in his native city, The Hague, until his death. He has been rightly called the father of modern midwifery, for his book, with its interesting plates, gives the first accurate description of the pelvis and its deformities, and the effect of the latter in complicating labor. At the same time it is a pioneer work in the delineation of deformities of the spine. There was nothing quite like it until "Das enge Becken" of Michaëlis was published, one hundred and fifty years later.

---

[1] The forceps was invented by Peter Chamberlen, Sr., about 1670; with it, Hugh Chamberlen failed to deliver a rachitic dwarf confided to him by Mauriceau.

[2] Portal: La pratique des accouchemens, Paris, 1685.

Hendrik van Roonhuyze (1625?–   ) was a champion of Cesarean section, which he seems to have performed several times with success, and his "Heelkonstige Aanmerkkingen" (1663) has been described as the first work on operative gynecology in the modern sense. It is illustrated with unique copper plates, showing his mode of incision in Cesarean section, and contains case reports of extra-uterine pregnancy and rupture of the uterus. Roonhuyze was otherwise a skilful operator, excising tumors, treating wounds of the head without trephining, and performing operations for wry-neck and hare-lip. Stromeyer says he was the first to practise orthopedic surgery. As Dr. Howard Kelly points out, he first proposed a scientific operation for vesico-vaginal fistula, the features of which were exposure of the fistula by a retracting speculum, with the patient in the lithotomy position, marginal denudation, exclusive of the bladder-wall, and approximation of the denuded edges of the fistula by means of quills fastened by silk threads.[1] He is not to be confused with his son, Rogier van Roonhuyze, to whom the elder Hugh Chamberlen is said to have sold the secret of his obstetric forceps about 1693.

Roonhuyze and Deventer did much to improve the status and education of midwives in Holland, in which they were followed by the former's successors in Amsterdam, Frederik Ruysch, and by Cornelis Solingen (1641–87).

A work which compares with Uffenbach's "Thesaurus Chirurgiæ" in size and shape is the huge "Hebammenbuch" of Gottfried Welsch (1652), consisting of nearly 2000 pages of translations, with commentaries, of the works of Mercurio, Pinæus, and Louise Bourgeois.

There was no printing press in the North American colonies before the year 1639, when one was set up at Cambridge, Massachusetts, its first publication being the Bay-State Psalm-Book of 1640. The only medical publication of the New England colonists in the seventeenth century was the "Brief Rule to Guide the Common People of New England how to Order themselves and theirs in the Small Pocks or Measels" (Boston, 1677), by Dr. Thomas **Thacher** (1620–78), an Englishman who settled in New England in 1635, and in 1669 became pastor of the Old South Church, at the same time practising medicine with success. He was a good Hebrew and Arabic scholar, and wrote a Hebrew lexicon and a catechism, which are like the "Brief Rule" in that each of them occupies, as Handerson slyly observes, "only a single sheet of paper."

[1] H. A. Kelly: Tr. Am. Gynæc. Soc., Phila., 1912, xxxvii, pp. 8–10.

14

CULTURAL AND SOCIAL ASPECTS OF SEVENTEENTH CENTURY MEDICINE

The age of the rise of England and Holland was a time of spiritual and intellectual uplift, and the effect of the continued battle for freedom of thought was to make it a period of individual scientific endeavor rather than of concerted advancement of science. The stirring events of this age—the burning of Bruno (1600), the Thirty Years' War, the Fronde, the English Revolution, the embarkation of the Pilgrims, the anathemas hurled at Spinoza, the suicide of Uriel Acosta—all go to show that the superior men of the time felt themselves "in the presence of high causes." Although the wars of the Fronde riveted the bonds of monarchy and ecclesiasticism upon France, and although Germany was ruined by the Thirty Years' War, yet England and Holland were free, and the barbarities of feudalism became tempered down into real governmental activities, largely from the growing interest in the study and application of the law. From the time of the perhaps legendary discovery of Justinian's Pandects at Ravenna, about 1135, there had been a gradual attempt to regulate national and civil government, as well as the intercourse of nations, by the Roman law, and this was brought to a focus through the labors of the two greatest jurists of the period, Hugo Grotius (1583–1645), of Delft, Holland, and Samuel von Pufendorf (1632–94), of Chemnitz, Saxony. With better legal regulations and restrictions, the social status of the physician was correspondingly improved, although the surgeon was still under the ban, unless needed in wartime. In Germany, the physician proper was styled *medicus purus*, and often held definite official positions, such as physician in ordinary to a potentate (*medicus ordinarius*), state or city physician (*physicus*), or plague doctor (*medicus pestilentiarius*), all at high salaries; while army surgeons were called *Feldscheerer* because they had to shave the officers. The general run of surgeons were still roughly classed with the horde of barbers, bath-keepers, executioners, and vagrant mountebanks.

The condition of medicine was further improved by the ambitions of princes to found new universities, and by the introduction of two new factors of great moment, viz., the scientific society and periodical literature.

The seventeenth century marks the rise of many famous Dutch and Germanic **universities**, notably Harderwijk (1600), Giessen (1607), Groningen (1614), Rinteln (1621), Dorpat (1632), Utrecht (1636), Åbo (1640), Bamberg (1648), Herborn (1654), Duisburg (1655), Kiel (1665), Lund (1666), Innsbruck (1672), and Halle (1694). The idea of **scientific societies** originated in Italy. Porta's Secret Academy at Naples (1560) was followed by the Academy of the Lynxes (*Accademia dei Lincei*), which was founded at Rome, August 17, 1603, by Prince Federigo Cesi, its seal bearing the image of a fox. This at first consisted of a closed corporation of four members, who met to discuss new experiments, mathematical problems, and "the ornaments of elegant literature and philology, which, like a graceful garment, adorned the whole body of science." Although it encountered much opposition from the Church, it lived to include Galileo as one of its members, and still survives, publishing handsome transactions in quarto. In 1657, a similar society, called the Accademia del Cimento (Academy of Experiment), was established at Florence. In 1645 an "Invisible Society," similar to Porta's Secret Academy, was founded in London by Haak, Hartlieb, Boyle, Wren, Pelty, and others, and, in 1662, was chartered by Charles II as the Royal Society, which began to publish its world-renowned "Philosophical Transactions" in 1665. The latter soon reached such a high level of merit as to include many important works of Leeuwenhoek and Malpighi. Richelieu, in France, founded the famous Académie Française at Paris in 1635, with the object of improving the French language and literature; and in 1665 Colbert founded the Académie des Sciences, which began to publish its transactions ("Histoire" and "Mémoires") in 1699. In Germany the Society of Scientific Physicians (Gesellschaft naturforschender Aerzte), founded at Schweinfurt in 1652 by Johann Lorenz Bausch and others, became in 1677 the Imperial Leopoldine Academy of Scientists (Kaiserliche leopoldinische Akademie der Naturforscher), which had begun to publish its "Ephemeridæ" in 1670. These were followed by the Acta medica Hafniensia, edited by Thomas Bartholinus (Copenhagen, 1671–79), and the Acta eruditorum (Leipzig, 1682–1754). Detached periodical literature had, meanwhile, taken an independent course. Following the Venetian Foglietti of 1600, a city newspaper, edited by Verhoeven, had already appeared at Antwerp in 1605, to be followed, in turn, by the first German newspaper (Frankfurter Postamtszeitung) in 1615, the London Weekley News, first issued on May 23, 1622, and followed by Marchamont Nedham's Mercurius Britannicus (August 16, 1643), the Gazette de France, issued at Paris by the physician Théophraste Renaudot (May 30, 1631, and, in America, the solitary number one of the Publick Occurrences, edited by Benjamin Harris, and published at Boston, September 25, 1690. The new tendency was represented in science by the Journal des Sçavans of Paris (1665) and, in medicine, by the Nouvelles Découvertes sur Toutes les Parties de la Medécine of Nicolas de Blegny (Paris, 1679–81), usually regarded as the first medical periodical in the vernacular. It was translated into Latin, and continued by Théophile Bonet as the Zodiacus medico-gallicus (Geneva, 1680–85). The abortive Journal de Médecine (1681–85) of the abbé J. P. de la Roque was continued (1686) by Claude Brunet, who also edited a monthly Progrès de la Médecine (1695–1709).[1] De Blegny was also the author of a series of satirical sketches of his contemporaries, which, published as the "Mercure savant" (1684), became the original of subsequent "city directories." Théophraste Renaudot was the originator of pawn-shops and intelligence offices. When we reflect that a postal service did not exist on the continent of Europe before the year 1516,[2] the value of these scientific societies, periodicals, and directories for the more rapid dissemination of knowledge will at once appear.

The great centers of **medical education** in the seventeenth century were Leyden, Paris, and Montpellier. At Leyden were Sylvius, Ruysch, Nuck and Bidloo; van Deventer and Cornelis Solingen were at The Hague; Roonhuyze and Swammerdam at Amsterdam; Duverney, Vieussens, Pierre Dionis, Mauriceau, Jules Clément, and Paul Portal at Paris; Giorgio Baglivi at Padua, and

---

[1] Sudhoff: München. med. Wochenschr., 1903, 1, 455.

[2] Marco Polo describes an extensive courier service among the Chinese of his time, and Louis XI, in 1464, established an official service of mounted messengers (chevaucheurs en poste) in France, but the first mounted postal service for purely public use was established between Vienna and Brussels in 1516 by Franz von Thurn und Taxis.

212 HISTORY OF MEDICINE

no less than Sydenham was a pupil of Charles Barbeirac at Montpellier. In Germany, however, medicine had little chance until
after the Peace of Westphalia (1648), and even after that time
many original scientific investigations all over Europe were made
by practising physicians detached from universities. It is not
without significance that the huge output of brilliant work in
anatomy and physiology followed directly upon the close of the
Thirty Years' War. In 1633, as Baas records, Ingolstadt had
only 3 students; in 1647, 2; but 16 in 1648; while Strassburg had
but 13 students during the entire period 1612–31, 4 in 1632–48,
and 6 in 1649–99. German medical instruction in this period
was, moreover, along the old medieval, scholastic lines, a mere
blind following of Galen and the Arabians, in opposition to the
folk-medicine of Paracelsus. A lively teapot-tempest was stirred
up by Thomasius in 1688, when he attempted to emulate the
example of Paracelsus by lecturing in the German language, and
the same prejudice was even encountered by Schönlein in 1840.
Sydenham, Glisson, and the Swiss physician, Theodore Turquet
de Mayerne, were the leading exponents of the bedside study of
disease in England, but, on the continent, the true clinical method,
introduced in Leyden as early as 1591 by Jan van Heurne (Heur-
nius)[1], was taught only by Sylvius, and perhaps by Barbeirac at
Montpellier. The usual method of teaching internal medicine
was to read off a perfunctory lecture in Latin, followed by a
number of prescriptions which were variously Galenical, Spagy-
rical, Iatro-Mathematical, Iatro-Chemical or Hermetic, and which
the students copied.

Dissecting as a means of teaching anatomy was more frequent
in Italy, Holland, and France than in Germany or England. In
the latter country, the material was usually obtained by grave-
robbing. In Germany, dissections, *longo intervallo*, were in the
nature of civic events attended by festivities. When Rolfink
began to have two annual dissections upon executed criminals at
Jena in 1629, the practice was held in holy horror by the peasantry,
who watched newly made graves lest they be "Rolfinked." A
skeleton for teaching purposes was a rarity, and although there
were anatomical theaters in most of the continental cities in course
of time, there was none in Edinburgh until 1697. The latter,
however, became the starting-point of the Edinburgh ascendancy
in anatomic teaching under the Monroe dynasty. In France,
Vieussens is said to have made as many as 500 dissections alone.
The popularity and frequency of dissecting in Holland are sufficiently evidenced in the canvases of the great Dutch artists of

---

[1] Janus, Amsterdam, 1912, xvii, 443.

the time. The earliest known of these is the "Anatomie" of Dr. Sebastian Egberts by Arend Pietersz (1603), in the Amsterdam Gallery, representing 28 physicians, with high ruffed collars and Vandyke beards, gathered around the demonstrator, who is about to insert the scalpel in the cadaver before him. Another "Anatomie" by Thomas de Keyser (1619), also in the Amsterdam collection, represents the same physician quizzically tickling the ribs of a hilarious skeleton, to the amusement of five of his friends. A superb document is the canvas of van Mierevelt in the Delft Hospital (1617), representing a body with exposed viscera, surrounded by Dr. van der Neer and 17 other figures, with all the accessories of dissecting. Rembrandt's famous Anatomy of Dr. Tulp (1632) at The Hague is sufficiently well known, and the same great master of realistic painting has, in the Amsterdam Gallery, a remarkable unfinished study of a foreshortened cadaver (1656), resembling Mantegna's picture of the Dead Christ, and styled the "Anatomie" of Dr. Johan Deyman. The finest of all these "Anatomies" are Adriaen Backer's, in the Amsterdam Gallery (1670), representing a dissection by Frederik Ruysch, and Johan van Neck's picture of the same master, demonstrating the viscera of an infant to five physicians, while a child toys with an infantile skeleton in the corner. As we survey the strong, valid faces of these Dutch physicians, richly clad in silk or velvet gowns, or jerkins with high ruffed collars, we get no bad idea of the dignity of the profession in the seventeenth century. In the Rembrandt pictures and two "Anatomies" of Frederik Ruysch the ruffed collars have already become Geneva bands. In Rembrandt's Doctor Tulp, as in Greenbury's "Anatomy" of Sir Charles Scarborough (1649) in the Barber's Hall, London, the short, lace-edged collar, which was evidently a token of wealth or worldly place, is in evidence.[1] An etching representing the Anatomical Theater at Leyden, of date 1610, shows a circular inclosure affording mere fence-rail accommodations for seats, the separate tiers of which are interspersed with stuffed birds, skeletons of animals, and human skeletons (one on horseback) bearing placards adorned with appropriate mortuary inscriptions. These skeletons and inscriptions were also a feature of Ruysch's famous anatomic museum at Leyden, which was purchased by Peter the Great in 1717 for 30,000 florins (about $75,000), and is still in a fair state of preservation in the Anatomical Museum of the Imperial Academy of Sciences at St. Petersburg. A second collection, which Ruysch afterward made, was, on the authority of Hyrtl, scattered and destroyed after his death.

---

[1] For reproductions and full descriptions of all these pictures see Eugen Holländer, Die Medizin in der klassischen Malerei, Stuttgart, 1903, pp. 34–60.

As the great Renaissance physicians had commonly followed botany or zoölogy as special lines of investigation, so we find the physician of the seventeenth century distinguishing himself as a mathematician and astronomer, a physicist, a microscopist, or a chemist. In university teaching, the most extraordinary versatility was sometimes displayed, Meibom, for instance, presiding over philosophy, philology, archeology, and geometry, as well as medicine (Baas). In physics, the work of Descartes, Kepler, Sanctorius, Hooke, Borelli, and Scheiner has been mentioned, and of physician-chemists we need refer only to van Helmont, who first used the term "gas," and knew the properties of hydrogen,

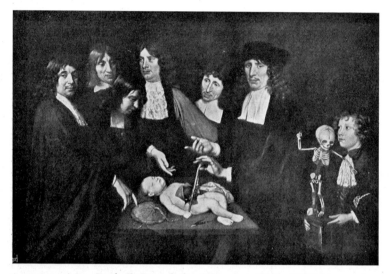

Anatomy of Dr. Frederik Ruysch by Johan van Neck (1683) (Amsterdam Museum), Hanfstaengl, Munich.

carbon dioxide, and sulphur dioxide; Leeuwenhoek and Redi, who were the first food chemists; Boyle, who first defined chemical "elements," founded analytical chemistry, and discovered that the pressure of a gas is proportional to its density (Boyle's law); John Mayow, who all but discovered oxygen; Minderer, who discovered ammonium acetate (spiritus Mindereri); Nicolas Lémery (1645–1715), who discovered iron in the blood; and Thomas Willis, who discovered the sweetish taste of diabetic urine. Johann Rudolph **Glauber** (1604–88), of Carlstadt, whose bust was used as a chemist's sign for nearly two hundred years, discovered sodium sulphate (Glauber's salt), made sulphate of copper, arsenic chloride, and zinc chloride, distilled ammonia from bones, and obtained hydrochloric acid by distilling sulphuric acid with sea-salt; investigated pyroligneous acid (acetum lignorum), did much for the chemistry of wines and spirits, and published a valuable encyclopedia of chemical procedures. He often sold "secrets" to manufacturers, was accused of selling the same secret several times, or of selling secrets which would not work, and his great secret, which he expressly declined to sell or publish, was the Alkahest, or Universal Solvent. Hence Oliver Cromwell said "This Glauber is an arrant knave"; but the latter was easily the greatest analyt-ical chemist of his time, and those of his calling who have had their discoveries stolen by their assistants have learned to appreciate his canny sense in keeping his business to himself. The secretive Glauber is particularly interesting, because he stands between the scientific chemists, like Boyle or Mayow, and those who deliber-ately followed alchemy. Although opposed by the Church in the famous bull, "*Spondent pariter,*" of John XXII (1317), alchemy became an intensive cult of extraordinary magnitude in the six-teenth and seventeenth centuries, because it appealed particularly to the lust of money, the love of life, and the corresponding fear of death. For the philosopher's stone, otherwise known as "the quintessence" or "grand magistery" was not only supposed to transmute the baser metals into gold, make precious stones, and a universal solvent, but also conferred perfect health and length of days. It was described by all who claimed to have seen it as of a reddish luster. Raymond Lully called it a carbuncle; Para-celsus likened it to a ruby; Berigard de Pisa, to a wild poppy with the smell of heated sea-salt; van Helmont, to saffron with the luster of glass (Thorpe).[1] The choral symphony in praise of its capacity for maintaining health resembled the testimonials of "Vin Mariani" and other nostrums of our time.

From the universal solvent it was but a step to a universal remedy, like that of Butler's French quack, who

> "Set up physic
> And called his receipt a general specific."

The effect of alchemy upon the medicine of the sixteenth and seventeenth centuries had been to create a number of offshoots of the Paracelsian or Spagyric School, which were variously termed Hermetic, Cabalistic, Zoroastrian, or Rosicrucian, according to

---

[1] The Alkahest, the name of Paracelsus' Universal Solvent, which could be prepared by the stone, was supposed to be derived from the Latin *alkali est,* from the German *all Geist* (all gas), or *Alles est* (it is all), but the chemist Johann Kunkel (1630–1704), who pointed out these derivations, said its true name was *Alles Lügen ist* (It's a lie); for "if it dissolved everything, no vessel could contain it." Sir E. Thorpe, History of Chemistry, London & New York, 1909, i, 46–56, 81.

the individual penchant for the doctrines of Hermes Trismegistus (the Egyptian Thoth), the Hebraic "oral tradition" or Cabala, the traditional "living word" (Zendavesta) of the Persian Zoroaster (Nietzsche's Zarathustra), or the cult of the mythical Christian Rosencreutz. The doctrine of the **Rosicrucians** emanated from three books of mystic and alchemistic jargon, which were published during the years 1614–16 and called the Fama Fraternitatis, the Confessio Fraternitatis, and the Chymical Marriage of Christian Rosencreutz. The supposititious author traveled in the East (as usual), where he learned necromancy, alchemy, and philosophy. Upon his return, he imparted the new knowledge to seven associates, forming the Brethren of the Rosy Cross, who were to follow science and to communicate their results to one another, to render free assistance to the sick poor, and to have no distinctive tokens of their cult except the letters "C. R." It goes without saying that they could manufacture gold, if so inclined, but, like the Spiritualists and Theosophists of our own time, disdained to make any practical use of their superior knowledge, which, they admitted, was obtained by direct illumination from God. It was subsequently discovered that the three basic texts of the Rosicrucian cult were written, not by Rosencreutz, but by the Württemberg pastor, Johann Valentin Andreas (1586–1654), who perpetrated this solemn piece of mystification in the same spirit in which Meinhold wrote "Sidonia the Sorceress." All the "six follies of science," viz., circle squaring, multiplication of the cube (fourth dimensional space or spiritism), perpetual motion (Cornelius Drebbel), judicial astrology, alchemy, and magic were rampant in seventeenth century medicine, and most of them were subjected to keenest ridicule by Butler, the archsatirist of his age. Prominent figures in the latter's "Hudibras" were Ralph, the Judicial Astrologer, who presumably purged and let blood by the signs of the zodiac, and was otherwise

"For profound
And solid lying much renowned."

And Sidrophel, the Rosicrucian and veterinarian

"To whom all people, far and near,
On deep importances repair:
When brass or pewter hap to stray,
And linen slinks out of the way:

. . . .

When cattle feel indisposition
And need the opinion of physician."

The dupes of astrologic physicians of this type were ridiculed in Congreve's "Love for Love" (1695), in the character of "Foresight, an illiterate old fellow, peevish and passive, superstitious, and pretending to understand Astrology, Palmistry, Physiognomy, Omens, Dreams, &c."; and Dr. Johnson, in his criticism of this play, assures us that "the character of Foresight was then common. Dryden calculated nativities; both Cromwell and King William had their lucky days; and Shaftesbury himself, though he had no religion, was said to regard predictions."[1] But the tendency was by no means confined to the learned laity. Minderer (of Spiritus Mindereri) advised the plague doctors to repeat the Twenty-second Psalm every time they approached a patient, just as the old Saxon Leechdoms urged the application of holy water and the intoning of Psalms LI, LXVII, and the Athanasian Creed over cattle afflicted with pleuropneumonia.[2] That able clinician, Daniel Sennert, believed in witchcraft and pacts with the devil. Sebastian Wirdig favored divining-rods and magic. Goclenius and Fabricius Hildanus were patrons of the weapon-salve, and, in 1658, the University of Montpellier heard Sir Kenelm Digby's celebrated discourse on the sympathetic powder, which Madame de Sévigné pronounced "a perfectly divine remedy" (January 28, 1685). **Digby,** an *Uebermensch* in his way, first leaped into prominence as a corsair in the Levantine sea-fight commemorated in Ben Jonson's droll couplet:

> Witness his action done at Scanderoon
> Upon his birthday, the eleventh of June.

Wealthy and courted, in spite of his father's imprisonment for treason, he dabbled in politics, religion, and science, got a hearing, although, according to Lady Fanshawe, "he enlarged somewhat more in extraordinary stories than might be averred," and wrote a unique autobiography. The sympathetic powder, his special hobby, consisted, it is said, of nothing more than green vitriol, first dissolved in water and afterward recrystallized or calcined in the sun. The Duke of Buckingham testified that Sir Kenelm had healed his secretary of a gangrenous wound by simply soaking the bloody bandage in a solution of the powder. Digby claimed to have got the secret remedy from a Carmelite monk in Florence, and attributed its potency to the fact that the sun's rays extracted the spirits of the blood and the vitriol, while, at the same time, the heat of the wound caused the healing principle thus produced to be attracted to it by means of a current of air—a sort of wireless therapy. Quite as amusing are the superstitions of the sympathetic or magnetic cure of wounds and the healing of disease by "stroking." The former originated with Paracelsus, and was exploited in 1608 by Rudolph Goclenius,

---

[1] Johnson: Lives of the Poets, *sub voce* Congreve.
[2] Cockayne: Saxon Leechdoms, i, 389.

one of his followers, in the tract, "De magnetica curatione vulneris." The treatment consisted in anointing the weapon which had inflicted the wound with the *unguentum armarium*, of the patient's blood and human fat, the wound itself being wrapped in wet lint. This doctrine was supported by Fabry of Hilden, Robert Fludd the Rosicrucian, and van Helmont, who attributed the cure to animal magnetism. The clergy held that the weapon cure was wrought by magic and the devil, and their view was set forth by William Foster in "Hoplocrisma Spongus, or a Sponge to Wipe away the Weapon-Salve" (1631). Robert Fludd (1619), van Helmont (1621), Kircher, in "Magnes" (1643), and William Maxwell (1679) were the early theorists about animal magnetism, which was carried into practice by Valentine Greatrakes (Greatorex) (1628–66), one of Cromwell's soldiers in Ireland, who achieved an enormous reputation in his "cures" of disease by laying on of hands (stroking) and the cure of scrofula with carrot poultices. The treatment of the latter disease was, however, the special prerogative of royalty. The King's Evil, or *morbus regius*, has recently been made the subject of an exhaustive and scholarly monograph by Dr. Raymond Crawfurd (1911), and the results of his original investigations of the medieval sources are briefly as follows:

> The personal power of healing, in the first instance, always an attribute of the gods, became, by natural association of ideas, a divine right of kings, and many instances of it are recorded by the Roman chroniclers and the fathers of the Church. Thus Helgald, a monk of the eleventh century, records that Robert the Pious (996–1031 A. D.) wrought cures by touch, and Guibert, Abbe de Nogent, bears witness that touching for scrofula (*scrophas circa jugulum*) was done by Philip I (1061–1108) of France, and his son Louis VI (1108–37). Shortly before his death, in 1066, Edward the Confessor touched for scrofula in England, on the authority of William of Malmesbury and a monkish chronicler of Westminster. The practice was continued by the French monarchs, even up to the time of Louis XVI, and was actually revived at the coronation of Charles X in 1824, no less than Dupuytren and Alibert presenting the 121 patients. In England, the Royal Touch fell into disuse among the Norman Kings after the Confessor, but was revived by Henry II, Henry III, and the three Edwards. Items in the wardrobe accounts of the latter show the payment of alms to the scrofulous poor. After Richard II's time, there is complete silence in the chronicles until 1462, when Henry VII revived the royal prerogative with an elaborate ritual, and, in 1465, the minting of a special coin, the gold Angel, as a touchpiece. The ceremonial and touchpieces were features of all subsequent reigns to the time of William of Orange, who treated the practice cavalierly; but Queen Anne revived it, even touching Dr. Johnson (without success). The exiled Stuarts "over the water" also upheld it, but it was practically discarded by George I.

It was in the seventeenth century that the practice of the Royal Touch reached its height. Richard Wiseman, one of the ablest surgeons of the time, wrote the classic account of the King's Evil, in which he bears ample witness to the healing power of Charles II. Shakespeare, in the time of James I (1607), describes (Macbeth, Act IV, sc. 3) how—

"strangely-visited people,
All swoln and ulcerous, pitiful to the eye,
The mere despair of surgery, he cures;
Hanging a golden stamp about their necks,
Put on with holy prayers."

The Royal Touch was not even subjected to ridicule in the *Pseu-dodoxia Epidemica; or Enquiries into Vulgar and Common Errors* (1646) of **Sir Thomas Browne** (1605–82), the old Norwich physician, whose delightful writings—*Religio Medici* (1643), *Urn Burial* (1658), and the rest—belong to literature proper, in the most exquisite sense. The "Religio Medici," with its quaint and original modes of expression, is an attempt to reconcile scientific skepticism with faith. The "Vulgar Errors," while nominally a critical onslaught upon superstition, displays the same delightful whimsicality through its author's credulous attitude toward many of the things he set out to ridicule.

Thus while the medical science of the seventeenth century was making rapid strides forward, its popular medicine was already in process of retrogression to the excesses of the Byzantine Period, which bears out our main thesis, that the folk-ways of medicine are inevitably the same and independent of time and place and circumstance. This can be easily verified by a glance at the **materia medica** of the period.

The first edition of the *London Pharmacopœia*, published in 1618, contains some 1960 remedies, of which 1028 were simples, 91 animal, 271 vegetable. Among these were worms, lozenges of dried vipers, foxes' lungs (for asthma), powders of precious stones, oil of bricks, oil of ants, oil of wolves, and butter made in May (for ointments). Among the 932 compounds, many of which had the names of their Greek and Arabian originators attached, were vegetable syrups, compound senna powder, Neapolitan (blue) ointment, Vigo's plaster (compounded of vipers' flesh, with live frogs and worms), and the celebrated antidote of Mattioli, made up of about 230 ingredients, including the multifarious mithridate (*confectio Damocratis*) and the theriaca Andromachi. The Pharmacopœia of 1650 contains cochineal, antimonial wine, the red and white mercurial precipitates, moss from the skull of a victim of violent death, and Gascoyne's powder, compounded of bezoar, amber, pearls, crabs' eyes, coral, and black tops of crabs' claws. In the Pharmacopœia of 1677, the names of the Greeks and Arabians disappear, showing that their influence had also declined, while jalap, cinchona bark, burnt alum, digitalis, benzoin, balsams of copaiba and tolu, steel tonics, and Irish whisky (*aqua vitæ Hibernorum sive usquebaugh*) make their appearance for the first time, as also human urine, so highly recommended by Madame de Sévigné (June 13, 1685).[1] Among the queer remedies contained in the three London Pharmacopœias of the period were the blood, fat, bile, viscera, bones, bone-marrow, claws, teeth, hoofs, horns, sexual organs, eggs, and excreta of animals of all sorts; bee-glue, cock's-comb, cuttlefish, fur, feathers, hair, isinglass, human perspiration, saliva of a fasting man, human placenta, raw silk, spider-webs, sponge, sea-shell, cast-off snake's skin, scorpions, swallow's nests, wood-lice, and the triangular Wormian

---

[1] The latter was also a warm advocate of viper meat, to "temper, purify, and refresh the blood," and gossip claimed that Sir Kenelm Digby poisoned his wife with too frequent doses of viper's wine, given in aid of preserving her good looks.

bone from the juncture of the sagittal and lambdoid sutures of the skull of an executed criminal (*ossiculum antiepilepticum Paracelsi*).[1] The Chinese materia medica itself could go no further than this toward demonstrating that the folk-mind is stationary or discontinuous. Yet Minderer prescribed oil of spiders and earthworms for plague, Robert Boyle recommended *album Græcum* as a homely but experienced remedy for dysentery, Nicolas Lémery, cat-ointment and oil of puppies boiled with earthworms, Mattioli, oil of scorpions, and Paracelsus, human ordure (*Zebethum occidentale*). Glauber alone, in an important treatise on salts (1658),[2] urged the employment of chemical preparations in lieu of animal excreta. Old Nicholas Culpeper, the arch herbalist and quacksalver of the time, indulged in a vast amount of scurrilous raillery at the expense of the London Pharmacopœias of 1618 and 1650, but, except for his herb-lore, he was himself only the credulous astrologer described by Nedham as "a frowsy-headed coxcomb" who had "gallimawfried the Apothecaries' Book into nonsense" in his aim to "monopolize to himself all the knavery and cozenage that ever an apothecary's shop was capable of."

Another curious feature of seventeenth century therapy was the large number of private or proprietary preparations. Prominent among these nostrums were the Scot's Pills (Grana Angelica), compounded by Patrick Anderson (1635) of aloes, jalap, gamboge, and anise (the modern pilulæ aloes et myrrhæ), which were, according to Wootton, successfully patented down to 1876, and are still asked for in the shops. The *Baume Tranquille*, compounded of herbs, by one of the Capuchins of the Louvre, was highly recommended by Madame de Sévigné (December 15, 1684). The *Baume Fioravanti*, another herbal tincture of the time, is still featured in the French Codex. Daffy's Elixir is still made. Dutch Drops, or Haarlem Oil, a mixture of oil of turpentine with other ingredients, has been used since 1672 as a "medicamentum" or routine preventive of disease. Charles II gave anywhere from £5000 to £15,000 for the formula of "Goddard's Drops," recommended by Sydenham, and said to have been made of raw silk. Carmelite water (*eau de Melisse des Carmes*), an aromatic cordial, made at the pharmacy of the Barefooted Carmelites near the Luxembourg in 1611, was patented in 1791, and sold up to 1840. Seignette's salts (*sal polychrestum*), devised 'about 1672, and a secret up to 1731, were Rochelle salts. Singleton's Golden Eye Ointment is described in Wootton's Chronicles as the oldest private remedy sold in England, and is still proprietary. Antimony, Basil Valentine's innovation, had an extraordinary vogue in the seventeenth century through the fact that tartar emetic cured Louis XIV of a dangerous illness in 1657. Tartar emetic was first described by Adrian Mynsicht in 1631, and may have been identical with the Earl of Warwick's Powder (1620). Kermes mineral, devised by Glauber in 1651, was a secret for which Louis XIV paid a high figure in 1720, under the guise of *poudre des Chartres*. Antimony cups (*pocula emetica*) were in common use in Germany, but disappeared toward the end of the century.[3]

Professional poisoning, as bad as that described in Livy and Cicero, was particularly rampant in Italy and France. Much of sixteenth and seventeenth century poisoning was, no doubt, intestinal obstruction, extra-uterine pregnancy, appendicitis, or what not. But the objects in the Musée de Cluny[4] and other data indicate that it was an ambition of the time

> To carry pure death in an earring, a casket,
> A signet, a fan-mount, a filigree basket,

---

[1] A. C. Wootton: Chronicles of Pharmacy, London, 1910, vol. ii, pp. 2–31.

[2] Glauber: Tractatus de natura salium, 1658.

[3] These nostrums are all described at length in Wootton's "Chronicles of Pharmacy," London, 1910, *passim*.

[4] For a description of these see L. Courtadon, in Æsculape, Paris, 1912, ii, 188–192.

and the scene in Swinburne's "Queen Mother," in which Catherine
de Medicis poisons her clown with a pair of gloves, is probably not
exaggerated. Such an Italian poisoner was Exili, who left Rome
for Paris, with a record of 150 cases against him, and came in contact with Sainte Croix, the paramour of the depraved Marquise de
Brinvilliers. From Exili, Sainte Croix is said to have learned of the
subtle compound with which his mistress disposed of her father,
two brothers, and many unfortunate patients in hospital. She
was caught up with by a love-making detective, tried, and hung
in 1676. The white powder she employed defied all analysis.
The affair led to a fashionable epidemic of secret poisoning, against
which Louis XIV instituted the celebrated "Chambre Ardente."
This was a kind of "third-degree" tribunal, and, through its official grillings, the female fortune-tellers, La Voisin and La Vigour-
eux, with their *poudre de succession*, were exposed and brought to
justice. Arsenic was probably the toxic principle of the Aqua
Tofana or Aquetta di Napoli of Teofania di Adamo, a diabolic
female who, in 1709, owned to having poisoned over 600 persons
with it, and was subsequently imprisoned or strangled.

Apothecaries' bills were exceptionally high in the seventeenth century,
and the cost of medicines was often exploited by physicians and surgeons as
an excuse for running up their charges. In London, Bucklersbury was not
only the great drug mart, but had become a fashionable highway of intrigue—
a sort of seventeenth century Bond Street. The grocers were the original drug
merchants, even after the apothecaries were duly incorporated by James I in
1606, but, in 1617, the druggists succeeded in shedding the grocers by means of a
new charter, after which time they had the physicians against them. The reason
of this was that the apothecaries set up as practitioners, not only selling drugs
but prescribing them. The long wrangle between physicians and apothecaries
which came to a head in Garth's "Dispensary" began about the time of the
Great Plague in London (1665), when the apothecaries made good in public
estimation by staying at their posts, while the physicians (even Sydenham)
fled for their lives. Extortion was the great failing of the apothecaries. In
two drug bills of 1633 and 1635, cited by Handerson, 4s. are charged for a glass
of chalybeate wine; "a purge for your worship" is listed at 3s. 6d.; "a purge
for your son" at 3s.; and a powder to fume the bed-clothes at 4s. High as
these charges were for the time, they are as nothing to the mulcting practised
in 1633 by George Buller, who charged 30s. apiece for pills and £37 10s. the
boxful. In the reign of James I, the College of Physicians prosecuted Dr.
Tenant for charging £6 each for a pill and an apozeme (decoction), and Pitt, in
1703, stated that apothecaries had been known to make between £150 and
£320 out of a single case, and that their prescription charges were at least 90
per cent. more than the shop prices. At this time, the average London physician's fee was about half a sovereign, while the apothecaries in ordinary to
Charles I and Charles II got £40 and £72 per annum respectively. In 1687,
the College of Physicians bound their fellows and licentiates to treat the sick
poor of London and its suburbs free of charge, which strained the situation still
further, and, in 1696, 53 influential physicians subscribed £10 each to establish
dispensaries for supplying drugs to the poor at cost price. War was now joined
not only between physicians and apothecaries, but an internecine wrangle
broke out among the dispensarians and anti-dispensarians, the latter being,
of course, favored by the apothecaries. A lively bout of scurrilous pamphlet-
eering ensued, and in 1699 Garth published *The Dispensary*, a satirical poem in
the meter of Pope, urging the injustice of the dilemma forced upon the physi-

cians, "to cheat as tradesmen or to fail as fools." It was described by Dr. Johnson as "on the side of charity against the intrigues of interest, and of regular learning against licentious usurpation of medical authority." Pope also had a slap at

> Modern pothecaries, taught the art
> By doctors' bills to play the doctor's part,
> Bold in the practice of mistaken rules.

But, in spite of the support of the men of letters, the physicians were in the end beaten by the apothecaries, for a test case against an apothecary who had exceeded his license, which was brought to trial in 1703, and at first decided in the physicians' favor, was subsequently reversed in a higher court. After this time, the English apothecaries became practitioners to all intents and purposes, and then began to make war upon those of their number who did not come up to certain standards of their own devising.

The purchasing power of money in the seventeenth century is said to have been some seven or eight times what it is now, and, with this ratio in mind, we may gain some idea of the **compensation and income** of the physician and surgeon of the time. The salary of a physician in ordinary was £100 annually, but Turquet de Mayerne got £400, with an annuity of £200 settled upon his wife. While the average fee of the English physician was, as stated, about 10s. (worth about $35 today), we find Richard Mead (1673–1754) charging a guinea a little later and half a guinea for coffee-house practice. Harvey, who was not a successful practitioner, left an estate of £20,000. The annual salary of the Professor of Physic in the University of Cambridge in 1626 was £40.

An old bill of 1665 gives 12s. as the fee for a twenty-mile visit; another, £1, and, for an outside visit of two days' duration, £1 10s. Bleeding a lady in bed cost 10s., as against 2s. 6d. for a man. A postmortem cost 3s. 4d.[1]

Thomas Arthur, a physician of Limerick, Ireland, although prevented by religious prejudice from practising among the wealthy, made an average income of about £250, or the equivalent of about $7000 today (Walsh). His fee for the management of a case of gonorrhea (1619) was £2 in advance, and, for a putrid sore throat, 8s. The Professor of Physick in the University of Cambridge got £40 per annum in 1626. In Germany the tariff was fixed by the ordinances of Hesse (1616), Frankfort on the Main (1668), and Prussia (1685). According to the Frankfort ordinance, an office visit was worth 40 pfennige (about 75 cents today), a house visit 1.35 marks, a night visit 1.70 marks, and a consultation one gold gulden (about $12.50). Foreigners were charged half as much again, and the wealthy paid what they liked. The family physician (*Hausarzt*) received a lump sum annually, as high as 100 marks in one case, for attendance on a Bavarian countess (Baas). A city physician got over 500 marks if he inspected the city pharmacies; a court physician, 850 marks; and a physician in ordinary, 900 marks. The pest-doctor of Prague received 2000 marks a month. In France, Seguin purchased the post of physician in ordinary from Guillemeau for 50,000 livres and sold it for 22,000 crowns (about 200,000 francs in present money), while Valot, in 1652, paid Cardinal Mazarin 30,000 crowns for the vacant post of royal physician. Buckle states that the average French doctor's fee was as low as that of an English farrier. According to the Levamen Infirmi (1700), cited by Handerson, an English surgeon's fee was 12

---

[1] See Brit. Med. Jour., London, 1870, ii, 169.

pence a mile, 10 groats for bone-setting, a shilling for blood-letting, and £5 for
amputation. Richard Wiseman got £150 as surgeon in ordinary in 1661, and
de Choqueux £80 in 1665. According to the Frankfurt tariff of 1668, a German barber surgeon got 10½ marks for setting a broken arm (20½ marks, if
two bones were broken), 30.85 marks for a dislocation of the elbow- or knee-
joint, or half as much if the result was poor. A surgeon charged 31 marks for
amputating an arm, 41 marks for a leg, 51 marks for a lithotomy, or half price
if the patient died. Herniotomy was rated at 51 marks, and cataract operation 17 marks for one eye, or 25 marks for both. According to Baas's tabula-
tion of the pay of army surgeons in Mark Brandenburg, a company surgeon
got about 11 to 15 marks monthly in the infantry, and in the cavalry, 11.40
marks in 1639, and 27 in 1655. A regimental surgeon got 30 marks in 1638,
15 marks in 1639, 27 marks in 1655, and 52.80 marks in 1685. During 1635–85
the surgeon of the exiled French mousquetaires got 90 marks monthly. The
pay of a Saxon Feldscheerer in 1613 was 33 marks a month. In England,
under the Commonwealth in 1650, army surgeons at the northern posts got
6s. 8d. per diem and £15 for horses and medicine chests, if mounted. An English naval surgeon got £8 1s. for one hundred and seventy-five days' services
in 1653 and £16 14s. for fifty-one days' service in 1654.

The old-time strife and rivalry which, as we have seen, had
always existed between the physicians, surgeons, and barbers, continued with unabated fervor in the seventeenth century. After the
incorporation of the English barbers and surgeons in one company
in 1540, the former continued to be a thorn in the side of the latter,
and the surgeons did not succeed in getting rid of them until 1745.
Meanwhile, this united Company of Barber Surgeons were permitted to have public dissections in their own hall, but nowhere else,
and the cause of their education was further advanced by the Arris
(1643) and Gale (1698) foundations for public dissections and lectures. In France, the medical profession had consisted for centuries of an aristocracy of physicians, a petite bourgeoisie of clerical
barber-surgeons, and a proletariate of laic barbers or outcast surgeons (barbitonsores), all hating and despising one another and ad-
hering to rigid caste distinctions. When, after the foundation of
the College de St. Côme, the surgeon was in a manner assimilated
to the status of the physician, he began to put on airs like the latter,
wearing the square cap and long robe, substituting the device of
three boxes of ointment upon his guild-banner for the traditional
three basins, arrogating to himself the right to examine the barbers,
and insisting that his apprentices be "grammarian-clerks." By
the seventeenth century, the physician had become a sterile pedant
and coxcomb, red-heeled, long-robed, big-wigged, square-bonneted,
pompous and disdainful in manner, making a vain parade of his
Latin, and, instead of studying and caring for his patients, tried
to overawe them by long tirades of technical drivel, which only concealed his ignorance of what he supposed to be their diseases.
Among themselves, the physicians were narrowly jealous of their
rights and privileges, regarding their fraternity as a closed corporation, yet eternally wrangling about fantastic theories of disease and current modes of treatment. The lay barber, although

an outcast and an outlaw, was, in some respects, the most worthy of all three, since he was driven to study nature at first hand. He showed little submission or respect toward his rivals, and out of his clan had come Franco and Paré. Thus, while the barbers were crowding the surgeons who, in servile imitation of the physicians, had formed a syndicate against them, the physicians themselves maintained a supercilious, Malvolio-like attitude toward both. The latter, as Forgue says,[1] would sometimes join with the barbers in an aristocrat-socialist combine against the surgeons, although sometimes teetering toward the latter's vows of precedence over the barbers, while barbers and surgeons would again solidify as a unit against the doctors. The result of all this intrigue and turmoil was that the barbers finally came into their own through the royal decree of 1660, which unified barbers and surgeons in one guild, but otherwise reduced them to the humblest status and drew down upon them the centupled wrath of the physicians. The curious isolation and sterile inefficiency of the French internists of the seventeenth century are strikingly revealed in the letters of Guy Patin (1601–72), Dean of the Paris Faculty, who regarded the surgeons as mere "booted lackeys . . . a race of evil, extravagant coxcombs who wear mustaches and flourish razors." In 1686, however, an event occurred which Michelet has deemed "more important than the work of Paré." Louis XIV suffered, it seems, from a fistula in ano, which, after remaining obdurate to the exhibition of all manner of ointments and embrocations, was successfully healed by operation at the hands of the royal surgeon, Félix. The latter received for his trouble 300,000 livres, three times more than the honorarium of the royal physician, and was ennobled, becoming the Seigneur de Stains. Félix was succeeded by Mareschal, and to the latter is due the elevation of the French surgeon's social condition in the eighteenth century. Louis XIV influenced French medicine in three curious ways: His attack of typhoid fever (1657) gave an immense vogue to the use of antimony; his anal fistula (1686) brought about the rehabilitation of French surgery; and the fact that his mistress was attended by Clément, the royal accoucheur, in 1663, did much to further the cause of male midwifery.

The best sidelight on the pedantic formalism and complacent ineptitude of the French internist of the period is afforded in the pensive mockery of **Molière** (1622–73). The great dramatist had no use whatever for the medical profession, whose ridiculous side early excited his derision and against whom he seems to have cherished a lasting grudge, partly because of their inability to do

---

[1] E. Forgue: Montpellier méd., 1911, xxxii, 601; xxxiii, 8.

anything for his own malady (consumption), and partly because he believed that they had killed his only son and one of his bosom friends with their eternal antimony. No less than five of his printed comedies abound in pungent raillery and light-barbed sarcasm, directed with unerring skill against the tribe of doctors.

The tendency is exhibited in his very earliest farces, such as *Le Docteur Amoureux*, *Les Trois Docteurs Rivaux*, *La Jalousie de Barbouille*, *Le Médecin Volant*. In *Le Médecin Volant*, Sganarelle, the valet, cleverly mimics the pedantries of the Paris Faculty. In *L'Amour Médecin*, we have an inimitable burlesque of professional consultations and discussions among five physicians of different types, one of the points brought out being the relative merits of the old-fashioned Episcopal mule and the new-fangled horse as a means of transportation. In the second act, a strolling drug-vendor chants the virtues of the popular opiate, *orviétan*. In *Le Médecin Malgré Lui*, Sganarelle is again impressed, by dint of drubbing, into playing the part of doctor, and, having a glib tongue, acquits himself exceeding well. In *Monsieur de Porceaugnac*, two physicians, who have been bribed to pronounce the latter insane, hold a solemn consultation *de lunatico inquirendo* over the pursy provincial, and their long scholastic tirades seem exactly in the spirit of the times. But the height of medical satire in Molière is achieved in his last great work, *Le Malade Imaginaire*, of which the central figure, Argan, the hypochondriac, forever drugging his imaginary ailments, is of the type portrayed by Butler in 'The Medicine Taker. The first act discloses Argan grumbling over his apothecary's accounts, the principal sources of medical revenue in those days. In order to have a physician at beck and call about his household, he is desirous of marrying his daughter, Angélique, to Thomas Diafoirus, a dense young medical graduate who is a good match, as matches go, but by no means the young lady's choice. To outwit this design, Toinette, the maid, disguises as a doctor, and through a clever stratagem succeeds in making Argan relent his purpose, as well as in restoring him to health and sanity. In the meantime, however, he is fairly bullied off the stage by M. Purgon, an irate member of the Faculty, who terrorizes him with the prospect of bradypepsia, dyspepsia, apepsia, lientery, dysentery, dropsy, and general decline. The doctors defeated, the intrigue is resolved by persuading Argan to become a physician himself. Then follows what is perhaps the choicest bit of medical satire ever penned, the intermezzo-ballet, a joyous burlesque of those ceremonies of medical graduation which John Locke described in his French diary. The French routine of medical examination and graduation in this period was portentous in length and pomp, and our description is taken from the admirable account by Maurice Raynaud.[1] The unfortunate candidate, drilled almost to extinction in the scholastic régime of the "naturals," anatomy and physiology, the "non-naturals," hygiene and dietetics, and the "contra-naturals," pathology and therapeutics, without any bedside teaching whatever, was put through his paces every two years by a long string of examinations and argumentation of theses which lasted a week. The latter disputations usually began at 5 or 6 A. M., lasting until mid-day, and woe to the luckless candidate who could not cope with the fire of absurd questions which were rained upon him. If he came through all this successfully and his name was one of those drawn by lot from the fateful urn, he became a licentiate for graduation. Hereupon the licentiates and bachelors proceeded in solemn array to request the presence of all prominent and influential personages at the graduation ceremonies. The feature of the latter was the Dean, the paranymph of the old Greek marriage ritual, who inducted the newly fledged licentiate into a sort of mystic union with the Faculty. At 5 in the morning of the momentous day, a preparatory session was held to determine questions of precedence, which were again decided by the urn. At 10, the hall was opened to visitors, the lists were proclaimed, and the successful candidates fell upon their knees to receive the apostolic bene-

---

[1] M. Raynaud: La médicine au temps de Molière, Paris, 1862.
15

diction. The chancellor then proposed a question of religious or literary character to the candidate, which the latter immediately took up. This completed,
the assembly proceeded in a body to the cathedral to thank the Holy Virgin for
her good offices. Then followed, after an interval of six weeks or longer, the
doctorate, the object of which was to introduce the candidate into the sanctuary
of the Faculty, as the licentiate had introduced him to the public. After a
close inquiry into his moral character the candidate was first admitted to the
Vesperie, which consisted in a solemn, intimate presidential discourse on the
dignity and importance of the medical profession, followed by the discussion
of another thesis, with speeches. Academic full-dress visits to the regents of
the Faculty occupied the next few days. On the final day, the candidate was
sworn to the three articles of medical faith, viz., to obey all laws and observe
all prescribed customs of the Faculty, to attend the mass for deceased physicians following St. Luke's Day, and to be unsparing in warfare against all illicit
practitioners. The candidate having taken oath to this in the single word,
Juro, the President (Præses), placed the square bonnet upon his head, after
making the sign of the cross with the latter, and, with the administration of a
slight tap or *accolade*, the doctor in embryo was born into the world. He immediately entered into his rights and privileges by proposing a thesis to be discussed by one of the physicians present, after which he delivered a florid, perfunctory discourse of thanks and praise. On the St. Martin's day following,
he presided at the *acte pastillaire*, a general discussion of a thesis of his own
choosing, and on the following day his name was inscribed on the registers as a
junior for the next ten years.[1] This lengthy ceremony, which was set off
everywhere by innumerable dinners, suppers, and banquets of old-time dimensions, forms the substance of Molière's immortal ballet. At the start, the
Præses burlesques, in mock Latin, the solemn discourse of the *Vesperie*. The
first doctor then propounds the nice question: Why does opium produce sleep?
To which the candidate replies

Quia est in eo
Virtus dormitiva,

to be greeted by the obligato chorus:

Bene, bene, bene, bene respondere,
Dignus, dignus est intrare
In nostro docto corpore.

The candidate is then plied with questions as to his probable line of treatment
in a string of diseases, for each of which he advances the incontestable merits of
the clyster, the lancet, and the purge—

Clysterium donare,
Postea seignare
Ensuita purgare,

followed by the constantly reiterated "Bene, bene." The famous Juro is then
administered, and after the Præses has conferred the bonnet, the candidate
delivers a flowery discourse, full of servile praises of his benefactors. The ballet
closes with festal dances and cheers, the physicians, surgeons, and apothecaries
filing out solemnly at the end.

The good-humored character of Molière's satire, and the apparent indifference with which it was received by the medical profession of his time and country, indicate that there was plenty of
human nature in the French physician of the seventeenth century,
in spite of his innocuous pedantry and sterile fanaticism. Across
the Pyrénées we find the same conditions, if we may trust the
Spanish romances of the *picaresco* type, and the medical scenes in

---

[1] These data have been taken from Maurice Raynaud's delightful study,
"La médecine au temps de Molière," Paris, 1862. Frank Baker, on The Faculty
of Paris in the 17th Century, 115–121, is an attractive presentation of the
subject in English. New York Med. Jour., 1913, xcviii.

Le Sage's Gil Blas, which, although published in 1715, is pure seventeenth century in its characters and local color. The droll consultation in the third chapter of its fourth book, in which Doctors Andros and Oquetos agree that the trouble in Don Vincent's case is "a mutiny of the humors," is fairly typical, the patient losing his life through the consequences of their dispute whether the Hippocratic expression ὀργασμός meant a fermentation or a concoction of these humors. Then there is the slap at the "fellows in this town calling themselves physicians, who drag their degraded persons at the Currus Triumphalis Antimonii, or . . . Cart's Tail of Antimony, apostates from the faith of Paracelsus, idolaters of filthy kermes"; and the side-light on the use of the seton afforded in the case of Dame Jacinta: "Though a little stricken in years," she cherished her bloom by depletions and "doses of all powerful jelly . . ." but "what perhaps contributed most to the freshness of this everlasting flower was an issue in each leg, of which I should never have known but for that blab Inesilla." But the medical interest of Gil Blas centers in the figure of Dr. Sangrado, "the tall, withered, wan executioner of the sisters three," whose name has, in fact, become a symbol for the kind of intensive blood-letting which was rife in the seventeenth century. Sangrado's procedure of reducing the old canon to death's door in less than two days by drawing off 18 good porringers of blood, with abundant drenches of warm water, may be paralleled by the actual experiences cited by Guy Patin, who bled his wife 12 times for a fluxion in the chest, his son 20 times for a continued fever, himself 7 times for a cold in the head, while his friends, M. Mantel and M. Cousinot, bled 36 and 64 times in a fever and a rheumatism respectively. It is now known that the rationale of this extraordinary therapy (in able-bodied people) lay in the copious drafts of water which were given with it, acting as a kind of blood-washing in the evacuation of peccant humors. In Italy, where the functions of the physician and surgeon had never been entirely separated, intensive blood-letting had continued in vogue since the days of Botallo. The technic of the practice had become highly specialized, as we see in the handsome copper-plates of such books as Malfi's "Il Barbiere" (1626). Costly bleeding-glasses of Venetian type were handed down in families as heirlooms. In Germany, perhaps for some temperamental reason, the degree of blood-letting seems to have been less intense,[1] although the practice was otherwise frequent enough, being a common detail in the numerous pictures of bathing scenes. At these bathing resorts, it was required to spend one hundred and twenty-four hours in the water as a cure, with frequent cupping and

---

[1] On this point, see France méd., Paris, 1912, lix, 365.

venesection, set off by the consumption of enormous quantities of food. Immorality was frequent, and the bath-keeper, plying his trade as a minor surgeon, is an index of the low status of the art in the Germanic countries, where Fabry of Hilden was almost the only educated surgeon. The German barbers were permitted to let blood, set broken bones, treat wounds and syphilis, but were not allowed to purge. Some of them went on voyages to the East Indies, or on whaling expeditions to Greenland, to learn what they could, and toward the end of the century we find another queer

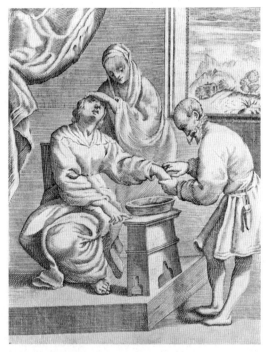

Blood-letting in the seventeenth century.   (From Malfi's Il Barbiere, 1626.)

substitute for the surgeon proper, namely, the headsman or executioner. That the ceremonies of medical graduation in seventeenth century Germany were as long and as expensive as those ridiculed by Molière is evidenced by an edict of the Elector of Brandenburg (1683), in which, to save the students' purses, banqueting was cut down to a single supper, limited to ten courses. "Ladies" and confectionery were excluded. In the case of needy students, the sumptuary features could be limited to the simple announcement of the candidate's graduation in the auditorium (at half price), the distribution of gloves and the convivium being omitted, unless the student saw fit to invite a few professors to a modest repast, at discretion (Baas). Although medical students have always borne a hard reputation for pranks and horseplay, the social customs of the German students, their hazing and "pennalism," were coarse and barbaric beyond belief. As in France, the junior student was a mere *bec jaune*, that is, a novice or aspirant, and treated as such. The lower strata of the profession were made up of all sorts of strolling quacks—tooth-drawers, uroscopists, magicians, rope-dancers, chiropodists, crystal-gazers—who were also common in the Low Countries, and a favorite theme of the Dutch and Flemish artists. Of the many pictures of vagabond dentists, the best are the spirited canvases of the Flemish artist Theodore Rombouts in the Prado at Madrid, and, among the Dutchmen, those of Gerard Honthorst (Dresden Gallery), Gerard Dow (Louvre, Dresden, and Schwerin Galleries), Adriaen Brouwer (Cassel Museum and Lichtenstein Gallery, Vienna), and the younger Teniers (Cassel and Dresden). All these tooth-drawers have costumes evidently designed to make the bravest showing consistent with their means, some of them highly fantastic, with fur-trimmed robes and Oriental turbans. The current methods of venesection are well represented by the younger Teniers (Musée du Draguignan), Frans van Mieris (Vienna), in the fainting woman by Eylon van der Neer, and in the Death of Seneca of Rubens, both in the Old Pinakothek at Munich. The pedicurists, or corn-cutters, were a favorite subject of such men as David Teniers, Jr. (Cassel, Budapest, Madrid), and Adriaen Brouwer (Pinakothek Prado, Schönborn Gallery, Vienna). The strangest of the Low Country itinerants were the quacks who pretended to cut stones from the head for the relief of insanity, idiocy, or other mental disorders. In the sixteenth and seventeenth centuries it was a common byword to describe a person mentally unbalanced as having "a stone in his head." The therapeutic imposture consisted in making a superficial incision in the scalp, and palming a stone or stones, which were cast into a convenient basket at stated intervals during the patient's struggles. The trick seems to have been a very old one, and some of its representations in art, such as those of van Bosch in Amsterdam, Jan Sanders in the Prado, or the etching of Pieter Breughel, Sr., in the Amsterdam Cabinet, go back to the fifteenth and sixteenth centuries. The most comic specimens of seventeenth century work in this field are the stone-drawers of Frans Hals, Jr., and Jan Steen in the Musée Boijmans at Rotterdam. The latter represents a quack incising the occipital region of a screaming fool who is tied in a chair, while an old woman holds the pail into which a giggling lad in the rear tosses the supposititious stones, one by one.

A red chalk drawing of the younger Teniers shows a quack, with feathered turban and sword, opening the head of a stoical patient, who sits with folded arms and compressed lips. Physicians of a higher grade are to be seen in the many Dutch pictures of water-casting. A solemn consideration of the appearance of the patient's urine seems to have been the favorite procedure in cases of the so-called *minne pyn* or *mal d'amour*, that is, the chlorosis of love-sick young women. To this theme Jan Steen devoted no less than nine canvases, Frans van Mieris, four, and Gabriel Metsu, two. In

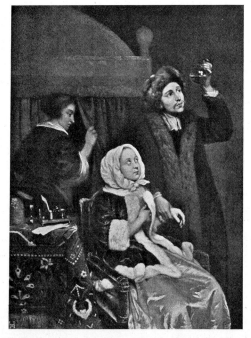

Mal d'Amour, by Gerard Dow.   (Buckingham Palace.)
Hanfstaengl, Munich.

these pictures, the fur-trimmed jackets and rich gowns of the women indicate the wealthier class, the attending physicians being correspondingly dressed in black velvet robes or doublet and hose, with flat bonnets or bell-crowned hats, according to their social or religious affiliations. The representation of the pallor and fever-ish discontent of the greensick, lovelorn maidens is very life-like, particularly in the fine canvas of Gabriel Metsu in the Preyer Collection at Vienna. The *clou* of this group of paintings is undoubt-edly the *Mal d'Amour* of Gerard Dow (Buckingham Palace), a charming picture, representing a handsome young doctor, in fur-trimmed pelisse and fur cap, earnestly scanning a urine flask, while he feels the pulse of a pretty *meisje*,whose upturned face reveals the all-important fact that her interest in his personality is in excess of her confidence in his professional skill.[1]

The seventeenth century marks the rude beginnings of two new phases of national medicine—the Russian and the American.

In the fifteenth century Ivan III (1468–1505), the first Russian ruler to bear the title of Czar, invited foreign physicians to settle in Moscow, with the not very alluring prospect of having their throats cut if they failed to cure. Under the reign of Ivan IV (1533–84), called the Terrible, many English physicians came to Moscow by invitation and some of these also acted as ambassadors or diplomatists. One of them founded an Apteka, or drug-store, in 1581. Under the Romanoff dynasty (1613–45), there was a great influx of adventurous foreigners which, through the encouragement of Peter the Great and Catherine, continued well into the eighteenth century. These undoubtedly did a great deal to stimulate an interest in medicine, although, like the Greeks in Rome, they were eyed with suspicion by the natives, who were always ready to sack their houses in popular uprisings. Upon their arrival, the foreign physicians took an oath of office, pledging themselves not to use poisonous drugs, and, after an audience with the Czar, were loaded with rich presents, money, provender, horses, and sometimes even acquired an estate of from 30 to 40 "souls." The Russian therapeutic superstitions of the time were identical with those we have found in other countries. There was the same elaborated polypharmacy, including extracts made from insects and parts of animals, and not even the critique of Ambroise Paré had dispelled the belief in the efficacy of the unicorn's horn, for three specimens of which 100,000 roubles ($30,000) were offered in 1655. Drugs were, however, imported from Germany and Holland, botanic gardens were started, and, in 1671, a brief account of native Russian simples was drawn up, "a sort of miniature Siberian pharmacopœia," based upon information gathered from the peasants by the Siberian *voyevods*, or military governors. Under the Romanoffs a Ministry of Medical Affairs was founded, also a central store (Apteka) for the distribution of drugs to the followers of the Moscow court. A later Apteka, of larger scope, which dispensed drugs to soldiers and civilians and looked after the prevention of infectious diseases, was the nucleus of the above-mentioned Aptekarski Prikaz (Ministry of Medical Affairs), the starting-point of the patriarchal public health service of Russia.[2]

---

[1] For a fuller account of all these pictures, with reproductions, see Eugen Holländer, "Die Medizin in der klassischen Malerei," Stuttgart, 1903.

[2] For further details, see the article on Russian medicine in Lancet, London, 1897, ii, 354–361.

Among the foreign physicians who visited Russia was John Tradescant, a Fleming, who journeyed to Archangel with Sir Dudley Digges in 1618, and made a unique collection of natural history specimens, coins, medals, and other objects of *virtù*, which became in time the present Ashmolean Museum at Oxford.

The new-world settlements of Jamestown, Virginia, in 1607, Plymouth Colony in 1620, and the New Netherlands in 1623, naturally drew to them a number of European physicians who, as in Russia, were active agents in advancing the interests of legitimate medicine in the colonies. Prominent among these were Dr. Lawrence Bohun, who became Physician General of Virginia in 1611, Dr. John Pot, the first physician to reside permanently in Virginia, and elected temporary governor of the state in 1628, Dr. Johannes La Montagne, a Huguenot, who was councillor of Wilhelm Kieft, Director General of the New Netherlands, Dr. Samuel Fuller, who came over in the Mayflower and practised in New England until his death in 1633, and Dr. John Winthrop, Jr., who was the first governor of Connecticut (Handerson). One of these emigrant physicians, Thomas Thacher, was, as we have seen, the author of the first and only medical publication printed in the North American colonies in the seventeenth century (1677). Meanwhile, higher education had a definite start with the foundation and endowment of Harvard College in 1636–38, and of William and Mary College in Virginia in 1693; and native-born students and practitioners soon acquired the habit of going to Leyden, Oxford, or Paris to complete their medical courses. The practice of physic was often combined with the preaching of the gospel. Giles Firmin, who, prior to 1647, delivered the first course in anatomy in New England, was one of these clerical physicians, and his probable scheme of treatment and instruction has been outlined in the witty imaginative sketch of Oliver Wendell Holmes.[1] His anatomy he got from Vesalius, Paré, Fallopius, and Spigelius; his internal medicine was a mixture of the Greeks, Fernelius, van Helmont, and Sir Kenelm Digby; his pathology was mythology.

"His pharmacopœia consisted mainly of simples, such as the venerable 'Herball' of Gerard describes and figures in abounding affluence. St. John's wort and Clown's All-heal, with Spurge and Fennel, Saffron and Parsley, Elder and Snake-root, with opium in some form, and roasted rhubarb and the Four Great Cold Seeds, and the two Resins, of which it used to be said that whatever the Tacamahaca has not cured, the Caranna will, with the more familiar Scammony and Jalap and Black Hellebore, made up a good part of his probable list of remedies. He would have ordered Iron now and then, and possibly an occasional dose of Antimony. He would perhaps have had a rheumatic patient wrapped in the skin of a wolf or wild cat, and in case of a malignant fever

---

[1] O. W. Holmes, Medical Essays, Boston, 1883, 278–283.

with 'purples' or petechiæ or of an obstinate king's evil, he might have prescribed a certain black powder, which had been made by calcining toads in an earthen pot. . . . Barbeyrac and his scholar Sydenham had not yet cleansed the Pharmacopœia of its perilous stuff, but there is no doubt that the more sensible physicians of that day knew well enough that a good honest herb-tea which amused the patient and his nurses was all that was required to carry him through all common disorders."

Two features of American medicine in the colonial period are especially worthy of note. First, the half-fledged youth, who studied with some physician under indentures of apprenticeship, received actual bedside instruction from the start, and, although serving as sweep and stable-boy to his master, was still learning how to bleed and cup, to prepare drugs and apply them. Second, under primitive, frontier conditions, the medieval antagonism between the physician and surgeon soon disappeared, for the necessary and sufficient reason that, while midwifery was in the hands of women, the open-country or backwoods doctor was liable to be called upon in any emergency, and, thrown upon his own resources, soon learned to enlarge such native skill as he had in bone-setting, treatment of arrow and gunshot wounds, reducing hernias and the like. Before 1769, according to Toner, the term "Doctor" was not even employed in the colonies. As Handerson says, "Many of these apprentices doubtless proved as successful physicians (and success is the usual test of merit) as some of their more fortunate colleagues who boasted an M.D. of Leyden, Aberdeen, or Cambridge and slew their patients *secundum artem.*"[1] We may agree with the same authority that, from this period on, American medicine acquired that eminently practical tendency which has been its chief merit and of which we have no reason whatever to feel ashamed. That the profession soon developed a certain *esprit de corps* is evident in that we find no records of strolling lithotomists, cataract-couchers, or other quacks among them, that the names of no New England physicians are connected with the scandal of Salem Witchcraft (1692), and that we find records of the latter giving service to the sick poor for a remittance of taxes. Such medical legislation as the colonies had in this period was, as in the Code Hammurabi, mainly concerned with the momentous question of fees. As early as 1636, the Assembly of Virginia passed an act providing that those who had served apprenticeships as surgeons and apothecaries should receive five shillings a visit and university graduates ten. Doctors' bills were usually paid, however, with such articles of barter as corn (in New England), tobacco (at the South), or wampum (among the Indians), and they soon became so exorbitant that, in 1638 and 1639, the Assemblies

---

[1] Baas: History of Medicine, New York, 1889, 582.

of Maryland and Virginia passed laws to moderate them. In 1649, the Massachusetts colony passed a law restricting the practice of medicine, surgery, and midwifery to such persons as might be judged competent by "some of the wisest and gravest," or most skilful in the same art, with the additional consent of the patient. A similar law was passed in New York in 1665, and in 1699 an act to prevent the spread of infectious diseases became a law in Massachusetts.

The first hospital in the New World was erected by Cortez in the city of Mexico in 1524. In 1639, a Hôtel Dieu was established in Canada by the Duchesse d'Aguilon, and ultimately located in Quebec. The Montreal Hôtel Dieu was established in 1644, and the General Hospital of Quebec in 1693. The first hospital in what is now the United States was established on Manhattan Island in 1663.

In the seventeenth century, as one of its poets sings, "Devouring Famine, Plague and War," those primal causes of human misery, were everywhere rampant. The mortality from wars and **epidemic diseases** was as great as in the Middle Ages.

The bubonic plague, while it did not sweep all Europe as formerly, struck with terrific force in some places. The Great Plague of London (1665) carried away 69,000; the Vienna visitation of 1679, 70,000; that of Prague (1681), 83,000; while the Italian epidemic of 1630 numbered 80,000 victims in Milan and over 500,000 in the Venetian Republic. In the opinion of Haeser, these losses, together with the Candian war, contributed materially to the downfall of Venice, whose great fleets once held "the gorgeous East in fee." The earliest visitations were those in Russia (1601–03), in which Moscow lost 127,000 souls from pest and famine. Through the century, England (1603–65), France (1608–68), The Netherlands (1625–80), Italy (1630–91), Denmark (1654), Germany (1656–82), Sweden (1657), Switzerland (1667–68), and Spain (1677–81) were all severely ravaged. As in the sixteenth century, the local epidemics were commemorated in coins and medals, some of which were used as amulets, while others, highly ornate, betokened the freeing of a city from the pest. Of these we may mention the Thuringian silver pennies of 1600, 1602, and 1611, the pest-dollars (of Wittenberg type) of 1619, the coins and medals struck off in memory of the epidemics incident to the Thirty Years' War at Urbino (1631), Venice (1631), Breslau (1631), Ingolstadt (1634), Frankfort on the Main (1635), Munich (1637), and the relics of the later visitations at Vienna (1679), Leipzig (1680), Würzburg (1681), Erfurt (1683), and Magdeburg (1683). All these have been described in detail by Pfeiffer and Ruland (*Pestilentia in nummis*, 1882). Famine, always in the train of war and plague, was commemorated in the Annona medals, in praise of the Papal regulation of the price of corn, which were struck off in honor of Popes Clement X (1671–73) and Alexander VIII (1690); and in the medals relating to inundation in Hamburg (1685), to the plague of grasshoppers in Silesia and Thuringia (1693), hard times in the German Empire (1694), and hunger and cold in Holland (1698). The intense popular animosity against the corn pedlars and factors, whose thrifty extortions were not unnaturally confused with the unthrift of bad harvesting as a cause of human misery, is strikingly shown in the curious *Kornjudenmedaillen*.[1] Silesian medals of this type were struck off in 1694–95 and

---

[1] The obverse of these famine medals commonly displayed a sorry looking pedlar, weighted down by a sack of corn which a devil is engaged in puncturing.

again copied in the eighteenth century. Besides grasshoppers and pedlars, comets were still regarded with superstitious awe as "God's postillions" (*Gottespostillione*), harbingers of war, pestilence and famine, although Shakespeare had said

"When beggars die there are no comets seen,"

and the astronomer von Littrow has latterly shown that there is no probable connection between the hundreds of comets known and the slightest possible variation in the atmosphere.   There were comet medals for the years 1618, 1677, 1680, and 1686, but the appearance of Halley's comet in 1682 was distinguished by the great English astronomer's calculation that it would reappear in 1758.   With the verification of this prediction, it was perceived that comets are, after all, like any other periodic phenomenon in nature, and the comet theory of disease disappears from medical history after 1758.[1]

State and city ordinances against the plague were many, and, while providing for special hospitals, attendance, and sanitary inspection, were sometimes extremely narrow and severe.   Not only were plague-stricken houses burned to the ground, after the wise old Mosaic method, but persons suspected of spreading the plague by smearing its virus about were put to torture and death.   A striking instance is afforded in an episode of the great plague of Milan in 1630, as described by the novelist, Alessandro Manzoni,[2] and latterly in the valuable paper of Dr. Robert Fletcher.[3]   On the morning of June 1, 1630, Guglielmo Piazza, a commissioner of health of Milan, was seen going down the street, writing from an ink-horn at his belt, and wiping his probably ink-stained fingers against the walls of houses.   Being accused by the ignorant women of the neighborhood of smearing the houses with deadly ointments, he was, upon motion of the council, haled to torture.   The latter barbarity, a survival of the ordeal of feudal times, had an elaborate ceremonial, prescribed by legal code, in which the accused was stripped, shaved to the scalp, and purged before going through his misery; and, if he survived the atrocities inflicted upon his body three times, God was supposed to have intervened in a miracle. The unhappy Piazza stood for two applications of this hideous rite, but yielding to the "third degree" suggestions of his tormentors, finally stated that he had obtained a poisonous ointment from a barber named Mora.   The latter, upon being apprehended, yielded to the first application of torture, and though both unfortunates recanted more than once, the clamors of the superstitious populace against them were such that, upon sentence, they were torn with red-hot pincers, had their right hands cut off, their bones broken, were stretched on the wheel, and, after six hours, burned.   Their ashes were then thrown into the river, their possessions sold, the house of the crime razed to the ground, and its site converted into a sort of Aceldama by the erection of a "column of infamy" (*colonna d'infamia*).   This was less than three centuries ago.

The physicians delegated to treat the plague wore a strange prophylactic garb, consisting of a long red or black gown of smooth material, often Morocco or Cordovan leather, with leather gauntlets, leather masks having glass-covered openings for the eyes and a long beak or snout, filled with antiseptics or fumigants, for the nose.   In his hand the pest-doctor carried a wand to feel the pulse.   In spite of this comic opera make-up, he was a highly esteemed functionary, often drawing a large salary.   In the Italian cities, immense pits for burying the dead had sometimes to be dug, the *apparitori* or summoners going before, ringing a bell notifying the people to bring out their dead, the *monatti* attending to the matter, and the *commissari* reporting upon

---

The other side bore a bushel measure, on the inner surface of which was inscribed (in German) the verse of Proverbs (xi, 26): "He that withholdeth corn, the people shall curse him," the outer surface reading: "But blessing shall be upon the head of him that selleth it."

[1] Pfeiffer and Ruland: Pestilentia in nummis, Tübingen, 1882, p. 19.

[2] Manzoni: Storia della colonna infame, 1840.

[3] R. Fletcher: Johns Hopkins Hosp. Bull., Baltimore, 1898, ix, 175–180.

the cases and supervising the whole. Sometimes the rude common graves became filled to overflowing, and the dead lay putrefying in the streets. This is shown in Micco Spadara's picture of the Pest in Naples (1656), in which the Piazza del Mercato is seen swarming with dead and dying bodies which the *monatti* are struggling to remove, under direction of sundry physicians on horseback, while, in the heavens, God with a drawn sword appears, apparently yielding to the entreaties of the Virgin.

Leprosy had so completely died out by the end of the sixteenth century that, in 1656 and 1662, Louis XIV was able to abolish the lazar-houses and devote their endowments to charity and general hospital construction. Relics of the disease in art are preserved in Rubens' painting of St. Martin (Windsor Castle) and Murillo's St. Elizabeth in the Prado. Syphilis had also ceased to be epidemic, and was treated by mercurial fumigation and inunction at the hands of the barber-surgeons. It broke out in Boston, Massachusetts, in 1646, sixteen years after the foundation of the city.[1] Beyond the illustrated books, such as Stephen Blancard's, and the views of Sydenham, who regarded it as a modified West-African yaws, the seventeenth century literature of lues is not important. Next to the plague, the typhus and typhoidal fevers, which were often vaguely described as "pest," had the highest mortality, especially in connection with the miseries engendered by the Thirty Years' War. Dysentery and scurvy also added their quota, and so great was the mortality occasioned by all these that, according to the Excidium Germaniæ (cited by Haeser), "one could wander for ten miles without seeing a soul, scarce a cow, only an occasional old man or child, or a pair of old women. In every village, there are houses filled with dead bodies and carrion; men, women, children, servants, horses, swine, cows, and oxen lying pell-mell together, throttled by plague and hunger, devoured by wolves, dogs, crows, and ravens, for want of decent burial." Add to this the sexual atrocities of soldiery, as depicted in Grimmelshausen.[2] In the cities, typhus fever was carefully studied by such observers as Stahl and Friedrich Hoffmann in Halle, or Schröckh in Augsburg. In England, Willis described the typhoid epidemic among the Parliamentary troops at the siege of Reading in the damp spring of 1643. Typhoid pneumonia was prevalent in Italy (1602–12, 1633, 1696), as described by Codronchi and others. Hochstätter described an Augsburg epidemic of 1624, and Switzerland was visited in 1652, 1685 (Lake Geneva), and 1694–95. Malarial fever was pandemic in the years 1657–69 and 1677–95 (Haeser). The English epidemics were described by Willis, Morton, and Sydenham, Morley and Lucas Schacht, the Italian by Cavallari (1602) and Borelli (1661), the Dutch by Sylvius (1677) and Fanois (1669), the French by Chirac (1694). The severe Italian epidemic of 1690–95 was described by Ramazzini and Lancisi. Dysentery was epidemic throughout the countries ravaged by the Thirty Years' War, notably Germany, Holland, and France (1623–25), and it reinvaded Germany in 1666 and the North in 1676–79. The English epidemics of 1668–72 were described by Morton and Sydenham. During the period 1583–1610, diphtheria was confined to Spain. In the latter year, it broke out in Italy, where it was again epidemic in 1618–30 and 1650, while Spain was revisited in 1630, 1650, and 1666. Cases occurred at Roxbury, Massachusetts, in 1659 (Jacobi). There were many epidemics of ergotism in the Sologne (1630–94), in various parts of Germany (1648–93), and in Switzerland (1650, 1674). Scurvy occurred at the siege of Breda (1625), at Nuremburg (1631), and at Augsburg (1632). Influenza was common through the century, both in the old world and the new; it was first reported in America in 1647.[3] Yellow fever appeared at New York in 1668, in Boston (1691–93) and Charleston, South Carolina, in 1699, but did not reach the old world until the following century. Of the exanthemata, small-pox was pandemic in Europe in 1614, epidemic in England

[1] Packard: History of Medicine in the United States, Philadelphia, 1901, 39.

[2] H. J. C. von Grimmelshausen: Der abentäuerliche Simplicius Simplicissimus, 1668.

[3] A. Jacobi: Jahrb. f. Kinderh., Stuttgart, 1913 (Baginsky Festschrift), 414.

during 1666–75, while in New England scattered outbreaks occurred all through the century, the disease reaching Pennsylvania in 1661, and Charleston, S. C., in 1699. The most important accounts were those of Sydenham. The first accounts of unmistakable scarlatina were those of Michael Doering and Daniel Sennert in 1627, but the disorder became generally known through the descriptions of Sydenham and Morton in 1661. Sydenham first clearly differentiated it from the "morbilli," in which the others had classed it. Measles, rubella and "the purples" (miliary fever) were usually grouped together and not sharply defined. Puerperal septicemia was first defined and differentiated by Willis in 1660.[1] Infantile conjunctivitis was first reported in America in 1658 (Jacobi).[2]

The seventeenth century, as we have seen, was the age *par excellence* of medical delineations in oil painting. Velasquez, the greatest portrait painter of all time, devoted some twelve canvases to the representation of cretinoid or hydrocephalic dwarfs, four to court fools, and three to idiots. Of these, the Prado contains ten, including the hydrocephalic Don Sebastian de Morra, El Primo, the achondroplasic and rachitic specimens in Las Meniñas, the buffoons of "silly Billy" type, and those wonderful figurations of idiocy, El Niño de Vallecas and the strabismic El Bobo de Coria. Ribera has a remarkable picture of unilateral paralysis in a boy (Vienna Gallery), showing the characteristic deformity in arm and leg, while a hand-bill carried by the lad shows that the speech center is also affected. A disorder of the pituitary may be inferred in the obese, myxedematous girl of Juan Careño de Miranda in the Prado. Rubens depicted a microcephalic dwarf in his painting of Count Thomas Arundel and wife (Old Pinakothek, Munich). His "Death of Seneca" and his crayon studies of muscular anatomy have already been mentioned. Rembrandt adhered rigidly to the normal, even in his etchings, in which he depicted every physiologic action of the human body. We have mentioned the success of the Dutch painters in representing chlorosis (*febris amatoria*), and in the same class belong Gabriel Metsu's Feverish Child (Steengracht Gallery, The Hague), Gerard Dow's Dropsical Woman (Louvre), and Frans van Mieris' Physician with a Melancholic Patient (Vienna Gallery). A remarkable painting by Simon Vouet, in the possession of Professor W. A. Freund, of Berlin, represents a case of suppurative osteomyelitis in a woman whose handsome appearance is in sharp contrast with her repulsive looking limb. The Dutch paintings of scenes of medical consultation and urine inspection are, for costumes and accessories, the finest in existence, in particular those of Gerard Dow in the Hermitage (St. Petersburg) and Vienna Gallery, Adriaen van Ostade and Gerard Terborch in the Old Museum at Berlin, the elder Teniers in the Uffizi (Florence), Ga-

[1] De febribus, 1660, ch. xvi.   [2] *Op. cit.*, 413.

briel Metsu in the Hermitage, Frans van Mieris in the old Pinakothek (Munich), and Teniers' village physicians in the Brussels
and Carlsruhe Galleries.[1] Returning to the normal, it is worthy of
remark that Rubens excelled all other artists in conveying the
charm of healthy infants and children. His handling of this
theme in oil reminds us of what Swinburne says about Andrea del
Sarto's "round-limbed babies in red-chalk outline, with full-blown
laughter in their mouths and eyes; such flowers of flesh and live
fruits of man as only a great love and liking for new-born children
could have helped him to render."[2]

---

[1] For reproductions of these pictures, see Eugen Holländer, Die Medizin
in der klassischen Malerei, Stuttgart, 1903.
[2] A. C. Swinburne: Essays and Studies, London, 1875, p. 356.

THE EIGHTEENTH CENTURY: THE AGE OF THEORIES AND SYSTEMS

THE best work of the seventeenth century, whether of Shakespeare or Velasquez, Rembrandt or Molière, Spinoza or Newton, Harvey or Leeuwenhoek, was either conceived from some deep source of original inspiration or else sprang from a fresh, naïve wonderment over the newly revealed marvels of nature, as when old Pepys declared himself "with child" to see any new or strange thing. The noble sacrifices of the heroes and martyrs of the preceding century had borne rich fruit in science as well as a great gain for spiritual and intellectual freedom. It was natural that the period preceding the outburst of political revolution should be as a lull before an approaching tempest, and indeed things veered far to the opposite extreme of exaggerated sobriety and apparent content with the old order of things. In the literature of France, at least, there is sometimes an undertone which seems to tell of the coming change:

> The day that dawns in fire will end in storms,
> Even though the noon be calm—

but, in the end, everything tended toward formalism, and every theory, however idealistic, soon hardened into a rational, methodistic "system." In this regard, the most characteristic figures of the age—Kant and Rousseau, Voltaire and Hume, Swedenborg and Wesley, Linnæus and Buffon, Racine and Pope—speak for themselves. Even the music of Mozart, Haydn, and Gluck, although in sheer beauty like something Greek strayed out of place and time, seems of precise and formal cut if compared with the sublime polyphony of Palestrina or the splendor in infinite detail of that seventeenth century giant Bach; while Händel is absolutely square-toed, silver-buckled and periwigged in style. The best scientific work of the period was still in physics and chemistry, as witness the names of Lagrange and Laplace, Cavendish and Priestley, Scheele and Lavoisier, Galvani and Volta, Franklin and Count Rumford, Fahrenheit, Celsius, and Réaumur, Watt, Fulton, and Stephenson. For medicine, aside from the work of a few original spirits like Morgagni, Hales, Hunter, Wolff, and Jenner, it was essentially an age of theorists and system-makers. Linnæus established the vogue of classification in medicine as well as his own science and seems to have set the pace everywhere. In this respect,

eighteenth century medicine is as dull and sober-sided as that of
the Arabic period.   We see the great theorists of the time, as Emerson has described the gods, each sitting apart in his own sphere,
"beckoning up to their thrones," yet somehow Hippocrates and
Sydenham, Vesalius and Harvey, Celsus and Paré, seem nearer
and more accessible to moderns than Stahl or Barthez, Bordeu
or Boerhaave, Brown or Reil.

The great Swedish botanist, Carl von Linné (1707–78), or
Linnæus, was himself a physician, having studied medicine in

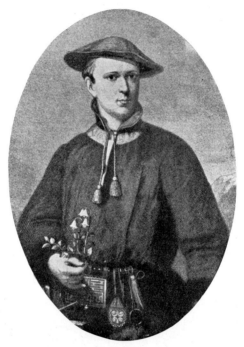

Carl von Linné (Linnæus) (1707–1778)

order to win the hand of a wealthy practitioner's daughter, the
father declining to consent to the match unless his prospective son-
in-law became a doctor.   Linnæus gave the most concise descriptions of plants and animals in all natural history, and originated
the binomial nomenclature in science, calling each definite natural
object by a generic or family name and a specific or given name,
and classifying man himself as *Homo sapiens* in the order of pri-
mates.   He believed, however, in the fixity of species (*nulla species
nova*), maintaining that "there are just as many species as issued

in pairs from the Creator's hands" and no more. His first work, the "Systema naturæ" (1735), consisting of twelve folio pages containing his classification of plants, animals, and minerals, became so popular that it passed through twelve editions in his lifetime. Specific names were first employed by Linnæus in his "Species Plantarum" (1753), for plants, and in the tenth edition of the "Systema Naturæ" (1758), for animals. The latter is, in consequence, the most highly prized of all the editions of his great work.

The medical writings of Linnæus include his materia medica (1749–52) and his scheme of nosology (Genera morborum, 1763). He had some notion of water-borne malarial fever and of the parasitic origin of disease. Hektoen says he gave good descriptions of embolism, hemicrania, and aphasia (1742).

Linnæus based his classification of plants upon characters derived from the stamens and pistils (the sexual organs of the flower), and his system, which exaggerated the importance of the flower at the expense of the whole plant, and which Linnæus himself admitted to be a faulty but convenient mode of indexing things, was called the "Sexual System." It dominated European botany for more than a century, and was further expanded by Michel Adanson (1727–1806), a physician of Aix in Provençe, whose "Familles des plantes" (Paris, 1763) comprised an arrangement of genera in 58 families; and by Antoine Laurent de Jussieu (1748–1836) of Lyons. Jussieu was the nephew of Bernard de Jussieu, a botanist who had applied the Linnæan system in arranging the plants in the Royal Garden of the Trianon, and when young Jussieu became demonstrator at the Jardin des Plantes, he was called upon to arrange the flora in this garden. He adopted a natural system of one hundred orders arranged in fifteen classes, harking back to the basic principles suggested by Ray,—Acotyledones, Monocotyledones, Dicotyledones,—further subdividing the latter according to the petals. His principal work is his "Genera Plantarum" (Paris, 1789), which was the source of authority until the Geneva botanist de Candolle introduced a morphologic system, based upon the form and development of the organs of plants as opposed to their physiologic functions. All these systems exerted a profound influence upon medical men in their attempts to classify disease, and the system of de Candolle, as we shall see, was the basis of the curious arrangements of pathologic phenomena which were made by Schönlein, Canstatt, Fuchs, Rokitansky, and other members of the German "Natural History" school in the early part of the nineteenth century.

The ludicrous side of the eighteenth century mania for sterile, dryasdust classifications of everything in nature or out of it was

16

keenly felt by Goethe, the ablest plant morphologist of his time, and his sentiments are voiced in the expressive lines in his Faust:

Grau, alter Freund, ist alle Theorie,
Und grün des Lebens goldener Baum.

We may dispose of the medical votaries of "gray theory" at once. First of all, Georg Ernst **Stahl** (1660–1734), of Ansbach, Bavaria, a stiff-necked bigoted pietist of excellent character, got himself into hot water with scientists and theologians alike by revamping van Helmont's idea of a "sensitive soul" as the source of all vital phenomena. As the Stahlian soul acted directly, without the intervention of archæi or ferments, its author maintained that both anatomy and chemistry are useless in medicine. He even doubted the efficacy of drugs like opium or quinine, and was so far behind his time that he still recommended castration in hernia. His conception of "life" was apparently identical with Imlac's definition of immortality in "Rasselas"—"a natural power of perpetual duration as a consequence of exemption from putrefaction." As Stahl regarded all this in the light of a divine revelation, we cannot wonder that he sank into abject melancholia toward the end of his days. Apart from his treatise on diseases of the portal system (1698),[1] which has won even the commendation of Virchow, and his original account of lachrymal fistula (1702),[2] he left nothing of value, and even his own generation grew weary of him. The tendency to confuse what the poet calls "the sublime and irrefutable passion of belief" with the purposes of scientific investigation is, indeed, one of the saddest things in the history of medicine. And Stahl was a well-meaning reactionary in still another direction—in his false theory of combustion which threw back the progress of chemistry for a hundred years. He assumed that when a body burns it is "dephlogisticated," that is, gives off a hypothetic substance, "phlogiston," although Mayow before him (as Black and Lavoisier after him) had shown experimentally that a burning substance gains rather than loses in weight.

The principal follower of Stahl was François Boissier de la Croix de Sauvages (1706–67), who considered the soul the cause of the mechanism of the body, but is better remembered by his "Nosologia methodica" (1768), which illustrates the taxonomic mania in a most ludicrous way. Sauvages endeavored to classify diseases as if they were specimens in natural history, subdividing them into 10 classes, with as many as 295 genera and 2400 species.

The "animism" of Stahl became finally merged into the vitalism

---

[1] Stahl: De venæ portæ porta malorum, Halle, 1698.
[2] Stahl: De fistula lachrymali, Halle, 1702.

of the "four B's," Bordeu, Barthez, Bichat, and Bouchut—to find a more recent avatar in the tedious "entelechies" of Driesch. Eighteenth century vitalism assumed a specially modern form in the "Bildungstrieb" of Johann Friedrich **Blumenbach** (1752–1840), which argues an innate impulse in living creatures toward self-development and reproduction. A great deal of theorizing in the eighteenth century was bound up with the Glisson-Haller doctrine of irritability as a specific property of living tissues. William **Cullen** (1712–90), a lucid spirit of attractive character, sought to remove some of the difficulties the theory encountered by considering muscle as a continuation of nerve and regarding life itself as simply a function of nervous energy. In this way, our modern phrase, "nerve force," became a substitute for the old Galenic "animal spirits," and, even today, when a doctor refers to some undetermined pathological condition as "probably nervous," he is unconsciously harking back to Cullen. Upon this sort of reasoning still another theoretic element was superimposed—the ancient Methodistic doctrine of the "strictum et laxum" of Asclepiades. Friedrich **Hoffmann** (1660–1742), of Halle, assumed a mysterious, ether-like fluid acting through the nervous system upon the muscles, keeping them in a state of partial tonic contraction, and also keeping the humors of the body in the motion necessary for life. Acute diseases should, therefore, be due to a spasmodic condition, chronic diseases to atony. Besides spasm and atony, Hoffmann admitted humoral changes and faulty excretions as causes of disease, the four to be relieved by sedatives, tonics, alteratives, and evacuants respectively. In Sir Clifford Allbutt's view, Hoffmann was the greatest of the iatromechanists and the first to perceive that "pathology is an aspect of physiology."[1] He left an original description of chlorosis (1730), and was one of the first to describe rubella (1740).

The Asclepiadean Methodism was published to an absurd and yet most logical limit by the celebrated John **Brown** (1735–88). "The disputatious and disreputable Brown," as Allbutt styles him, was a coarse man of low habits, whom Cullen had taken up and launched, but who, like Colombo, Borelli, and other ingrates of medicine, turned against his quiet teacher with the plebeian's usual tactics of reviling his intellectual betters in order to exalt himself. Yet the Brunonian theory, as it was called, actually held the attention of Europe for a quarter-century, and, as late as 1802, a *rixa*, or students' brawl, between Brunonians and non-Brunonians at the University of Göttingen lasted two whole days and had finally to be put down by a troop of Hanoverian horse. As

---

[1] Allbutt: Brit. Med. Jour., London, 1900, ii, 1850.

far as it went, the theory was absolutely consistent and complete
in all its parts. Brown regarded living tissues as "excitable"
in lieu of the Hallerian "irritability," and life itself as non-existent, except as a resultant of the action of external stimuli upon
an organized body. Diseases are then "sthenic" or "asthenic,"
according as the vital condition or "excitement" is increased or
diminished. The essentials of diagnosis are simply whether a disease is constitutional or local, sthenic or asthenic, and in what degree, and the treatment consists in either stimulating or depress-
ing the given condition. To this end opium, and, of course, alcohol, were Brown's favorite agents. Hippocrates said that no
knowledge of the brain can tell us how wine will act upon any
particular individual, and Brown proceeded to apply this experimental idea *in propria persona* to elucidate his theory, using successive doses of five glasses at a time. Abuse of opium and alcohol
eventually killed him. His therapeutic ideas, Baas asserts, destroyed more people than the French Revolution and the Napoleonic wars combined, and we will not dispute the same historian's
pronouncement that he was "morally deserving of the severest
condemnation."

Another ludicrous phase of theoretic medicine in the eighteenth
century was the so-called "doctrine of the infarctus" of Johann
Kämpf, the supposititious *causa causans* of most human ills being
simply fecal impaction. This fine theory, of course, fell in with
the vogue of clysters, then fashionable, the memory of which is
preserved in Molière and in the indescribable fantasies of the
artists of the period.

The leading physician of the age was the founder of the "Eclectic School," Hermann **Boerhaave** (1668–1738), who is especially
remarkable through his pupils, Haller, Gaub, Cullen, Pringle, and
the leaders of the "Old Vienna School," van Swieten and de Haen.
At first a follower of Spinoza, Boerhaave was educated along the
broadest lines, but while he was the leading practitioner of his
time, he is now principally remembered as a great teacher and especially as a chemist. His "Elementa chemiæ" (Leyden, 1732)
was easily the best book on the subject all through the eighteenth
century. In medicine, as Allbutt says, he made no experiments,
and "seems to have contented himself with hashing up the partial
truths and the entire errors of his time."[1] An examination of his

---

[1] Allbutt: *Op. cit.*, p. 1850. The only experiment credited to Boerhaave is
his attempt to ascertain the effect of extreme heat upon animals. He had
his pupils, Prevoost and Fahrenheit, put a dog and a cat in an oven heated up
to 63° C.; it was found that they died in twenty-eight minutes, while a sparrow,
under the same conditions, lasted seven minutes. This, surely, is a kind of
experimentation that we could get along just as well without.

"Aphorismi" (Leyden, 1709), which immediately suggests his reputation as the "Batavian Hippocrates" (the sedulous de Haen aping Galen as commentator of the great man), also suggests that this reputation has evaporated very considerably of recent years. Baas (a good critic) says that many of his Delphic utterances seem today "ambiguous rather than profound," while his maxim, *simplex sigillum veri*, "was never manifested in his treatment," and "his prescriptions were less effective than his personal appearance." Yet his writings had an enormous reputation in their day, and his "Institutiones" (1708) were translated even into

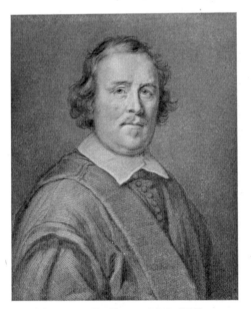

Hermann Boerhaave (1668–1738).

Turkish and Arabic.[1] The anecdotes about his fame reaching to China and his capacity for making monarchs wait only go to show that his influence was largely one of personality, a personality which was kindly, dignified, and unassuming. Boerhaave was perhaps the earliest of the great physicians who have loved music and frequently assembled performers at his house. As a clinician, he is credited with being the first to describe rupture of the esophagus and the aura-like pain which precedes hydrophobia. It is said that he was the first to establish the site of pleurisy exclusively in the pleura, and to prove that small-pox is spread exclusively by

---

[1] See Janus: Leyden, 1912, xvii, 295–312, 2 pl.

contagion. His scientific reputation today rests largely upon the idea of "affinity" between substances which he introduced into chemistry, together with an improved method of making vinegar (1732).

The theories just reviewed, with the single exception of Hoffmann's perhaps, are not entitled to the respect which we accord to the ideas of an Asclepiades, a van Helmont, or a Sydenham, for it is just these eighteenth century men who have given currency to the notion, so active in the lay mind, that the progress of medicine itself is only a "succession of forgotten theories." Far abler work was done by a very different group, the systematists, and we may now approach, with all due reverence, the greatest systematist after Galen, and one of the most imposing figures in all medical history, Albrecht **von Haller** (1708–77), the master physiologist of his time. Haller came out of the old bourgeois aristocracy of Bern, Switzerland, and was an infant prodigy, writing Latin verses and a Chaldee grammer at ten, and at sixteen, worsting his senior, Professor Coschwitz, in the latter's contention that the lingual vein was a salivary duct (1727).[1] After graduating at Leyden, having for his teachers men like Boerhaave, Albinus, Winslow, and (in mathematics) John Bernouilli, his fame as a poet and botanist soon drew him away from his native city to the newly established university at Göttingen, where he remained for seventeen years, teaching all branches of medicine, establishing botanic gardens and churches, writing some 13,000 scientific papers, and incidentally doing his best experimental work. In 1753, at the age of forty-five, he was seized with an attack of *Heimweh*, and retired to Bern for the rest of his days, leading a life of most varied activity as public health officer and savant, with a touch of "Lord High Everything Else." He was equally eminent as anatomist, physiologist, and botanist, wrote poems and historic novels, carried on perhaps the most gigantic correspondence in the history of science, and was the principal founder of medical and scientific bibliography, his patient, arduous labors in this field being marvels in their kind.[2] The Hallerianum at Berne is a symbol of his chief title to fame as the founder of recent physiology, the forerunner of Johannes Müller, Claude Bernard, and Carl Ludwig. His greatest single contribution to the subject is his laboratory demonstration of Glisson's hypothesis that irritability (*e. g.*, in an excised muscle)

[1] A. von Haller: Experimenta et dubia circa ductum salivalem novum Coschwizianum, Leyden, 1727.

[2] Bibliotheca botanica, Zürich, 1771–72; Bibliotheca anatomica, Zürich, 1774–77; Bibliotheca chirurgica, Bern, 1774–77; Bibliotheca medicinæ practicæ, Basel, 1776–78.

is the specific property of all living or organized tissues. This classic research, based upon 567 experiments, of which he himself performed 190, was made at Göttingen in 1757,[1] where he also laid the foundation for his "Elementa physiologiæ corporis humani" (Lausanne, 1759–66). Of this great work, Sir Michael Foster says truly that to open it is to pass into modern times. Read Professor Kronecker's "Haller redivivus"[2] and see how many apparently "new" discoveries of modern observers had already been accounted for by this great master and are now forgotten, doubtless because humanity does not take kindly to the theorist on his pedestal. They include a reassertion of the myogenic theory of the heart's

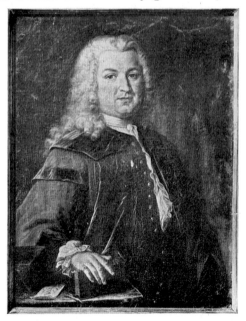

Albrecht von Haller (1708–77). (From an oil-painting by Studer.)

action (1736), a recognition of the use of bile in the digestion of fats (1736), and the first experimental injections of putrid matter into the living body (1765). Akin to the French Encyclopedists in his grasp of detail, Haller was the best historian of medicine[3] after Guy de Chauliac, and his literary judgments are veritable *lumina*

---

[1] "De partibus corporis humani sensilibus et irritabilibus," in Comment. Soc. reg. Gottingæ (1752), 1753, ii, 114–214.

[2] Mitth. d. naturf. Gesellsch. in Bern (1902), 1903, No. 1519–1550, pp. 203–226.

[3] Haller: Methodus studii medici, Amsterdam, 1751.

sententiarum. In embryology, he was something of a reactionary, and successfully wet-blanketed the correct ideas of Wolff, as will appear. He lectured and wrote on surgery, and made a superb bibliography of the subject,[1] but never performed an operation in his life. In private life, Haller was modest, sensible, kindly, and charitable, and—rare trait—not afraid to affirm his ignorance when he could not explain a phenomenon. As he was complacent about his own infallibility, however, and did not like to have it questioned, he left no school of followers behind him. To his contemporaries he seemed a *"vir gloriosus,"* living apart on a high eminence; but

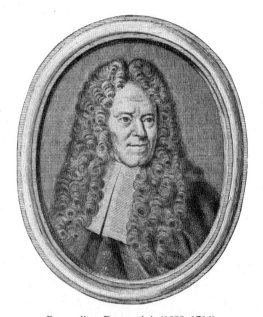

Bernardino Ramazzini (1633–1714).

he was probably not the "pursy, play'd-out Philistine" of some of his portraits. As a youth he was singularly fine-looking. In the history of German literature, Haller has a substantial, honorable place, and his *Versuch schweizerischer Gedichte* (1732) was the subject of the famous literary quarrel between Bodmer and Gottsched as to the relative merits of the natural and the artificial in poetry. His poem, *Die Alpen* (1729), first drew attention to the glorious beauties of Swiss mountain scenery, and its influence may be seen in Klopstock, in Schiller, and even in Coleridge. By

[1] Bibliotheca chirurgica, Bern, 1774–75.

some irony of fate Haller, the poet, is now chiefly remembered by the following commonplace expression of bourgeois materialism:

Ins Innre der Natur dringt kein erschaffener Geist,
Zu glücklich, wann sie noch die äussre Schale weist.

In Nature's inmost heart no spirit doth abide,
Happy indeed the wight who knows its outer side—

which so excited the derision of Goethe.[1] With Haller, the systematist, we may class the works of a group of very original men, beginning with the "De morbis artificium diatriba" (Modena, 1700) of Bernardino **Ramazzini** (1633–1714), which opened up an entirely new department of modern medicine, the diseases and hygiene of occupations. Ramazzini was the first after Paracelsus to call attention to such conditions as stone-mason's and miner's phthisis (pneumonokoniosis). Italy has done eponymic honor to his memory in the medical periodical which bears his name.

"The Divine Order" (1742)[2] of the old Prussian army chaplain, Johann Peter **Süssmilch** (1707–77), is an epoch-making work in the development of vital and medical statistics, bringing together many data of capital importance in public hygiene, life insurance, and national polity. Although the old theologian's view is entirely teleologic, basing everything upon a divine order in nature, and although the English statist, John Graunt, had long before noticed (1662) that the population can be estimated from an accurate death-rate, yet the importance of Süssmilch to medical men is of a higher order than the mere casting up of figures. He it was who insisted upon the moral and political significance of statistics and affirmed that the true wealth of any nation consists in an industrious, healthy native population, and not merely in material and financial resources. The intelligent application of this humane, broad-minded principle is the secret of the industrial and military power of the mighty German Empire today.

In connection with the name of Süssmilch three other German systematists may be mentioned, viz., Johann Friedrich **Blumenbach** (1752–1840), of Göttingen, and Pieter Camper, the founders of anthropology and craniology, and Johann Peter Frank, the founder of public hygiene. Although Blumenbach's thesis, "On the Native Varieties of the Human Race" (1776),[3] was preceded

---

[1] The lines occur in Haller's apostrophe to Newton, which, of course, stirred the ill-will of Goethe, on account of his own opposition to Newton's theory of colors.

[2] J. P. Süssmilch: Die göttliche Ordnung in denen Veränderungen des menschlichen Geschlechts, Berlin, 1742.

[3] Blumenbach: De generis humani varietate nativa, Göttingen, 1776.

by the essays of Bernier (1684) and Linnæus (1735), yet it may fairly be considered the starting-point in modern ethnology, since he bases his classification upon the shape of the skull and the facial configuration, as well as the color of the skin. In describing his large collection of crania, in an atlas of 70 plates (1790–1820), he used the vertical aspect from above downward as a norm in classification, but because a female Georgian skull was the most symmetric, he introduced the unfortunate term, "Caucasian," to represent the Aryan race. He is also remembered by the *clivus Blumenbachii* in the pons. Blumenbach was followed by Pieter **Camper** (1722–89), an artist in training, who illustrated his own

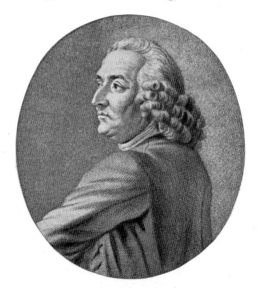

Pieter Camper (1722–89).

works and introduced the "facial angle" as a criterion of race (1760).

A rare and happy mixture of German thoroughness with French intelligence was the Bavarian, Johann Peter **Frank** (1745–1821), the four volumes of whose "Complete System of Medical Polity" (*System einer vollständigen medicinischen Polizey*), published at Mannheim in 1777–88 by Schwann, the printer of Schiller's "Robbers," are the very foundation of modern public hygiene, and a noble monument of a life-long devotion to humanity. The author was a poor waif, almost cast adrift at a street door, who made himself one of the greatest teachers and practitioners of his time by his own industry. He was the first physician to signalize the impor-

tance of diseases of the spinal cord (1792),[1] defined diabetes insipidus (1794), and wrote an important treatise on therapeutics (1792–
1821).[2] His great work on public hygiene, as covering the whole
subject of man's life "from the womb to the tomb"—sewerage,
water-supply, even school-hygiene, sexual hygiene, and suitable
benches and meals for the children, as well as the ideal of a
scientific "medical police"—really leaves little for Pettenkofer and
the moderns. In the preventive medicine of the future, the name
of Frank will loom larger with meanings, for he was himself a
true modern.

After Haller, the principal landmark of eighteenth century

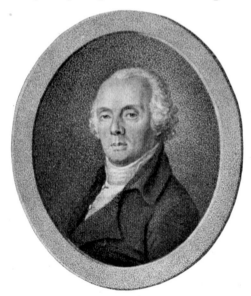

Johann Peter Frank (1745–1821).

physiology is undoubtedly the *Statical Essays* (1731–33) of Stephen
Hales (1677–1761), an English clergyman of inventive genius, who
enriched practical science in many ways, particularly as the originator of artificial ventilation (1743). In the first part of these
essays Hales investigates the movement of sap in plants. The
second part, entitled *Hæmadynamics* (1733), contains his most
important work, on the mechanical relations of blood-pressure,
marking the first real advance in the physiology of the circulation

---

[1] Frank: "De vertebralis columnæ in morbis dignitate," in his Delect.
opusc. med., Ticini, 1792, xi, 1–50.

[2] "De curandis hominum morbis epitome," Vienna, 1792–1821.

between Harvey and Poiseuille. By fastening a long glass tube inside a horse's artery Hales devised the first manometer or tonometer, with the aid of which he made quantitative estimates of the blood-pressure, the capacity of the heart, and the velocity of the blood-current, which in tendency are essentially modern.

The **physiology of digestion** was materially advanced by the experiments of René-A.-F. **de Réaumur**[1] (1683–1757) upon a pet kite, in which he succeeded in isolating the gastric juice and demonstrating its solvent effect upon foods (1752).[2] These results were very ably confirmed and extended by the work of the Abbé Lazaro **Spallanzani** (1729–99), of Scandiano, Italy, an in-

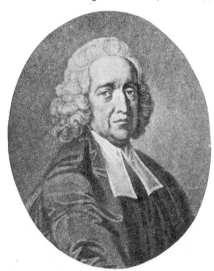

vestigator of singular power. Spallanzani discovered the digestive power of saliva, and reaffirmed the solvent property of the gastric juice,[3] showing that it will act outside the body, and that it can not only prevent putrefaction, but will inhibit it when once begun. He failed, however, to recognize the acid character of the gastric juice, a point which was to be brought out by the American physiologist Young. In 1768,[4] Spallanzani founded the doctrine of the regeneration of the spinal cord through his dis-

Stephen Hales (1677–1761).

covery of its new-growth during regeneration of the tail in the lizard. He also showed that the sexual posture in the frog is maintained as a spinal reflex after decapitation or after section of the two brachial nerves, fore and aft (1768).[5] He made important investigations of the respiratory exchanges in warm- and cold-blooded animals,[6] showing that hibernating animals can live comfortably for

---

[1] The inventor of the 80 degrees thermometer.

[2] Réaumur: "Sur la digestion des oiseaux," Mém. Acad. roy. d. sc., 1752, Paris, 1756, 266–307.

[3] Spallanzani: Della digestione degli animali, in his: Fisica animale, Venice, 1782, vol. i, 1–312, ii, 1–83.

[4] Prodromi sulle riproduzione animale: Riproduzione della coda del girinc, Modena, 1768.

[5] Ibid.   [6] See the memoirs on respiration in his collected works.

a time in carbon dioxide gas, where ordinary warm-blooded creatures die at once; that cold-blooded animals can live in hydrogen and continue to give off CO_2; and, most important of all, that living tissues, excised from a freshly killed animal, will take up oxygen and give off CO_2 in an atmosphere of air or hydrogen or nitrogen. His experiments on the bat proved that it is very slightly dependent on vision, so that its known deficiency in visual purple (Kühne) may be due to disuse. A most important investigation of Spallanzani's bore upon the doctrine of spontaneous generation. In 1748 Walter Needham, an English Catholic priest in residence on the continent, published certain experiments on boiled meat-juices, inclosed in vials and sealed with mastic, the subsequent presence of microorganisms in these liquids leading him to the conclusion that they were produced by spontaneous generation. Spallanzani refuted all this by using glass flasks with slender necks, which could be hermetically sealed in flame, immersing them in boiling water prior to the test; and he also overthrew Needham's subsequent objection to the boiling feature by showing that exposure of the sealed fluids to the air again would renew the presumable germinative or "vegetative force" in the liquids, which, Needham maintained, had been destroyed by the flame. Finally, Spallanzani was, with Réaumur, Trembley, and Bonnet, one of the pioneers of experimental morphology in the strictly modern sense. Réaumur, in 1712, produced regenerations of the claws and scales of lobsters and crabs.[1] In 1740–44,[2] Abraham Trembley cut hydras into several pieces, producing new individuals, and got a third generation by cutting up the latter. In this he was followed by Bonnet,[3] who experimented on fresh-water worms (1741–45), and by Spallanzani, who produced regenerations of the heads, tails, limbs, and tentacles of earthworms, tad-poles, salamanders, and snails (1768).[4] These experiments were not taken up again until the end of the nineteenth century, but they contain all the essentials of the modern work of Roux, Driesch, Morgan, Loeb, and others.

An English physiologist, whose work was long forgotten but has now come to the front on account of its essential importance, is William **Hewson** (1739–74), of Hexham, Northumberland. Hewson was a pupil of the Hunters, and John Hunter left him in charge of his dissecting-room when he went abroad with the army. He afterward went into partnership with William Hunter in anatomic

---

[1] Réaumur: Mém. de l'Acad. de sc., Paris, 1712, 223–242, 1 pl.

[2] Trembley: Mémoires pour servir à l'histoire d'un genre de polypes d'eau douce, Leyden, 1744.

[3] Bonnet: Traité d'insectologie, pt. 2. Paris, 1745.

[4] Spallanzani: Prodromo di un'opera sopra le riproduzioni animali, Milan, 1829.

teaching, sharing his profits, and later assisting him at the school in Great Windmill Street from 1769 on. When Hewson married, William Hunter, who seems to have had a natural aversion to Benedicts, abruptly broke off the partnership, much to Hewson's pecuniary disadvantage. He soon retrieved himself, however, having made his reputation through his Royal Society memoir on the lymphatics, which got him the Copley medal in 1769 and the honor of F.R.S. in 1770. Hewson's discovery of the existence of lacteal and lymphatic vessels in birds, reptiles, and fishes was esteemed of capital importance in its day, because the two Hunters

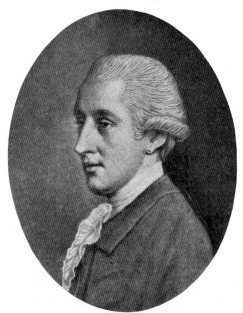

William Hewson, F.R.S. (1739–74).

maintained that absorption is an exclusive function of the lymphatics, against which it was objected that there are animals which have neither lacteals nor lymphatics. Magendie's demonstration that the blood-vessels have an absorbent function of course threw this phase of Hewson's work into the background, and present interest is centered on his "Experimental Inquiry into the Properties of the Blood" (1771). This work, a fine example of the experimental method taught by the Hunters, establishes the essential features of the coagulation of the blood in an entirely modern spirit. Before Hewson's time, coagulation was ascribed to the supposed cooling off of the blood, to the fact that it had ceased to move, or to the idea that its corpuscles had solidified into rouleaux. Hewson showed that when the coagulation of the blood is delayed, as by cold, neutral salts, or otherwise, a coagulable plasma can be separated from the corpuscles and skimmed off the surface, and that this plasma contains an insoluble substance which can be precipitated and removed at a temperature a little over 50° C. Coagulation, in Hewson's view, was due to the formation in the plasma of this insoluble substance, which he called "coagulable lymph," and which we now know to be fibrinogen. Hewson's experiments were soon forgotten, even after Andrew Buchanan had shown, in 1845, that a substance can be extracted from the lymphatic glands, the buffy coat of the blood, and other tissues which will coagulate not only blood, but serous fluids not in themselves coagulable. The modern discovery that fibrinogen is a nucleoproteid, and that in coagulation it is converted into fibrin, threw the work of Hewson into stronger relief. He also made the important observation that air is contained in the lungs in pneumothorax (1767), and was one of the first to perform the operation of paracentesis, although in this he was preceded by Monro *secundus*. Hewson, a man of genius, died of a dissection wound in 1774.

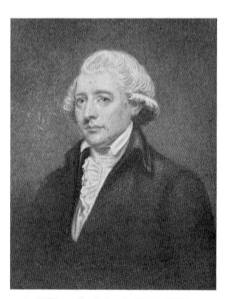

William Cruikshank (1745–1800).

William Cumberland **Cruikshank** (1745–1800), of Edinburgh, who succeeded Hewson as William Hunter's assistant, gave the latter such satisfaction that he was made a partner in the Great Windmill Street School, which, after Hunter's death, he took charge of, in conjunction with Matthew Baillie. Cruikshank investigated the reunion and regeneration of divided nerves (1776),[1] the passage of the impregnated ovum through the Fallopian tube (1778),[2] the physiology of absorption (1778–86), and in his "Ex-

[1] Phil. Tr., London, 1795, lxxxv, 177–189, 1 pl.
[2] *Ibid.*, 1797, lxxxvii, 197–214, 1 pl.

periments Upon the Insensible Perspiration of the Human Body
(1778) he demonstrated that the skin gives off carbon dioxide, as
well as the lungs. His "Anatomy of the Absorbing Vessels
of the Human Body" (1786) embodies the results of his
labors with William Hunter.[1] Cruikshank had a large practice,
turning his private office into a public dispensary for the poor on
occasion, which won him the warm regard of his friend, Dr. Johnson, whom he treated in his last illness and who described him, in
the Scottish phrase, as "a sweet-blooded man."

Robert **Whytt** (1714–66), of Edinburgh, a pupil of Monro
primus, Cheselden, Winslow, Boerhaave, and Albinus, is memorable for his work on the physiology and pathology of the nervous
system. In his memoir, "On the Vital and Other Involuntary
Motions of Animals" (Edinburgh, 1750), he demonstrated for the
first time that the integrity of the spinal cord as a whole is not necessary for reflex action, and that the preservation of only a small
fragment of it will suffice for this purpose. He also discovered
that destruction of one of the anterior corpora quadrigemina
will abolish reflex contraction of the pupils to light (Whytt's
reflex, 1768), and was one of the first to notice the phenomena
of spinal shock. In all these observations, he was moved to
discard the current hypothesis of Stahl that a "rational soul"
is the cause of involuntary movements. In his "Observations
on the Dropsy in the Brain" (1768) Whytt first described
tubercular meningitis in children, and his book, "On Nervous,
Hypochondriacal, or Hysterical Diseases" (1764), was an
important contribution to neurology in its day.

The cerebrospinal fluid was discovered by Domenico Cotugno
(1736–1822) in 1784.

Electrophysiology had its origin in the epoch-making experiments on muscle-nerve preparations, summarized in 1792[2] by
Luigi **Galvani** (1737–98) of Bologna. Animal electricity had
been observed in the torpedo by John Walsh in 1773, and in
John Hunter's studies of other electric fishes, but Galvani's discovery of the electric properties of excised tissues, which he happened upon in his laboratory by sheer accident, is the starting-
point of modern work. It was followed up, with rare skill and insight, by Alessandro **Volta** (1745–1827), in his "Letters on Animal
Electricity" (1792). Volta divided conductors of electricity into
metallic and liquid (electrolysis), devised the famous Voltaic pile,
and showed that a muscle can be thrown into continuous (tetanic)

---

[1] Hunter was accustomed to say that the anatomy of the lymphatic system was developed by himself, his brother John, Hewson, and Cruikshank.

[2] Galvani: De viribus electricitatis in motu musculari, Modena, 1792.

contraction by successive electric stimulations. Meanwhile Benjamin Franklin, Kratzenstein, Schaeffer (1752), G. F. Rössler (electric bath, 1768), Manduyt (1777), William Henly (1779), and many others were already utilizing electricity in the treatment of disease.

The Abbe Felice Fontana (1730–1803) was the author of a treatise on the venom of the viper (1767),[1] which was the starting-point of the modern investigation of serpent venoms.

But perhaps the best piece of physiologic work in the eighteenth century was the completion of the modern **theory of respiration,** which turned upon the discovery of the different gases in the atmosphere, viz., carbon dioxide by Black (1757), hydrogen by Cavendish (1766), nitrogen by Rutherford (1772), oxygen by Priestley and Scheele (1771) and Lavoisier (1775). The great Scottish chemist Joseph **Black** (1728–99) is known to physicists for his original definitions of "specific heat" and "capacity for heat," and for his subtle criterion of "latent heat" —that the temperature of a body and the amount of heat it possesses are two entirely different things. In his *Dissertatio de humore acido a cibo orto* (1754) he made a distinction equally important for chemistry and physiology. Chemists of Black's day, following Stahl, believed that when lime is heated it gains phlogiston, and when quicklime is slaked it loses phlogiston. Black's experiments exploded Stahl's theory by showing that, in reality, quickened lime loses something ($CaCO_3 = CaO + CO_2$), and quicklime, when slaked, gains something ($CaO + 2H_2O = Ca(OH)_2$). He also noted that the gas or "fixed air" given off by quickened lime and alkalis is also present in expired air, and is physiologically irrespirable, although not necessarily toxic.

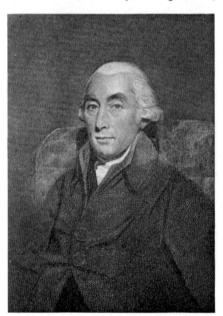

Joseph Black (1728–99).

---

[1] Fontana: Ricerche fisiche sopra il veleno della vipera, Lucca, 1767.

17

Thus Black had again isolated the carbonic acid gas which Van Helmont had, over a hundred years before, noted in fermentation as *gas sylvestre*. A few steps further and he would have arrived at the conclusion of the whole matter. Joseph **Priestley** (1733–1804) had the truth in his grasp when he isolated oxygen (1772)[1] and saw that vegetating plants renew vitiated air, but being a confirmed Stahlian, he only made matters worse by seeing respiration as "the phlogistication of dephlogisticated air." It was reserved for the genius of Antoine-Laurent **Lavoisier** (1743–94) to discover the true nature of the interchange of gases in the lungs, and to demolish the phlogiston theory by his introduction of quantitative relations in chemistry.

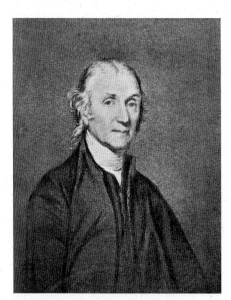

Joseph Priestley (1733–1804).

As Sir Michael Foster maintains, "he and he alone discovered oxygen" (1775),[2] for Mayow, Priestley, and Scheele had only isolated it. Priestley, deceived by the specious label, "phlogiston," had explained the facts of respiration in an inverted order. But Lavoisier proved that inspired air is converted into Black's "fixed air," the nitrogen or "azote" (which he also discovered) alone remaining unchanged. Further, in conjunction with the astronomer **Laplace** (1780–85),[3] he demonstrated that respiration is in every way the analogue of combustion, the chemical products being carbon dioxide and water. But Lavoisier, whose life was lost to science through the fanaticism of the French Revolutionists, had adopted the erroneous theory that the oxidation of carbon and hydrogen takes place in the tubules of the lungs. This was corrected in 1791 by **Lagrange,** the author of the *Mécanique analytique*, who maintained, through his pupil Hassen-

---

[1] Priestley: Observations on Different Kinds of Air, Phil. Tr., London, 1772, lxii, 147–264, 1 pl.

[2] Lavoisier: Hist. Acad. roy. d. sc. 1775, Paris, 1778, pp. 520–526.

[3] *Ibid.*, 1780, Paris, 1784, 355–408.

fratz,[1] that the dissolved oxygen of the inspired air slowly takes up carbon and hydrogen from the tissues as the blood courses through them. The finishing touch was added when Gustav Magnus, in 1837,[2] showed, with the aid of a Sprengel's air-pump, that venous and arterial blood both contain oxygen as well as CO_2, demonstrating—what Cruikshank toward the end of his life had partly elucidated—that all the tissues respire in the sense of assimilating oxygen and giving up CO_2. Thus the development of the physiology of respiration, from Borelli to Magnus, was almost exclusively the work of three mathematicians, two physicists, and five chemists.

The great center of **anatomic teaching** in the seventeenth century was Leyden; at the beginning of the eighteenth century, Paris. The rise of Edinburgh as a center of medical teaching was due to the following train of circumstances. In 1700 John **Monro,** a Scotch army surgeon of good family, settled in Edinburgh, and, knowing of the superiority of continental training in medicine, conceived the idea of starting a medical school in the northern

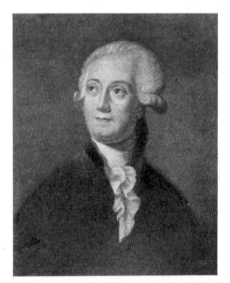

Antoine-Laurent Lavoisier (1743–94).

capital, mainly out of a great affection for his only son, Alexander, whom he desired to leave well established in this world. In accordance with this plan, young Alexander Monro received a careful medical education at London, Paris, and Leyden, becoming a warm friend of Cheselden and Boerhaave, and, on returning to Edinburgh in 1719, was duly examined and qualified by the Surgeon's Guild, and, in 1720, on recommendation of the Town Council, was elected professor of anatomy in the newly established university at the age of twenty-two. Being a teacher of marked ability, his courses were soon followed by enthusiastic students in large numbers, the roster climbing from 57, in 1720, to 182, in

[1] Hassenfratz: Ann. d. chim., Paris, 1791, ix, 275.
[2] Magnus: Ann. d. Phys. u. Chem., Leipzig, 1837, xli, 583–606.

1749, this steady arithmetic progression being interrupted only by the Rebellion of '45. Alexander Monro followed his father's plan for his own son, and the latter extended the same policy to the grandson, both of whom were also named Alexander, so that the three Monros, *primus, secundus,* and *tertius,* as they were called, held the chair of anatomy at Edinburgh in uninterrupted succession, like an estate in gavelkind, for a period of one hundred and twenty-six years (1720-1846). The men of the Monro dynasty were, all of them, original characters of unusual attainments, authors of many valuable works, morbid on the subject of controversy, it is true, but in every way worthy of the confidence placed in them

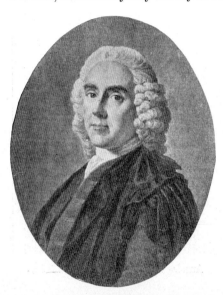

Alexander Monro *primus* (1697-1767).

by their fellow-townsmen. During the period 1720-90, some 12,800 students were taught by Monro *primus* and *secundus* alone, and it was largely due to them that Edinburgh became the great center of medical teaching that it was in the "last century." Anatomical research in this period did not attain the brilliancy it had in the preceding century, nearly every year of which was distinguished by some new discovery. Many of the best anatomists of the eighteenth century, such as Cheselden, Pott, the Monros, the Hunters, Desault, Scarpa, were so-called surgeon-anatomists, and the studies of the time were mainly topographic and inconographic. Surgical anatomy, in fact, begins properly with the writings of Joseph Lieutaud (1703-80) and, after this time (1724), a great number of fine atlases were published, such as Cheselden on the bones (1733),[1] Albinus on the bones and muscles (1747-53),[2] Eisenmann on the uterus (1752),[3] Zinn on the eye (1755),[4] Scarpa

---

[1] Cheselden: Osteographia, London, 1733.

[2] B. S. Albinus: Tabulæ sceleti et musculorum corporis humani, Leyden, 1747.

[3] G. H. Eisenmann: Tabulæ anatomicæ quatuor uteri (etc.), Strassburg, 1752.

[4] J. G. Zinn: Descriptio anatomica oculi humani, Göttingen, 1755.

on the ear (1772–99),[1] Soemmerring on the cranial nerves (1778),[2] Sandifort on the duodenum (1780),[3] or Mascagni on the lymphatics (1787).[4]   These and many others were all gathered together in the great collection of Caldani (Icones Anatomicæ, Venice, 1801–13).   The surgeons Pierre Dionis and William Cheselden wrote anatomic text-books which were both of them popular in their day, but probably the best all-around treatise on the subject between Vesalius and Bichat was the "Exposition anatomique" (1723) of the Danish teacher Jakob Benignus **Winslow** (1669–1760), a pupil of Duverney, who did much to condense and systematize what was known, especially in regard to such matters as the origin and insertion of the different muscles.   His work was the authoritative text-book for nearly a century. There was a fair showing of those specialized investigations of physiological import which added so much luster to seventeenth century anatomy.   Duverney's work on the ear (1683) was very ably supplemented by the investigations of Valsalva (1704) and Cotugno (1774), and with these may be mentioned the monographs of Cowper on the urethral glands (1702),[5] of Abraham Vater on the ampulla of the bile-duct (1702),[6] of Lieberkühn on the intestinal glands,[7] of James Douglas on the peritoneum (1730),[8] of the elder Meckel (1748)[9] and Wrisberg (1777)[10] on the vagus nerve, of Zinn on the ciliary ligaments (1753),[11] and the varied researches of Santorini (1724).[12]

Toward the end of the century, Samuel Thomas von **Soemmerring** (1755–1830), a native of Thorn, Western Prussia, wrote a monumental treatise on anatomy (1791–96), which was reissued

---

[1] A. Scarpa: De structura fenestræ rotundæ auris et de tympano, Modena, 1772. De auditu et olfactu, Pavia, 1789. De penitiorum ossium structura, Leipzig, 1799.

[2] Soemmerring: De base encephali et originibus nervorum cranio egredentium, Göttingen, 1778.

[3] E. Sandifort: Tabulæ intestini duodeni, Leyden, 1780.

[4] P. Mascagni: Vasorum lymphaticorum corporis humana historia et iconographia, Siena, 1787.

[5] W. Cowper: Glandolarum quarundam, nuper detectarum . . . descriptio, London, 1702.

[6] A. Vater: Diss. anat. qua novum bilis diverticulum circa orificium ductus choledochi [etc.], Wittenberg, 1720.

[7] J. N. Lieberkühn: De fabrica et actione intestinorum tenuium hominis, Leyden, 1745.

[8] J. Douglas: A description of the peritonæum, London, 1730.

[9] J. F. Meckel: De quinto pare nervorum cerebri, Göttingen, 1748.

[10] H. A. Wrisberg: Observationes anatomicæ de quinto pare nervorum encephali, Göttingen, 1777.

[11] J. G. Zinn: De ligamentis ciliaribus, Göttingen, 1753.

[12] G. D. Santorini: Observationes anatomicæ, Venice, 1724.

nearly half a century later by Rudolf Wagner, Henle, and others.[1] He made most important researches on the brain, the eye, the ear, nose and throat, hernia, the anthropology of the negro (1785),[2] and the injurious effects of corsets (1793),[3] but is now best remembered for his remarkable accuracy in anatomic, illustration and by his classification of the cranial nerves (1778),[4] which eventually superseded that of Willis. Soemmerring was also one of the inventors of the electric telegraph (1809).

A remarkable family of Prussian anatomists were the Meckels, father, son, and two grandsons. Johann Friedrich **Meckel**, the

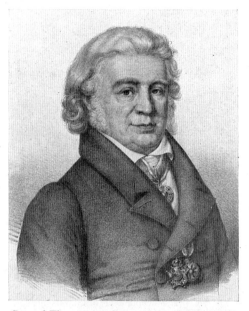

Samuel Thomas von Soemmerring (1755-1830).

elder (1724-74), of Wetzlar, graduated at Göttingen with his above-mentioned noteworthy dissertation on the fifth nerve (Meckel's ganglion) in 1748, became professor of anatomy, botany and obstetrics at Berlin in 1751, and was the first teacher of midwifery

---

[1] S. T. von Soemmerring: Vom Baue des menschlichen Körpers, Frankfort on the Main, 1791-96.

[2] Ueber die körperliche Verschiedenheit des Negers vom Europäer, Cassel, 1784.

[3] Ueber die Wirkung der Schnurbrüste, with copper-plate, Berlin, 1793.

[4] De basi encephali et originibus nervorum cranio egredentium libri quinque, Göttingen, 1778.

at the Charité. He was the first to describe the submaxillary ganglion (1748), and made important investigations of the nerve-supply of the face (1751) and the terminal visceral filaments of the veins and lymphatics (1772). His son, Philipp Friedrich Theodor Meckel (1756–1803), of Berlin, graduated at Strassburg in 1777, with an important dissertation on the internal ear, was professor of anatomy and surgery at Halle in 1779, and editor of the "Neues Archiv der praktischen Arzneykunst" (Leipzig, 1789–95). He was a favorite and highly honored obstetrician at the Russian court. His son, Johann Friedrich Meckel (1781–1833), of Halle, called the younger Meckel, was an eminent pathologist, and the greatest comparative anatomist in Germany before Johannes Müller. He has been called the German Cuvier. His most important works are his treatises on pathologic anatomy (1812–18), normal human anatomy (1815), his atlas of 33 plates representing human abnormities (1817–26), and his great system of comparative anatomy (1821–30), in which he sets forth the view that the development of the higher animals is an epitome of the ancestral stages which preceded it. He translated Wolff's monograph on the development of the intestines in 1812, and is memorable as the discoverer of the Meckel diverticulum in the intestines. His younger brother, August Albrecht Meckel (1790–1829), of Halle, became professor of anatomy and forensic medicine at Bern in 1821, and was a specialist in the latter branch.

The starting-point of modern **embryology** was the *Theoria Generationis* (1759) of Caspar Frederich **Wolff** (1733–94), of Berlin, one of the most original spirits of his time, who is eponymically remembered by his discovery of the Wolffian bodies. Wolff revived Harvey's doctrine of epigenesis or gradual building up of parts, and took a firm stand against the current theory that the embryo is already preformed and incased in the ovary (*emboîtement*), but his negation of germinal continuity and the opposition of Haller prevented his evolutionary ideas from gaining any ground until 1812, when the younger Meckel translated his great monograph on the development of the intestines in the chick (1768–69), one of the acknowledged classics of embryology. While the plates and the argument of the *Theoria Generationis* (1759) are far inferior to Malpighi's work, Wolff surpassed himself in the memoir of 1768, described by von Baer as "the greatest masterpiece of scientific observation that we possess." Wolff's view, that the organs are formed from "leaf-like (blastodermic) layers," comes as near as possible to the germ-layer theory of von Baer himself. In 1767, from investigations of the buds of cabbages, beans, and other plants, Wolff arrived at the conclusion that "all parts of the plant except the stem are modified leaves."

This conclusion was reached independently by Johann Wolfgang von Goethe (1749–1832), in his essay on plant metamorphosis (1790),[1] in which he argued deductively the fundamental unity of leaf, flower, and fruit, and the descent of all plants from an archetypal form (*Urpflanze*). Like more recent botanists, he was unable to decide whether the direction of evolution was from foliage-leaf to reproductive leaf, or *vice versâ*, and he was painfully surprised when Schiller observed, "This is not an observation, it is an idea." The great poet was, however, one of the pioneers of evolution, the first to use the term "morphology," and the discoverer of the intermaxillary bone (1786).[2] Independently of Oken (1790), he stated the theory that the skull is made up of modified vertebræ, and, before Savigny, he saw that the jaws of insects were modified limbs. In connection with Goethe's botanical work, a passing mention should be made of Christian Konrad Sprengel (1750–1816), the old Prussian pastor who was thrown out of his rectorate at Spandau because he neglected his congregation for botany, and whose "Newly Discovered Secret of Nature" (1793) was brought to the front by Darwin. Sprengel pointed out that the colored markings, shapes, nectar, etc., of plants are adaptations to secure cross-fertilizations by insects, and that the latter process is the rule, not the exception. The teleologic significance of cross-fertilization was afterward proved by Herbert, Gärtner, and others, and utilized by Darwin. Other forerunners of Darwin were the naturalist Buffon (1707–88), whose Histoire Naturelle (1749–1804), although a popular descriptive work, contained many casual denials of the fixity of species and a veiled suggestion of a possible common ancestor for horse and ass, ape and man; and Erasmus Darwin (1731–1802), whose 'Loves of the Plants" (1789) and "Zoönomia" (1794) emphasized the gradual evolution of complex organisms from simple primordial forms, the struggle for existence in animals and plants, sexual selection, protective mimicry, and the indirect influence of environment in producing transformations which may modify species.

Perhaps the greatest comparative anatomist of the eighteenth century was Felix **Vicq d'Azyr** (1748–94), permanent secretary of the Paris Academy of Medicine, whose studies of the flexor and extensor muscles of man and animals, and the morphology of the brain, the vocal cords, and the structure of birds and quadrupeds, were the best of the period.

The best specimens of **anatomic illustration** in the eighteenth century show the gradual passage from the copper-plate, through the "taille-douce" to the steel-plate period, as seen in such splendid folios as Cheselden's "Osteographia" (1733), Haller's "Icones Anatomicæ" (1743–56), or William Hunter's "Anatomia Uteri Humani Gravidi" (1774), and the masterpieces of Santorini, Albinus, Soemmerring, and Scarpa. Colored copper-plates were introduced in the eighteenth century by Jacques-Christophe Le Blon (1667–1741), who left only one anatomic specimen of his handiwork, a little plate of the genital organs made for the 1719 edition of Cockburn's treatise on gonorrhea, now exceedingly rare. It was followed by six anatomic plates of his pupil, Jan Ladmiral, and by the many fine atlases of Jacob-Fabian Gaultier d'Agouty (1717–86).

One of the greatest anatomic illustrators of his time was Bern-

---

[1] Goethe: Versuch die Metamorphose der Pflanzen zu erklären, Gotha, 1790.

[2] Goethe: Ueber den Zwischenkiefer des Menschen und der Thiere. Nova Acta Acad. Leopold-Carol., Halle, 1831, xv.

hard Siegfried **Albinus** (1697–1770), of Frankfort on the Oder, who had studied under Bidloo, Boerhaave, and Duverney, and held the chairs of anatomy and surgery (1718) and medicine (1745) at the University of Leyden. Albinus edited the works of Harvey, Vesalius, Fabricius, and Eustachius, and in illustrating these, as well as his own works, he employed the best artistic talent. His atlases of the bones (1726, 1753), the muscles (1734), the veins and arteries of the intestines (1736), the fetal bones (1737), the skeleton and skeletal muscles (1747, 1762), the gravid

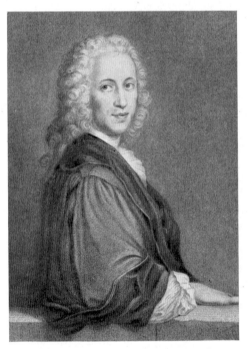

Bernhard Siegfried Albinus (1697–1770).

uterus (1749), are all justly renowned for their beauty and accuracy of illustration and for the elegant style of the accompanying text. Albinus was also held to be an incomparable lecturer, and was a master of the art of anatomic injection.

Of all medical men who have illustrated their own books, probably none have ever exhibited such striking artistic talent as that brilliant Venetian, Antonio **Scarpa** (1747–1832). In appearance like the youthful Napoleon, Scarpa was a virtuoso in the most varied sense, a great anatomist and surgeon, equally skilled as orthopedist and ophthalmologist, an irreproachable

Latinist, a master of sarcasm, yet a most attractive teacher, and a draftsman of the first order. In anatomy he is remembered for his discovery of the membranous labyrinth, the nasopalatine nerve, and the triangle in the thigh which bears his name; he was the first to regard arteriosclerosis as a lesion of the inner coats of the arteries; he wrote important treatises on hernia and eye diseases, and originated the procedure of iridodialysis; he made a shoe for club-foot which is still the model for orthopedists; but his greatest work is undoubtedly the magnificent "Tabulæ Nevrologicæ" (Pavia, 1794), which gives the first proper delineation

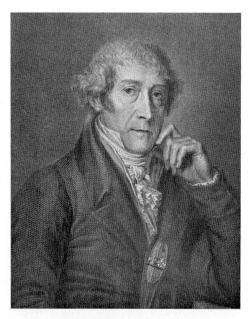

Antonio Scarpa (1747–1832).

of the nerves of the heart. Executed with the force of genius, and irreproachable in accuracy of detail, Scarpa's illustrations are the crown and flower of achievement in anatomic pen-drawing, while Anderloni's masterly steel-plates of the same are comparable in *brio* with the work of Sharp, the Drevets, and other masters of the best period of line-engraving.

In Great Britain anatomic study received a mighty impulse from the teaching of the brothers Hunter, and the name of William Hunter is inseparably connected with the advancement of **obstetrics.** During the eighteenth century, the care of labor cases began to pass from the midwife proper to the trained male obstetrician. In Paris, the pace for this was already set during the preceding century through the circumstance that Jules Clément was called upon to attend La Vallière, mistress of the "Grand Monarque," in her confinement in 1663, receiving the title of "accoucheur" for his trouble; whereupon, in due course, male midwifery became the fashion among the great ladies of the court. Progress in this matter was, of course, slow, and when a certain obstetrician told Joseph II that the Viennese women were too modest to have men as midwives, that moral monarch replied, with fitting irony: *Utinam non essent adeo pudicae.*[1] At first, as in some court circles today, the obstetrician simply supervised or "assisted at" the conduct of labor among those who could afford his services; but, as soon as women began to permit physicians to examine the parts as well as deliver them, inductive knowledge of the complex details of midwifery began to make rapid strides. In London, this change was principally due to the teaching and influence of two Lanarkshire men, William Smellie, and his pupil, William Hunter, to Sir Fielding Ould in Dublin, and to Charles White in Manchester. On the continent, the cause of male midwifery was upheld by Röderer in Göttingen, Camper in Amsterdam, Baudelocque and Levret in Paris, Boër in Vienna, and Saxtorph in Copenhagen.

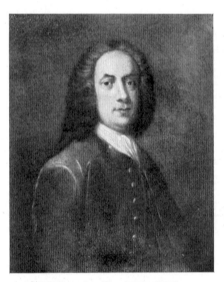

William Smellie (1697–1763).

William Smellie (1697–1763), the friend and teacher of Smollett, learned his obstetrics in Paris, and, settling in London in 1739, conceived the idea of teaching the subject at his own house, using a leather-covered manikin supported by actual bones, and charging three guineas for the course. In spite of the bitter opposition of Mrs. Nihell, the Haymarket midwife, and of his own un-

---

[1] "Would they were not modest to that extent." (Cited by Moll.) Perhaps the Emperor was thinking of the advice which Van Swieten gave to his father.

cultivated bearing, he acquired a large practice, and to him William Hunter came as resident pupil in 1741. Smellie's Midwifery (1752) was the first book to lay down safe rules for using the forceps and for differentiating contracted from normal pelves by actual measurement. It was deemed worthy of the honor of a special reprint by the Sydenham Society in 1876–78.

William Hunter (1718–83) had five years' training at Glasgow University and three as a pupil of Cullen's, and followed the example of his London teachers, Smellie and Douglass, by giving, in 1746, a course of private lectures on dissecting, operative sur-

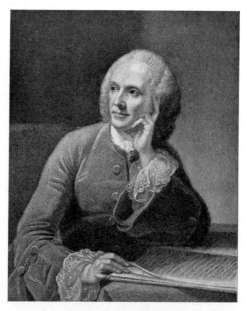

William Hunter (1718–83).

gery, and bandaging. He soon advanced in practice and public esteem, through his refined and courtly ways and his sagacious disposition, and eventually became the leading obstetrician and consultant of London. In 1768, he built the famous anatomic theater and museum in Great Windmill Street, where the best British anatomists and surgeons of the period, including his brother John, were trained. Here he labored with ardor to the end of his days, and few men have shown such austere devotion to science. We may contrast his noble gift of a museum worth £100,000 to the city of Glasgow with the Scotch tenacity of purpose and the self-denying stoicism of his private life, as summed up in the terse phrases of Mr. Stephen Paget: "He never married; he had no country house; he looks, in his portraits, a fastidious, fine gentleman; but he worked till he dropped and he lectured when he was dying." In relation to his colleagues, William Hunter was a jealous, sensitive, thin-blooded, high-strung man, who embittered his own life by needless controversy with contemporaries whom he easily overshadowed. His greatest work is his atlas of the pregnant uterus (London, 1774), the only medical publication of the celebrated Baskerville Press, illustrated by Rymsdyk at an enormous expense to the author, and representing the labor of thirty years. His special discovery of the "decidua reflexa" and the separate maternal and fetal circulation, in which his brother had a part, is the foundation of modern knowledge of placental anatomy. William Hunter also wrote papers of permanent value on old dislocations of the shoulders (1762),[1] symphysiotomy (1778),[2] the jurisprudence of infanticide (1783),[3] and the history of anatomy (1784).[4] He was the first to describe arteriovenous aneurysm (1761)[5] and retroversion of the uterus (1770),[6] and one of the first to recommend the tapping of ovarian cysts (1757);[7] but, unlike Smellie, he opposed the use of the forceps, and sometimes exhibited his own instrument, covered with rust, in evidence of the fact that he never used it.

The obstetric treatise of the Manchester surgeon, **Charles White** (London, 1773), stands out in its time as a pioneer work in aseptic midwifery.

The mechanism of labor was first considered by Sir Fielding Ould (1710–89), of Dublin, in his "Treatise on Midwifery" of 1742.

Prominent continental obstetricians of special note were Jean Palfyn (1649–1730), who reinvented or reintroduced the forceps in 1720;[8] Guillaume Mauquest de La Motte (1665–1737), who extended the use of podalic version to head presentations (1721); Pieter Camper (1722–89), who first proposed symphysiotomy, and Jean Réné Sigault, who first performed it successfully upon Mme. Souchot in 1777; Jean Louis Baudelocque, sr. (1746–1810), who invented a pelvimeter and advanced the knowledge of the mechanism of labor,

---

[1] Med. Obs. & Inquiries, London, 1762, ii, 373–381.

[2] "Reflections on dividing the Symphysis of the Ossa Pubis." Published as a supplement to the second edition of J. Vaughan's "Cases and Observations on the Hydrophobia," London, 1778.

[3] "On the uncertainty of the signs of murder in the case of bastard children," in Med. Obs. & Inquiries, 1778–83, London, 1784, vi, 266–290.

[4] Two Introductory Lectures, London, 1784.

[5] Med. Obs. & Inquiries, London, 1753–57, i, 340; 1762, ii, 390.

[6] Med. Obs. & Inquiries, London, 1771, iv, 409; 1776, v, 388.

[7] Med. Obs. & Inquiries (1757–61), London, 1762, ii, 44, 45.

[8] For further details about the history of the forceps in the eighteenth century, see Alban Doran's papers in Jour. Obst. and Gynæc., Brit. Empire, London, 1912, xxii, 119; 203: 1913, xxiii, 3; 65.

but overspecialized in his enumeration of possible positions of the fetus (1781); André Levret (1703–80), who improved the forceps and extended its use (1747); Carl Caspar Siebold (1736–1807), who performed the first symphysiotomy in Germany (1778); and Lucas Johann Boër (1751–1835), who was the ablest German obstetrician of his time and the pioneer of "natural obstetrics" (1791–1806). Before the time of Boër, pregnancy had been regarded as a sort of nine months' disease. He was the first to treat the condition as a physiologic process, and was a forerunner of Ramsbotham in tilting against "meddlesome midwifery."

Operative **gynecology,** as an independent specialty, had no real existence before the first half of the nineteenth century. Of stray contributions in the eighteenth century, we may mention Robert Houstoun's treatment of an ovarian dropsy (1701) by tapping the cyst (etymologically an "ovariotomy," but in no sense an excision of the ovary); William Hunter's proposal of excision for ovarian cyst in 1757, and his description of retroversion of the uterus (1770); Sigault's symphysiotomy (1777); Matthew Baillie's description of dermoid cysts of the ovary (1789), and Sömmerring's essay on the injurious effects of corsets (1793). Georg Ernst Stahl (1660–1734) wrote a lengthy monograph on the diseases of spinsters in 1724, and Jean Astruc (1684–1766) achieved a six-volume treatise on diseases of women in 1761–65.

Up to the time of John Hunter, **surgery** was entirely in French hands, and Paris was the only place where the subject could be properly studied. In Germany, as a consequence of the great setback of the Thirty Years' War, general surgery was practised mainly by the executioner and the barber (*Chirurgus*), or else by the wandering incisors, couchers, and bone-setters, while the army surgeon was called a "Feldscherer," because it was his duty to shave the officers. Even with such talent as that of Heister, von Siebold, and Richter, the art had no real status before the time of Frederick the Great. In England, there were only two clinical surgeons of first rank before Hunter's time, William Cheselden and Percival Pott. The whole period before Hunter was one of enterprise in respect of new amputations, excisions, or other improvements in operative technic, most of which are associated with French names.

As early as 1673 Pierre **Dionis** (died 1718) was giving courses on operative surgery on the cadaver, and his treatises on anatomy (1690) and surgery (1707) were, both of them, standard works for half a century, and translated even into Chinese. Dionis' "Cours d'opérations" is now valued for its anecdotes and pictures of the surgery of the day, in particular the story of the wandering lithotomist, Frère Jacques, who began as a bungling experimenter and became a master through his study of anatomy.

Jean-Louis **Petit** (1674–1750), of Paris, the leading French surgeon of the early eighteenth century, was the inventor of the screw-tourniquet, gave the first account of softening of the bones and of the formation of clots in wounded arteries, and made improvements in amputations and herniotomy. He was the first to open the mastoid process, an operation which he describes in this surgical treatises.[1] Petit's pupil, Dominique **Anel** (1628–1725), of Toulouse, is remembered by his operation for lacrimal fistula (1712), and by the fact that, like Guillemeau in the sixteenth century, he treated a traumatic aneurysm by single ligature (1710) before John Hunter's time. Pierre **Brasdor** (1721–97) is also remembered for his suggestion that aneurysms be treated by distal ligation, which was made an accomplished fact by Wardrop in 1828.

Pierre-Joseph **Desault** (1744–95), the teacher of Bichat, was the founder of an important surgical periodical, the *Journal de Chirurgie* (1791–92) did much to improve the treatment of fractures, and developed the technic of ligating blood-vessels for aneurysms.[2] Nicholas **André** (1658–1742) coined the term "orthopedics" in his treatise of 1741, and was the first to describe infra-orbital neuralgia (1756). The true founder of surgical orthopedics was, however, Jean-André **Venel** (1740–91), of Geneva, Switzerland, who, in 1780, founded the first orthopedic institute at Orbe, Canton de Vaud, where he achieved many successful results. He was the author of monographs on the treatment of foreign bodies lodged in the esophagus (1769), and on the correction of lateral curvatures and torsion of the spine by mechanical devices (1788). The name of François **Chopart** (1743–95), of Paris, is associated with his method of amputating the foot (1792), and that of P.-F. Moreau with the earliest excisions of the elbow (1786–94).[3]

The leading German surgeons of the age were Lorenz **Heister** (1683–1758), whose "Chirurgie" (Nuremburg, 1718) is of unusual historic interest on account of its instructive illustrations, and August Gottlieb **Richter** (1742–1812), who wrote a good history of surgery (1782–1804), which he left uncompleted, edited an important surgical journal (*Chirurgische Bibliothek*, 1771–96), and wrote a treatise on hernia (1777–1779),[4] which is still an acknowledged classic. With Richter's book on hernia may be grouped the important works on the same subject by Percival Pott (1756), Antonio de Gimbernat (1793), Pieter Camper (1801), and Antonio Scarpa (1809).

Johann Ulric **Bilguer** (1720–96), one of Frederick the Great's surgeon generals, was the author of a monograph *De amputatione membrorum rarissime administranda aut quasi abroganda* (1761), which was translated into French by Tissot in 1764, and

---

[1] J. L. Petit: Traité de mal. chir., Paris, 1774, pp. 153, 160.

[2] P. J. Desault: Œuvres chirurgicales, Paris, 1801, 553–580.

[3] P. F. Moreau: Observatione pratiques relatives à la résection des articulations affectées de carie, Paris thesis, an. xi (1803).

[4] Richter: Abhandlung von den Brüchen, Göttingen, 1777–79.

is indeed the most important plea for conservative surgery of the joints before the time of Fergusson, Brodie, and Syme.

Of English surgeons before the time of Hunter, we may consider the names of Cheselden, and his pupil, Sharp, Charles White, of Manchester, and Percival Pott.

William **Cheselden** (1688–1752), of Somerby, Leicestershire, a pupil of Cowper's, became surgeon to St. Thomas's Hospital in 1718. On publishing his "Treatise on a High Operation for Stone" in 1723, he was assailed with violent abuse by James Douglass, on the score of alleged plagiarism from the latter's "Lithotomia Douglassiana" (1720). Cheselden accordingly dropped the pro-

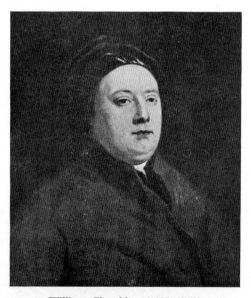

William Cheselden (1688–1752).

cedure he had described, and went on to modify the method of Frère Jacques into a "lateral operation for stone," which he performed March 27, 1727, and which has hardly been improved upon since. In 1728, he introduced a new operation for artificial pupil, consisting of a simple iridotomy with a needle.[1] His anatomy (1713) was popular in its day, and his atlas of osteology (1733), illustrated by Van der Gucht, is a work of permanent value. Cheselden was a genial, kind-hearted, versatile man, not unlike Hogarth in appearance. He was a patron of boxing, and a good

---

[1] W. Cheselden: Phil. Tr., London, 1728, xxxvi, 447.

draftsman; prepared the plans for Old Putney Bridge and the Surgeon's Hall in the Old Bailey, and assisted Van der Gucht in sketching bones for his "Osteographia" under the camera obscura. He was perhaps the most rapid of all the pre-anesthetic operators, performing a lithotomy in fifty-four seconds, which equals or outpaces the time record of even a Langenbeck or a Pirogoff. His social and professional status is embalmed in Pope's couplet:

"I'll do what Mead and Cheselden advise,
To keep these limbs and to preserve those eyes."

Charles **White** (1728–1813), of Manchester, one of the pioneers of aseptic midwifery (1773), first excised the head of the humerus

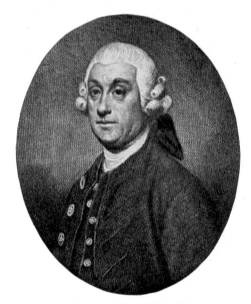

Percival Pott (1714–88).

in 1768,[1] gave the first account of "white swelling," or phlegmasia alba dolens (1784),[2] and introduced the method of reducing dislocations of the shoulder by means of the heel in the axilla. De Quincey called him "the most eminent surgeon by much in the North of England."

Percival **Pott** (1714–88), of London, was surgeon at St. Bartholo-

---

[1] C. White: Phil. Tr., London, 1769, lix, 39–46, 1 pl.

[2] White: An inquiry [etc.], Warrington, 1784; also London M. J., 1785, v, 50–57.

mew's Hospital from 1744–87, having, in his own words, served it "man and boy for half a century." Through a fall in the street, he sustained the particular fracture of the fibula which bears his name, and, taking up authorship while confined to his bed, he began to produce in rapid succession such masterpieces as his treatises on hernia (1756), head injuries (1760), hydrocele (1762), fistula in ano (1765), fractures and dislocations (1768), and, above all, the epoch-making pamphlet on palsy from spinal caries (1779).[1] Toward the end of the century Pott had the largest surgical practice in London. Like Cheselden, he was a man of kindly, charitable nature, and his lectures drew many foreign pupils to St. Bartholomew's.

All the operators before Hunter's time were clinical surgeons, of the stamp of Paré or Richard Wiseman, and knew nothing of pathology. Even long after the publication of Morgagni's great work (1761), the latter science had no real existence. For example, the first case of localized appendicitis on record was operated on and reported by **Mestivier** in 1759,[2] and the pathologic appearances clearly described in the autopsy, yet it made no impression upon practice whatever.

With the advent of **John Hunter** (1728–93), surgery ceased to be regarded as a mere technical mode of treatment, and began to take its place as a branch of scientific medicine, firmly grounded in physiology and pathology. Hunter came up to London in 1748, a raw, uncouth Scotch lad, fonder of taverns and theater galleries than of book-learning. He was taken in hand by his brother, the refined and accomplished William, and put at dissecting. Here he soon found himself, and, at a year's end, was teaching anatomy on his own account and following surgery under Cheselden and Pott. After some experience as staff surgeon with the expedition to Belle Isle (1761), where he gained his unique knowledge of gunshot wounds, he settled down in London to a life of ardent original investigation, diversified by extensive surgical practice and a commanding influence as a teacher. In personality, Hunter was very like Ruskin's description of Carlyle,— a Northern god struck by lightning,—in other words, a Norse or Saxon Scot crossed by Celtic emotionalism and whimsicality. His nature was kindly and generous, though outwardly rude and repelling, and, if crossed or thwarted, he was apt to paw the air like a restless, high-spirited horse. Late in life, for some private

---

[1] Although spinal caries is now termed "Pott's disease," Pott did not describe the disease or its tubercular nature, but only the deformity and the sequelæ of the latter.

[2] See Howard A. Kelly: Les débuts de l'histoire de l'appendicite en France, Presse médical, Paris, 1903, 437–441.

or personal reason, he picked a public quarrel with the brother who had formed him and made a man of him, basing the dissension upon a quibble about priority entirely unworthy of so great an

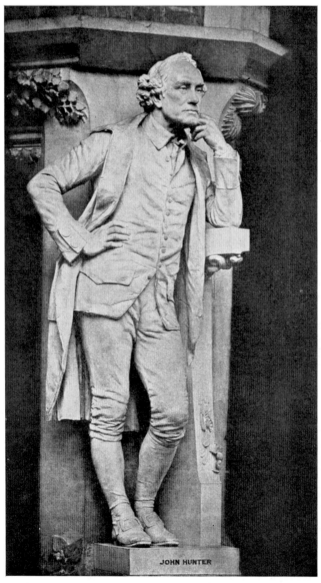

Statue of John Hunter ("The Queen's Hunter"). (Courtesy of Professor William Stirling, Manchester, England.)

investigator. Yet three years later, he lived to mourn this brother's death in tears. Of a piece with this was the pathos of John Hunter's own end. Being a victim of angina pectoris, he had said: "My life is in the hands of any rascal who chooses to annoy and tease me," and so it fell out. He was something of a scornful Ishmaelite among his professional colleagues, and being contradicted by one of these in a public discussion, was overtaken by the fatal malady and led out of the room. In a few minutes, the strong, imperious man had passed away. Many years after his death, his brother-in-law, Sir Everard Home, consigned himself to oblivion by burning Hunter's manuscripts after using them as the groundwork for sundry Croonian lectures and other alleged scientific contributions of his own devising. As Hunter was a composite character, so his work was many-sided, and we sense its magnitude not merely in his writings, many of which were destroyed, but in the great museum of over 13,000 specimens which he collected; and by the influence such pupils as Jenner, Astley Cooper, Abernethy, Cline, Clift, Parkinson, Blizard, Wright Post, and Physick. His permanent position in science is based upon the fact that he was the founder of surgical pathology and a pioneer in comparative physiology and experimental morphology. As the phlogiston-chemistry of his day was sadly muddled, he was fortunate in knowing nothing about it. He got up no elaborate experiments, and his mode of questioning nature has been justly praised for its simplicity. Thus his observations of the collateral capillary circulation in the antlers of deer in Richmond Park led to his method of treating aneurysms. His studies on the repair of tendons began with an accident he sustained while dancing. He accidentally inoculated himself with lues, and purposely delayed treatment in order to study the disease in his own person. As a surgical pathologist, he described shock, phlebitis, pyemia, and intussusception, and made epoch-making studies of inflammation, gunshot wounds and the surgical diseases of the vascular system. He differentiated clearly between hard (Hunterian) chancre and the chancroid ulcer, but his auto-inoculation seems to have confused gonorrhea with syphilis, a confusion which obtained until the time of Ricord. His greatest innovation in surgery was the establishment of the principle that aneurysms due to arterial disease should be tied high up in the healthy tissues by a single ligature (1786),[1] which displaced the old Antyllus method of securing the aneurysm between two ligatures and evacuating its contents. The novel feature was not the single

---

[1] Tr. Soc. Improvement Med. & Chir. Knowledge, London, 1793, i, 138–181; 1800, ii, 235–256.

ligature, which had already been employed by Guillemeau (1594) and Anel (1710), but the sound pathologic reasoning upon which its use was based. Not credited in Hunter's day, it has since saved "thousands of limbs and lives." As a biologist, Hunter dissected and described over 500 different species of animals, but, unlike many modern systematists, declined to publish any monographs on a single animal, aiming to connect morphology with physiology by studying the relation between structure and function. He held that the blood is alive, that structure is the ultimate expression of function, and not *vice versâ*, that abnormities are an expression of "arrested development," and that the embryo in each successive stage of its existence resembles the completed form of some order lower than itself, leading to the basic principle of comparative physiology, that the functional activities of the lower forms of life are, as it were, simplifications of those in the higher. In all this, Hunter was sound and modern. His defective education crops out in his various references to the fluid parts of the body as sentient beings, endowed with consciousness, and in such expressions as "the irritation of imperfection," "the stimulus of death," "the blood's consciousness of its being a useful part of the body." Phrases like these not only outvitalize the vitalists, but indicate Hunter's complete ignorance or wilful disregard of the work of his predecessors. In his dispute with the Abbé Spallanzani about digestion he was hopelessly at fault. His reasoning about phlebitis and pyemia was wrong, since he regarded the former condition as the cause of thrombosis, a theory which was demolished by Virchow in 1856. But, when all is said, Hunter remains one of the great all-around biologists like Haller and Johannes Müller, and, with Paré and Lister, one of the three greatest surgeons of all time. Only a passing reference can be made to his observations on vital heat in animals and vegetables, fetal smallpox, free martins, superfetation, electric fishes, postmortem digestion of the stomach, and his experiments on pathologic inoculations and on regeneration and transplantation of tissues, in which he is, in some sort, a forerunner of the experimental morphologists and extra-vital tissue-growers of our own time. His four masterpieces are the "Natural History of the Human Teeth" (1771); the treatise "On Venereal Disease" (1786); the "Observations on Certain Parts of the Animal Œconomy" (1786); and the "Treatise on the Blood, Inflammation and Gun Shot Wounds" (1794). Although Hunter was the first to study the teeth in a scientific manner, and the first to recommend complete removal of the pulp in filling them, his work was preceded by a French and a German classic, Pierre **Fauchard**'s "Le Chirurgien Dentiste" (1728), and Philipp **Pfaff**'s "Abhandlung von den

Zähnen" (1756), these three books being the most important in the history of dentistry. The second edition of Fauchard's work (1746) contains (pp. 275–277) the first account of pyorrhœa alveolaris, familiarly called Riggs's disease, after the American dentist, John M. Riggs, who, in 1876,[1] introduced the modern heroic treatment of the condition by scraping the teeth to the roots. Fauchard was also the first to employ orthodontal procedure in the treatment of malocclusion.

Hunter's immediate successor in London was his devoted pupil, John **Abernethy** (1764–1831), who constituted himself a

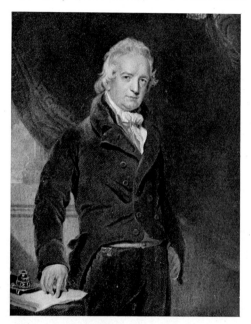

John Abernethy (1764–1831).

sort of champion of his master's physiologic theories, which he dramatized in the lecture room by his poetic imagination and vigorous style of delivery. Abernethy was the first to ligate the external iliac artery for aneurysm (1796), an operation which he performed four times, twice with success.[2] He ligated the common carotid for hemorrhage in 1798, and improved the treatment of lumbar abscesses by incision, admitting as little air as possible. He also described an anomaly of the viscera which is not unlike the

---

[1] J. M. Riggs: Penn. J. Dent. Sc., Phila., 1876, iii, 99–104.
[2] J. Abernethy: Surgical Observations, London, 1809, 234–292.

Eck fistula (1793).[1] He believed that local diseases are either of constitutional origin or due to digestive disturbances, and, in practice, treated nearly everything by calomel and blue-mass. Although kind-hearted and generous at bottom, he affected a brusque, downright manner with his patients on the ground that masterful rudeness wins confidence, where amiability might suggest weakness and so diminish respect—

> "Die recht zur Zeit ertheilten Hiebe
> Erwachen Furcht, Vertrauen und Liebe."

Of pioneer operations by American surgeons in the eighteenth century, a passing notice may be taken of an amputation of the shoulder-joint by John Warren, of Boston, in 1781, three cases of laparotomy for extra-uterine pregnancy by John Bard, of New Jersey, in 1759,[2] and by William Baynham, of Virginia, in 1791 and 1799;[3] and Wright Post's operation for femoral aneurysm by the Hunterian method in 1796.[4]

The **surgery of the eye** received an important uplift in 1752 at the hands of Jacques **Daviel** (1696–1762), the originator of the modern treatment of cataract by excision of the lens. In the early part of the century Brisseau (1706) and Maître-Jan (1707) had brought out the important fact that true cataract is, in effect, a clouding and hardening of the lens. Before this time it had been regarded as a sort of skin or pellicle immediately inside the capsule. Daviel was a Norman by birth. After studying surgery with an uncle at Rouen, and showing his courage and humanity in fighting the plague at Toulon and Marseilles, he settled in Paris in 1746, where he soon succeeded in surgical practice, being appointed eye surgeon to Louis XV in 1749. In 1752 he sent to the Royal Academy of Surgery his only literary production, the memoir on the cure of cataract by excision of the crystalline lens,[5] giving statistics of 100 successful operations out of 115. By 1756 he had a record of 434 extractions, with only 50 failures, and from that time on his method became a permanent part of ophthalmic procedure, the principal modification being the addition of iridectomy by von Graefe.[6]

Other ophthalmic contributions of note were Georg Ernst

---

[1] J. Abernethy: Phil. Tr., London, 1793, 59–68, 2 pl.

[2] Bard: Med. Obs. & Inq., 1757–61, London, 1762, ii, 369–372.

[3] Baynham: New York Med. & Phil. Rev., 1809, i, 160–172.

[4] Post: Am. Med. & Phil. Reg., New York, 1814, iv, 452.

[5] J. Daviel: "Sur une nouvelle methode de guérir la cataracte par l'extraction du cristallin" in: Mém. Acad. roy. de chir., Paris, 1753, ii, 337–354.

[6] Even in the employment of iridectomy, Daviel was a pioneer, as is shown in his letter to Haller (J. de méd., chir., pharm. [etc.], Paris, 1762, xvi, 245–251).

Stahl's original description of lacrimal fistula (1772),[1] Heberden's account of nyctalopia or night-blindness (1767),[2] and John Dalton's account of color-blindness (1794).[3]

Of equal rank with Daviel in ophthalmology was Thomas **Young** (1773–1829), of Milverton, England, a Quaker physician and one of the greatest men of science of all time. Learning Latin and many Oriental languages at an early age, he began to study medicine in 1792 under John Hunter, Matthew Baillie, and William Cruikshank, graduated at Göttingen in 1796, took his M.B. and M.D. at Cambridge in 1803 and 1808, and practised in London from 1799 to 1814. Young was thus the most highly educated physician of his time, and held many scientific positions of honor. Tscherning calls him "the father of physiologic optics," and Helmholtz, "one of the most clear-sighted men who ever lived."

In 1792, he read to the Royal Society his paper showing that visual accommodation of the eye at different distances is due to change of curvature in the crystalline lens,[4] which, however, he erroneously attributed to some muscular structure in the latter. In this memoir, "On the Mechanism of the Eye" (1801),[5] he gave the first description of astigmatism, with measurements and optical constants. He also stated the now famous Young-Helmholtz theory that color vision is due to retinal structures corresponding to red, green, and violet, color-blindness being deficient response of these to normal stimuli. In his Croonian lecture of 1808, he clearly stated the laws governing the flow of blood in the heart and arteries. His "Introduction to Medical Literature" (1813) gives his classification of diseases. His essay on consumption (1815) summarizes the knowledge of his time. In physics, Young is most famous as the author of the wave theory of light (1801–03), that it is due to undulations of the ether. In 1809, he showed its application to crystalline refraction and dispersion phenomena, which led to the Fresnel theory of double refraction (1821) and the Helmholtz theory of dispersion for absorbent media. He introduced the modern physical concepts of "energy" and "work done," showing that they are proportional to each other, and in 1804 he stated the theory of capillary attraction, founded upon the doctrine of energy, which was independently advanced by Laplace in 1805. He also defined the "modulus of elasticity" (Young's modulus); regarded heat as the "mechanical vibrations of particles larger and stronger than those of light"; and his theory of tides (1813) is said to have explained more tidal phenomena than any other hypothesis before the time of Airy. Young was also an accomplished Egyptologist, one of the earliest decipherers of hieroglyphics (Rosetta Stone), and his discovery that the demotic characters are not alphabetic but symbols derived from hieroglyphs and that the latter are not words but phonetic signs, was soon adopted by Champollion. His extraordinary versatility is also evidenced in his reports on ship-building, gas-lighting, standardization of the seconds pendulum and the imperial gallon, longitude, and life insurance.

Young was fond of dancing and good society, but was not regarded as a successful practitioner because he studied symptoms

[1] Stahl: De fistula lachrymali, Halle, 1702.

[2] Heberden: Med. Tr. Coll. Phys. London, 3, ed., 1785, i, 60: 1806–13, iv, 56.

[3] Dalton: Mem. Lit. & Phil. Soc., Manchester, 1798, v, pt.1, 28–45.

[4] Young: Phil. Tr., London, 1793, 169–181, 1 pl.

[5] *Ibid.*, 1801, xci, 23–88, 5 pl.

too closely, although his treatment was admitted to be effective. In person, he was probably the handsomest of all the great physicians. His fine open countenance was of classic contour, expressing great kindliness and good will, and with that sign of the mathematic mind which the old French poet has also esteemed a criterion of beauty—

"Eyes wide apart and keen of sight."[1]

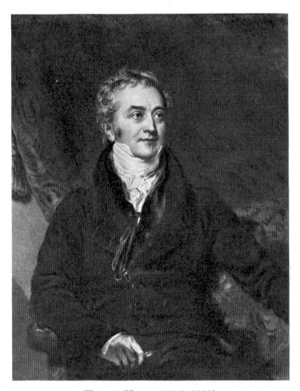

Thomas Young (1773–1829).

Otology was very materially advanced in the eighteenth century. Among the contributions of capital importance were the studies of the structure and physiology of the ear by Valsalva (1717),[2] Scarpa (1772–89),[3] and Cotugno (1774),[4] and the morpho-

---

[1] François Villon, Swinburne's translation.

[2] Valsalva: De aure humana tractatus, Utrecht, 1717.

[3] Scarpa: De structura fenestræ rotundæ auris, Mutinæ, 1772; and his: Anatomicæ disquisitiones de auditu et olfactu, Ticini, 1789.

[4] Cotugno: De aquæductibus auris humanæ internæ, Vienna, 1774.

logical essays of Geoffroy (1778)[1] and Comparetti (1789).[2] Catheterization of the Eustachian tube was first attempted by the French postmaster Guyot in 1724[3] and subsequently performed by Archibald Cleland in 1741.[4] Eli, a strolling quack, is credited with the first perforation of the tympanic membrane for deafness (1760),[5] and, in 1755, Jonathan Wathen had treated catarrhal deafness by means of injections into the Eustachian tube through a catheter inserted in the nose.[6]

More important still, the mastoid process was opened for the first time in the history of surgery by Jean-Louis Petit in 1774,[7] and by the Prussian army surgeon Jasser in 1776.[8]

The salient features of **clinical medicine** in the eighteenth century were the introduction of postmortem sections, of new methods of precision in diagnosis, and of preventive inoculation, none of which, however, were much appreciated until the following century. In the year 1761 there were published two works which have exerted a profound influence upon the medicine of our own period, viz., the *Inventum Novum* of Auenbrugger and the *De Sedibus et Causis Morborum* of Morgagni.

Leopold **Auenbrugger** (1722–1809), a Styrian by birth, became physician-in-chief to the Hospital of the Holy Trinity at Vienna in 1751, and there he tested and tried out the value of the discovery which afterward made him famous. His little book is the first record of the use of immediate percussion of the chest in diagnosis, based upon observation verified by postmortem experiences. Our author's first proposition is that the chest of a healthy subject sounds, when struck, like a cloth-covered drum. He then proceeds to outline his special method of eliciting information by striking the chest gently with the points of the fingers brought together (stretched out straight and afterward flexed), the patient holding his breath; a muffled sound or one of higher pitch than usual indicating the presumable site of a diseased condition. This great discovery was slighted and even snubbed by de Haen, Sprengel, and other contemporary writers, and remained unnoticed until Corvisart took it up in 1808, one year before its

---

[1] Geoffroy: Dissertations sur l'organe de l'ouie, Amsterdam, 1778.

[2] Comparetti: Observationes anatomicæ de aure interna comparata, Padua, 1789.

[3] Guyot: Hist. Acad. roy. d. sc., 1724, Paris, 1726, 37.

[4] Cleland: Phil. Tr., 1732–41, London, 1747, ix, 124, 1 pl.

[5] A. Politzer: Gesch. der Ohrenheilk., Stuttgart, 1907, i, 336.

[6] Wathen: Phil. Tr., 1755, London, 1756, xlix, 213-222, 1 pl.

[7] Petit: Traité d. mal. chir., Paris, 1774, 153; 160.

[8] Jasser: In Schmucker's Vermischte chirurgische Schriften, Berlin, 1782, vol. iii, pp. 113–125.

author's death. Although Corvisart might easily have revamped the idea of percussion as his own discovery, he says with fine feeling that he would not sacrifice the name of Auenbrugger to personal vanity: "It is he and the beautiful invention which of right belongs to him that I wish to recall to life." Auenbrugger himself was too well poised and serene by nature to worry about his posthumous reputation. Grave, genial, inflexibly honest, unassuming and charitable, loving science for its own sake, composing a little opera for the delectation of Maria Theresa,[1] and modestly waiving her request that he repeat the experiment on the ground that "one was enough," caring more for the society of his beautiful wife, good music, and *Gemüthlichkeit* generally

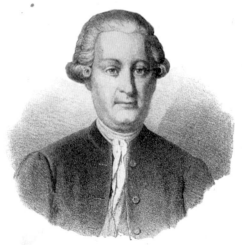

Leopold Auenbrugger, Edler von Auenbrugg (1722–1809).

than for any notoriety, he is, indeed, a noble example of the substantial worth and charm of old-fashioned German character at its very best.[2]

Giovanni Battista **Morgagni** (1682–1771), of Forlì, a pupil of Valsalva and later a professor at Padua (1715–71), published the results of his life-work in his seventy-ninth year. It consists of 5 books of letters, 70 in number, written in an engagingly communicative manner, and constituting the true foundation of modern pathologic anatomy, in that, for the first time, the records

---

[1] It was called "The Chimney Sweep" (Der Rauchfangkehrer).

[2] For the finest appreciation of Auenbrugger in medical literature, see Dr. S. Weir Mitchell's beautiful tribute in Tr. Cong. Am. Phys., 1891, New Haven, 1892, ii, 180, 181.

of postmortem findings are brought into correlation with clinical records on a grand scale. In the preface, Morgagni modestly disavows any special claim to originality, and gives all due credit to the works of his predecessors, such as the "Sepulchretum" of Bonnet (1679). But while others, like Benivieni or Bonetus, may have looked at diseased viscera in the dead body with some intelligence, it was by the vast scope of his work and his many descriptions of new forms of disease that Morgagni made pathology a genuine branch of modern science, even if the seed sown, as Sir Clifford Allbutt contends, fell "upon hard and sterile

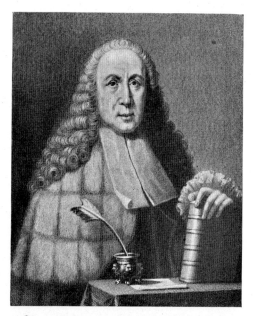

Giovanni Battista Morgagni (1682–1771).

ground." Morgagni gave the first description of syphilitic aneurysm and disease of the mitral valve; early cases of acute yellow atrophy of the liver and tuberculosis of the kidney, and the first recorded case of heart-block (Stokes-Adams disease)[1]; identified the clinical features of pneumonia with solidification of the lungs, emphasized the extreme importance of visceral syphilis, and was the first to show that intracranial suppuration is really a sequel of discharge from the ear, a phenomenon which even Valsalva had conceived the other way around. Morgagni also described

[1] De Sedibus, Venice, 1761, i, 70. Cited by Sir William Osler.

what is now known as "Morgagnian cataract." The "De Sedibus" gave "the death-blow" to humoral concepts in pathology.
A worthy follower of Morgagni was Matthew **Baillie** (1761–
1823), who, like Smellie, Cullen, and the Hunters, was a native
of Lanarkshire, Scotland. He received a good classical education
at Balliol College, was advised by his uncle, William Hunter, to
study medicine, and, in due course, became a pupil and house-
intimate at Windmill Street. He was physician to George III,
and is said to have ruined his health by devoting sixteen hours
a day to his extensive practice. Baillie's *Morbid Anatomy* (London,

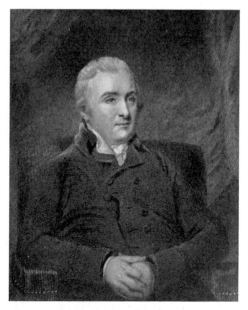

Matthew Baillie (1761–1823). (From the painting by John Hoppner.)

1793), illustrated with beautiful copper plates by William Clift,
John Hunter's famulus, differs from Morgagni's work in that it
is the first attempt to treat pathology as a subject in and for itself,
describing the morbid appearances of each organ in systematic
succession, as in a modern text-book. In each instance, the autopsy
is correlated with a full case-history, and the author seems to
have grasped the idea that postmortem appearances are only
end-results, although such results "may then become again the
cause of many symptoms." He wisely limited his descriptions,
as a rule, to such naked-eye appearances as he actually understood,—those in the brain and the viscera,—and he did not at-

tempt to deal with the nerves or the spinal cord. Baillie described transposition of the viscera,[1] hydrosalpinx, and dermoid cysts of the ovary[2]; gave the first accurate definitions of cirrhosis of the liver and of "hepatization" of the lungs in pneumonia; distinguished renal cysts from renal hydatids; described endocarditis, gastric ulcer, and the ulceration of Peyer's patches in typhoid fever (without understanding the latter); and showed that death from "polypus of the heart" is really due to a clot of fibrin, and that pulsation of the abdominal aorta is not necessarily a sign of internal disease. In consultation, Baillie had the same gift of

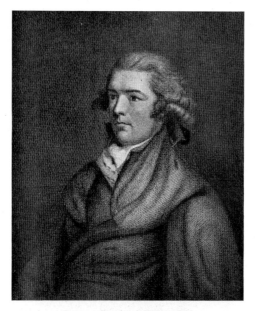

James Currie (1756–1805).

clear, concise expression which distinguished his writings. He was the last inheritor of the "Gold-headed Cane," and his bust is in Westminster Abbey.

During the eighteenth century there were some noteworthy attempts to employ instruments of precision in **diagnosis.** In 1707, Sir John **Floyer** (1649–1734), of Staffordshire, published his "Physician's Pulse Watch," which records the first effort in a century to revive the forgotten lore of Galileo, Kepler, and Sanctorius. Floyer, in Haller's phrase, "broke the ice," in that he tried to get

---

[1] Baillie: Phil. Tr., Lond., 1788, lxxvii, 350–363.
[2] London Med. Jour., 1789, x, 322–332.

the pulse-rate by timing its beats with a watch, which ran for exactly one minute. He tabulated his results, but his work was neglected or its intention even vitiated by a revival of the old Galenic doctrine of specific pulses, *i. e.*, a special pulse for every disease. Of the pulse lore of the eighteenth century, Dr. Weir Mitchell, the historian of instrumental precision in medicine, says: "It is observation going minutely mad; a whole Lilliput of symptoms; an exasperating waste of human intelligence," and he adds that "it was not until a later day, and under the influence of the great Dublin school, that the familiar figure of the doctor, watch in hand, came to be commonplace."

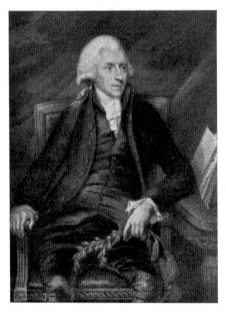

William Withering (1741–1799). (From a painting by C. F. Breda.)

The clinical thermometry dreamed of by Sanctorius, and coquetted with by Boerhaave, Haller, and de Haen, was revived in the classic "Essays and Observations" (1740) of George **Martine** (1702–41), of Scotland, which is the only scientific treatment of the subject before the time of Wunderlich. Martine's ideas were carried into practice in the "Medical Reports" (1798) of James **Currie** (1756–1805), another Scot, who, after an adventurous experience in America, attained eminence as a practitioner in Liverpool. Long before Brand of Stettin, Currie used cold baths in typhoid fever and checked up his results with the clinical thermometer.   He used sea-water, as a rule, pouring it over the patient's body and making the douches colder and more frequent, the higher the temperature, as measured by the thermometer. Dr. S. Weir Mitchell finds "absolute genius" in Currie's book, which, like those of Floyer and Martine, was neglected, if not soon forgotten.

One of the ablest clinicians of his time was William **Withering** (1741–99), of Shropshire, England, memorable as the pioneer in the correct use of digitalis.   An Edinburgh graduate of 1766, afterward enjoying a large and lucrative practice at Birmingham, Withering was not only an admirable observer of the English school,

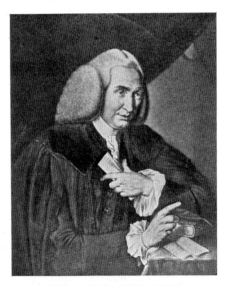

William Cullen (1712–1790).

but a man of unusual versatility.   He described the epidemics of scarlatina and scarlatinal sore throat in 1771 and 1778, and in 1793 recommended an admirable modern treatment for phthisis. He was one of the greatest of medical botanists, wittily called "the flower of physicians," and his "Botanical Arrangement of all the Vegetables" (1776) is esteemed his masterpiece.   He also made analyses of minerals and mineral waters, was an opponent of phlogiston, a member of the famous "Lunar Society," a climatologist, a breeder of dogs and cattle, and solaced his leisure hours with the flute and harpsichord.   In 1776, Withering learned from an old grandame near Birmingham that foxglove was good for dropsy.   He immediately set about trying it in heart diseases, afterward recommending its use where he could, and by 1783 it was introduced into the Edinburgh Pharmacopœia. His *Account of the Fox-glove* (1785), a pharmacological classic, was incidentally a protest against the abuses of digitalis, which were already creeping in. In Withering's time, dropsy was regarded as a primary disease, and he did not know of the distinction between cardiac and renal dropsy, which was afterward made by Bright. He was disappointed to find that "cerebral dropsy" (hydrocephalus) and ovarian (cystic) dropsy did not yield to the drug. Withering was buried in the old church at Edgbaston, and the foxglove adorns the monument over his grave.

Among the English clinical teachers of the eighteenth century there is no name more justly and highly esteemed than that of William **Cullen** (1710–90). A pupil of Monro *primus*, he was instrumental in founding the medical school of Glasgow in 1744, and, during his long life, held the chairs of medicine and chemistry at both Glasgow and Edinburgh. He was one of the first to give clinical or infirmary lectures in Great Britain, and his lectures were the first ever given in the vernacular instead of Latin (1757). Having a mind of philosophic bent, he was probably greater as an inspiring teacher than as a clinician, and was noted for his kindness in assisting needy students. Although he introduced some new remedies into practice, Sir William Hamilton was not far from right when he said that "Cullen did not add a single new fact to medical science." His "Synopsis nosologiæ methodicæ" (1769), which divides diseases into fevers, neuroses, cachexias, and local disorders, even including gout among the neuroses, is now forgotten, although it made his reputation; but his "First Lines of the Practice of Physic" (1776–84) was for years authoritative on medical practice, even among the pioneers and "forty-niners" in the Far West.

The names of many English physicians of Queen Anne's time, such as Radcliffe, Mead, Garth, Arbuthnot, Sloane, and Blackmore, have a literary and social, rather than a scientific, interest.

A typical practitioner of the period, whose lifetime covered nearly the whole century, was the distinguished William **Heberden** (1710–1801), of London, Soemmerring's "medicus vere Hippocraticus," whom Dr. Johnson called "ultimus Romanorum, the last of our great physicians." A Cambridge graduate of superior attainments, Heberden was esteemed as one of the finest Greek and Hebrew scholars of his time, and he resembles the classical writers in his careful portrayals of disease. His *Commentaries* (1802), written in Latin, are the result of a lifetime of conscientious note-taking,

19

and contain his original descriptions of varicella (1767),[1] angina pectoris (1768),[2] and the nodules in the fingers which differentiate rheumatic gout (1802).[3] He also described "night-blindness,[4] or nyctalopia" (1767).[5] As Sir Dyce Duckworth points out, Heberden's Commentaries are rich in the subtle notation of such clinical minutiæ as the diminished liability to diphtheria after adolescence, the lightning flashes before the eyes in hemicrania, or the tendency of phthisis to rebate in pregnancy, but not after it. An actual case of angina pectoris was described in

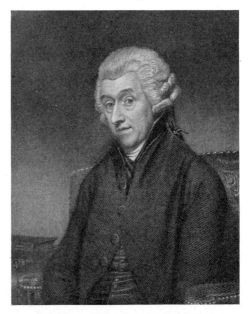

William Heberden (1710–1801).

the memoirs of the Earl of Clarendon (1632) in the person of his own father, but it was Heberden's classical account that put the disease upon a scientific basis, and his work was soon confirmed by the observations of Parry (1799) and Edward Jenner. In his "Essay on Mithridatium and Theriaca" (1745), Heberden did a most important service to therapeutics by dispelling current super-

[1] Heberden: "On the chicken-pox," Med. Tr. Coll. Phys., London, 1767, 3d ed., 1785, i, 427–436.

[2] Ibid., 1768–70, ii, 59–67.

[3] Heberden: Commentarii, London, 1802, Cap. 28, p. 130.

[4] St. Bartholomew's Hosp. Rep., 1910, London, 1911, xlvi, 1–12.

[5] Med. Tr., Coll. Phys., London, 3d ed., 1785, i, 60; 1806–13; iv, 56.

stitions about these curious concoctions, and banishing them forever from the pharmacopœia. This little book is one of the shining monuments of medical scholarship.

A group of men who resembled Heberden in character, if not in learning, were Fothergill, Lettsom, and Parry.

John **Fothergill** (1712–80), of Carr End, Yorkshire, a Quaker pupil of Monro *primus*, became a very successful and wealthy London practitioner, was noted for his generous philanthropies, his magnificent botanic garden, his splendid collections of shells, insects, and drawings, which after his death fell into the hands of his friend, William Hunter. He was a true follower of Syden-

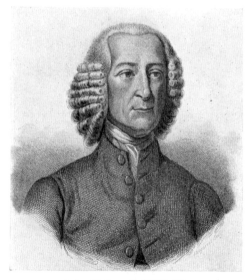

John Fothergill (1712–80).

ham in his "Observations on the Weather and Diseases of London" (1751–54), and his original descriptions of diphtheric sore throat (1748) and facial neuralgia (1773).

John Coakley **Lettsom** (1744–1815), of Little Vandyke (Virgin Islands), also a Quaker, and, like Fothergill, lavish in expenditure and munificent in philanthropy, was one of the original founders of the Medical Society of London, which commemorates his name, with Fothergill's, in the Lettsomian and Fothergillian lecture foundations. Lettsom was a prolific writer on such subjects as tea, chlorosis in boarding-schools, effects of hard drinking (1791), and the like, but his only contribution of value to modern medicine is his original account of alcoholism, which is incidentally the first paper on the drug habit (1789).[1]

Caleb Hillier **Parry** (1755–1822), a highly esteemed practitioner of Bath, who, like Heberden, acquired a lifelong habit of taking notes, described the first recorded case of facial hemiatrophy (1814),[2] and, in 1786, left an account of exophthalmic goiter[3] so complete and original that it more justly entitles him to the honor of its discovery than either Flajani (1800), Graves (1835), or Basedow (1840).

The work of these men illustrates the eminently practical ten-

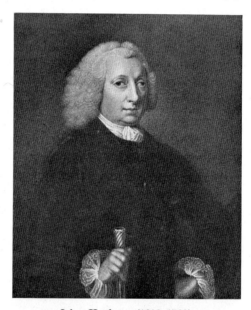

John Huxham (1692–1768).

dencies of English physicians since the time of Sydenham, and, as careful, common-sense observers, studying their patients' symptoms rather than books, they were true followers of the master. The same thing may be said of two physicians of a more provincial stamp, Huxham and Baker. John **Huxham** (1692–1768), of Totnes, Devon, one of Boerhaave's pupils who had studied Hippocrates in the original, made meteorologic observations like Fothergill's, won the Copley medal for his essay on antimony (1755), and in

[1] Lettsom: Mém. Med. Soc., London, 1779–87, i, 128–165.

[2] Parry: Collected Works, London, 1825, i, 478–480.

[3] *Ibid.*, iii, 111–128.

his "Essay on Fevers" (1755) gave careful and original observations of many infectious diseases, differentiating, in particular, between the "putrid malignant" and the "slow nervous" fevers, that is, between typhus and typhoid. Huxham devised the familiar tincture of cinchona bark with which his name is associated, and in 1747 recommended that 1200 sailors of Admiral Martin's fleet, who had been disabled by scurvy, be put upon a vegetable diet.[1] In his essay on malignant sore throat (1757), he was the first to observe the paralysis of the soft palate which attends diphtheria, although he confused the latter with scarlatina. In 1739, he described Devonshire colic[2] (from cider-drinking), without, however, ascertaining its true cause. This cause was discovered in 1767[3] by Sir George **Baker** (1722–1809), another Devonshire man, who noticed that the cider-time colic, endemic in Devon, was connected with large pieces of lead used in the vats and cider presses, which were not so employed in other counties of England. He completed his chain of induction by extracting lead from the Devonshire cider, and proving that none could be found in the cider of Herefordshire. Although he was denounced from the pulpit as a "faithless son of Devon" for his pains, yet, in course of time, the colic disappeared from the county and Baker extended his investigations of lead-poisoning to iron pipes, glazed earthenware, and the linings of iron vessels. Public service of the same high character was rendered by Sir John **Pringle** (1707–82), the founder of modern military medicine and the originator of the Red Cross idea. Pringle, a Scotch pupil of Boerhaave and Albinus, and a friend of van Swieten's, was a surgeon on the continent in the mid-century wars, and surgeon general of the English army from 1742 to 1758. In his "Observations on the Diseases of the Army" (London, 1752) he lays down the true principles of military sanitation, especially in regard to the ventilation of hospital wards. Both Pringle and Stephen Hales were instrumental in securing better ventilation for those confined in ships, jails, barracks, and mines. Pringle was also a pioneer of the antiseptic idea; gave a good description of typhus fever; showed that jail fever and hospital fever are one and the same; correlated the different forms of dysentery, and named influenza. It was about the time of the battle of Dettingen (1743) that he made the historic suggestion to the Earl of Stair that the military hospitals of both the French or the English sides should be regarded as

---

[1] See his "De scorbuto," Venice, 1766.

[2] De morbo colico Damnoniensi, London, 1739.

[3] Baker: An essay concerning the cause of the endemial colic of Devonshire, London, 1767.

neutral and immune from attack. The rule remained loosely in force until it was put upon an absolute basis through Henri Dunant, in the Geneva Convention in 1864.

In connection with Pringle's work in **military medicine** mention should be made of van Swieten's monograph on camp diseases (1758),[1] and Hugues Ravaton's treatise on military surgery (1768).[2] Prominent contributions to naval medicine were James Lind's essay on the hygiene of sailors (1757), and Thomas Trotter's "Medicina nautica" (1797–1803). The important feature of this subject in the eighteenth century was the study of scurvy, which

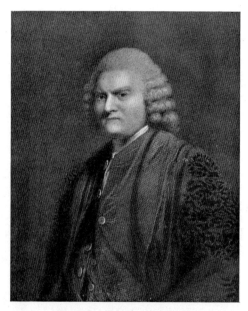

Sir John Pringle (1707–82).

first came into prominence through its ravages among the sailors of Lord Anson's expedition in 1740, and which was also the subject of monographs by Lind (1753) and Trotter (1786). Against the disease, Huxham, as we have seen, recommended a vegetable diet for Admiral Martin's sailors in 1747, and Sir Gilbert Blane (1749–1834) recommended lime-juice in his "Observations on the Diseases of Seamen" (1785).

---

[1] Van Swieten: Kurze Beschreibung und Heilungsart der Krankheiten welche am öftesten in dem Feldlager beobachtet werden, Vienna, 1758.

[2] Ravaton: Chirurgie d'armée, Paris, 1768.

The epoch-making reforms of **John Howard** (1726–90) in relation to the management of the prisons, hospitals, and lazarettos of Europe (1777–89)[1] had much to do with the suppression of that vermin-carried disease, typhus fever. The work of Johann Conrad Amman (1669–1724), on the education of deaf-mutes (1692–1700),[2] the efforts of the Abbe de L'Épée (1712–90) to get an alphabet of communication for the deaf and dumb (1771),[3] and Pestalozzi's work in the cause of popular education (1781–1803), are remarkable features of social medicine in this period.

There was little of value in the clinical medicine of France in the eighteenth century. Its principal representative, **Théophile de Bordeu** (1722–76), the founder of the Vitalistic School of Montpellier, is now remembered as a theorist pure and simple. He graduated at Montpellier in 1794, was director of the baths in the Pyrénées, but spent the greater part of his life in Paris, where he held a high reputation in spite of his wrangles with the Faculty. Like most medical leaders of his time, Bordeu maintained a rigid, dogmatic "system," which was not unlike that of van Helmont. He held that the organs of the body, with their several functions, are federated with and dependent upon each other, but presided over and regulated by the stomach, the heart, and the brain, which he called the "Tripod of Life." Next in importance were the nerves and the glands, the former centralizing the different functions of the body into a *vita propria*, and consequently governing the secretions of the latter. Bordeu first stated the doctrine that not only each gland, but each organ of the body, is the workshop of a specific substance or secretion, which passes into the blood, and upon these the integration of the body as a whole depends. Thus Bordeu, as Neuburger has shown,[4] was very close upon the modern theory of the internal secretions and "hormonic equilib-

---

[1] Howard: The State of the Prisons in England and Wales, Warrington, 1777; and his "An Account of the Principal Lazarettos in Europe," Warrington, 1789.

[2] Amman: Surdus loquens, Amsterdam, 1692.

[3] De L'Épée: Institution des sourds et muets par la voie des signes méthodiques, Paris, 1776. It is said that the idea of a mode of communication for deaf-mutes originated with Ponce de Leon, of Fountain of Youth fame; but, from the sign-language of the North American Indians to the "Gebärdensprache" of the Southern Italians, the thing itself, apart from deaf-mutism, is widely known among primitive peoples.

[4] M. Neuburger in Janus, Amst., 1903, viii, 26–32; and Wien. klin. Wochenschr., 1911, xxiv, 1367. Neuburger cites the following from Bordeu's "Analyse médicinale du sang" (1774): " J'en conclus que le sang roule toujours dans son sein des extraits de toutes les parties organiques . . . chacun (des organes) aussi sert de foyer et de laboratoire à une humeur particulière qu'il renvoie dans le sang après l'avoir préparée sans son sein, après lui avoir donné son caractère radical," p. 943, 948.

rium," but, as he made no experiments, his ideas can be regarded as only theoretical. Disease he regarded as passing through the stages of irritation, coction, and crisis, dependent upon the glandular and other secretions of the blood. In consequence, he classified diseases, not according to their clinical or pathological manifestations, but arbitrarily as *cachexias*. Of these he unrolled an extraordinary list, corresponding to the different organs and secretions, as bilious, mucous, albuminous, fatty, splenic, seminal, urinary, stercoral, perspiratory, and so on, with an equally complex classification of the pulse as critical, non-critical, simple critical, compound critical, nasal, tracheal, gastric, renal, uterine, seminal, etc. The most interesting part of his theory is his observation of the effects of the testicular and ovarian secretions upon the organism. He regarded the *aura seminalis* of the sexual secretions as giving a "male (or female) tonality" to the organism, "setting the seal upon the animalism of the individual," and, in effect, "the particular stimulus of the machine (*novum quoddam impetum faciens*)." In this connection, he made clever studies of the obesity, retiring disposition, and other characteristics of eunuchs, capons, and spayed animals, suggesting some phases of the modern "pluriglandular syndromes."

Bordeu's successor, Paul-Joseph Barthez (1734–1806), of Montpellier, who was successively a theologian, physician, soldier, editor, lawyer (even a counselor of justice), philosopher, and again a physician, is memorable for his introduction of the term "vital principle" (*vitalis agens*) to denote the cause of the phenomena in the living body. The vitalism of Bordeu and Barthez underwent a third transformation in the nineteenth century as the "seminal vitalism," of Bouchut.

The rise of the **Old Vienna School,** under Gerhard **van Swieten** (1700–72), of Leyden, was a feature of the ascendancy of Austria under Maria Theresa and Joseph II. Van Swieten, who was in special favor with the Empress, did much to advance Austrian medicine, particularly in regard to medical education. He was a great friend of the poor, and wrote an important work upon the hygiene of troops in camp (1758). As a clinician, he noted such things as the aura in hydrophobia, and the occurrence of symmetrical gangrene in spinal affections, was instrumental in bringing about the internal use of corrosive sublimate in syphilis, and left a commentary upon the aphorisms of Boerhaave (1741–76), which occupied him for over thirty years. Besides van Swieten, the Vienna group included such prominent figures as the quarrelsome, pragmatic Anton de Haen (1704–76), of The Hague, who wrote a treatise on hospital therapeutics in 15 volumes (1758–69), and occasionally used the thermometer; the bureaucratic Anton Stoerck (1731–1803), of Swabia, who did some careful work in pharmacology and toxicology, notably his investigations of hemlock (1760–61), stramonium, hyoscyamus, and aconite (1762), colchicum (1763), and pulsatilla (1771); the epidemiologist, Maximilian Stoll (1742–87), of Swabia, who wrote well upon medical ethics; Marcus Anton von Plenciz, Sr. (1705–86), who advanced the idea of a *contagium animatum*, with a special *seminium verminosum* for each disease; the dermatologist, Joseph Jacob von Plenck (1732–1807), who

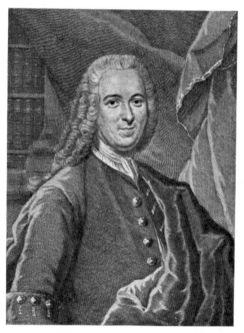

Paul Gottlieb Werlhof (1699–1767).

followed the method of Linnæus in classifying diseases of the skin (1776); and, above all, the sterling figures of Auenbrugger and Frank.

The leading practitioners in Germany were Stahl, Hoffmann, Kämpf, Werlhof, Zimmermann, Wichmann, Senckenberg, Reil, and Heim. Of these, Paul Gottlieb **Werlhof** (1699–1767), of Helmstedt, court physician at Hannover, was a great friend of Haller, and, like him, wrote poems in the German language and medical works in Latin. He is now remembered by his original description of purpura hæmorrhagica, or morbus maculosus Werlhofii (1735).[1]

The snobbish Johann Georg **Zimmermann** (1728–95), of Brugg, Switzerland, a practitioner of great repute, who succeeded Werlhof as ordinarius at Hannover, was the author of an important monograph on "Epidemic Dysentery in the Year 1765,"[2] and of the famous "Treatise on Solitude," which so tickled the sentimental palates of our grandfathers.

Johann Ernst **Wichmann** (1740–1802), a contemporary of Werlhof's at Hannover, is notable for his monograph on scabies (1786);[3] and Johann Christian Senckenberg (1702–72), for his public-spirited endowment of the Senckenberg Foundation at Frankfort on the Main.

Johann Christian **Reil** (1759–1813), of Eastern Frisia, professor of medicine at Halle (1787) and Berlin (1810), was the original editor of the *Archiv für die Physiologie* (Halle, 1795–1815), the first periodical to be devoted to the science. It eventually passed into the elder Meckel's hands, and became in the course of time the epoch-making Müller's Archiv. Reil is especially memorable for his description of the "island of Reil" in the brain (1809),[4] and for his "Rhapsodies" on the psychic treatment of the insane (1803).[5] His trite physiological theory (life-matter in motion) is unimportant.

Ernst Ludwig **Heim** (1747–1834), a wealthy, witty, very honest, and very independent practitioner of Berlin, is said to have introduced Jennerian vaccination into that city in 1798, and as *"der alte Heim,"* is remembered for his many sharp sayings.

Simon-André **Tissot** (1728–97), the famous practitioner of Lausanne, was one of the leading propagandists of variolation (1754), wrote considerable treatises on epilepsy (1770) and nervous diseases (1782), and became widely known through his popular writings on onanism (1760), the hygiene of literary men (1766), and the diseases of men of the world (1770). His best known achievement in this kind was the *Avis au peuple sur la santé* (1760), a tract on popular medicine which ran through ten editions in less than six years, and was translated into every European language.

Théodore **Tronchin** (1709–81), of Geneva, Boerhaave's favorite pupil, Voltaire's favorite physician, and one of the wealthiest

---

[1] Werlhof: Opera omnia, Hannover, 1775, ii, 615–636. (Dissertation published at Brunswick, 1735.)

[2] J. G. Zimmermann: Von der Ruhr unter dem Volke im Jahr 1765, Zürich, 1767.

[3] Wichmann: Aetiologie der Krätze, Hannover, 1786.

[4] Reil: Arch. f. Physiol., Halle a. S., 1809, ix, 136; 195.

[5] Reil: Rhapsodieen (etc.), Halle, 1803.

and most fashionable practitioners of his time, is remembered by his compilation "De colica Pictonum" (1757), in which he showed that "Poitou colic" was caused by lead used to sweeten wine. He introduced inoculation into Holland (1748), Switzerland (1749), and France (1756), having 20,000 successful cases to his credit; and was a pioneer of the open-air cult, of psychotherapy, and of suspension in spinal curvature (1756).

The greatest Italian clinician of the period was Giovanni Maria **Lancisi** (1655–1720), of Rome, who was physician to several popes, one of whom (Clement XI) placed in his hands the forgotten 47 copper plates of Eustachius, executed in 1552, which Lancisi edited with marginal notes and published, with a title page vignette by Pier Leone Ghezzi, in 1714. Lancisi was the author of two works of capital importance on sudden death (1707)[1] and on aneurysm (1738),[2] in the latter of which he clearly established the part played by syphilis in the causation of aneurysm.

Francesco **Torti** (1658–1741), professor at Modena, and a good pharmacologist, wrote an important treatise on the pernicious malarial fevers (1712,),[3] which practically introduced the employment of cinchona bark into Italian practice.

Pellagra was originally described by Gaspar Casal (1691–1759), a Spanish physician, in a book written by him in 1735, but not published until 1762.[4] At court, Casal met Francois Thiéry, who, from what he had seen or heard of Casal's description, published an account of the disease in 1755,[5] antedating him in priority of publication, but not of first-hand description. Both Casal and Thiéry called the new disease "rose sickness" (*mal de la rosa*). In 1771,[6] Francesco Frapolli, an Italian physician, published a careful account of pellagra, in which he gave the malady its present name.

Connected with the history of internal medicine on the continent is the revival of Athanasius Kircher's hypnotic idea, under the guise of "animal magnetism," by Franz Anton **Mesmer** (1734–1815), of Itznang, Switzerland. Mesmer's graduating dissertation had been upon the subject of the influence of the planets on man (1771), and, in experimenting with the magnet, he got the idea that a similar power is possessed by the human

---

[1] Lancisi: De subitaneis mortis, Rome, 1707.

[2] Lancisi: De motu cordis et aneurysmatibus, Naples, 1738.

[3] Torti: Therapeutice specialis ad febres quasdam perniciosas, Modena, 1712.

[4] Casal: Historia natural y medica de el principado de Asturias, Madrid, 1762.

[5] Thiéry: Jour. de méd., chir. et pharm., Paris, 1755, ii, 337–346.

[6] Frapolli: Animadversiones in morbum, vulgo pelagram, Milan, 1771.

hand. Attempting to practise mesmerism in Vienna, his private séances were investigated by one of Maria Theresa's "commissions," and he was compelled to leave the city inside of twenty-four hours. Arriving in Paris in 1778, after some failures at Spa, he at length gained a foothold, and in a very short time he was making a great deal of money by his hypnotic séances. In these he appeared clad in a lilac suit, playing upon a harmonica, touching his patients with a wand, staring into their eyes, and attending them in a private chamber in case of a "crisis." A prominent feature of the mesmeric treatment was a number of so-called magnetic tubs, or *baquets*, containing a *mixtum compositum* of hydrogen sulphide and other ingredients, and provided with iron conductors from which depended a ring for purposes of contact with the patients, who stood around the tubs, joining hands. Being investigated by another committee, Mesmer was again driven from the field, and, after the Revolution, dropped out of sight. His book, containing his ideas on mesmerism, was published in 1779.[1] Although the subject did not gain a scientific foothold until the time of Braid, mesmerism, like Lavater's ideas on physiognomy (1772),[2] attracted a great deal of public and private notice and was exploited in various mystic forms by d'Eslon, a pupil of Mesmer's, the brothers Puységur, Lavater, the novelist Justinus Kerner, and by Baron Karl von Reichenbach, whose concept of "odic force" still survives in the ouija-boards and odic telephones of the present time. In London, Mesmer's charlatanry cropped out in the notorious "Temple of Health" (1780) of the quack James Graham, in the ministrations of which Emma Lyon, the future Lady Hamilton, played a prominent choreographic part.

With all its lack of instrumental precision, the internal medicine of the eighteenth century, as a whole, was far superior to its surgery, because the systematic tendencies of the age led to the composition of specialized text-books, the introduction of new drugs, and the accurate description of many new forms of disease. Among these **isolated clinical discoveries** we may mention Friedrich Hoffmann's descriptions of chlorosis (1730)[3] and rubella (1740)[4]; |Freke's case of myositis ossificans progressiva (1736)[5]; Fothergill's accounts of diphtheria (1748)[6]; facial neuralgia (1773),[7] and sick headache (1784)[8]; Nicolas André

---

[1] Mesmer: Mémoire sur la découverte du magnétisme animal, Geneva and Paris, 1779.

[2] Joh. Caspar Lavater: Von der Physiognomik, Leipzig, 1772.

[3] F. Hoffmann: De genuina chlorosis indole, 1730.

[4] Opera omnia, Geneva, 1748, ii, 63.

[5] J. Freke: Phil. Tr., 1732–44, London, 1747, ix, 252.

[6] J. Fothergill: An account of the sore throat, London, 1748.

[7] Med. Obs. Soc. Phys., London, 1771–76, v, 129–142.

[8] Med. Obs. & Inquiries, London, 1784, vi, 103–107.

on infra-orbital neuralgia (1756)[1]; the description of pellagra or "mal de la rosa" by Francois Thiéry (1755),[2] William Hunter on arteriovenous aneurysm (1757)[3]; Tronchin on lead colic (1757)[4]; Mestivier's operated case of appendicitis (1759)[5]; Robert Hamilton on orchitis in mumps (1761)[6]; Heberden on varicella (1767)[7] and angina pectoris (1768)[8]; Robert Whytt's clinical picture of tubercular meningitis (1768)[9]; Rutty's account of relapsing fever (1770)[10]; Cotugno on sciatica (1770)[11]; Van Swieten on the paralytic type of rabies (1771); Werlhof on purpura hæmorrhagica (1775)[12]; Matthew Dobson's demonstration of sugar in diabetic urine (1776)[13]; Bylon and Benjamin Rush on dengue (1779–80); Pott on pressure paralysis from spinal caries (1779)[14]; Lettsom on the drug habit and alcoholism (1786)[15]; Parry on exophthalmic goiter (1786)[16]; Hezekiah Beardsley's case of congenital hypertrophic stenosis of the pylorus (1788)[17]; Sömmerring's case of achondroplasia (1791)[18]; Wollaston's discovery of urates in gouty joints (1797)[19]; Nikolaus Friedreich's description of peripheral facial paralysis (1797)[20]; and John Haslam's description of general paralysis (1798).[21] Besides this brilliant array of original work, which would honor any century, there were many admirable treatises or textbooks on special branches of internal medicine, such as Astruc (1736), Girtanner (1788–89), and Benjamin Bell (1793) on venereal diseases, Senac on diseases of the heart (1749), Plenciz on scarlatina (1162), Zimmermann on dysentery (1767), Lind on tropical diseases (1768), Millar on asthma and whooping-cough (1769), Walter on peritonitis (1785), Chabert on anthrax (1780), Malacarne (1788) and Foderé (1792) on cretinism and goiter, and John Rollo on diabetes (1797). There was a great increase in the literature bearing on the diseases of children, as evidenced in the pediatric treatises of Cadogan (1748), Rosén von Rosenstein (1752), Armstrong (1767), Mellin (1783), Underwood (1784), and Girtanner (1794). Gout and scurvy were favorite subjects of the English practitioners of the period, notably George Cheyne (1720) and Cadogan (1764) on the former, Lind (1753) and Thomas Trotter (1785) on the latter. Of all these special monographs, the best was unquestionably the treatise of Robert Willan (1757–1812) on diseases of the skin (1796–1808), which marks an epoch in the history of **dermatology,** but belongs essentially to the modern period. Of original contributions to descriptive dermatology, we may

---

[1] N. André: Observations pratiques sur les maladies de l'urétre, Paris, 1756.

[2] F. Thiéry: J. de méd., chir. et pharm., Paris, 1755, ii, 337–346.

[3] W. Hunter: Med. Obs. & Inquiries, London, 1757, i, 340.

[4] T. Tronchin: De colica Pictonum, Geneva, 1757.

[5] Mestivier: J. de méd., chir. et pharm., 1759, x, 441.

[6] Tr. Ry. Soc. Edinb. (1773), 1790, ii, pt. 2, 59–72.

[7] Heberden: Med. Tr. Coll. Phys., London, third edition, 1785, i, 427–436·

[8] Heberden: Med. Tr. Coll. Phys., London, 1768–70, ii, 58–67.

[9] Whytt: Observations on the Dropsy in the Brain, Edinburgh, 1768.

[10] Rutty: A chronological history (etc.), London, 1770.

[11] Cotugno: De ischiado nervosa, Vienna, 1770.

[12] Werlhof: Opera omnia, Hannover, 1775, ii, 615–636.

[13] Dobson: Med. Obs. & Inq., London, 1776, v, 298–316.

[14] Pott: Remarks on that kind of palsy (etc.), London, 1779.

[15] Lettsom: Mem. Med. Soc. London, 1779–87, i, 128–165.

[16] Parry's works, London, 1825, ii, 111.

[17] Beardsley: Cases & Obs. Med. Soc., New Haven County, 1788, 81–84.

[18] Soemmerring: Abbildungen . . . einiger Missgeburten, Mainz, 1791, 30, pl. xi.

[19] Wollaston: Phil. Tr., London, 1797, lxxxvii, 386–400.

[20] Friedreich: Med. chir. Ztg., Salzburg, 1798, i, 415.

[21] Haslam: Observations on insanity, London, 1798.

mention John Machin's observation of ichthyosis hystrix in the Lambert family (1733),[1] which was followed through successive generations by Henry Baker (1755),[2] and Tilesius (1802)[3]; the observation of scleroderma in Curzio's clinic at Naples by William and Robert Watson (1754)[4]; Wichmann on the parasitic origin of scabies (1786),[5] and Sir Everard Home's description of cutaneous horns (hyperkeratosis) in 1791.[6] The subject of **medical jurisprudence** was carefully systematized in the eighteenth century, and the leaders in this field were the Germans, who were the first to found professorships of forensic medicine and turned out the most important treatises. The earliest of these was the "Corpus juris medico-legale" of Michael Bernhard Valentini (1657–1729), published in 1722, a huge storehouse of well-arranged facts. It was followed in 1723 by the "Institutiones" of Hermann Friedrich Teichmeyer (1685–1746), which was for a long time the standard authority, and, in 1736–47, by the "System" of Michael Alberti (1682–1757) of Halle, a six-volume work, not unlike Valentini's in scope and thoroughness. In France, Antoine Louis (1723–92) was the pioneer in applying medical knowledge to court-room practice. He wrote an important memoir on hanging, with reference to the differential signs of murder and suicide in cases of hanging (1763), and, in his discussion of the celebrated Villebranche case (1764), he ridiculed the possibility of extremely protracted pregnancy, endeavoring to set the time-limits of normal gestation, which, under the Code Napoleon, were finally fixed at three hundred days, as in the Roman laws of the Twelve Tables. Fodéré's great treatise on legal medicine (1798) belongs to the modern period of the science. The first English work was the "Elements" of Samuel Farr (1788), but William Hunter's essay on the signs of murder in bastard children (1783) is probably the most important English contribution in the eighteenth century.

Medical ethics was treated in Friedrich Hoffmann's "Medicus politicus" (1738) and by Stoll.

Medical history was systematically treated in the works of Freind (1725–27), Daniel Leclerc (1729), Blumenbach (1786), and Kurt Sprengel (1792–1803). Of these, John **Freind** (1625–1728), of Croton, Northamptonshire, who was highly educated at Oxford in the humanities and in medicine, and delivered the Ashmolean lectures on chemistry in 1704, was an intellectual light of considerable prominence in his day. He accompanied the Earl of Peterborough on his Spanish campaign of 1705, as physician to the English forces, and subsequently mixing in politics as a partisan, was committed to the Tower on the charge of high treason in March, 1722–23; but was soon released through the good offices of Mead, and became physician to Queen Caroline in 1727. During his short imprisonment, he planned his "History of Physick from the time of Galen to the beginning of the Sixteenth Century" (London, 1725–26), dedicated to Mead, and intended as a continuation of Leclerc. This is usually regarded as the best English work on the period of which it treats, although, as Sir Clifford Allbutt says, the author "spread his net too widely" and produced a general survey "from the time of Galen," where he might have done better by confining himself to English medicine in detail. Haller's 1751 edition of the "Methodus Studii Medici" of Boerhaave is an introduction to medical literature similar to that compiled by Thomas Young more than half a century later, and is remarkable for those sententious critical aperçus for which Haller is so justly famous.

An important three-volume treatise on **medical geography** was published by Leonhard Ludwig Finke (1747–1828) in 1792–95.[7]

---

[1] Machin: Phil. Tr., London, 1733, xxxvii, 299–301, 1 pl.

[2] Baker: Phil. Tr., London, 1755, xlix, pt. 1, 21–24.

[3] Tilesius: Ausführliche Beschreibung . . . der beiden sog. Stachelschweinmenschen, Altenburg, 1802.

[4] Watson: Phil. Tr., London, 1754, xlviii, 579–587.

[5] Wichmann: Aetiologie der Krätze, Hannover, 1786.

[6] Home: Phil. Tr., London, 1791, lxxxii, 95–105.

[7] L. L. Finke: Versuch einer allgemeinen medicinisch-praktischen Geographie, Leipzig, 1792–95.

Toward the end of the century came one of the greatest triumphs in the history of medicine—the successful introduction of **preventive inoculation** by Edward **Jenner** (1749–1823), son of a Gloucestershire clergyman, who, in 1770, became a friend and pupil of John Hunter's, and helped him a good deal in his experiments. It had long been a countryside tradition in Gloucestershire that dairy-maids who had contracted cow-pox through milking did not take smallpox, and similar observations had been noted in Germany and France. On learning of this fact from a milkmaid, Jenner early conceived the idea of applying it on a grand

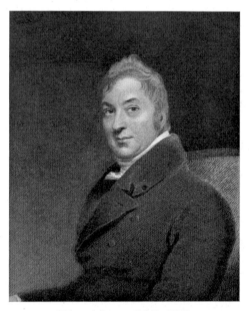

Edward Jenner (1749–1823).

scale in the prevention of the disease. On communicating his project to Hunter, the latter gave him the characteristic advice: "Don't think, try; be patient, be accurate." On returning to his home at Berkeley he began to collect his observations in 1778, and on May 14, 1796, performed his first vaccination upon a country boy, James Phipps, using matter from the arm of the milkmaid, Sarah Nelmes, who had contracted cow-pox in the usual way. The experiment was then put to the test, by inoculating Phipps with smallpox virus on July 1st, and the immunization proved successful. By 1798 he had 23 cases, which he embodied in his work, *An Inquiry into the Causes and Effects of the Variolæ*

Vaccinæ, a thin quarto with four colored plates, printed in 1798, and dedicated to Parry of Bath. This book establishes his main thesis that a vaccination with cow-pox matter protects from small-pox, and was followed, during the years 1799–1806, by five successive pamphlets, recording his subsequent experiments and improvements in technic up to the stage of recommending ivory points as the best vectors in inoculation. Jenner's work was rapidly taken up on the continent and in America; good statistics began to pour in, in less than a year's time, and, by 1800, as many as 6000 people had been vaccinated. In 1802 and 1807, Parliament voted grants amounting to £20,000 to Jenner in aid of prosecuting his experiments. At the same time, he met with bitter opposition from jealous contemporaries, like Ingen-Housz, Woodville, and Pearson, who either claimed priority or acted upon the parliamentary principle that the duty of the opposition is to oppose. The mere idea of inoculation is apparently as old as the hills. Human inoculation of variolous virus is said to be mentioned in the Atharva Veda (Baas) and certainly in the Flos of the School of Salerno, and was known to most Oriental peoples. The idea was introduced into England by Timoni's and Pilarini's communications to the Royal Society in 1713–16, and was afterward taken up by Sir Hans Sloane (1717). On March 18, 1718, Lady Mary Wortley Montague had her three-year-old son inoculated in Turkey, and her five-year-old daughter was inoculated in England in April, 1721. During the sixth epidemic of smallpox in Boston, Massachusetts, Zabdiel Boylston (1679–1766) courageously inoculated his son and two negro slaves on June 26, 1721, and had inoculated 244 persons before its close, exciting great opposition and even threats of hanging. In the Boston epidemic of 1752, 2109 were inoculated, and nearly 20,000 in England, under Daniel Sutton in 1764–65.[1] Apart from the huge eighteenth century literature on inoculation, one of the most important items of which is the proposal of preventive inoculations against the plague (1755) by the Hungarian physician, Stephan Weszprémi (1723–99), there had been successful cow-pox inoculations by the Dorset farmer, Benjamin Jesty, in 1774–89, and by Plett of Holstein in 1791. All these efforts were, however, "as an arrow shot in the air or a sword-stroke in the water." The merit of Jenner's work rests upon the fact that, like Harvey, he started out with the hope of making his thesis a permanent working principle in science, based upon

---

[1] See Reginald H. Fitz, on Zabdiel Boylston in Bull. Johns Hopkins Hospital, Baltimore, 1911, xxii, 315–327, and A. C. Klebs: *Ibid.*, 1913, xxiv, 69–83, *passim*. Inoculation was a common preventive measure in America during the War of the Revolution.

experimental demonstration, and he succeeded to the extent of carrying his inoculations successfully through several generations in the body, and, above all, in overcoming the popular aversion to vaccination. In short, Jenner transformed a local country tradition into a viable prophylactic principle, and, although he was preceded by really scientific experts in inoculation (variolation), his reputation in his own field is fairly safe from the priority-mongers. Faults of diffuseness and lack of skill in marshaling facts have been imputed against the "Inquiry," but, on the whole, it remains an unimpeachable record of careful scientific work, the effect of which is seen today in the rapid strides that preventive medicine is making and in the results of compulsory vaccination in Prussia and Holland, where the mortality curve of smallpox approaches zero as its limit. Striking, indeed, were the vaccination statistics of the Franco-Prussian War in 1870–71, in which the unvaccinated French army lost over 20,000 men from smallpox, while the Germans, who had been revaccinated within two years, lost 297. Kitasato's statistics of vaccination in the Russo-Japanese war (1911)[1] show that, with smallpox endemic in Japan, there were only 362 cases and 35 deaths in an army of over a million soldiers. Jenner's monograph of 1798 has loomed into especial prominence of late through the fact that it contains an early reference and a clear explanation of anaphylaxis or allergy. In case 4, he notes that inoculation of variolous matter in a woman who had had cow-pox thirty-one years before, produced a palish red efflorescence of the skin, which he regards as almost a criterion of whether the infection will be received or not, attributing the phenomenon to the dynamic effect of a permanent change in the blood during life.[2] In the later years of his life, Jenner lived in London, of which city he was made an honorary citizen. He died there of apoplexy in 1823, and his monument, erected in 1858, is in Trafalgar Square. In personality Jenner was the typical English country gentleman, blond, blue-eyed, of handsome figure. A well-known account describes him ready for a mount, in blue coat, nankeen riding-breeches, and top-boots, with whip and silver spurs. He was a bird-fancier, played the flute and violin, botanized, and wrote clever verses, of which the "Address to a Robin" and the "Signs of Rain," redolent of the English countryside, deserve a place in any anthology of minor poets. Jenner's kindness of heart is seen in

---

[1] Cited by Osler in his Principles and Practice of Medicine, eighth edition, New York, 1912, p. 330.

[2] Jenner: Inquiry, 1798, footnote to p. 13, cited by L. Hektoen in Jour. Am. Med. Ass., Chicago, 1912, lviii, footnote to p. 1087.

20

his regard for his first vaccination patient, James Phipps, for whom he built a cottage, planting the roses in the garden with his own hands. Like Newton, Harvey, Sydenham, Darwin, and Lister, he is one of the great men of purely Saxon genius, a happy combination of rare common sense with extreme simplicity of mind and character.

In Germany, Jenner's work was immediately taken up about 1798–99 by Hugo von Wreden in Hannover, by Heim and Brenner in Berlin, by Hirt in Saxony, and by de Carro and Ferro in Austria, the former being also the first to introduce Jennerian vaccination into Asia. Pinel and Thouret in France, Vrancken in Holland, Demanet in Belgium, Sacco in Italy, Heinrich Callisen in Denmark, Amar and others in Spain, were among the earliest promoters of the practice. In the United States, the Harvard professor of medicine, Benjamin Waterhouse (1754–1846), made the first vaccinations upon his four children in July, 1800,[1] procuring his virus from Dr. Haygarth of Bath, England. He was speedily followed by Crawford and Smith in Baltimore, James Jackson in Boston, David Hosack in New York and John Redmond Coxe in Philadelphia. The first Vaccine Institute was organized in Baltimore by James Smith in 1802 and a national Vaccine Agency was established by Congress under his direction in 1813. Waterhouse said that, before the introduction of vaccination, the fear of smallpox compelled the New Englanders, "the most democratical people on the face of the earth,"to endure "restrictions of liberty such as no absolute monarch could have enforced.[2] The early American tracts of the colonial pamphleteers on inoculation such as Benjamin Colman (1721–22), Isaac Greenwood (1721), Cotton Mather (1722), William Douglass (1722–30), Zabdiel Boylston (1726), Adam Thomson (1750), Nathanael Williams (1752), Lauchlin MacLeane (1756), Benjamin Franklin (1759), John Morgan (1776), and Benjamin Rush (1781), with the Waterhouse pamphlets on vaccination (1800–02), are now among the rarest and most highly prized of medical curiosities.

There was no **American medical literature** to speak of until long after the American Revolution. The first medical book to be published on the North American continent was printed by the Spaniards in the city of Mexico in 1570, and the first medical school was founded by them in 1578. Thacher's "Brief Rule" (Boston, 1677) was the only medical publication of the New England Colonies in the seventeenth century.

"At the commencement of the Revolutionary War," says Billings, "we had one medical book by an American author, three reprints, and about twenty pamphlets"; and of the book in question, John Jones's "Plain, Concise, Practical Remarks on the Treatment of Wounds and Fractures" (New York, 1775), he goes on to say that "it is simply a compilation from Ranby, Pott, and others, and contains but one original observation."[3] The book contains, however, an appendix on camp and military hospitals, and was of great use to the young military and naval surgeons of the Revolution, for whom it was primarily designed, being, in fact, the first American book on military medicine. Of the pamphlets, there were some now curious colonial productions on the various anginas and eruptive fevers of the time by John Walton (1732), Cad-

---

[1] In the "Columbian Sentinel" of March 12, 1799, Waterhouse refers to vaccination, in down-East phrase, as "Something curious in the medical line."

[2] Cited by Dock.

[3] J. S. Billings in "A Century of American Medicine," Philadelphia, 1876, p. 293.

wallader Colden (1735), William Douglass (angina ulcusculosa, 1736), and Jabez Fitch (1736) and the tracts on inoculation, already mentioned. The early inaugural dissertations of the students Elmer, Potts and Tilton at the University of Pennsylvania in 1771, the latter a product of the celebrated Bradford Press, are now only collectors' curiosities, and the same thing applies to the oration "Antiqua novum orbem decet medico-philosophica," delivered at the University of Virginia, June 12, 1782, by Jean-François Coste (1741–1819), medical director of the French forces in America, published at Leyden in 1783 and dedicated to Washington. Better than these are the essays on yellow fever by John Bard, Colden (1743), Mitchell (1741), John Lining (1753) and William Currie (1792); and, more important still, the clinical studies of Thomas Cadwalader (1708–79) of Philadelphia on the ileac passion (1740) and the West-Indian dry-gripes (lead-poisoning), the latter printed by Benjamin Franklin at Philadelphia in 1745; John Bard on malignant pleurisy (1749), and the essay of Samuel Bard (1742–1821) on diphtheria or "angina suffocativa" (1771), which is spoken of by Osler as "an American class of the first rank." The "Cases and Observations of the Medical Society of New Haven County," founded in 1784, contains the first recorded case of congenital hypertrophic stenosis of the pylorus (1788)[1] by Hezekiah Beardsley (1748–90), of Stratford, Connecticut, which Osler rescued (in Lessing's sense of the term) by reprinting it in 1903.[2] The history and geography of yellow fever in the United States were treated of by William Currie (1792) and Noah Webster (1796–99), and the work of Matthew Carey (1760–1839) on the Philadelphia epidemic of yellow fever in 1793 stands with that of Benjamin Rush as the most graphic, realistic, and complete account of the disease that had yet appeared.[3]

Some good botanical works were printed abroad, notably a first account of senega and its uses by John Tennant, of Virginia, in 1736, John Clayton's "Flora Virginica" (Leyden, 1739), probably the first work on American botany; "An Experimental Inquiry into the Properties of Opium," by John Leigh of Virginia (Edinburgh, 1786), which gained the Harveian prize in 1785; and the still more interesting "Materia medica Americana" (Erlangen, 1787) of the old Anspach-Bayreuth surgeon, Johann David Schoepf (1752–1800), who came out to America with the Hessian troops in 1777, remained over after the war, and recorded his experiences in his "Travels in the Confederation" (1788), which was translated and published in Philadelphia in 1911.

The War of the Revolution was the making of medicine in this country, and it was in the nature of things that it should bring to the front the three leading American physicians of the time, Morgan, Shippen and Rush. The War found us in a state of "unpreparedness," with nothing of military, still less of medical, organization. Every one was on the fighting line, and there was little time for building hospitals, making instruments or obtaining drugs. After drafting the Declaration, the ablest members of the Continental Congress were called, like every one else, to immediate and pressing duties in their several states; and Congress itself became, by all accounts, a feeble, bungling, almost impotent thing, accomplishing very little in aid of the medical administration of the war, in some respects the

---

[1] Beardsley: *Loc. cit.*, pp. 81–84.

[2] Arch. Pediat., New York, 1903, xx, 355–357.

[3] Charles Brockden Brown's novel of Arthur Mervyn contains another interesting account of this epidemic.

most important feature of all. As Mumford says, there was but one man who was found "steadfast, patient, imperturbable," and that was Washington.[1] All honor belongs to the two army surgeons who were associated with him and who did so much for the organization of American medical education, John Morgan and William Shippen. Besides these, only brief mention can be made of other physicians, many of whom played a noble and self-sacrificing part, such as John and Joseph Warren of Massachusetts, the latter serving in the ranks and losing his life at Bunker Hill;

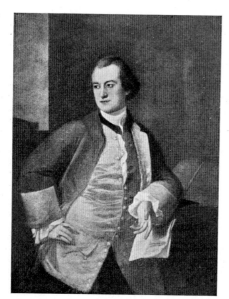

John Morgan (1735–89).

Benjamin Church, the first Surgeon General of the American Army; Hugh Mercer, of Virginia, who was killed at Princeton in 1777; James Thacher, the first American medical biographer, whose "Military Journal" (Boston, 1827) gives a picturesque account of the struggle and perhaps the best word-picture of the personality of Washington; and James Tilton, whose "Observations on Military Hospitals"(Wilmington, 1813) is a contribution of permanent value to his subject.

John **Morgan** (1735–89), a native of Philadelphia, was a student of John Redman's, served as surgeon in the French wars, and graduated at Edinburgh in 1762, where he was trained by such masters as William Hunter, the Monros, Cullen and Whytt. Returning to his native city in 1765, he published, in the same year, his "Discourse upon the Institution of Medical Schools in America," which files the first brief for adequate medical education in this country and commemorates the organization, at the College of Philadelphia (founded in 1740), of the Medical Department of the University of Pennsylvania, of which Morgan was, with Shippen, the principal founder and in which he held the first chair of practice of medicine.

---

[1] J. G. Mumford: A Narrative of Medicine in America, Philadelphia, 1903, p. 122.

THE EIGHTEENTH CENTURY 309

In 1775 Congress appointed Morgan "Director General and Physician in Chief" of the American Army, to succeed Church. He entered upon his duties with vigor, insisting upon rigorous examinations for medical officers and subordinating the regimental surgeons to the hospital chiefs, but the enmity of his subalterns and the shiftiness of politicians led to his unjust dismissal by Congress in 1777 and Shippen was appointed in his place. Morgan thereupon published his spirited "Vindication" (1777), in which he ably defends himself, with all loyalty to the cause and his great chief, demanding at the same time a court of inquiry. After two years' deliberation, the latter met and honorably acquitted him of all the charges in 1779. Broken in spirit, poor, and injured in health, Morgan retired to private practice and died twelve years later.

William **Shippen,** Jr. (1736–1808), of Philadelphia, who succeeded Morgan as Surgeon General in 1777, was also an Edinburgh graduate (1761), coming under the Hunters, Cullen and Monro *secundus*. Returning to America in 1772, he began to give private and public instruction in anatomy and obstetrics, and was, indeed, the first public teacher of obstetrics in this country, where he greatly advanced the cause of male midwifery. In 1765, he collaborated with Morgan in organizing the Medical Department of the University of Pennsylvania, in which he was, at the same time, appointed professor of anatomy and surgery. Upon his accession to the surgeon-generalcy in 1777, Shippen proved himself more practical, less sensitive, better off in worldly wisdom than Morgan, and was consequently more successful. He resigned in 1781, to devote his entire attention to medical teaching, which he had kept up intermittently during his period of military service. With this his name is best associated, for he left no literary contributions of moment.[1]

Benjamin **Rush** (1745–1813), of Pennsylvania, was of English Quaker stock and a graduate of Princeton (1760) and Edinburgh (1768), his graduating thesis in medicine being "De coctione ciborum in ventriculo." In 1769, he was elected professor of chemistry in the College of Philadelphia and succeeded Morgan as professor of practice in the same institution in 1789, attaining the chair of institutes of medicine, when the latter was merged into the University of Pennsylvania, in 1791. He was also physician to the Pennsylvania Hospital (1783–1813), the chief founder of the Philadelphia Dispensary (the first in this country) in 1786, and Treasurer of the United States Mint (1799–1813). Rush was a man of highly

---

[1] Shippen's graduating dissertation at Edinburgh, "De placentæ cum utero nexa" (1761) is now only of bibliographic interest.

original mind, well read, well trained in his profession, an attractive, straightforward teacher, of wide human interests, sometimes wrong-headed as well as strong-headed.   A signer of the Declaration and sometime surgeon general for the Middle Department under Shippen (1776–78), he deserted Washington at Valley Forge to join the infamous "Conway Cabal" against the latter's "Fabian policy."   As a medical theorist, he opposed Cullen's solidism and his elaborate classification of diseases for a modified Brunonianism. His own therapeutic scheme was upon the most arbitrary basis. He looked upon inflammation as the effect rather than the cause of

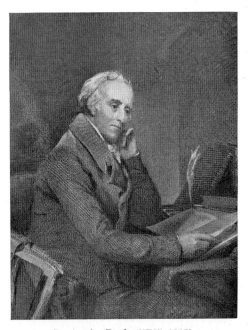

Benjamin Rush (1745–1813).

disease, and in regard to his statement that "Medicine is my wife and science my mistress," Dr. Holmes has added the caustic comment: "I do not think that the breach of the seventh commandment can be shown to have been of advantage to the legitimate owner of his affections."   A typical eighteenth century theorist, and a man whose social propagandism against war, slavery, alcoholism, and the death penalty was perhaps not entirely dissociated from a personal interest in increasing his practice, Rush was easily the ablest American clinician of his time, and his writings and reputation won him golden opinions abroad.   Lettsom called him the American Sydenham, where effusive but more uncritical compatriots had dubbed him the Hippocrates of Pennsylvania, and he was the recipient of a diamond and various medals from royalty. He belongs to the school of Sydenham in his adherence to blood-letting and in his careful accounts of the diseases under his observation. Of these, he described cholera infantum in 1773; he was the first, after Bylon, of Java (1779), to describe dengue (1780),[1] and perhaps the first to note the thermal fever occasioned by drinking cold water when overheated. His monograph on insanity (1812) has been pronounced by Mills[2] to be, with that of Isaac Ray, the only systematic American treatise on the subject before the year 1883. His account of the Philadelphia epidemic of yellow fever in 1793 is only approached by that of Matthew Carey for its realism. In fighting this epidemic, Rush played a distinguished part, breaking down his health by treating 100 to 150 patients a day, and incurring civic and professional hatred through insisting that the disease was not imported from without but arose *de novo* in the city. His line of treatment was the exhibition of large doses of calomel and jalap, copious blood-letting, low diet, low temperature in the sick-room, and abundant hydrotherapy, within and without. As a blood-letter, Rush has been likened to Sangrado, but he saved many patients and, when sick, as he thought, of yellow fever, consistently submitted to his own line of treatment. Apart from his clinical memoirs, Rush wrote a valuable pamphlet on the hygiene of troops (1777), and his papers on the diseases of North American Indians (1774) and their vices (1798), with his account of the German inhabitants of Pennsylvania (1798), are perhaps the earliest American contributions to anthropology. The original bent of his mind is shown in his inquiries into the effects of ardent spirits on the mind, the cure of diseases by the extraction of decayed teeth, and the effect of arsenic in cancer. Like Shippen and Physick, Rush was a well-featured man of aquiline profile, suggesting native shrewdness and penetration.

The name of **Benjamin Franklin** (1706–90), of Boston, is intimately connected with American medicine through his invention of bifocal lenses (1785)[3] and a flexible catheter, his treatment of nervous diseases by electricity (Franklinism), his letters on lead-poisoning, and his observations on gout, the heat of the blood, sleep, deafness, nyctalopia, infection from dead bodies, death-rate in infants, and medical education. He was the principal

---

[1] Rush: Medical Observations and Inquiries, Philadelphia, 1789, v, 104–121.

[2] C. K. Mills: Benjamin Rush and American Psychiatry, 1886. Cited by Mumford.

[3] In his letter to Whately of London, 1785.

founder and the first president of the Pennsylvania Hospital (1751), of which he wrote a history, by request, printed at his own press in 1754. Of special bibliographic interest are his "Dialogue with the Gout" and his pamphlet on inoculation in small-pox (London, 1759), which was accompanied by William Heberden's directions for performing the operation.

Thomas **Cadwalader** (1708–79), of Philadelphia, a pupil of Cheselden, was a pioneer of inoculation (1730), a founder of the Philadelphia Library (1731) and its director (1731–39), and the first to teach anatomy by dissections in the city (1730–31). His "Essay on the West-India Dry-Gripes," printed by Benjamin Franklin in 1745, and sometimes wrongly catalogued as an "Essay on the Iliac Passion," is

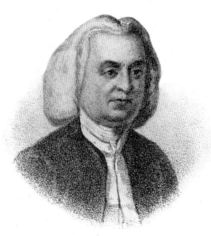

Thomas Cadwalader (1708–79).

an account of lead colic and lead palsy from the habitual use of Jamaica rum distilled through leaden pipes. It contains his autopsy of a case of mollities ossium (1742), and ranks with the essays of Huxham (1739), Tronchin (1757), Bordeu (1761–63) and Baker (1767) as one of the classical accounts of lead poisoning in the eighteenth century.

Apart from the work of Morgan, Rush and Shippen, the writings of the colonial pamphleteers on inoculation, the clinical observations of Cadwalader, Samuel Bard, Beardsley, Rush and Carey, and the pioneer exploits in pelvic and vascular surgery by John Bard, William Baynham and Wright Post, most of the productions of American medicine in this period, although of a respectable character, are aside from the main current of scientific progress. As Sainte Beuve said to Matthew Arnold about Lamartine's poems, they are "important to *us*," in the sense of having a definite local and historic interest.

THE EIGHTEENTH CENTURY 313

CULTURAL AND SOCIAL ASPECTS OF EIGHTEENTH CENTURY MEDICINE

The rise of Prussia and Russia and the American and French revolutions are perhaps the only historic events which exerted much influence upon the condition of medicine in the eighteenth century, and then only in relation to the development of surgery. The tendencies of the age were artificial and theoretic rather than sincere or realistic. This periwigged period is conceded to have been the "Golden Age," alike of the successful practitioner and the successful quack. The reason of this is to be sought in the stationary condition of society prior to the French Revolution, which kept all occupations in a definite groove; so that the internist or physician proper was in every sense of the word a family doctor (*Hausarzt*), who was given a voluntary annual honorarium for his continuous services during the year, thus relieving him of the necessity of competing with his fellow practitioners or of struggling for his existence beyond a certain point. Practice was inherited from father to son or passed on to favorite pupils, and, in this way, a certain elegant leisure was acquired by the well-to-do members of the profession, giving them exceptional opportunities for the acquisition of culture. Haller, William Hunter, Scarpa, Heberden, and Thomas Young yield to none in scholarship and variety of attainments. Arbuthnot, Garth, and other physicians of Queen Anne's reign were coffee-house intimates of the wits and poets of the period.[1] Lessing had studied medicine. Goldsmith and Schiller were medical graduates; and such men of letters as Garth, Arbuthnot, Blackmore, Akenside, Haller, Zimmermann, and Werlhof were practitioners. There is plenty of evidence that the social status of the eighteenth century physician was as good as, if not better than, it is now. In some countries he wore a sword, his color was the "austere scarlet," and people commonly took off their hats to him, even when he bore a muff, to preserve his delicacy of touch in diagnosis. In England, the fashionable physician wore a powdered wig, a handsome coat of red satin or brocade, short breeches, stockings and buckled shoes, a three-cornered hat, and bore a gold-headed cane. Werlhof, at Hannover, on the occasion of his second marriage, wore a violet velvet coat. Toward the end of the seventeenth century, ruffled collars gave place to Geneva bands, an appropriate

[1] Every reader of Pope will recall his grateful tribute to Arbuthnot:

"Friend to my life; (which did you not prolong,
The world had wanted many an idle song),
. . . .
The muse but serv'd to ease some friend, not wife,
To help me through this long disease, my life,
To second, Arbuthnot! thy art and care,
And teach the being you preserved to bear."

symbol of the clerical origin of the medical profession. The summit of its grandeur, in costume at least, is to be seen in the portrait of the elder Baron, the pleasant-faced dean of the Paris Faculty (1730–34), which is reproduced in the beautiful album of its artistic collections published in 1911.[1] The handsome dean wears a long, carefully curled wig, an ermine cape, a delicate, transparent *rabat* in place of the stiff Geneva band, a red ecclesiastical cope (the "regal dalmatic") with lace ruffles at the sleeves,

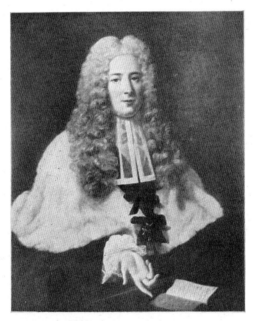

Hyacinthe-Théodore Baron père (1710–58), Dean of the Paris Medical Faculty, 1730–34.   (Courtesy of M. Noé Legrand, Paris, from his "Les Collections Artistiques de la Faculté de Médecine de Paris," 1911.)

and, over his breast, a decoration suspended by a long black ribbon. Solemn elegance could go no further.   Careless elegance as well as political sympathies were sometimes evinced in the loosely knotted "Steenkirk tie."[2]

Except in caricature, the art of the eighteenth century throws

---

[1] Les collections artistiques de la Faculté de médecine de Paris.   Inventaire raisonné par Noé Legrand et L. Landouzy, Paris, 1911.

[2] So called from the disordered condition of rich cravats at the battle of Steinkirk (1692).   After this event, the studiously disarranged tie became fashionable in France, and, if we may trust the Restoration dramatists, even in England.   See Vanbrugh's Relapse, act 1, sc. 3, and Scott's Rob Roy, ch. xxxi.

little light upon the status of the medical profession. Reynolds and Gainsborough, Fragonard and Watteau, are unusually reticent about medicine in their canvases, although a few portraits of physicians were, of course, painted by Raeburn and others, with Sir Joshua's great portrait of John Hunter at the head of the list. Hogarth's "Company of Undertakers" (1736), with the legend, *Et plurima mortis imago*, represents twelve hard-featured individuals, all bewigged and armed with gold-headed canes, who are

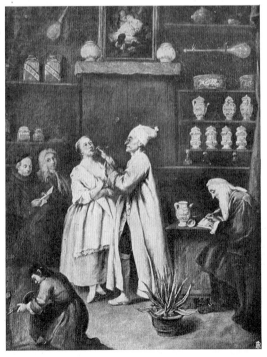

The Apothecary, by Pietro Longhi (1702–85).   (Italian interior of the eighteenth century.)

supposed to represent Spot Ward, the Chevalier Taylor, Madame Mapp (in a zany's coat of many colors), and other quacks of the period.   Hogarth also made two pictures of Maria Toft's miraculous birth of rabbits, a celebrated imposture of the eighteenth century, and has various broad or slanting allusions to prostitution, pregnancy, alcoholism, and insanity in his copper plates, including the quack with the poor syphilitic child in Mariage à la Mode (Plate III).   Gillray and Rowlandson, those masters of the coarse and grotesque, indulged their animal spirits abundantly at the ex-

pense of medicine, but their plates belong mostly to the Georgian
period. Those on The Dying Patient, or the Doctor's Last Fee
(Rowlandson, 1786), Transplantation of Teeth (Rowlandson,
1787), The Gout (Gillray, 1799),The Midwife (Rowlandson,1800),
and Metallic Tractors (Gillray, 1801), are all true eighteenth century in implication. Animal magnetism, vaccination, clysters, Macassar oil, men-midwives, metallic tractors, phrenology, and other
foibles of the period were all abundantly caricatured in the fugitive anonymous plates of the time. That prolific Danzig artist,
Daniel Chodowiecki, the illustrator of the *Zopfzeit*, has some
clever etchings of German interiors, representing inoculation,
animal magnetism, dissecting, fashionable physicians (*Mode-*

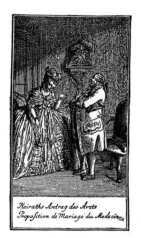

Heiraths Antrag des Arts
Proposition de Mariage du Medecin

A proposal of marriage.
Etching by Daniel Chodo-
wiecki (1726–1801).

doctoren), miraculous healers (*Wunder-*
doctoren), Frederick the Great having a
vein opened, a sick person receiving extreme unction, an absurd proposal of
marriage by a corpulent physician to an
equally stout patient, and a plate showing Prussian police in the act of ordering
patients to the Charité. Boucher's cartoon of the orviétan-vendor (1736), was
reproduced in Gobelin tapestry. A clever
painting by Pietro Longhi represents an
Italian apothecary shop of the period.

In the secular literature of the eighteenth century, the physician was especially satirized by Smollett (Count Fathom),
Sterne (Dr. Slop), and Le Sage (Gil Blas).
In Smollett's Count Fathom, the adventurous knave takes it into his head to en-
roll himself among "the sons of Pæan," and
his experiences give an amusing purview
of the "solemnities of dress and address," the trade tricks (being
called out of church or riding aimlessly about in a chariot) which
were resorted to, even by practitioners of better repute. The
capable Huxham, a butcher's son, who first practised among non-
conformists and afterward went over to the Established Church,
often had himself summoned out of conventicle at stated intervals,
whereupon he would gallop through the town to create the impression of an extensive practice. He usually stalked about in a scarlet
coat, flourishing a gold-headed cane, a footman bearing his gloves
at a respectful distance. Le Sage throws much light upon medicine
in Spain, where blood-letting and cathartics were almost the only
known remedies, where cleaning the streets of offal was opposed
for a fantastic reason, where there was not a single apothecary for

over half a century, and where, as late as 1795, permission to practise outside of Madrid cost only $45 (Baas). The ignominious position of the army surgeon in Germany before the time of Frederick the Great is alluded to in the early writings and poems of Schiller. In Roderick Random, Smollett describes the exceedingly low status of the medical profession on board ship and the humbuggery and corruption which attended the competitive examinations for the position of surgeon's mate. His picture of M. Lallemant, the shabby, nimble-shilling apothecary, is equally significant. In an age in which caste distinctions were on an iron-clad basis (witness the French Revolution), it is obvious that the imposing dress and manners of the upper-class physicians should lend themselves readily to imitation at the hands of unscrupulous impostors. The eighteenth century was the age *par excellence* of successful quacks, and it only yields to the nineteenth century in respect of those patented or secret preparations of which the poet Crabbe, the satirist of quacks, laments:

"From the poor man's pay
The nostrum takes no trifling part away."

Quackery, if not universal, was at least, in Thoreau's phrase, "universally successful." Rolling stones, like Cagliostro and Mesmer, managed to ply their trade for a long while without interruption. Casanova paid a decorous visit to Haller at Bern, and his stay with the great man was supposed to be not so much "the homage which vice pays to virtue" as a manifestation of genuine esteem, for Casanova not only affected to enjoy the commerce of the learned, but had written Latin dissertations or had someone write them for him. In England, there was a long line of successful medical charlatans of both sexes. The earliest of these was Sir William Read, who started out as a tailor, but in 1694 set up in the Strand as an oculist, having hired some one to write a book on eye diseases under his name and a Grub Street poet to praise him in verse. His success in this specialty attracted the attention of Queen Anne, whose bad eyesight made her an easy victim of such impostors, and, gaining her good graces, he was actually knighted, subsequently becoming oculist to George I. He frequented the society of Swift and the other coffee-house wits, who made fun of him while accepting his lavish hospitality, and he is even mentioned in the Spectator (September 1, November 27, 1712). Other quack oculists of importance in their day were Dr. Grant, who was also patronized by Queen Anne, and the Chevalier Taylor. The latter, the son of a female apothecary of Norwich, had actually worked with Cheselden at St. Thomas's and had invented a cataract needle and other instruments, but, failing of success in

London, decided for the adventurous career of a roving oculist. It has been remarked that even Daviel, in the early part of his career, did practically the same thing, trumpeting his praises abroad after the fashion of the wandering eye-couchers of the Middle Ages, but with this difference that Daviel was really a great ophthalmic surgeon in the making, where Taylor was only a clever buffoon. Clad in black, with a long flowing wig, possessed of a good address and undoubtedly of some skill in eye surgery, Taylor went about, lecturing like a mountebank at a fair, expressing himself in queer sentences with inverted syntax, in imitation of Latin, which style he called "true Ciceronian." He numbered even Gibbon and Händel among his patients, but did not impose upon Horace Walpole or Dr. Johnson. The latter says of him (Boswell, 1779): "Taylor was the most ignorant man I ever knew, but sprightly: Ward, the dullest. Taylor challenged me once to talk Latin with him [laughing]. I quoted some of Horace, which he took to be a part of my own speech. He said a few words well enough." The Ward to whom Dr. Johnson refers was Joshua Ward, another famous quack, also known as "Spot" Ward, on account of a claret mark on one side of his face. Ward was originally a drysalter who had tried politics without success, but soon made his fortune by the sale of antimonial pills and drops, a "liquid sweat," a "dropsy purging powder," and other nostrums. His "essence for headache" and "Ward's paste" (for fistula and piles) afterward appeared in the Pharmacopœia as compound camphor liniment and confection of pepper. He won the absolute confidence of George II by reducing a dislocated thumb with a sharp wrench, after which he was given a room in Whitehall and liberally patronized by the great, numbering Chesterfield, Walpole, and Gibbon among his patients. He was specially exempted from the penalties of the Parliamentary Act of 1748, restricting the practice of medicine, and, in his will, had the impudence to request burial in Westminster Abbey. Pope has embalmed him in a couplet:

"Of late, without the least pretence to skill,
Ward's grown a famed physician by a pill."

Famous female impostors of the period were Mrs. Mapp, a bonesetter, who was so successful that she could drive in from Epsom in a chariot and four, with gorgeously liveried servants, and Joanna Stevens, a widow, who, in 1739, actually succeeded in having her remedy for stone purchased *pro bono publico* by Act of Parliament. Her philanthropy went to the extent of agreeing to part with this valuable recipe for £5000, but even a titled subscription list could not raise this sum in the first instance, and powerful influence was brought to bear upon Parliament, even

Cheselden, Sharp, and Cæsar Hawkins vouching for her merits. The recipe was published in the London Gazette of June 19, 1739, and turned out to be a set of mixtures of egg-shells, garden-snails, swines' cresses, soap, and such vegetable ingredients as burdock seeds, hips, and haws. In each one of her certified "cures," the stone was found in the bladder after death.

Of secret or proprietary medicines patented in England, Timothy Byfield's *sal oleosum volatile* (1711) was the first to take advantage of the old Statute of Monopolies of 1624. It was followed by Stoughton's Great Cordial Elixir (1712), Betton's British Oils (1742), John Hooper's Female Pills (1743), and a long list of other nostrums, down to Ching's Worm Lozenges (1792) and Della Lena's Powder of Mars (1799). The most famous of these were the antimonial fever powder (1747) and analeptic pills (1794) of Dr. Robert James, a physician of solid ability, who wrote a bulky Dictionary of Medicine and a Pharmacopœia Universalis, and was an esteemed friend of Dr. Johnson. The original James's powder was, in the opinion of Christison, more effective than its antimonial substitute in the Pharmacopœia. Among the therapeutic fads of the time were quassia-cups, anodyne necklaces for pregnant women and teething children, Macassar oil (for the hair), and the metallic or magnetic tractors patented by Elisha Perkins of Connecticut in 1798. These were compass-like affairs, with one blunt-pointed and one sharp-pointed arm, made of combinations of copper, zinc, and gold, or iron, silver, and platinum. Cures were effected by stroking, and their principle of action was supposed to be analogous to that of galvanism or animal magnetism. Perkins's tractors had a remarkable vogue in England, were abundantly satirized in the colored prints and pamphlets like "A Terrible Tractoration," until John Haygarth, a Bath physician, showed that similar cures could be effected with wooden tractors, whence it was perceived that they were due to imagination. Electricity and animal magnetism were used as a special mode of appealing to the baser passions by James Graham of Edinburgh, who was the coryphæus of "celestial beds" for rejuvenating senility. Graham was a man of handsome physique, aquiline features, and pontifical manner, who had half studied medicine and picked up some knowledge of electricity from hearing about Franklin's experiments in America. His "Temple of Health," opened in London in 1780, consisted of a sumptuously appointed apartment, with all the implications and accessaries of a strictly Oriental interior, including mysterious perfumes, soft music, and bacchantic poses. The entrance fee was six guineas, and, in a plain-spoken lecture which "tickled the ears of the groundlings," immediate conception was guaranteed to the child-

less for a £50 banknote. The fraud did not last long, and when the
crash came, in 1782, Graham was driven to preach mud-baths
(fangotherapy), evincing his sincerity by remaining in them for
hours at a time each day. "Half knave, half enthusiast," as
Robert Southey called him, he did not profit by his hygienic
theories, and died at an early age. More respectable and hardly
to be classed among quacks, pure and simple, were the "Whitworth doctors," otherwise the Taylor brothers, two village farriers
who took up human ailments, buying Glauber's salts by the ton,
and dispensing it in proportion, bleeding the poor free of charge
on Sunday mornings, setting broken bones and treating cancers,
apparently with some show of success. Although the elder Taylor
cared more for horse-doctoring than for human patients, Whitworth was crowded with the visiting sick, who were treated strictly
as they came, without preference or deference for rank. Even
royalty had to taste the same rustic independence. The "Whitworth red bottle" and "Whitworth drops" were famous a century
ago. When John Hunter asked Taylor the composition of one of
his ointments, he replied, "No, Jack, that's not a fair question.
I'll send you as much of it as you like, but I won't tell you what it's
made of."[1]

Toward the close of the century, a Mr. and Mrs. Loutherbourg
acquired an enormous following by reviving the old method of
Valentine Greatrakes of curing disease by touch, in other words,
faith cure. They were besieged by great crowds of patients
whom they professed to treat gratis, declining to take any fee
whatever, but it was discovered that they were in collusion with
certain agents who sold their "free" tickets for whatever they
could get. Dr. Katterfelto, another sharp practitioner, traveled
about the north of England in a van drawn by six horses, containing a number of black cats and attended by many outriders in gay
liveries. Dr. Myersbach, in spite of Lettsom's opposition, continued to make a large income out of fashionable people. On
the continent, Villars had enormous success with a five-franc
nostrum of niter and water, and Ailhaud, whose powders are said
to have destroyed as many people as Napoleon's campaigns,
though he was put out of business by Tissot in his Avis au Peuple
(1803), had already attained to three baronies and was known as
the Baron de Castelet.[2]

---

[1] For further information about the English quacks of the eighteenth
century see the admirable quackery number of the British Medical Journal for
May 27, 1911 (vol. i, 1264–1274); Wootton's Chronicles of Pharmacy, London, 1910, vol. ii, 203–219, and the separate biographic notices in Leslie
Stephen.

[2] J. C. Jeaffreson: A Book about Doctors, New York, 1861, ch. vi, pp. 101–
114.

In Farquhar's Recruiting Officer (act iv, sc. 3), there is a scene in which Sergeant Kite whiles away his time by passing himself off as a conjurer. Assuming the power of prediction, he tells a butcher that, from his skill in swinging the cleaver, he will some day become surgeon general of the army. This was at the beginning of the century, and, only a little while before, the witty and dissolute Earl of Rochester is said to have diverted himself by hiring a stall on Tower Hill, where he practised as a quack doctor, delivering himself of truly Paracelsian tirades,[1] and selling cosmetics and remedies for female complaints. It is obvious that the great army of adventurers, card-sharpers, quacks, and other financial crooks who flourished in the eighteenth century succeeded, then as now, by the kind of assurance which the Germans call *imponiren*. They dared to be themselves with a vast amount of swagger and with the trait of clever brutality which is always an asset among rogues. Yet the same aplomb was noticeable in more honorable branches of activity, and, as Jeaffreson says, "the physician, the divine, the lawyer, the parliament-man, the country gentleman, the author by profession—all had peculiarities of style, costume, speech, or intonation, by which they were well pleased that they should be recognized . . . The barrister's smirk, the physician's unctuous smiles, the pedagogue's frown, did not originate in a mean desire to be taken for something of higher mark and esteem than they really were."[2] Indeed, Thomas Sergeant Perry maintains that the uneasy sense of inferiority and concern about the opinion of others which is snobbery first made its appearance in literature in the episode of Mrs. Tibbs in Goldsmith's "Citizen of the World" (1762).[3] The eighteenth century physician of better type was in position to make large sums of money without using his profession as a trade and enjoyed social and cultural advantages far above the average. Let us glance for a moment at some of the fashionable London practitioners of the period. In England, Garth was the idol of the Whigs, Arbuthnot, of the Tories. Sir Samuel **Garth** (1661–1719) was the only physician who belonged to the famous Kit-Kat Club, and, while making a name for himself in literature and taking an occasional hand in politics, had no mean success as a practitioner. John **Arbuthnot** (*"Martinus Scriblerus"*) (1667–1735), the author of "The History of John Bull," was the friend and familiar of Pope and Swift and eventually became physi-

---

[1] For an amusing speech by Rochester, see Wootton's Chronicles of Pharmacy, London, 1910, ii, 204–205.

[2] Jeaffreson: Op. cit., 83.

[3] T. S. Perry: The Evolution of the Snob, Boston, 1887, pp. 57–60.

21

cian to Queen Anne. Sir Richard **Blackmore** (–1729), although a total failure as a poet, was accounted one of the most
successful men in the medical profession, the oracle of the wealthy,
whom he emulated in "style." Sir Hans **Sloane** (1660–1753),
the first physician to be made a baronet, enjoyed the highest
scientific and professional reputation, was a founder and later
secretary and president of the Royal Society, and his museum and
library, after his death, became the nucleus of the present British
Museum collections. John **Radcliffe** (1690–1729), although of
humble origin, was appointed physician to Princess Anne of Denmark, which position he lost through his arrogant demeanor.
He had financial luck from the start, commencing practice about
the time that Richard Lower was losing ground, and was making
more than twenty guineas a day at the end of his first year. He
was a Jacobite, and, says Jeaffreson, "contrived by his shrewd
humor, arrogant simplicity, and immeasurable insolence to hold
both Whigs and Tories in his grasp. The two factions of the
aristocracy bowed before him." His disposition was somewhat
soured by the fact that he had been once jilted and once rejected
in a proposal of marriage, yet, though he pretended to be miserly,
he was frequently generous with his money . After liberally providing for his relatives in his will, he left funds to Oxford for the
present foundations known as the Radcliffe Library, the Radcliffe
Infirmary, and the Radcliffe Observatory. Toward the close of
his life, he took a fancy to young Richard **Mead** (1673–1754),
who flattered his vanity and so inherited his practice. "Mead,
I love you," said Radcliffe, "and I'll tell you a sure secret to make
you a fortune—use all mankind ill." Mead was a complete contrast to his predecessor—a scholar where Radcliffe was ignorant
of books, courtly and polished where Radcliffe was crude and overbearing. "Dr. Mead," said Dr. Johnson, "lived more in the broad
sunshine of life than almost any man." Through Radcliffe's
influence, he was summoned to the death-bed of Queen Anne, and
he became the most prosperous practitioner of his time, making
in one year as much as £7,000. Upon moving into Radcliffe's
house in Bloomsbury Square, he inherited the latter's famous gold-
headed cane, which passed successively through the hands of
Askew, Pitcairn, and Baillie, and is now in the Library of the Royal
College of Physicians. Mead afterward moved into a handsome
establishment in Ormond Street and lived to be eighty-one.
After him came such men as Heberden, Lettsom, Fothergill,
Parry, and the Hunters. On the continent we find Werlhof,
court physician at Hannover, and, after the battle of Dettingen
(June 27, 1743), physician in ordinary to George II. He was suc-
ceeded by Zimmermann and Wichmann, who, says Baas, flourished

a barber's bowl before he entered the gymnasium. In Leyden, Boerhaave was preëminent; in Halle, Stahl and Hoffmann; in Berlin, Heim; in Jena, Hufeland; in Vienna, Van Swieten and de Haën; in Paris, Théophile de Bordeu; in Modena, Torti; in Geneva, Tronchin; and in Laussanne, Tissot. All these physicians were fortunate above the average, and one characteristic seems common to most of them. As they were not specially exposed to commercial competition and the petty human traits it brings forth, they could afford to be charitable in the best sense. No other single group of physicians was probably so generous to the poor. Take, for example, this little note which Garth scribbled to Sir Hans Sloane:

"Dear Sir Hans:
"If you can recommend this miserable slut to be fluxed, you'll do an act of charity for, dear sir,
"Your obed[t] ser[t]
"S[l] Garth."

or this of John Hunter to his brother William:

"Dear Brother:
"The bearer is very desirous of having your opinion. I do not know his case. He has no money, and you don't want any, so that you are well met.
"Ever yours,
"John Hunter."

Rough kindness this, yet it shows a degree of fraternal confidence between physicians which seldom exists today, and toward the humble poor the sentiment of Empedocles:

"Thou art my friend, to thee
All knowledge that I have,
All skill I wield are free."

That this sentiment was reciprocated by the mass of mankind we need no better evidence than the experience of Jenner, or the extraordinary popularity of such books as Tissot's *Avis au Peuple* or Hufeland's *Makrobiotik*.

Another side-light on the social status of eighteenth century physicians is afforded by the incomes they made and the **fees** some of them received. Mead commonly charged a guinea as an office fee, two guineas or more for a visit to patients in good standing, and, like Radcliffe, he wrote half-guinea prescriptions for the apothecaries while sitting in his coffee-house, without seeing the patient. His average income was between £5000 and £6000 per annum, which had a purchasing power of over three times its value in modern money. Later on, we find Fothergill making £5000 a year and Lettsom £12,-000. Baas considers 3000 to 4000 marks ($2250 to $3000 in present value) as a mediocre eighteenth century income in a city of size, and he states that, in 1782, Heim, in Berlin, got 4200 marks from 784 patients, 6600 marks from 393 patients in 1784, 26,400 marks from 1000 patients in 1790, and by 1805, his annual income had gone up to 36,000 marks. Orräus, in Moscow, was making 90,000 marks in a short time.[1] The phenomenal fee of the period was that acquired by

---

[1] Baas: Op. cit., pp. 745, 751, 763.

Thomas Dimsdale for inoculating Catherine of Russia and her son, viz., $50,-
000, with $10,000 additional for traveling expenses, a pension of $2500 for
life, and the rank of baron of the empire.   Quarin got a pension of $10,000 per
annum and was made a baron for his consultation with Joseph II.   University
professors were also well paid.   Baas assumes an average salary of 3000–7500
marks for the North German universities, but points out that the cost of comfortable living was about 6000 marks annually in Hannover and 7500 in Berlin.
De Haen got 10,000 and Johann Peter Frank 9000 marks in Vienna, Morgagni
about $4500 in Padua.   Frank got 342 marks as court physician at Baden,
1370 marks and many perquisites as physician in ordinary to the Bishop of
Speyer, and 9600 marks as imperial physician in Russia.

Three new editions of the London Pharmacopœia were issued during the
eighteenth century, each of them characterized by changes which show the
status of **therapeutics** and the gradual advance of pharmacology.[1]   The
fourth Pharmacopœia (1721), edited by Sir Hans Sloane, drops many of the
old syrups and waters, but retains theriac, the extracts of excreta and other
animal products, and introduces stramonium, gamboge, Secale cornutum,
senega, ipecac, tartar emetic, lunar caustic, lime-water, Ethiops mineral, spirit
of sal volatile, iron sulphate, tincture of perchloride of iron, and other inorganic
preparations.   The fifth London Pharmacopœia (1746), revised by Mead, Heberden, Freind, and others, professes to condemn the old astrological and folk
remedies, and while it drops human fat, spider-webs, moss from human skulls,
unicorn's horn, virgin's milk, bones from the stag's heart, and the like, still
retains mithridate, theriac, crabs' eyes, wood-lice, pearls, bezoars, vipers,
coral, etc.   Syrups and medicated waters diminish in number, but there are
many new tinctures, including those of valerian and cardamoms.   Glauber's salts, sweet spirits of niter, syrup of squills, liquor potassæ, and potassium
acetate are added.   One year before this pharmacopœia was printed, William
Heberden published his famous essay, "Antitheriaka" (1745), in which he
showed that the belief in the efficacy of theriac and mithridate was based upon
a tissue of absurdities, since the actual formula for theriac found in the cabinet
of Mithridates after his death called for 20 leaves of rue, 1 grain of salt, 2 nuts,
and 2 dried figs, a striking contrast to the long-winded recipes for its composition which had been imagined by later authorities.   Heberden successfully
ridiculed these nostrums out of existence, but it was too late to make any
changes in the Pharmacopœia of 1746.   The effect of his destructive criticism appears to advantage in the sixth Pharmacopœia (1788), in which practically all the animal materia medica has disappeared, along with theriac and
mithridate; while among the new drugs and compounds added are aconite,
arnica, castor oil, colombo, cascarilla, kino, quassia, magnesia, senega, sima-
ruba, ether, tartrate of iron, oxide of zinc, Dover's powder, Hoffmann's anodyne, Huxham's tincture, James' powder, spiritus Mindereri, sarsaparilla de-
coctions, compound tincture of benzoin, extract of chamomile, tincture of
opium, and "tinctura opii camphorata" (paregoric).   Of these, kino and cate-
chu were introduced by Fothergill, colombo by Gaub, quassia by Daniel Ro-
lander, senega by John Tennent of Virginia.   Dover's powder was introduced by
the famous buccaneer physician, Thomas Dover (1660–1742), who was once
in residence with Sydenham, and, in 1709, rescued Alexander Selkirk (Robinson Crusoe) from the island of Juan Fernandes.   Dover's formula for his "dia-
phoretic powder" is given in his "Ancient Physician's Legacy to His Country"
(1732).   Digitalis was introduced by William Withering in 1785, but did not
appear in the London Pharmacopœia until 1809.   Stoerck of Vienna made
careful studies of conium, stramonium, hyoscyamus, colchicum, pulsatilla,
clematis, and recommended their use (1760).   Thomas Fowler introduced his
solution of arsenic in 1706.   Compound licorice powder was the invention of
E. G. Kurella of Berlin, and first appeared in the Prussian pharmacopœia in
1799.   In 1724, Friedrich Hoffmann discovered a mineral spring at Seidlitz,
Bohemia, which owed its medicinal properties to a combination of magnesium
and sodium sulphates; but of "Seidlitz powders" only the name remains attached

---

[1] Wootton: Op. cit., ii, pp. 65–67.

to the present formula, which was patented by the Bond Street chemist Savory in 1815. Many physicians of the eighteenth century, including Hoffmann, Stahl, Sloane, and Mead, made money by selling preparations with secret formulas, and a token of the popular faith in drugs was the large-sized medicine spoon which often formed part of a bride's dowry. In this period, both physicians and surgeons compounded and dispensed their own remedies, and, as the practitioners themselves were usually "family doctors," their incidental charges were made for their prescriptions and not for their visits. This largely accounts for the terribly long-winded prescriptions which abound in the eighteenth century, and, as Billings remarks, the surgeons "kept on prescribing and using their oils, ointments, plasters, vulnerary drinks, etc.," for similar reasons.[1]

Except in France, the status of **surgery,** during the greater part of the eighteenth century, was exceedingly low. The French surgeon owed the improvement in his social condition to the fistula of Louis XIV and its successful treatment by Félix, which made the latter, and his successor, Mareschal, royal surgeons. In 1724, Mareschal obtained from Louis XV the creation of five chairs of surgical instruction at St. Côme. The Paris Faculty immediately went into revolt and, in spite of the king's order, made a public demonstration against St. Côme.[2] Decked out in their scholastic robes, the physicians, headed by the dean of the Faculty, preceded by a beadle and an usher, marched to St. Côme in solemn array, in spite of the bitter cold weather, the snow and sharp sleet, which made their red robes almost unrecognizable. Cheering one another on with cries and oaths and followed by a great crowd of people, they at length ranged themselves in a long line against the wall, while the dean presented himself at the door of the College accompanied by the only anatomist of the Faculty, who stood behind him holding a skeleton. Cries and imprecations, knocks, and threats to break down the door, were only greeted by the jeers of the students from within, and, when an usher tried to make himself heard in the matter of what the surgeons owed to the physicians, the people suddenly turned against these formalities, which they had once respected like a religion, and drove the doctors away without regard for their furs and costly raiment. Two steps more put the surgeons on a social and scientific level with the doctors, viz., the foundation of the Academy of Surgery, the first session of which was held in 1731, and the ordinance of Louis XV (1743), delivering the surgeons from further association with barbers and wig-makers, who were forbidden to practise, and declaring that no one could be a master in surgery without being a master of the arts. This was the French surgeon's declaration of independence. Henceforth, he was a

---

[1] J. S. Billings: The History and Literature of Surgery (in Dennis's "System"), New York, 1895, i, 70.

[2] E. Forgue: Montpellier méd., 1911, xxxiii, 10, 11.

lettered man, prepared for his life-work by a special scientific education. The King was inspired to make this wise move by La Peyronie, the eminent Montpellier surgeon, who, with Mareschal, had founded the Academy of Surgery and, in fact, devoted his entire fortune to the advancement of his beloved art. In addition to Mareschal's five surgical professorships of 1724, La Peyronie founded a sixth at his own expense, with an assistant to each professor, and also obtained four chairs of surgery for Montpellier, laying upon each incumbent the obligation of lecturing on obstetrics to both surgeons and midwives. In his will, he left a legacy of annual prizes in surgery, his two houses in the Grande Rue, and 100,000 francs to build the amphitheater of St. Côme, now the Bourse and the Chamber of Commerce. It was due to La Peyronie that Paris became the surgical center of the world in the eighteenth century. During the French Revolution, the 18 medical faculties and 15 medical colleges of France were abolished by vote in 1792, and along with them the Société royale de médecine (founded 1776) and the Académie de chirurgie (1731). This was modified in 1794, by the creation of Écoles de santé, the title of "health officer" (officier de santé) being substituted for that of "doctor." All distinction between physicians and surgeons as separate guilds or cliques was broken down, and practice was thrown open to everybody who could pay for a license. Hospital internes, externes, physicians, and "ordinary professors" were appointed by competitive trials (concours), and medical societies became "Sociétés libres de médecine." The Écoles de santé were created to supply the urgent need for military surgeons for the armies of the Republic, and the schools at Paris, Montpellier, and Strassburg were, in reality, schools of military medicine. It was soon found that this chaotic scheme was fatal to further progress, and with the reëstablishment of the Empire, the medical and surgical faculties were restored (1803–4), with the revival of examinations and diplomas. The concours were finally abolished by the Bourbons after 1821.[1]

In eighteenth century England, there were no surgeons of first rank before the time of Pott and Cheselden, Hunter and Abernethy. In 1745, through the good offices of Mr. Ranby, serjeant surgeon to the king, the surgeons were formally separated from the barbers as the "Masters, Governors, and Commonalty of the Art and the Science of Surgeons of London," and it was declared to be a penal offense for any one to practise surgery in London or within a radius of seven miles from it, without being duly examined and licensed by ten of their number. In getting rid of the barbers, the surgeons

---

[1] Baas: Op. cit., pp. 749, 760, 774. For a specimen "examination" of 1803, with the illiterate answers given, see, E. Wickersheimer: Paris méd., 1912–13. suppl., 749.

left them the hall, library, and plate, only appropriating to themselves the Arris and Gale endowments. By 1790, the company of surgeons had a local habitation, but Mr. Gunning, the master, reminded them that "Your theater is without lectures, your library room, without books, is converted into an office for your clerk, and your committee room is become his parlor."[1] In 1800, the Corporation of Surgeons was rechartered by George III as the present Royal College of Surgeons of London. Cheselden began to lecture at St. Thomas's Hospital about 1720, Pott at St. Bartholomew's in 1763, and there had been some haphazard lecturing on anatomy in the latter institution from the year 1734 on. The London Hospital began to take in students in 1742, and was fully organized in 1785. When Guy's Hospital was opened to students in 1769, it was agreed that all surgeons of the hospital should lecture on their subject now and then. Surgical teaching in Edinburgh began vaguely with the Monro dynasty, whose whole concern was anatomy. The only Edinburgh surgeons of prominence were Benjamin and John Bell. The latter's unfortunate passion for controversy kept him out of the Royal Infirmary and thus deprived students of the only surgeon who could have taught them properly. In Ireland, the guild of barbers chartered by Henry VI in 1446 was combined with the surgeons by the charters of Elizabeth (1572) and James II (1687), but they began to break asunder in 1745, and in 1784 the surgeons were given their own autonomy through the creation of the Royal College of Surgeons in Ireland. Through a bequest of Sir Patrick Dun, president of the College of Physicians in Ireland, medical and surgical teaching was begun in Dublin in 1744.

In Germany, there was little advancement of the surgeons' status before the time of Frederick the Great. Heister's illustrated treatise, printed in the vernacular (1743), was, it is true, the most popular surgical work in the eighteenth century, but Haller lectured and wrote on the subject without having performed an operation in his life, and there was no adequate teaching until Richter began to lecture at Göttingen in 1766 and von Siebold at Würzburg in 1769. Surgical practice was mainly in the hands of the barber, the executioner and the strolling bone-setters, cataract-couchers, herniotomists and lithotomists, of whom the famous Dr. Eysenbarth was the type. In Goethe's Autobiography, the barber who shaved his father is styled "der gute Chirurgus." Even Theden, Surgeon General of the Prussian Army, was once a barber. The barber's apprentice was usually an illiterate lad, practically a servant in the household, advertised for as a bond slave if he ran away. Superstitious belief in charms and magic prevailed, and the

---

[1] Cited by Billings, op. cit., p. 83.

executioner was believed to have a compact with the devil, power to deal with diseases caused by witchcraft, and, from his occasional duty of breaking bones upon the wheel, he was credited with a special talent for setting fractures and dislocations. Even Frederick the Great, in 1744, allowed the Prussian executioners to treat wounds, ulcers, and fractures on the ground that, if competent, they were better for the uncared masses than bungling surgeons or no surgeons at all. Judicial torture was, in fact, still very common in the eighteenth century, and approved of, for instance, by Maria Theresa.[1] Indeed, owing to the great need for competent surgeons in the Prussian army, the Theatrum Anatomicum at Berlin (founded in 1713) was expanded in 1724 to include a Collegium medico-chirurgicum, and the Charité Hospital at Berlin was founded, in 1727, by Friedrich Wilhelm I to furnish clinical instruction to the students at the Collegium. But Frederick the Great, in his Silesian campaigns, still found his army sadly deficient in surgeons, and not only sent medical cadets to Paris and Strassburg to complete their surgical education, but, in 1743, engaged 12 French surgeons, with assistants, to look after his troops. The Prussian army surgeon of the day was ranked above a drummer and beneath a chaplain. Being a barber's apprentice, he had to shave the officers, and if he proved delinquent in line of duty, he could be beaten with sticks at their instance. The general ignorance and incompetence of these army surgeons gave so much dissatisfaction that, in 1785, under Surgeon General Görcke, the Collegium Medico-Chirurgicum was converted into a Medico-Chirurgical Pepinière, devoted exclusively to the education of army surgeons and retaining its connection with the Charité. This institution was also known as the Friedrich-Wilhelms Institut and, since 1895, has been called the Kaiser-Wilhelms Akademie. The leading Prussian army surgeons of this period were Holtzendorf, the first surgeon general (1716); Schmucker, who left some valuable collections of surgical cases (1774–82); Bilguer, who filed the first brief for a conservative attitude toward amputation (1761); Theden, who was an early advocate of methodical bandaging, and Görcke, who reorganized the Prussian army medical department. In October, 1810, the University of Berlin was opened with such men as Hufeland, Reil, Ernst Horn, Rudolphi, and the elder

---

[1] Her codification of laws, the Constitutio criminalis Theresiana (1768), was as iron-clad in this respect as the earlier code of torture of Guazzini (1612), and while the practice was abolished by Frederick in Prussia in 1740–54, and in Saxony in 1770, it was not until 1776 that Maria Theresa consented to do away with it. Austria owes this advance to the humanitarian writings and efforts of Ferdinand von Leber and Joseph von Sonnenfels. See Max Neuburger: Wien. klin. Wochenschr., 1909, xxii, 1075–1078, and H. Schneickert: Arch. f. Krim.-Anthrop., Leipzig, 1907, xxvii, 341–345.

Graefe in the medical faculty, and here many of the young army surgeons of the Pepinière, including Helmholtz, were educated. In 1748, a similar Collegium medico-chirurgicum was established at Dresden, and in 1785, under Joseph II, the Medico-Chirurgical Academy or Josephinum was founded at Vienna, in charge of Brambilla, for instruction in military medicine, with permanent military hospitals at Prague, Budapest, Brünn, and other cities. The pupils at the Josephinum, like those in Berlin, were usually barbers or sons of poor officials, but these institutions undoubtedly did most to elevate the status of surgery in Prussia, Saxony, and Austria. In Russia, Peter the Great, who visited Boerhaave and Ruysch, tried to nationalize medicine, and to this end built the first hospital and medical school in Russia (copied from the Greenwich Hospital) in 1707. Being of wood, this structure was often burned down and as often rebuilt, in spite of the grumbling of the ecclesiastics who "had to find the funds." There were 50 pupils in 1712, but the constant disputes between Synod and Senate about finances led to the neglect of the hospital, and it gradually fell into ruins. In 1754, under Elizabeth, it passed into the hands of the Military Collegium, the War Department of the period. The students were clad in a caftan or long cloak, a camisole, and breeches. There were much brawling and drunkenness among them, they were often subjected to imprisonment or beating with the knout, and from various side-lights upon this period in literature and painting, some of them may have answered to the thumbnail sketch of the Russian poet:

> "Buried in his cravat, his coat reaching down to his heels,
> Heavily mustached, with a dull look and a falsetto voice."

Peter the Great opened the St. Petersburg Admiralty Hospital in 1716, and, in 1717, the Dry Land Hospital, which was rebuilt in 1733. In 1799, the Russian Army Medical Academy was founded, and the ancient hospital and medical school became the purely military institution which it is today. In 1763, the seventeenth century Apeteka became a Collegium medicum under an "Archiater," the first of these being a Scotchman, Robert Erskine, who was also "Leib-medik" of Peter the Great. A prominent feature of the bureaucratic machinery founded by the latter was the institution of the "tchins" in 1722, consisting of a series of grades of nobility conferred upon the *tchinovniks* or public servants, a very complicated scheme of degrees of gentility and precedence. Under this system, still in vogue, medical men may rise to almost any rank.[1]

---

[1] Lancet, London, 1897, ii, 354–361.

The principal advances made in **medical education** in the eighteenth century were in anatomy and clinical medicine. Before the time of John Hunter, surgery was well taught only at Paris; before the time of the Monros, anatomy flourished principally on the continent. Berlin and Strassburg seem to have had the best opportunities for obtaining material for dissection. A Theatrum anatomicum was founded at Berlin in 1713, was specially favored by medical legislation, and, by 1786, was supplied with some 200 dead bodies of suicides and work-house paupers. It was much frequented by foreigners. In Strassburg, under Salzmann, there were daily dissections and thrice weekly demonstrations as early as 1708, and he is said to have had 30 cadavers in 1725, and 60 in 1760, affording opportunities even for surgical work on the cadaver. At Tübingen, however, Haller, the student, did most of his dissecting on dogs, and, in Paris, he had to flee for his life for body-snatching. At Leyden, Albinus got only one cadaver a year and Friedrich Hoffmann, at Halle, only twenty bodies in twenty-four years. In Prague, there were only three dissections during the period 1692–1712; in Vienna, there was hardly a dissection as late as 1741, although an anatomic theater had been opened in 1718. In Great Britain, chairs of anatomy were established at Edinburgh (1705), Cambridge (1707), Glasgow (1718), Oxford ("lecturer on anatomy," 1750), Dublin (1785), and the four cadavers allotted to the Company of Surgeons (1540) and the College of Physicians (1565) had been increased by Charles II to six. The first professor of the subject was Robert Elliot, who assumed his Edinburgh chair in 1705, at an annual salary of £15, and resigned in favor of Monro *primus* in 1720. Yet, even under the Monro dynasty, instruction was very rudimentary, the whole demonstration being done upon a single cadaver, while the vessels and nerves were studied in a fetus and surgical operations taught upon a dog. John Bell,[1] in his reply to Gregory's diatribes, gives some grim details of bungling, incompetent surgery as a result of anatomical ignorance. In one operation for stone (1808), the patient was kept in intense suffering for over thirty minutes, and, even then, the stone could not be extracted, although the normal time limit for a lithotomy in those pre-anesthetic days was about five minutes, and Cheselden usually did it in three. In Italy, before the time of Scarpa, Fontana's wax preparations[2] were used in lieu of cadavers for teaching purposes, and in Spain, until the middle of the century, there was no anatomic teaching at all.

With such a great leader as Linnæus, it was natural that botany should have been extensively cultivated in this period. In England, Fothergill, Cruikshank, and others had private botanical gardens of their own. Kew Gardens was established about 1730, and a Physic Garden was added to it in 1759; other gardens were established at Madrid (1763) and Coimbra (1773), and the garden of the Royal Dublin Society at Glasnevin was opened about 1796. It is said that there were about 1600 botanic gardens in Europe at the end of the eighteenth century. The interest in botany in the New World is sufficiently evidenced by the generic names Claytonia, Coldenia, Kuhnia, Gardenia, Mitchella, Bigelowia, Marshallia, Bartonia, etc., which were bestowed upon colonial

---

[1] John Bell: Letters on Professional Character and Manners, Edinburgh, 1810, pp. 590–592.

[2] The Museum of the Abbé Felice Fontana (1730–1803) was the most famous anatomical collection of its kind in the eighteenth century, containing over 1500 preparations in wax. These still exist, "beautiful to look at, but inaccurate and of little scientific value" (J. S. Billings).

plants by Linnæus and others in honor of American botanists (H. A. Kelly).[1]

Except at Leyden, there was no **clinical instruction** until 1745, when an ambulatory clinic was established at |Prague, which lasted about one year. In 1745, van Swieten organized a clinic at Vienna, consisting of twelve beds at the Bürgerspital, in charge of de Haën, who published clinical reports of the work. The example was followed by Borsieri de Kanilfeld at Pavia in 1770, at Prague under von Plenciz in 1781, at Göttingen under Frank in 1784, at Jena under Hufeland about 1793. Bedside instruction was introduced into France by Desbois de Rochefort in 1780. In England, chairs of clinical medicine were established at Edinburgh in 1741, at Oxford in 1780, and, about 1757, Cullen began to lecture on medicine in English instead of Latin. The English physician, no doubt, got a great deal of his early clinical knowledge from his association with a patron or preceptor, as we have seen in the case of Mead, who inherited his practice from Radcliffe. The special feature of modern English clinical instruction, the hospital medical school, had its beginnings in such institutions as Guy's Hospital (1723), the Edinburgh Hospital (1736), or the Meath Hospital (Dublin, 1756), and attained a definite status at the London Hospital Medical School (1785), and at St. Bartholomew's under Abernethy (1790). Private instruction, such as that of Smellie in obstetrics, Cullen in internal medicine, Black in chemistry, or the Hunters in anatomy, surgery, and obstetrics, was the feature of the period. The private medical school of Sir William Blizard and Maclaurin became, in 1785, the London Hospital Medical School. Private instruction in midwifery was first given by Grégoire, Sr., in Paris in 1720, but, in 1797, there was a school for midwives at the Maternité under Baudelocque. Obstetric instruction was first given at Strassburg in 1728, followed by a school for midwives in 1737, and at Vienna in 1748. The first German institution for the instruction of male obstetricians was founded under Röderer at Göttingen in 1751, to be followed by schools for midwives and obstetricians at Berlin (1751), at Tübingen (1759), at Bern, under Venel (1782), at Cassel about 1760, at Jena (1788), at Marburg (1790), and at Würzburg under von Siebold (1778–99). In Edinburgh, instruction for midwives was given by Joseph Gibson in 1726, in England by John Maubray (1724) and Richard Manningham (1736), in Dublin by John Mosse (1746), and, his successor, Sir Fielding Ould (1759). Mosse's private lying-in hospital at Dublin, enlarged by Ould, became the Rotunda Lying-in Hospital in 1745. Chairs of midwifery were established at Edinburgh (1739), at Dublin (1743), and at Glasgow (1815). The British Lying-in Hospital was founded in 1749, the City of London Lying-in Hospital in 1750, the Queen Charlotte Hospital in 1752, and an obstetric polyclinic was opened at Meath Hospital (Dublin) by Fleury in 1763. In Italy, schools for midwives were opened at Piedmont (1728), Padua (1769), and Rome (1786).

Many new **hospitals** were built in the eighteenth century, but, in respect of cleanliness and administration, these institutions sank to the lowest level known in the history of medicine. The principal London hospitals were the Westminster (1719), Guy's (1725), St. George's (1733), the London (1740), the Middlesex (1745), and the Small-pox Hospital (1746), and there were provincial hospitals at York (1710), Salisbury (1716), Cambridge (1719), Bristol (1735), Windsor (1736), Northampton (1743), Exeter (1745), Worcester (1745), Newcastle (1751), Manchester (1753), Chester (1755), Leeds (1767), Stafford (1769), Oxford (1770), Leicester (1771), Norwich (1771), Birmingham (1778), Nottingham (1782), Canterbury (1793), and Stafford (1797). In Scotland hospitals were founded at Edinburgh (1736), Aberdeen (1739), Dumfries (1775), Montrose (1780), Glasgow (1794), and Dundee (1795); in Ireland, at Cork (1720–22), Limerick (1759), and Belfast (1797), while the earliest of the Dublin hospitals were the Jervis Street (1726), Steevens's (1733), Mercer's (1734), and the Meath Hospital (1756). The Charité at Berlin (1710), the Albergo dei poveri at Naples (1751), the Allgemeines Krankenhaus at Vienna

---

[1] H. A. Kelly: Jour. Am. Med. Ass., Chicago, 1911, lviii, 437–441.

(1784), the Necker (1779), Cochin (1780), Beaujon (1785), and St. Antoine (1795) at Paris were among the larger hospitals founded on the continent. To Catherine II, Moscow owed the Catherine, Pavlovski, and Golitzin Hospitals, an insane asylum and a foundling asylum (1764); St. Petersburg the Obuk- hovski Hospital (1784), a Foundling Hospital (1770), and a "Secret Hospital" for venereal diseases (1763), the linen of which was marked "Discretion."

In 1788, J.-R. Tenon published a series of memoirs on the hospitals of Paris,[1] containing his famous description of the old Hôtel Dieu, which was at that time a veritable hot-bed of disease. There were some 1220 beds, the most of which contained from four to six patients, and about 486 beds for single patients. The larger halls contained over 800 patients crowded on pallets, or often lying about miserably on heaps of straw, which was in vile condition. Acute contagious diseases were often in close rela- tion to mild cases, vermin and filth abounded, and the ventilation was often so abominable that the attendants and inspectors would not enter in the morning without a sponge dipped in vinegar held to their faces. Septic fevers and other contagia were the rule; the average mortality was about 20 per cent., and recovery from surgical operations was, in the nature of things, a rarity. The same thing was true of the Allgemeines Krankenhaus of Vienna, the Moscow Hospital, and many other institutions of size, and it was not until John Howard had made his exhaustive studies of the condition of European hospitals, prisons and lazarettos (1777–89), and Tenon had published his report, that any attempts at reforms were made. Baas says that, in Frankfurt am Main and other cities, "even physicians declined hospital service as equivalent to a sen- tence of death." Under Louis XVI and Joseph II, reforms were finally made in Paris and Vienna, with a very creditable and sig- nificant reduction of mortality. When the Czar Paul came to the throne, he was so horrified with the condition of the Moscow Hos- pital that he ordered its reconstruction in 1797, with the result that the new Moscow Hospital, with accommodations for 1280 patients, was completed in 1802. But hospitals remained no- torious for uncleanliness and general danger to life well into the nineteenth century, and many persons alive today can recall the horror in which they were held. The real angel of purity and cleanliness was Florence Nightingale, and there was no such thing as surgical cleanliness before the time of Lister.

Bad as was the management of hospitals, the **treatment of the insane** was even worse. They were either chained or caged when housed, or, if harmless, were allowed to run at large, the Tom o' Bedlams of England or the wizards and warlocks of Scotland (Lochiel in Campbell's poem). The earliest insane asylums in the

---

[1] Tenon: Mémoires sur les hôpitaux de Paris, Paris, 1788.

northern countries were St. Luke's in London (1751), the Quaker Asylum near York (1792), and the *Narrenthurm*, or "Lunatics' Tower" (1784), one of the show places of old Vienna, where, as in ancient Bedlam, the public were allowed to view the insane, like animals in a menagerie, on payment of a small fee. The latter institution was described by Richard Bright in 1815 as a fanciful, four-story edifice having the external appearance of a large round tower, but, on the inside, consisting of a hollow circle in the center of which a quadrangular building arose, joined to the circle by each of its corners. The inclosed structure afforded residence for the keepers and surgeons. The circular part contained three hundred patients, "whose condition," says Bright, "is far from being as comfortable as in many of the establishments for the insane which I have visited."[1] Mönkemöller's researches on German psychiatry in the eighteenth century, based on the records of an asylum at Celle,[2] go to show that the theoretical part of the science in this period was nebulous philosophic speculation, insanity being still attributed to yellow and black bile or to heat in the dog days, while symptoms like exaggerated self-esteem, jealousy, envy, sloth, self-abuse, etc., were regarded as causes. The cases treated were all of the dangerous, unmanageable, or suicidal type, and no hope of recovery was held out. There was an extensive exhibition of drugs and unconditional belief in their efficacy. A case that did not react to drugs was regarded as hopeless. Melancholia was treated by opium pills, excited states by camphor, pruritus by diaphoresis, and a mysterious power was ascribed to belladonna: if it failed, everything failed. Other remedies were a mixture of honey and vinegar, a decoction of "Quadenwurzel," large doses of lukewarm water, or, if this failed, "that panacea of psychiatry, tartarus tartarisatus." The costly aqua benedicta Rolandi, with three stout ruffians to administer it, a mustard plaster on the head, venesection at the forehead and both thumbs, clysters, and plasters of Spanish fly, were other resources. Barbarities were kept in the background, but the harsh methods of medieval times were none the less prevalent. A melancholic woman was treated with a volley of oaths and a douche of cold water as she lay in bed. If purgatives and emetics failed with violent patients, they came in for many hard knocks, with a régime of bolts and chains to inspire fear. A sensitive, self-conscious patient was confined in a cold, damp, gloomy, mephitic cell, fed on perpetual hard bread, and otherwise treated as a

[1] Bright: Travels . . . through Lower Hungary, Edinburgh, 1818, 87, 88.

[2] Mönkemöller: Psychiat.-neurol. Wochenschr., Halle, 1911–12, xiii, 211; 220; 232.

criminal. The diet—soup, warm beer, a few vegetables and salad —was of the cheapest. There were some attempts at open-door treatment, such as putting the patients to mind geese, sending them to the mineral baths at Meyenburg and Pyrmont, or sending them as harvest hands to Holland (*Hollandgeherei*). Marriage was also recommended as a cure.

The Quaker retreat, founded by the Tukes in 1792 at York, England, was the first attempt at humane treatment of the insane before the time of Pinel.

Outbreaks of **epidemic diseases** were more scattered and isolated than in former centuries. Malarial fever, influenza and scarlatina were often pandemic; small-pox, diphtheria, and whooping-cough were widely diffused, but plague, syphilis, ergotism were far less malignant, and with the return of Halley's comet in 1758, people began to get rid of various superstitious theories in regard to the origin of epidemic diseases. During 1702–05, southern Italy was visited by a series of earthquakes (described by Baglivi) which destroyed some 20,000 lives, and the winter of the year 1708–09 was beset with such intense cold that even Venice was icebound. Lancisi said that this winter was as fatal to life as the pest, and the general destruction of vegetation and consequent shortening of the food-supply brought on famine, diseases of cattle, and ergotism. Inundations and fluctuations of heat and cold were followed by epidemics of malarial and typhus fevers in the first quarter of the century, and during 1720–50 these gave place to diphtheria and the exanthemata. At the beginning of the century, the principal focus of the plague was in Turkey and the Danube region; by 1703, it was devastating the Ukraine, whence, through the war of Charles XII with Russia, it gradually spread to the Baltic Sea and the Scandinavian countries. Danzig sustained a mortality of 32,599 from January 5, to December 7, 1709, and Prussia and Lithuania lost 283,733 during 1709–10. The epidemic suddenly disappeared after a hurricane which swept over all Europe on February 27, 1714; but it was again introduced, this time in the south of France, devastating Provence during 1720–22. It was again prevalent along the Danube and in the Ukraine (1734), and, in 1743, cost Messina (Sicily) 30,000 lives. The most severe epidemic was that at Moscow in 1770–71, in which the total mortality was 52,000 out of a population of 230,000. This epidemic was checked through the prophylactic measures of Orräus, but matters were further complicated by the outbreak of a revolution. Typhus or camp fever was, of course, especially prevalent during all the wars of the century, in particular the long contest between Frederick the Great and Maria Theresa (1740–48), the Seven Years' War (1756–63), and the French Revolution (1789–99), with the events preceding it. One Prussian outbreak of typhus (1757) was described by the statistician Süssmilch, who was one of Frederick's army chaplains. Typhus was particularly fatal at Prague (1742), around Mainz (1760), and, as "famine fever," in Ireland (1740), where a failure of the potato crop cost 80,000 lives, in Saxony (1778), and Italy (1783). Malarial fever and dysentery also played havoc in camps and were clearly defined and distinguished in the careful observations of Pringle. Typhus and typhoid fevers were, of course, confused, and were variously termed "putrid," "gastric," or "nervous." Baglivi described typhoid as "mesenteric fever"; Huxham, during the Plymouth epidemic of 1737, clearly distinguished between "putrid" (*febris putrida*) or typhus, and "slow nervous fever" (*febris nervosa lenta*) or typhoid fever. During the heavy epidemic of typhoid fever at Göttingen in 1757–63, a careful account of the disease was published, in 1762, by Johann Georg Roederer, professor at the Göttingen clinic, and his assistant Wagler, who made autopsies of the cases. The intestinal lesions were carefully noted, but the authors regarded the disease as identical with intermittent fever and dysentery. Perhaps for this very reason the classic monograph was soon forgotten, although Cotugno is said to have made similar postmortem observations in Italy. The old theory of epidemic constitutions was still in the ascendant, and Stoll of Vienna thought that the diseases of "bilious" type, which had been prevalent since 1760, began to take on a "putrid" character about 1779–82, a view which won much consideration in Germany and Italy. Malarial fever was spread by inundations, pollution of streams, and the unsanitary condition of streets and sewers. Dysentery was widely prevalent on the continent throughout the century, and a classic description of the Swiss epidemic in the cantons of Bern and Thurgau was published by Zimmermann in 1762. Scarlatina was common, and, from 1776 on, spread over both hemispheres. The monograph of Plenciz (1762) ascribes the disease to a *contagium animatum*. It was still confused with measles, which also caused a high mortality in the French and German cities and in Brazil (1749). Experimental inoculations of measles were made by Francis Home in 1759. There were several pandemics of influenza in both the old world and the new; diphtheria, yellow fever, whooping-cough, and epidemic pneumonia were wide-spread; croup and erysipelas were occasionally epidemic. Puerperal fever was often confused with "miliary" or sweating fever (*Schweiss-friesel*). Small-pox was so common everywhere that it was taken for granted and only the heavier epidemics were recorded, e. g., in Paris (1719), Sweden (1749–65), Vienna (1763; 1767), Tuscany (1764), and London (1766, 1770). It was especially destructive in the East Indies (1770–71), and among the Indians of the new world.[1] The great success of Jennerian vaccination has obscured the early history of the other preventive measure which it eventually displaced, viz., inoculation of human virus or **variolation**. Dr. Arnold C. Klebs, in his interesting study of variolation,[2] divides its history into an introductory period (1713–21), a period of stagnation (1727–46), a second revival (1746–64), and a scientific and experimental period (1764–98). The practice was introduced into Europe by Emanuel Timoni and Pylarini, who published accounts of it in 1713 and 1716 respectively. Timoni's daughter was inoculated in 1717, and the inoculation of the children of Lady Wortley Montague followed (1718–21). In the latter year, Boylston began to inoculate in Boston, Massachusetts, and, by 1752, had 2124 inoculations, with 30 deaths, while in Charleston, South Carolina, Kirkpatrick had inoculated between 800 and 1000 in 1743, with only 8 deaths. By 1728, there had been 897 inoculations in England and Scotland, with 17 deaths. In 1760, Robert and Daniel Sutton introduced inoculation by puncture, with dietetic preparation, and had some 30,000 cases, with about 4 per cent. mortality, while in Paris, Angelo Gatti, of Pisa, was given permission to inoculate by the scientific method of preparatory treatment and puncture inoculations in 1769. Prior to this, the great danger of inoculation had been the large amount of virus used and the extensive sores, which tended to make the subject a veritable small-pox carrier. The success of the Suttons and Gatti was such that in 1768, at the instance of Voltaire, Catherine of Russia permitted herself and the Grand Duke Paul to be inoculated by Dimsdale, and, in the same year, Ingen Housz inoculated three of the imperial family of Austria after preliminary experiments upon 200 children of the Viennese suburbs. In 1770, George Motherby was inoculating at Königsberg, but, by 1774, Benjamin Jesty had performed his first vaccination. The subsequent success of Jenner's experiments soon swept inoculation from the field, although it had well-nigh attained the status of a modern preventive injection. The success of vaccination was due to its relative harmlessness, there being little mortality and no possibility of convection of the disease by the vaccinated person. In England, variolation was declared a felony by Act of Parliament in 1840.

The leaders in the literature of **American medicine** in the colonial and revolutionary period have already been referred to, and, until after the Revolution, there was little advance upon the seventeenth century. Before 1800, there were five good medical

---

[1] Haeser. [2] Johns Hopkins Hosp. Bull., Baltimore, 1913, xxiv, 69–83.

schools established, viz., those of the University of Pennsylvania (1765), King's College, New York (1767), Harvard University (1782), the College of Philadelphia (1790), and the Medical School of Dartmouth College (1798). Medical societies were organized in Boston (1735), Philadelphia (1765), and New York city (about 1769), and state medical societies in New Jersey (1766), Massachusetts (1781), South Carolina (1789), Delaware (1789), New Hampshire (1791), Connecticut (1792), and Maryland (1798). Of these, the College of Physicians of Philadelphia (1787) and the Medical and Chirurgical Faculty of Maryland (1789, incorporated 1799), are especially remarkable for their ancient lineage and long descent. The societies of New Jersey (1766), Massachusetts (1790), and the College of Physicians of Philadelphia (1793) issued transactions and, in 1788, the Medical Society of New Haven County, Connecticut (instituted 1784), published a thin little volume of "Cases and Observations" containing, among other good papers, Hezekiah Beardsley's "Case of a scirrhus in the pylorus of an infant." The first medical periodical of the period was the "Medical Repository" of New York (1797–1824), edited by Samuel L. Mitchell, Elihu H. Smith, and Edward Miller. It was followed by a single number of a translation of the "Journal de médecine militaire" of Paris (1790), and by John Redman Coxe's "Philadelphia Medical Museum" (1804). The Memoirs of the American Academy of Arts and Sciences were begun in Boston in 1785. The hospitals of the early period were the Pennsylvania Hospital of Philadelphia, organized in 1751, and opened in a permanent building in December, 1756, the Philadelphia Dispensary (1786), the New York Dispensary (organized 1791, incorporated 1795), and the New York Hospital, which was begun in 1773, destroyed by fire in 1775, and not rebuilt until 1791. The first lying-in hospital was Shippen's private institution of 1762, and the first insane hospital, the Eastern Lunatic Asylum at Williamsburgh, Virginia, which was chartered in 1772 and opened in 1773. Medical libraries were founded in the Pennsylvania Hospital (1762), the New York Hospital (1776), and the College of Physicians of Philadelphia (1788), the latter being now one of the finest in the country. The favorite text-books of the period were Albinus, Cowper, Cheselden, Monro, and Winslow in anatomy, Haller's First Lines of Physiology, Boerhaave and van Swieten on internal medicine, Heister's surgery, Smellie's midwifery, and, of course, Sydenham, Huxham, Pott, and other well-known authors. There was strong prejudice against dissecting, and material was usually obtained by body-snatching. There was little study of physiology or pathology, but surgery was ably taught by such men as John Jones, William Shippen, Jr., Thomas

Bond, John Warren, Richard Bayley, and Wright Post. Obstetric cases were usually handled by midwives, and the first male obstetricians were pupils of Smellie and Willam Hunter. William Shippen, Jr., first lectured on the subject in Philadelphia in 1762. There were a few strolling dentists and oculists here and there, but, with the exception of Perkins's tractors, we hear little of quackery in the colonial period, for the simple reason that no very rich harvest was held out to its practitioners. Acts to regulate the practice of medicine and surgery were passed in New York city (1760) and New Jersey (1772), a special ordinance for midwives in New York city (1716), quarantine acts in Pennsylvania (1700), Massachusetts (1701), Virginia (1722), New York (1758), and other States, and a general quarantine act by Congress on February 23, 1799.

THE NINETEENTH CENTURY: THE BEGINNINGS OF ORGANIZED ADVANCEMENT OF SCIENCE

In the evolution of modern medicine, as in the development of pure science of which it was a part, three factors seem of especial moment. First of all, the great industrial or social-democratic movement of civilized mankind, which, following close upon the political revolutions in America and France, intensified the feeling for intellectual and moral liberty and upheld the new idea of the dignity and importance of all kinds of human labor, as exemplified in Napoleon's famous device: "The tools to those who can handle them" (*La carrière ouverte aux talens*). Some immediate corollaries of this proposition were the removal of the civil disabilities oppressing the Jews, and the opening out to talented womankind of occupations and modes of thought which had hitherto been closed to them. Second, the publication of such works as Helmholtz's "Conservation of Energy" (1847) and Darwin's "Origin of Species" (1859) did away forever with many of the silly anthropomorphisms and appeals to human conceit which have always hampered the true advancement of medicine in the past. Third, as an inevitable consequence, physics, chemistry and biology came to be studied as objective laboratory sciences, dissociated from the usual subjective human prepossessions. Hardly any one today doubts the theorem sustained by Emile Littré that the real advancement of biological and medical science has nothing to do with theological dogma or metaphysical speculation, but simply depends upon collateral improvements in physical and chemical procedure. Medicine owes much to the great mathematicians and physicists of the seventeenth and eighteenth centuries, who developed the theory of vision and almost the whole physiology of respiration. In the nineteenth century, the extension of the three fundamental branches of pure science has not been surpassed in variety by the work of any preceding age.

Of modern mathematicians, we need only mention the names of Euler, Gauss, Riemann, Jacobi, Abel, Weierstrass, Cayley, Sylvester; of physicists, Young, Carnot, Fourier, Kirchhoff, Clausius, Helmholtz, Ohm, Maxwell, Lord Kelvin, Boltzmann, Gibbs, J. J. Thomson, Edison, Tesla, Arrhenius; of chemists, Dalton, Dumas, Chevreuil, Berzelius, Liebig, Wöhler, Berthollet, Mendeleff, Ostwald, van't Hoff, Ramsay, Rutherford, and the Curies.

The physical principle of Conservation of Energy was demonstrated by Robert Mayer (a physician of Heilbronn) and James Prescot Joule in 1842, and applied to the whole field of chemistry and physics by Helmholtz in 1847. The principle of Dissipation of Energy was first stated by Sadi Carnot in 1824, developed by Clausius (1850) and Lord Kelvin (1852), and applied to all physical and chemical phenomena by the Yale professor, Willard Gibbs, in 1872–78. The generalization of Gibbs is now seen to be so complete and far-reaching as to make engineering, geology, biology, medicine, and every other phase of science that deals with states of substance, a branch of chemistry. The immediate consequence of the same generalization was the development of the new science of physical chemistry by Ostwald, Le Chatellier, van't Hoff, Roozeboom, and the chemists of the Dutch school. In physical or thermody-namic chemistry, all changes of substance are treated as rigid consequences of the laws of dynamics.

In 1859, Kirchhoff and Bunsen devised spectrum analysis. Faraday (1821–54) and Maxwell (1865) worked out the whole theory of electricity and electromagnetism, upon which followed such practical consequences as electric lighting, heating, and motor power, telephonic communication, and the reali-zation of wireless telegraphy by Hertz (1887) and Marconi (1895). The Röntgen-rays were discovered in 1895, and the Curies isolated radium chloride in 1898. Among physicians, Thomas Young described astigmatism in 1801, stated the wave theory of light in 1802, and the surface tension theory of capil-larity in 1805; John Dalton stated the chemical law of multiple proportions in 1802; Helmholtz invented the ophthalmoscope and the ophthalmometer in 1850, and elaborated the theories of vision (1853–67) and of tonal percep-tion (1856–63). Another physician, William Charles Wells (1757–1817), a native of Charleston, S. C., developed the theory of dew and dew-point in 1814. Photography was developed by Niepce (1814), Daguerre (1839), Draper (1840), and Fox Talbot (1840). Amici (1812), Chevalier (1820) and Joseph Jackson Lister (1830) devised the improved achromatic lenses of the compound microscope to which Amici had given the idea of water-immersion and Chevalier the compound objective, Purkinje stereopticon effects and re-agents, and E. Abbé the modern illuminating apparatus, apochromatic objec-tive, oil immersion and compensating ocular (1886).

It will be seen, from the dates of these discoveries, that the modern scientific movement did not attain its full stride until well after the middle of the century. The medicine of the early half was, with a few noble exceptions, only part and parcel of the sta-tionary theorizing of the preceding age. Up to the year 1850 and well beyond it most of the advancements in medicine were made by the French. After the publication of Virchow's "Cellular Pathology" (1858), German medicine began to gain its ascendancy. The descriptions of new forms of disease, and the discoveries of anesthesia (1847) and antiseptic surgery (1867), were the special achievements of the Anglo-Saxon race.

On the continent of Europe, the ideas of Immanuel Kant had little effect upon medical theories, but the so-called "Nature Philosophy" of Schelling, which aimed to establish the subjective and objective identity of all things, and the system of Hegel, which, like evolution today, regarded everything as in a state of becoming something else (Werden), exerted a very baneful effect upon German medicine by diverting mental activity away from the investigation of concrete facts into the realm of fanciful specula-tion. The "therapeutic nihilism" formulated by Skoda put a decided limitation upon Austrian medicine, and, in France and Italy, a vast deal of energy, and even of human life, was wasted over the doctrines of Broussais and Rasori. It took a long time to demonstrate that the advancement of **internal medicine** as a science can never be accomplished by hugging some pet theory out of a regard for its author's personality, but only through the performance of a vast amount of chemical, physical and biological research by thousands of willing workers. The first step in this direction was taken by Broussais, who did away with metaphysical conceptions of disease only to substitute something worse.

François-Joseph-Victor **Broussais** (1772–1838), the son of a Breton physician, had been a sergeant in the Republican Army in 1792, had swung a cutlass as a privateersman in 1798, and, after

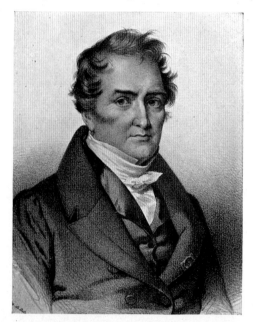

François-Joseph-Victor Broussais (1772–1838).

graduating in medicine in 1803, served for three years as an army surgeon in Napoleon's campaigns. He carried his rough schooling into his medical teaching, in which his methods were Napoleonic and his therapeutics sanguinary. Broussais modified the Brunonian theory by saying that life depends upon irritation, but, in particular, upon heat, which excites the chemical processes in the body. Disease, however, depends upon localized irritation of some viscus or organ, *e. g.*, the heart, or, above all, the stomach and intestines. Specific morbid poisons, such as the syphilitic virus, were to Broussais non-existent. The only merit in his reasoning was that he substituted the diseased organ for the hazy concept "fever" as the all-important factor, the *foyer de maladie*. Gastro-enteritis he thought the "basis of all pathology," as Cullen thought that nearly everything was a neurosis. Nature had no healing power and it was necessary to abort disease by active measures. To this end, he adopted a powerful antiphlogistic or weakening régime, the main features of which were to deprive the patient of his proper food and to leech him all over his body. As many as 30 to 50 leeches were applied at once, even 5 to 8 being prescribed in cases of extreme debility. Of the scarcity of leeches in Broussais' time, Baas records that "in the year 1833 alone 41,500,000 leeches were imported into France, and only nine or ten million exported. Yet in 1824–25 two or three million were sufficient to supply all demands." As he approached his dotage, which Dr. Holmes has so humorously described, Broussais, a "vieux mili-taire" by training, scolded, bullied, and wrangled with the vigor of Paracelsus, and although his follower, Bouillaud, was moved to let even greater torrents of blood, students began gradually to edge away from him, until his theories were firmly exploded by the good sense and temperate judgment of the clinician Chomel and the statistical inductions of his pupil Louis. Broussais' doctrine of irritation was taken up in Germany by Roeschlaub, and occa-sioned a pale temporary reflex in the writings of Benjamin Travers, Pridgin Teale, and other English physicians of the period, who ascribed many diseases to "spinal irritation." In Italy, about 1807, Giovanni Rasori, in his clinic at Milan, began to revamp the Asclepiadean theory of constricted and relaxed conditions (which Brown had called sthenic and asthenic and Hoffman tonic and atonic) by considering diseases as states of stimulus or contra-stimulus. Diagnosis of these conditions was effected by means of venesections which were supposed to turn out beneficially in over-stimulated conditions or *vice versâ*. Overstimulus was then opposed by sedatives, opium, and copious blood-letting; contra-stimulus by huge doses of gamboge, aconite, ipecac, nux vomica, and the like. This method, which did as much harm as that of Broussais', had to run its course, and like the latter, eventually died out.

The arbitrary doctrines of Broussais were finally overthrown by Pierre-Charles-Alexandre **Louis** (1787–1872), the founder of medical, as distinguished from vital, statistics. After passing six years in Russia, where his despair over the impotence of medicine in a diphtheria epidemic convinced him of the necessity of deeper study, he returned to Paris to complete his medical education, and, entering Chomel's clinic, devoted the rest of his life to teaching, combined with incessant dissecting and hospital practice. His principal works are his researches on phthisis (1825),[1] based upon 358 dissections and 1960 clinical cases, and pointing out the frequency of tubercle in the apex of the lung; his work on typhoid fever (1829),[2] which gave the disease its present name ("fièvre typhoïde"), and his polemics against Broussais (1835),[3] which finally demolished the latter's "system," and, by a statistical proof that blood-letting is of little value in pneumonia, did away with its abuse in that disease. Louis thought that the fallacies of an *a priori* theory, like that of Broussais, can easily be brought out and thrown into relief by good statistics and that the latter

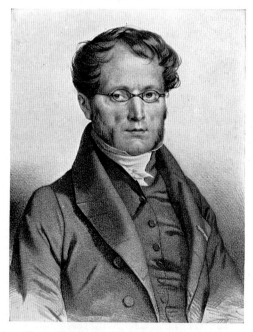

Pierre-Charles-Alexandre Louis (1787–1872).

can sometimes be used as an instrument of precision in cases where proper experimental methods are wanting. This idea met with no special support in his lifetime, but it has since proved its own worth in testing etiologic and hereditary data or the value of different therapeutic methods, especially through the great increase in medical periodicals, with corresponding improvements

[1] Louis: Recherches anatomico-physiologiques sur la phthisie, Paris, 1825.
[2] Recherches . . . sur la maladie connue sous les noms de gastro-entérite (etc.), Paris, 1829.
[3] Recherches sur les effets de la saignée (etc.), Paris, 1835.

in bibliography and census-taking, which, of course, furnish the materials for good statistics. Its value was shown by Fournier and Erb in demonstrating the causal nexus between tabes, paresis and syphilis; and by others, in testing the value of hydrotherapy in typhoid, of antitoxin in diphtheria, of operative intervention in appendicitis and other abdominal or pelvic diseases, or in trying out new drugs, such as "606." Louis was the first, after Floyer, to use the watch in timing the pulse, in which he was followed by the clinicians of the Irish, English and American schools. Through his American pupils, Holmes, Gerhard, the Jacksons,

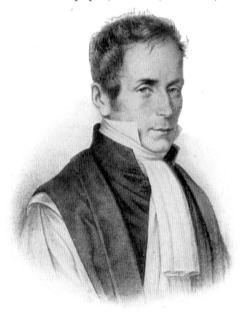

Réné-Théophile-Hyacinthe Laënnec (1781–1826).

the Shattucks, and others, he exerted a powerful influence upon the advancement of medical science in the Eastern United States. The strong stand which Louis took in favor of facts and figures as against the sterile theorizing of the past appealed especially to the keen, practical common sense of these northern physicians.

The most distinguished and important internist of the early French school was Réné-Théophile-Hyacinthe Laënnec (1781–1826), a native of Quimper (Brittany), who, like Bichat, was a regimental surgeon in the revolution, and was also, like him, an early victim of phthisis. He was physician to the Hôpital Beaujon in 1806 and to the Hôpital Necker in 1816. Laënnec made his name immortal by his invention of the stethoscope in 1819 (at first only a cylinder of paper in his hands), and by the publication of the two successive editions of his *Traité de l'auscultation médiate* in 1819 and 1823. This work placed its author among the greatest clinicians of all ages, and, unlike Auenbrugger's, was immediately taken up and translated everywhere. It is the foundation stone of modern knowledge of diseases of the chest and their diagnosis by mediate exploration. In the first edition (1819), Laënnec pursues the analytic method, giving the different signs elicited by percussion and auscultation, with the corresponding anatomic lesions (he was an expert pathologist). In the second edition (1823), the process is turned about and the method is synthetic, each disease being described in detail in respect of diagnosis, pathology and (most intelligent) treatment, so that this edition is, in effect, the most important treatise on diseases of the thoracic organs that was ever written. Laënnec not only put the diagnostic sounds of cardiac and pulmonary disease upon a reliable basis, but was the first to describe and differentiate bronchiectasis (first noted by his assistant Cayol in 1808), pneumothorax, hemorrhagic pleurisy, gangrene, and emphysema of the lungs, œsophagitis and that form of cirrhosis of the liver which is now termed "chronic, diffuse interstitial hepatitis." He left masterly descriptions of bronchitis and pneumonia, with a full account of the pathologic appearances, and his accounts of pulmonary gangrene and emphysema needed only the retouching of Rokitansky's microscope to make the pictures classic. Laënnec was also the first to discover and describe the "anatomical tubercle" or postmortem wart,[1] which McCall Anderson, in 1879, showed to be identical with lupus verrucosum; and he was the originator of such terms as "ægophony," "pectoriloquy," the sonorous and sibilant "râles," and other well-recognized signs of moment in the exploration of the chest. Personally, he was a slight, nervous, aquiline figure, of generous, tolerant, unaffected nature and refined feelings. Like Auenbrugger, he was modest about his work and cared more for his proficiency in horseback riding than for fame.

Among the prominent French internists contemporary with Louis and Laënnec were Bretonneau, Bouillaud, Corvisart, Pinel, Andral, Piorry, Rayer, and Ricord.

Pierre **Bretonneau** (1771–1862), of Tours, wrote important monographs on the contagion of typhoid fever (1819–29),[2] which he called "dothienenteritis," and on diphtheria (1826),[3] giving the

---

[1] Also noted by Sir Samuel Wilks as "verruca necrogenica," in 1862.

[2] Bretonneau: Arch. gén. de méd., Paris, 1829, xxi, 57–78.

[3] Des inflammations spéciales du tissu muqueux et en particulier de la diphthérite, Paris, 1826.

disease its present name; and performed the first successful tracheotomy in croup.

Jean-Baptiste **Bouillaud** (1796–1881), of Angoulême, although a furious blood-letter, was one of the ablest diagnosticians of his time. He was the first to point out that aphasia is correlated with a lesion in the anterior lobes of the brain (1825);[1] and he established a "law of coincidence" between the occurrence of heart disease and acute articular rheumatism (1836).[2] These researches

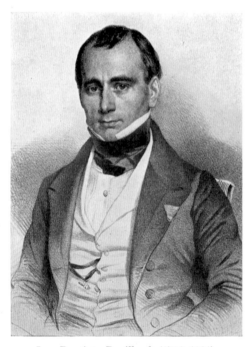

Jean-Baptiste Bouillaud (1796–1881).

were further extended in his important clinical treatise on articular rheumatism of 1840.[3]

Jean-Nicolas **Corvisart** (1755–1821), Napoleon's favorite physician, and the teacher of Dupuytren, Laënnec and Cuvier, is now remembered chiefly through his revival of Auenbrugger's work on percussion, a translation of which he appended to the third

---

[1] Arch. gén. de méd., Paris, 1825, viii, 25–45.

[2] Bouillaud: Nouvelles recherches sur le rhumatisme articulaire (etc.), Paris, 1836.

[3] Traité clinique du rhumatisme articulaire, Paris, 1840.

edition of his "Essay on the Diseases and Organic Lesions of the Heart and the Great Vessels" (1818).

The noble-minded Philippe **Pinel** (1745–1826), of Saint-Paul (Tarn), stands high in medical history as the first to treat the insane in a humane manner. At the risk of his own life and liberty, he initiated the reforms of striking off their chains, placing them in hospitals under lenient physicians, and doing away with the abuses of drugging and blood-letting to which they were subjected. In this regard he is the real founder of the modern "open-door" school of psychiatry, although his classifications of insanity and

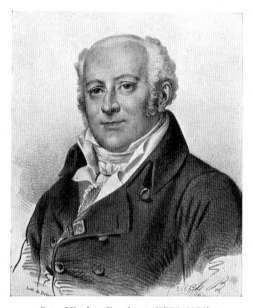

Jean-Nicolas Corvisart (1755–1821).

disease are now forgotten. His *Traité médico-philosophique sur l'aliénation mentale* (1801) is one of the most important of medical classics, and it was followed by such psychiatric milestones as Reil's Rhapsodies on the Psychic Treatment of Insanity (1803), Heinroth's books on insanity (1818), the jurisprudence of insanity (1825), and the psychology of lying (1834);[1] Calmeil, on general paralysis of the insane (1826);[2] Prichard's Treatise on Insanity, containing the first description of moral insanity (1835); Es-

---

[1] J. C. A. Heinroth: Die Lüge, Leipzig, 1834.

[2] L.-F. Calmeil: De la paralysie générale (etc.), Paris, 1826.

quirol's great work (1838),[1] Falret's original description of circular insanity (1853),[2] and John Conolly on "The Treatment of the Insane without Mechanical Restraints" (1856).

Gabriel **Andral** (1797–1876), of Paris, was a clear, methodical, analytical spirit who opposed all scholastic eccentricity and fanaticism, edited the works of Laënnec, joined hands with Louis in his propaganda against blood-letting, favored cold baths in typhoid and other fevers, and is to be especially remembered as the first

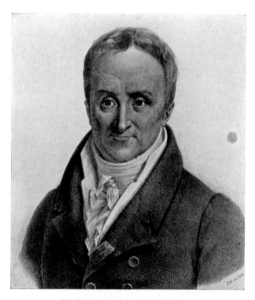

Philippe Pinel (1745–1826)

to urge a chemical examination of the blood in morbid conditions (1843).[3]

Pierre-Adolphe **Piorry** (1794–1879), of Poitiers, was the inventor of the pleximeter and the pioneer of mediate percussion (1828).[4] He wrote much, including a treatise on pleximetry (1866), and, although a "poet," affected an exaggerated and pedantic nomenclature, employing such high-sounding terms as "cardiodysneuria," "hypersplenotrophy," and so forth.

Pierre-François-Olive **Rayer** (1793–1867), of Calvados, was the author of a number of works of capital importance, including his

[1] J.-E. D. Esquirol: Des maladies mentales, 2 vols. and atlas, Paris, 1838
[2] J.-P. Falret: Bull. acad. de méd., Paris, 1853–4, xix, 382–400.
[3] Andral: Essai d'hématologie pathologique, Paris, 1843.
[4] Piorry: De la percussion médiate, Paris, 1828.

treatise on skin diseases, with atlas (1826–27), his classic monograph on glanders and farcy in man (1837),[1] his three-volume treatise on diseases of the kidney, with atlas (1837–41), which marks
an epoch in the development of the subject, and his memoir on
endemic hematuria (1839).

   Philippe **Ricord** (1799–1889), born of French parents in Baltimore, Md., and a graduate of the Paris Faculty, was the greatest
authority on venereal diseases after John Hunter. His treatise
on the subject (1838)[2] is memorable in the history of medicine for

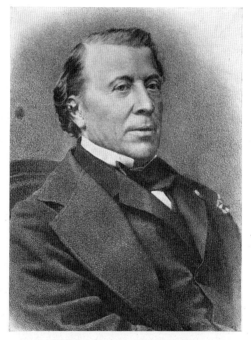

Philippe Ricord (1799–1889).

overthrowing Hunter's erroneous ideas as to the identity of gonorrhea and syphilis, establishing the autonomy of these diseases.
Ricord wrote on such subjects as the use of the speculum (1833),
gonorrhea in women (1834), epididymitis (1839), gonorrheal
conjunctivitis (1842), and he is credited with a vast number of
risky *bons mots* and anecdotes (Ricordiana) relating to his specialty.   Dr. Oliver Wendell Holmes styled him "the Voltaire of

---

[1] Rayer: De la morve et du farcin chez l'homme, Paris, 1837.
[2] Ricord: Traité pratique des maladies vénériennes, Paris, 1838.

pelvic literature—a skeptic as to the morality of the race in general, who would have submitted Diana to treatment with his mineral specifics, and ordered a course of blue pills for the vestal virgins."

Modern **dermatology** derives from the work of Willan, and his pupil Bateman, as continued and carried forward by the French and the New Vienna schools. Robert **Willan** (1757–1812), a Yorkshire Quaker who had studied the pathological work of Matthew Baillie to advantage, did much to clear up the nature of eczema and lupus, and divided cutaneous diseases, according to their objective appearances, into eight classes: the papular, squamous, exanthematous, bullous, vesicular, pustular, tubercular, and macular. By collating all the Greek, Latin, and Arabic terms, he established a definite classic nomenclature. His classification, which was awarded the Fothergillian gold medal in 1790, was the starting-point of modern dermatology, and is still more or less in use. Willan's great work *On Cutaneous Diseases* (1796–1808), published in parts, was left unfinished at his death, and was completed by Bateman. It contains original descriptions and figurations of prurigo, pityriasis, and ichthyosis, while psoriasis (the Biblical "leprosy" of Gehazi and Naaman), sycosis, tinea versicolor, lupus, and impetigo are more clearly defined and differentiated. Willan also defined erythema iris as a species of his original genus "iris" (herpes iris), and separated out the forms of eczema due to external irritation (eczema solare, impetiginodes, rubrum, mercuriale). This part of his work is included in the *Delineations of Cutaneous Diseases*, an atlas of 72 colored plates published in 1817 by Thomas **Bateman** (1788–1831), of Whitby, Yorkshire. Bateman was the first to describe lichen urticatus, molluscum contagiosum, and ecthyma, which Willan had depicted as "phlyzacia." Ecthyma terebrans was first described by Whitley Stokes of Dublin (1807), and xanthoma by Addison and Gull (1851).

The founder of the modern French school of dermatology was Jean-Louis **Alibert** (1766–1837), of Villefranche de l'Aveyron, Dr. Holmes' "jolly old Baron Alibert, whom I remember so well in his broad brimmed hat, worn a little jauntily on one side, calling out to the students in the court-yard of the Hospital St. Louis, *Enfans de la méthode naturelle, êtes-vous tous ici?*" This "natural method" of classifying diseases was, in fact, the passion of Alibert's life. A picture of his "family tree" of dermatoses, standing grim and solitary in the foreground of a barren, uninviting landscape, forms the initial plate of his principal work.[1] Alibert was the first to describe mycosis fungoides

[1] Alibert: Monographie des dermatoses, Paris; 1842, vol. i, plate opposite p. 1.

(*pian fungoïde*) in 1806 and keloid (*cancroïde*) in 1810 (later as "keloide" or "kelis") (1835). He also described, as "pustule d'Alep" (1829),[1] the endemic ulcer which has lately become so important in connection with the Leishman-Donovan bodies. Alibert's family tree was discarded by his pupil Biett for the system of Willan, and the ideas of Biett were further extended by Rayer (1826) and by Cazenave and Schedel (1828), who made the first classification of skin diseases upon an anatomic basis, e. g., inflammations, hypertrophies, disorders of secretion and sensation, hemorrhagic manifestations, etc. This classification was the forerunner of the second phase of modern dermatology, the pathologic or histologic period inaugurated by von Hebra and his followers, which will be considered in connection with the New Vienna School.

Laënnec's teaching had an immediate outcome in Great Britain in the brilliant clinical work of two physicians of the **Irish school.** The founders of the Dublin school were John Cheyne (1777–1836), who described acute hydrocephalus,[2] or "dropsy in the brain" (1818);[3] the surgeon Abraham Colles (1773–1843), who stated "Colles' law"; and Robert Adams (1791–1875), who left classical accounts of essential heart-block (1826)[4] and rheumatic gout (1857).[5] Other important members of this school were Corrigan (of "Corrigan's pulse"), William Wallace (1791–1838), who introduced the use of potassium iodide in syphilis (1836), and Francis Rynd (1801–61), who first employed hypodermic injections, by a gravity device (of his invention), for the relief of pain (1845–61).[6] The true leaders of the Dublin school, however, were Graves and Stokes.

Robert James **Graves** (1796–1853), the son of a Dublin clergyman, took his medical degree in 1818, and, while making the usual continental tour, had such adventurous experiences as being arrested as a German spy in Austria on account of his fluency as a linguist, and of successfully putting down a mutiny on board ship during a storm in the Mediterranean, afterward assuming command and saving the vessel through his pluck. Returning to Dublin in 1821, he became chief physician to the Meath Hospital

[1] Alibert: Rev. med. franc. et étrang., Paris, 1829, iii, 62–71.

[2] Cheyne: An essay on hydrocephalus acutus, Edinburgh, 1808.

[3] Cheyne: Dublin Hosp. Rep., 1818, ii, 216. *See also*, "The case of the Honourable Colonel Townshend" in George Cheyne's "English Malady" (London, 1733, 209–212).

[4] Adams: Dublin Hosp. Rep., 1827, iv, 396.

[5] Adams: Treatise on rheumatic gout, London, 1857.

[6] Rynd: Dublin M. Press, 1845, xiii, 165; and description of instrument in Dublin Quart. Jour. Med. Sc., 1861, xxxii, 13. For a full account of Rynd's invention see Pfender, Wash. Med. Ann., 1912, x, 346–359.

and one of the founders of the Park Street School of Medicine. Here he immediately went in for the widest reforms, introducing the continental methods of clinical teaching, such as making his advanced students handle and report on clinical cases, and suppressing the maltreatment and abuse which hospital patients had to endure from the rough-spoken Irish M.D.'s of the day. Tall, dark and *distingué*, Graves had a warm heart, in spite of his sarcastic speech, and once even did a stint of literary work for a poor student. His *Clinical Lectures* (1848), which Trousseau read and re-read with highest admiration, introduced many novelties,

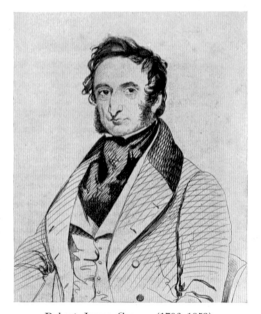

Robert James Graves (1796–1853).

such as the "pin-hole pupil," timing the pulse by the watch, and discarding the old lowering or antiphlogistic treatment of fevers. He requested that the phrase "He fed fevers" should be his epitaph. Graves also left early accounts of angioneurotic edema and scleroderma, and, in 1835, he published a description of exophthalmic goiter so admirable that the disease still goes by his name.[1]

William **Stokes** (1804–78), Graves's colleague at Meath Hospital, was the son of Whitley Stokes, Regius Professor of Medicine at

---

[1] Graves: London Med. & Surg. Jour., 1835, vii, pt. 2, pp. 516, 517.

Dublin, and succeeded his father in this position in 1845. As early as 1825, he put himself on record as a disciple of Laënnec by the publication of his "Introduction to the Use of the Stethoscope." During the Dublin epidemic of typhus fever in 1826, he worked hard for the poor, and had an attack of the disease himself in 1827. He reported the first case of cholera in the Dublin epidemic of 1832, and, in 1846, published his celebrated account of the Stokes-Adams disease.[1]   His treatises on diseases of the chest (1837) and diseases of the heart and aorta (1854) won him lasting fame. He was one of the few physicians who ever received the Prussian order *"pour le mérite."*

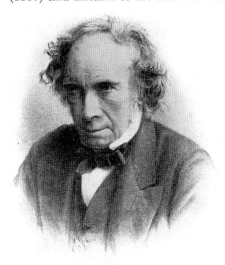

William Stokes (1804–1878).

Sir Dominic John **Corrigan** (1802–80), who described the "famine fever" of 1847, also wrote upon diseases of the heart, and, in 1832, published an original description of insufficiency of the aortic valve (with a superb plate) which is accepted as the classical account of the disease,[2] although the latter had been earlier noted by Cowper (1705), Vieussens (1715), and H o d g k i n (1829). Corrigan was the first to throw into relief the characteristic receding or "water-hammer" pulse in aortic regurgitation (Corrigan's pulse), and suggested that a flagging heart may be stimulated by tapping the precordial region with a hot spoon (Corrigan's hammer). He also noted the "cerebral breathing" of typhus and the expansile pulsation of aneurysm (Corrigan's sign), and described cirrhosis of the lungs or fibroid phthisis, which, like aortic incompetency, sometimes goes by his name.

The **English clinicians** of the early nineteenth century assimilated the ideas of Laënnec and Bichat in their practice, and, like Heberden, Parry, Fothergill and Huxham, showed themselves true followers of Sydenham in their descriptions of disease. Of special importance is the clinical and pathologic work which was

[1] Stokes: Dublin Quart. Jour. Med. Sc., 1846, ii, 73–85.

[2] Corrigan: Edinb. Med. & Surg. Jour., 1832, xxxvii, 225–245, 1 pl. (Hodgkin: London Med. Gaz., 1828–29, iii, 433–443).

done by the long line of brilliant workers at Guy's Hospital—the "great men of Guy's." Of these, Richard **Bright** (1789–1858), of Bristol, had studied under Astley Cooper and James Currie, and was physician at Guy's for twenty-three years (1820–43), where he worked for six hours a day in the wards and postmortem room, besides lecturing on materia medica and clinical medicine. His experience was further widened by extensive continental travel, in the course of which he came to know and admire Johann Peter Frank. He was the leading consultant of London in his day.

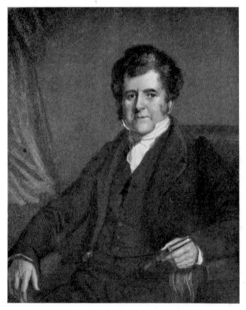

Richard Bright (1789–1858).

His *Reports of Medical Cases* (1827), containing his original description of essential nephritis, with its epoch-making distinction between cardiac and renal dropsy, at once established his reputation all over Europe. White clouds in the urine had been noticed even by Hippocrates;[1] Saliceto, the Italian surgeon, had pointed out the association of dropsy, scanty urine and hardened kidneys (*durities in renibus*) in 1476;[2] and the correlation between dropsy

---

[1] For instance, in the case of Thasus, wife of Philinus, in Epidemic Diseases, Book I, §13, Case iv.

[2] "Signa duritiei in renibus sunt, quod minoratur quantitas urinæ, et quod est gravitas renum et spinæ cum aliquo dolore; et incipit venter inflari post tempus et fit hydropicus secundum dies. Et ut plurimum fit talis durities post apostema calidum in renibus et post febrem ejus." Saliceto: Liber in scientia medicinali, 1476, ch. 140.

23

and albuminous urine had been established by William Charles
Wells (1811)[1] and John Blackall (1813);[2] but Bright was the first
to connect these symptoms with the peculiar inflammation of the
kidneys which he found in so many postmortems, and his epoch-
making synthesis soon made its way everywhere, on account
of its immense importance in medical practice.   In work of this
kind, he is one of the greatest of modern pathologists, and as an
original delineator of disease, he ranks next to Laënnec.   "Bright
could not theorize," says his biographer, Wilks, "but he could see,
and we are struck with astonishment at his powers of observation,
as he photographed pictures of disease for the study of posterity."
He advanced no special views of pathology and affixed no particular labels to his many descriptions of morbid states, but he
collected an extraordinary number of facts and knew how to use
them.   Thus, he gave original accounts of pancreatic diabetes
and pancreatic steatorrhea (1832),[3] acute yellow atrophy of the
liver (1836),[4] unilateral convulsions or Jacksonian epilepsy (1836),[5]
and "status lymphaticus" (1838),[6] which, had they been tagged
with appropriate names, would have been better known before our
day.   His Medical Reports contain accurate accounts of such
novelties as scarlatinal otitis, otitic abscess of the brain, laryngeal
phthisis, pressure paralyses, the cerebral hemiplegias, the hysterical
equivalents of disease, and striking plates of the pathologic
appearances in typhoid fever, nephritis, acute yellow atrophy of
the liver and cerebral disease.   Sir Samuel Wilks further records
that he was one of the first, if not the first, to describe pigmentation
of the brain in melanemia, condensation of the lung in whooping-
cough, small echinococci in the interior of hydatid cysts, and the
bruit of the heart in chorea.   Bright was a capable and accomplished artist, a collector and connoisseur of engravings, and his
early volume of Hungarian travels is illustrated with charming
pictures drawn by himself.   This great physician was also an able
botanist and geologist, and personally a simple, unprejudiced,
truth-loving man.

   Thomas **Addison** (1793–1860), of Longbenton, Cumberland,
Bright's colleague at Guy's, was more the brilliant pathologist,
lecturer, and diagnostician than the successful practitioner.   On
account of a haughty, repellent manner which, on his own showing,
concealed excessive shyness and sensibility, he never had a large

---

[1] Wells: Tr. Soc. Improve. Med. & Chir. Knowledge, 1804–12, London,
1812, iii, 194–240.
[2] Blackall: Observations on the nature and cure of dropsies, London, 1813.
[3] Bright: Med. Chir. Tr., London, 1832–33, xviii, 1–56.
[4] Guy's Hosp. Rep., London, 1836, i, 36–40.
[5] *Ibid.*, 604–637.   [6] *Ibid.*, 1838, iii, 437.

practice and lived almost entirely for his pupils and hospital work. He attached so little importance to drugging that (it is said) he sometimes forgot to prescribe; yet "Addison's pill," of calomel, digitalis, and squills, for hepatic dropsy in syphilis, is still used. He was also the first to employ static electricity in the treatment of spasmodic and convulsive diseases (1837), and, in collaboration with John Morgan, wrote the first book in English on the action of poisons on the living body (1829). In 1849, Addison read a paper before the South London Medical Society,[1] in which he described pernicious anemia (twenty years before Biermer) and disease of the suprarenal capsules ("melasma suprarenale").

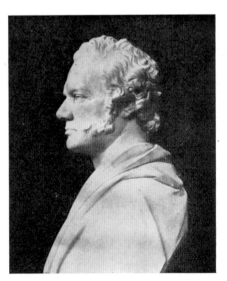

These clinical notations were afterward expanded at full length in his great monograph *On the Constitutional and Local Effects of Disease of the Suprarenal Capsules* (London, 1855). This book was regarded merely as a scientific curiosity in Addison's time, but it is now recognized as of epoch-making importance, since, in connection with the physiologic work of Claude Bernard, it inaugurated the study of the diseases of the ductless glands and of those disturbances of chemical equilibrium known as "pluriglandular syndromes." It was Trousseau who first proposed to call the suprarenal syndrome "Addison's disease." In 1851, Addison and Sir William Gull described the skin disease "vitiligoidea," now known as xanthoma. "Addison's keloid" is a circumscribed form of scleroderma.

Thomas Addison (1793–1860). (Courtesy of Dr. Herbert L. Eason, Guy's Hospital, London.)

The pathologist Thomas **Hodgkin** (1798–1866), of Tottenham, England, a member of the Society of Friends, always wearing their characteristic dress, was a philanthropist and reformer by nature and was driven away from Guy's, says Wilks, by his eccentric independence of spirit. His reputation rests upon his original description of

---

[1] London M. Gaz., 1849, xliii, 517.

that simultaneous enlargement of the spleen and lymphatic gland or lymphadenoma (1832)[1] which, as he himself records, was vaguely outlined by Malpighi in 1665, and which Wilks, in 1865, called "Hodgkin's disease." He also wrote an account of insufficiency of the aortic valve (1829),[2] which antedated Corrigan's classical paper by five years. His essay on medical education (1823) is an interesting contribution, and his "Lectures on the Morbid Anatomy of the Serous and Mucous Membranes" (1836–40) is one of the earliest English treatises on pathology. Being generous to

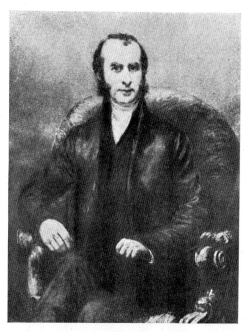

Thomas Hodgkin (1798–1866).

his patients and careless about collecting fees, Hodgkin gradually fell out of practice and devoted the rest of his life to various philanthropies. He died at Joppa, while traveling in the East with Sir Moses Montefiore, who erected the monument over his grave.

Three eminent English clinicians of the early period were Parkinson, Wells, and Hodgson.

James **Parkinson** (1755–1824), of London, one of John Hunter's

---

[1] Med. Chir. Tr., London, 1832, xvii, 68–114.
[2] Lond. M. Gaz., 1828–29, iii, 433–443.

pupils, is remembered today by his unique and classic description of paralysis agitans or "Parkinson's disease" (1817),[1] and by the fact that he reported the first case of appendicitis in English (1812),[2] this case being also the first in which perforation was recognized as the cause of death (H. A. Kelly). Parkinson was a radical, a reformer and political agitator, some time in hot water with the government, and what little is known of his life is almost entirely due to the recent interesting researches of L. G. Rowntree (1912).[3] He wrote political and controversial pamphlets, a number of small treatises on domestic medicine, and a good book on medical education (The Hospital Pupil, 1800); but his most important contributions outside of medicine are his works on fossil remains (1804–22). An able geologist and palæontologist, he is memorable, with Avicenna, Fracastorius, Stensen, Hutton, Wollaston, Owen, and Huxley as one of the medical men who have contributed something of permanent value to these sciences.

William Charles **Wells** (1757–1817) was born in South Carolina, but his people being Tories in the Revolutionary period, he must be accounted, by his own choice, a British subject. Wells was a highly original observer, both in medicine and physics, his most important contribution to the latter science being his well-known "Essay on Dew" (1814). He described the albuminous urine of dropsy in 1811,[4] and, in 1810, published perhaps the earliest clinical report on the cardiac complications of rheumatism.[5]

Joseph **Hodgson** (1788–1869), of Birmingham, a successful lithotomist, wrote an important *Treatise on Diseases of the Arteries and Veins* (1815), in which he gave the first description of aneurysmal dilatation of the aortic arch, which the French writers call *maladie d'Hodgson*. This book is a wonderful storehouse of knowledge on the subject of vascular disease, and contains a great many valuable historic data about aneurysms and the early ligations of important arteries. In connection with it, we may mention Allan Burns's "Observations" on Heart Disease (1809).

The most important English treatise on the practice of medicine in the first half of the nineteenth century was the "Lectures on the Principles and Practice of Physic," published in 1843 by **Sir Thomas Watson** (1792–1882). For more than a quarter century, this work continued to pass through many editions and

[1] Parkinson: An Essay on the Shaking Palsy, London, 1817.

[2] Med. Chir. Tr., London, 1812, iii, 57.

[3] Rowntree: Bull. Johns Hopkins Hosp., Baltimore, 1912, xxiii, 33–45.

[4] Wells: Tr. Soc. Improve. Med. and Chir. Knowledge, 1804–12, London, 1812, iii, 194–240.

[5] Wells: Tr. Soc. Improve. Med. and Chir. Knowledge, 1804–12, London, 1812, iii, 372–412.

enjoyed a well-deserved popularity on account of its author's attractive and elegant style and his clear presentation of his subject.

The treatise on practice by Bright and Addison, of which only the first volume was ever published (1800), is a strictly scientific production, in which the phenomena of disease are treated in rigid categories, as in a work on mathematical physics. It is remarkable for its frankly agnostic spirit in regard to obscure phenomena, such as the nature of fever. Most of the text is said to have been written by Addison.

Other clinical treatises of the period, now almost forgotten, were Scudamore on gout (1816), Thackrah on the blood (1819), Sir Charles Hastings on inflammation of the lungs (1820), Sir James Clark on phthisis (1835), Francis Sibson on position of the internal organs (1844), Golding Bird on urinary deposits (1845), and the works of James Hope (1832), Peter Mere Latham (1845), Alison (1845), and Chevers (1851) on heart disease.

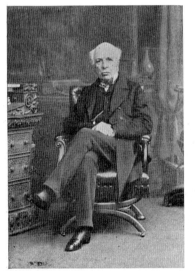

Sir Thomas Watson (1792–1882).

A prominent feature of English medicine in this period was the publication of admirable systems and encyclopedias of medicine, such as those of Forbes (1833–35), Todd (1835–59), Tweedie (1840), South (1847) and Reynolds (1866–79). These, with Panckoucke's sixty-volume "Dictionnaire des sciences médicales" (1812–22) and the forty-one volume "Encyclopédie" of Dechambre (1834–46),[1] were the forerunners of such later works as Quain's Dictionary of Medicine and the systems of Ziemssen, Eulenburg, Allbutt and Osler. A remarkable compiler of the day was James Copland (1791–1870), of the Orkney Islands, a "polyhistorian" of the type ridiculed in Germany, who made his living by hack work, and whose "Dictionary of Practical Medicine" (1834–59) consists of 3509 double column pages, all written by himself. Norman Moore likens it to the "Continent" of Rhazes, adding that our own generation leaves it "as undisturbed on the shelves as the Continent itself." As president of the Pathological Society of London, Copland excited many a chuckle of derision when he claimed various modern discoveries as his own.

A most important feature of British medicine in the nineteenth century was the work of the **Anglo-Indian surgeons.** The East India Company was chartered by Queen Elizabeth in 1600 and established its first trading station in 1612. Even in the early days, two surgeons, Gabriel Boughton, who, in 1645, was sent from Surat to the court of Shah Jahan at Agra, and William

---

[1] The seventeenth century encyclopedias of medicine were really anthologies. The modern idea of dictionary compilations originated in such works as the Konversations-Lexika of Hübner (1704) and Brockhaus (1796–1808), the encyclopedias of Ephraim Chambers (1728), Diderot (1751–72), and Voltaire (*Dictionnaire philosophique*, 1764), and the Encyclopædia Britannica (1768–71). For a good list of early medical encyclopedias, see Brit. Med. Jour., London, 1913, i, 725.

Hamilton, who accompanied the mission to Delhi in 1714–17, were both of them instrumental in securing trading concessions and charters for the company, leading up to the establishment of the three great centers at Bombay, Calcutta and Madras; but it was not until well after Clive's victory at Plassey in 1757 that we see the Indian Medical Service playing much of a part in colonial and tropical medicine. The earliest treatise on tropical medicine was, in fact, published in 1768 by James Lind (1716–94), whose important work was followed in due course by an imposing array of books on the Indian climate and diseases, notably those of John Peter Wade (1791–93), William Hunter (1804), Sir James Annesley (1825), William Twining (1832), Sir James Ranald Martin (1841), Allan Webb (1848), and Charles Morehead (1856), not to omit Goodeve's perennial little treatise on tropical pediatrics (1844). Aside from the development of tropical medicine, the organization of hospitals, of medical education, of public hygiene and other administrative duties connected with the building up of the Indian Empire, the most important achievements of these army surgeons were their remarkable first-hand accounts of heat stroke (those of Green, Barclay, Longmore et al., being among the closest to fact that we have), the descriptions of various forms of snake-bite, of native modes of poisoning and of the properties of far eastern drugs, the many contributions to Indian botany, zoölogy, geology and ethnography, the original accounts of cholera, beri-beri, scurvy, dysentery, leprosy and filarial elephantiasis, and the introduction of such novelties as mesmeric anesthesia, the British Army bamboo splint and the Hindu method of teaching surgical incision upon plants.

The literary organ of the Indian Medical Service at this time was the *India Journal of Medical Science* (1834–45), which was edited up to 1842 by Frederick Corbyn. The earlier volumes contain interesting engravings of some of the medical nabobs of the period.

Two of the Anglo-Indian surgeons will always hold a high place in the history of serpent venoms, viz., Patrick **Russell** (1727–1805), of Braidshaw, Scotland, whose "Account of Indian Serpents" (four volumes, 1796–1809) was the earliest venture in the field, containing the original description of the celebrated Russell's viper (Daboia Russellii); and Sir **Joseph Fayrer** (1824–1907), who played a spirited part in the Mutiny, and whose *Thanatophidia of India* (1872) is one of the great classics of zoölogy, describing all the venomous snakes of the Indian Peninsula, with magnificent life-size plates from drawings by Hindu pupils in the Government School of Art in Calcutta; and original experiments on the venoms, which were, however, preceded by the early work of the Abbe Fontana and Weir Mitchell (1870). The greatest of the Anglo-Indian zoölogists was Thomas Caverhill Jerden, whose accounts of the birds (1844–64) and mammals (1854) are famous. Among the many botanical works were William Roxburgh's "Plants of the Coromandel Coast" (1795–1819) and "Flora Indica" (1820–24), Nathaniel Wallich's "Tentamen Floræ Nepalensis" (1824–26) and "Plantæ Asiaticæ Rariores" (1830–32), Robert Wight's "Icones Plantarum Indiæ Orientalis," six volumes with over 2000 plates (1838–53), William Griffith's "Icones Plantarum Asiaticorum" (1847–51), and Thomson and Hooker's "Flora Indica" (1855). Important original monographs on tropical diseases were John Peter Wade on fever and dysentery (1791–93), John MacPherson's "Annals of Cholera" (1839), Edward Hare on the treatment of remittent fever and dysentery (1847), N. C. MacNamara's "History of Asiatic Cholera" (1876) and the original investigations of Henry Vandyke Carter (1831–97) on mycetoma (1874), leprosy, and elephantiasis (1874) and spirillosis (1882), and of Leonard Rogers on Indian fevers (1897–1908). Beri-beri had already been described in the seventeenth century by Bontius (1642) and Tulp (1652), but the treatise of John Grant Malcolmson (1835) will always be accounted the classical source of recent knowledge of the disease. Some of the Indian surgeons, who left the service early, attained distinction in other fields of activity, notably Murchison, Esdaile, Playfair, whose midwifery passed through nine editions (1876–98), Ireland, memorable for his writings on insanity, and Edward John Waring (1819–91), who compiled the first official

Indian pharmacopœia (1868), a bilingual work on Bazar Medicines (1860), also a Haller-like "Bibliotheca Therapeutica" (1878), and afterward did good service in public hygiene.

Charles **Murchison** (1830–79), born in Jamaica of Scotch parentage, entered the Bengal army in 1853, and published a treatise on the climate and diseases of Burmah in 1855.   Returning to England, he became a prominent physician at the London Fever Hospital (1856–70) and St. Thomas's Hospital (1871–79), in connection with his wonderful special knowledge of fevers; and, in 1873, he was presented with a testimonial by the residents of West London for tracing an epidemic of typhoid to a polluted milk supply.   He was noted for his solid accuracy, promptitude and decision in diagnosis, and although he opposed the bacterial theory of infection, his "Treatise on the Continued Fevers of Great Britain" (1862) is as important a work for England as Drake's Diseases of the Mississippi Valley is for the United States. Murchison translated Frerichs' book on diseases of the liver in 1861 and wrote a number of important monographs on the same subject himself.   Like his famous brother, he was an able geologist.

The name of Esdaile, of the Indian Medical Service, is prominently associated with the history of **hypnotism,** particularly of hypnotic anesthesia in surgical operations.   After the time of Mesmer, hypnotism was only a peg for arrant charlatanry. The great pioneer of scientific hypnosis was James **Braid** (1795– 1861), a surgeon of Fifeshire, Scotland, who settled in Manchester and became attracted to the subject of animal magnetism about 1841.   Braid at first believed that the phenomena produced by professional mesmerists were due to "collusion and illusion"; but he soon became convinced, upon experimentation, that there can be a genuine self-induced sleep brought about by a fixed stare at a bright inanimate object (Braidism).   The importance of Braid's work is that he proved that the mesmeric influence is entirely subjective or personal, and that no fluid or other influence passes from the operator to the patient.   This subjective trance he called neurohypnotism or hypnosis (1842), and his important treatise on the subject was entitled *Neurypnology, or the Rationale of Nervous Sleep* (1843).   Braid's ideas met with violent opposition, especially from the professional mesmerists, who wished to keep their exhibits upon a miraculous basis, but his ideas were taken up by Azam, Broca, Charcot, Liébeault, Bernheim, and became the true starting-point of the French school.[1]   Hypnotism was first used in surgical operations by John **Elliotson** (1791–1868), a professor of practice in the University of London and president

---

[1] Wilhelm Preyer translated Braid's complete works into German in 1882.

of the Royal Medical and Chirurgical Society, who, in 1843, published a pamphlet describing "Numerous Cases of Surgical Operations Without Pain in the Mesmeric State." Dispute about this led to his resignation from his various offices. A far more impressive record was made by James **Esdaile** (1808–59), of Montrose, Scotland, who, in 1845, began to try hypnotism in operating on Hindu convicts. He performed over 100 such operations with success, having been put to a severe test by the Deputy Governor of Bengal, and eventually had a record of 261 painless operations with a mortality of 5.5 per cent., which he described in his book, "Mesmerism in India" (1846). On returning to Scotland, Esdaile found that, except in disease, the self-contained Europeans differed from the impressionable, neurotic Hindus in not being specially susceptible to the hypnotic trance.

German medicine, in the first half of the nineteenth century, labored under the disadvantage of being split up into schools. Exhausted by the Napoleonic wars, and existing mainly as a set of petty principalities, with only a vague racial and political solidarity, the German people had to endure a long period of brutal military régime, as a natural sequel of the previous struggle against foreign invasion. In consequence, the best minds of the time were driven into various idealistic modes of thought, a fermentation which came to a head in the Revolution of 1848. During this period of idealism, the gods of their worship were Schelling and Hegel; and clinical medicine was dominated by the fanciful reveries of the **Nature-Philosophy School,** of which Schelling himself was, indeed, the founder. Its principal spirit was the Bavarian naturalist, Lorenz **Oken** (1779–1851), editor of the journal "Isis" and a founder of the first German Congress of Naturalists and Physicians (1822), in whom great originality of thought went hand in hand with much ineptitude. He accepted and expanded Goethe's vertebrate theory of the skull (in 1806), regarded the flesh as a conglomeration of infusoria (cells), and glorified the male element in nature to the extent of declaring that "Ideally every child should be a boy." Other members of the school, such as Döllinger, Görres, Treviranus and Steffens, drifted into a maze of incomprehensible jargon and fanciful distinctions as to the real and the ideal, identity, imponderables, polarities, irritability, metamorphosis, and the like. Hard upon the Nature-Philosophy School followed the Natural History School, which aimed to name and classify diseases after a rigid system, as in botany or zoölogy. This was succeeded by the rational or physiologic teaching of Roser and Wunderlich, Henle and Pfeufer, the forerunners of the scientific movement of German medicine, which was headed by the pupils of its prime mover, Johannes Müller. Apart from these, many strayed into such devious by-paths as Phrenology, Homœopathy, Rademacherism, Baunscheidtism, Hydropathy, Odic Force, Animal Magnetism, and other narrow and exclusive ways of conceiving the facts of medicine. The tendency of all these hole-and-corner schools was toward wholesale contempt for the scientific achievements of men like Bichat and Magendie, Laënnec and Louis, or the practical sense of such clinical workers as Bright, Stokes or Graves; and this tendency reached the limit of exaggeration in the doctrines of the New Vienna School, as stated by Skoda, Hamernijk and Dietl. Skoda said that while we can diagnose and describe disease, we dare not expect by any means to cure it. Dietl, in an oft-quoted utterance of 1851, announced that a physician must be judged, not by the success of his treatment but by the extent of his knowledge: "As long as medicine is art, it will not be science. As long as there are successful physicians there will be no scientific physicians." These ingenious paradoxes, which amounted virtually to a plea of impotence, made up the "therapeutic nihilism" of the New Vienna School. The Revolution of 1848 dissipated the silly doctrines of the Nature-Philosophy School into space, but the New Vienna School died hard, and Rokitansky had to be overthrown by Virchow, and Semmelweis had to sacrifice his life in proving his thesis before German medicine could finally emerge from the Happy Valley of speculation to gain the tableland of reality.[1]

The first to break away from the jargon of the Nature-Philosophy School was Johann Lucas **Schönlein** (1793–1864), of Bamberg, the founder of the so-called **Natural History School,** the ambition of which was, as we have said, to study medicine as descriptive botany and zoölogy are studied. Schönlein, his pupil, Carl Canstatt, and Conrad Heinrich Fuchs, all of them inspired by de Candolle's classification of plants, proceeded to make arbitrary classifications of disease, based, in each case, upon a very hazy *fundamentum divisionis,* not unlike those of Boissier de Sauvages in the eighteenth century. Schönlein, in particular, indulged in such whimsies as forcing gangrene of the uterus into the class "neurophlogoses" and cholera into the catarrhs. The real merits of Schönlein, however, are of a different order. In his clinic at the Charité, in Berlin, he was the first to lecture on medicine in German instead of Latin (1840), and was the founder of modern clinical teaching in Germany, introducing examinations of the blood and urine, chemical analysis, auscultation, percussion and

---

[1] For a brilliant and effective exposition of the intellectual follies of this period see Dr. A. Jacobi's account of his student days in Germany, in New York Med. Jour., 1901, lxxiii, 617–623.

microscopical investigations. He wrote little, his only contributions of importance being his description of peliosis rheumatica (Schönlein's disease) in 1837,[1] his discovery of the parasitic cause of favus (achorion Schönleinii) in 1839,[2] and his proposal of the terms "typhus abdominalis" and "typhus exanthematicus" to differentiate the latter diseases (1839). Schönlein was a man of peculiar character. During his later years in Berlin, he often affected the eccentricities of a recluse, denying himself to patients when it suited his whim, and otherwise treating them with the "godlike coarseness" of demeanor (göttliche Grobheit)[3] which was then the vogue. His scientific abilities have been ably set forth in the well-known eulogy of Virchow (1865),[4] but he seemed, alike to the delicate perception of Fanny Hensel and the plain common sense of Augustin Prichard, something of a boor.

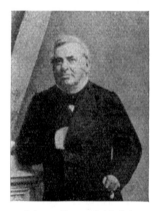

Johann Lucas Schönlein
(1793–1864).

Schönlein's pupil, Carl Friedrich **Canstatt** (1807–50), of Ratisbon, wrote a sterling text-book on practice, absolutely free from metaphysical dogma, which, says Jacobi,[5] was the "Bible of German medicine" until it was superseded by Niemeyer, as the latter was, in due course, by Strümpell.

The scientific movement in modern German medicine was started and kept in pace mainly through the medium of four important periodicals which stood out for exact investigation and exerted great influence upon the younger spirits in the speculative period, viz., Müller's *Archiv für Anatomie, Physiologie und wissenschaftliche Medicin* (1834), Henle and Pfeufer's *Zeitschrift für rationelle Medicin* (1841–69), Roser and Wunderlich's *Archiv für physiologische Heilkunde* (1842–59), and Virchow's *Archiv für pathologische Anatomie* (1847–1913). Of these able editors, Müller, Henle, and Virchow were the leaders in Germany

---

[1] Schönlein: Allg. u. spec. Path. u. Therap., Herisau, 1837, ii, 1848.

[2] Müller's Arch., Berlin, 1839, 82, 1 pl.

[3] The Homeric phrase occurs for the first time in Friedrich Schlegel's celebrated romance of "Lucinde." Virchow gives one (perhaps apocryphal) instance of Schönlein's rudeness. The latter was once consulted by an elderly physician, who, disconcerted by his brusque manner, pointed to his gray hairs. Schönlein retorted: *Auch die Esel sind grau!*

[4] Virchow: Gedächtnissrede auf Lucas Schönlein, Berlin, 1865.

[5] Jacobi: *Op. cit.*, p. 622.

of comparative, histologic and pathologic anatomy respectively, and Müller, in particular, was the greatest German physiologist of his time. Wunderlich was perhaps the most original clinician. Carl Reinhold August **Wunderlich** (1815–77), of Württemberg, graduated at Tübingen in 1837 and taught medicine there until 1850, when he succeeded to Oppolzer's chair at Leipzig (1850–77). He wrote a good treatise on practice (1858) and an excellent history of medicine (1859), but his masterpiece is undoubtedly his treatise on the relations of animal heat in disease (1868),[1] which is the very foundation of our present clinical thermometry. About 1850,

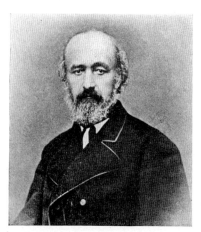

Clausius, Helmholtz, and Sir William Thomson had worked out the mathematical relations of the laws governing heat-transformations, and, in 1849, Thomson (Lord Kelvin) had established his "absolute scale of temperature," without which no thermometers could be reliable. Upon this hint, Wunderlich made many careful observations of temperature in disease, tabulating his results, and, after the true significance of the thermal changes in the body were better understood,

Carl R. A. Wunderlich (1815–1877). (By kind permission of Frau Geheimrat Franz Hofmann-Wunderlich, Leipzig.)

thermometry became a recognized feature in clinical diagnosis, and new studies were made of fever and other pathologic problems in which the idea of temperature is involved. Before the time of Clausius, heat (caloric) was still regarded by many as a material substance, an idea which threw back the progress of medicine as much as did its parent and forerunner, the phlogiston theory of Stahl.[2] By utilizing the advanced thermodynamic knowledge of his time, Wunderlich made his book a permanent scientific classic.

---

[1] Wunderlich: Das Verhalten der Eigenwärme in Krankheiten, Leipzig, 1868.

[2] It is now charitably supposed that when Stahl and his followers maintained that if a body undergoes combustion, it gives off something (becomes "dephlogisticated"), they were clumsily groping in the direction of Carnot's principle that "Heat cannot flow from a colder to a warmer body." Even as late as 1865, we find such an able engineer as the hard-headed Rankine still believing that heat is an indestructible substance.

Josef **Skoda** (1805–81), of Pilsen, Bohemia, was the leading clinician of the **New Vienna School** and the exponent of its therapeutic nihilism. He was the first medical teacher in Vienna to lecture in German (1847), and taught nearly all his life in the Allgemeines Krankenhaus. His principal contribution to medicine is his treatise on percussion and auscultation (1839),[1] in which he attempts to classify the different sounds in the chest by categories, ranged according to musical pitch and tonality, and alternating from full to hollow, clear to dull, tympanitic to muffled, high to deep. Skoda's resonance, the drum-like sound heard in pneu-

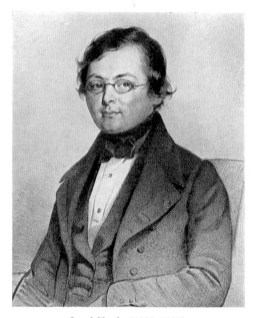

Josef Skoda (1805–1881).

monia and pericardial effusion, is a permanent part of modern diagnosis. Although little was known of the physics of sound in Skoda's time, his acoustic refinements were, in some respects, an improvement upon the loose descriptive terms used by the French clinicians of the period, so wittily exemplified in the "Stethoscope Song" of Dr. Holmes:

> "The *bruit de râpe* and the *bruit de scie*
> And the *bruit de diable* are all combined;
> How happy Bouillaud would be,
> If he a case like this could find."

---

[1] Skoda: Abhandlung über Perkussion und Auskultation, Vienna, 1839.

None the less, such an effective expression as Laënnec's "ægophony" still means a great deal to the ear of the modern practitioner. In recent times, Skoda's work has found further elaboration in the complicated instruments with Helmholtz resonators which some clinicians use to analyze the sounds of the chest for teaching purposes. Skoda was a whimsical, top-heavy old bachelor, who, as Baas relates, put up with queer clothes all his life for fear of offending his tailor (a personal friend), yet once sued a clergyman to obtain payment of a fee.[1] He looked upon his patients as objects of investigation merely, and, when it came to

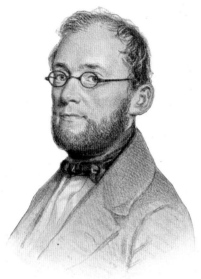

Carl Rokitansky (1804–1878).

treatment, said, with a shrug: *Ach, das ist ja alles eins!* This set a bad example. A diagnosis confirmed by a postmortem came to be a sort of shibboleth in Vienna, and snap-diagnoses (*Schnell-Diagnosen*) the fashion, even among practitioners who could not have differentiated the pitch and tonality of a heart-sound from a band of music.

Carl **Rokitansky** (1804–78), Skoda's colleague, was also a Bohemian, but a man of different type, genial and unassuming, where Skoda was pragmatic and pedantic; a graceful and witty writer, where Skoda was dry and dull. His Viennese *bonhomie* is sensed in his jest about his four sons, two of whom were physicians, the other two singers: *Die Einen heilen, die Anderen heulen*. Rokitansky did an enormous amount of pathologic work, and, it is said, had the disposal of between 1500 and 1800 cadavers annually. He made over 30,000 postmortems in his life. He was the first to detect bacteria in the lesions of malignant endocarditis, and to differentiate between lobar and lobular pneumonia, as also between Bright's disease and "Speckniere" (Virchow's amyloid degeneration of the kidney). He left a classic account of the pathologic appearances in acute yellow atrophy of the liver, giving the disease its present name (1843); described and defined the bronchitic and pulmonary complications of typhoid as broncho-

---

[1] Baas: *Op. cit.*, foot-note to p. 954.

typhus and pneumotyphus; and completed Laënnec's picture of emphysema of the lungs by describing the microscopic appearances of the same. In obstetrics and orthopedics, he is memorable as the first to describe the spondylolisthetic deformities (1839).[1] The value of the first edition of Rokitansky's treatise on pathological anatomy (1842–46)[2] was seriously impaired by his doctrine of "crases" and "stases," in which chemical states of substance were actually conceived of as being susceptible to "disease," and which was mercilessly chaffed out of existence by Virchow (1846).[3] The latter intimated that Rokitansky was in reality an adherent of the Natural History School, since he employed a bizarre terminology to describe things of which he had no ken, his chemical hypotheses of tissue changes being susceptible of a simpler and more purely mechanical explanation, while his attempt to revamp the ancient drivel about solidism and humoralism was a monstrous anachronism (*ein ungeheurer Anachronismus*). Virchow knew more chemistry than Rokitansky, but he cordially admitted that in picturing what was actually before him on the postmortem table his jolly Viennese rival was the ablest descriptive pathologist of his time. It is said that when the latter read Virchow's criticism, he could never bring himself to look at his unfortunate first edition again. Rokitansky's finest productions are unquestionably his monograph on diseases of the arteries (1852),[4] illustrated with 23 folio plates; and his great memoir on defects in the septum of the heart (1875),[5] the result of fourteen years' labor, giving his transposition theory of the deviation of the aortic septum. These works have been the subject of deep study by modern pathologists, in connection with the English classic of Thomas Bevill Peacock (1812–82) on malformations of the human heart (1866).

Johannes **von Oppolzer** (1808–71), also a Bohemian, was a clear-headed, extremely competent practitioner who steered clear of all haphazard theorizing, and, as professor at Leipzig, did much to popularize the Viennese innovations in Germany. He was noted for his quickness in offhand diagnosis. Hamernijk of Prague and Dietl of Cracow were the extremists in therapeutic

---

[1] Rokitansky: Med. Jahrb. des österreichischen Staates, Vienna, 1839, xix, 41; 195.

[2] Rokitansky: Handbuch der pathologischen Anatomie, Vienna, 1842–46.

[3] Virchow: Kritik des Rokitansky'schen Handbuchs der pathologischen Anatomie. Med.-Ztg. (Verein f. Heilk. in Preussen), Berlin, 1846, xv, Lit. Beilage, Nos. 49, 50, pp. 237, 243.

[4] Rokitansky: Ueber einige der wichtigsten Krankheiten der Arterien, Denkschr. d. k. Akad. d. Wissensch., Vienna, 1852, iv, 1–72.

[5] Die Defekte der Scheidewande des Herzens, Vienna, 1875.

nihilism, and the latter is now remembered only by the painful symptoms in floating kidney (Dietl's crises), attributable to a kink in the ureters or renal vessels, which he described in 1864.

Perhaps the most brilliant name of the New Vienna School, after Skoda's and Rokitansky's, was that of **Ferdinand von Hebra** (1816–80), of Brünn in Moravia, a pupil of both these masters, and the founder of the histologic school of **dermatology,** the second phase in its modern development. Hebra's classification of skin diseases (1845)[1] was based upon their pathological anatomy, and while complicated and artificial, lacking the simplicity of Willan's, it opened out new lines of investigation, in which his pupils, Kaposi, Neumann and Pick, played a prominent part. Hebra regarded most cutaneous disorders as purely local, and, from this viewpoint,

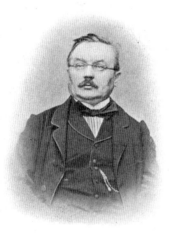

Ferdinand von Hebra (1816–1880).

devised many effective modes of treatment. Yet, as a champion of nihilistic therapy, he is said to have followed Skoda in feigning treatment in some cases in order to demonstrate to his own satisfaction that they could get well of themselves. Hebra revived the use of mercurials in syphilis and gave the classical accounts of lichen exsudativus ruber (1857)[2] and eczema marginatum (1860).[3] He also did much to clear up obscure points in classification and nomenclature, and was the first to describe impetigo herpetiformis (1872),[4] although the final account of the latter disease was completed by his son-in-law, Kaposi, in 1887.[5] Hebra's clinic was one of the most popular in Vienna, on account of his genial, offhand style of lecturing, and his keen, often sarcastic, humor.

The greatest single achievement of the New Vienna School was the determination of the true cause and prophylaxis of **puerperal fever.** In the eighteenth century, Charles White, of Manchester,

---

[1] F. von Hebra: Versuch einer auf pathologischer Anatomie gegründeten Eintheilung der Hautkrankheiten. Ztschr. d. k. k. Gesellsch. d. Aerzte zu Wien, 1845, i, 34; 142, 211.

[2] Allg. Wien. med. Ztg., 1857, ii, 95.

[3] Handb. d. spec. Path. u. Therap. (Virchow), 1860, iii, 31, 1. Abth., pp. 361–363.

[4] Wien. med. Wochenschr., 1872, xxii, 1197–1201.

[5] Kaposi: Vrtljschr. f. Dermat., Vienna, 1887, xiv, 273–296, 5 pl.

England, had enlarged upon the advantages of scrupulous cleanliness in these cases, and on February 13, 1843, **Oliver Wendell Holmes** (1815–94) read to the Boston Society for Medical Improvement his paper *On the Contagiousness of Puerperal Fever*,[1] in which he announced that women in child-bed should never be attended by physicians who have been conducting postmortem sections or cases of puerperal fever; that the latter disease may be conveyed in this manner from patient to patient, even from a case of erysipelas; and that washing the hands in calcium chloride and changing the clothes after leaving a puerperal fever case was held to be a preventive measure. Holmes's essay stirred up violent opposition on the part of the Philadelphia obstetricians, Hodge and Meigs, and, in 1855, he returned to the charge in his monograph on "Puerperal Fever as a Private Pestilence," in which he reiterated his views and stated that one "Senderein" had lessened the mortality of puerperal fever by disinfecting the hands with chloride of lime and the nail-brush. This Senderein was Ignaz Philipp **Semmelweis** (1818–65), a Hungarian pupil of Skoda's and Rokitansky's, who, in 1846, had become an assistant in the first obstetric ward of the Allgemeines Krankenhaus in Vienna. This ward had acquired such a high mortality in puerperal cases that women begged in tears not to be taken into it. Semmelweis had noticed that the first ward differed from the second (which had a lower mortality-rate) in that students came into it directly from the dissecting-room for instruction, often making vaginal examinations with unclean hands, while in the second ward, devoted to the instruction of midwives, much greater attention was paid to personal cleanliness. With this idea in mind, he also made a careful study of the autopsies in the fatal puerperal cases. In 1847,

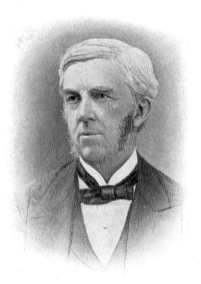

Oliver Wendell Holmes (1815–94).

---

[1] Holmes: N. Engl. Quart. Jour. Med. and Surg., Boston, 1842–43, i, 503–530.

24

Kolletschka, Rokitansky's assistant, died of a dissection-wound, and Semmelweis was present at the postmortem. As he stood beside the body of his former instructor, he noticed that the pathologic appearances were the same as in the unfortunate puerperæ of the first ward, and he now had his chain of evidence complete. He immediately instituted such precautions in the handling of labor cases that the mortality curve sank from 9.92 to 3.8 per cent. In the following year, he had a mortality as low as 1.27 per cent., and all through the simple expedient of washing the hands in a calcium chloride solution in connection with pregnancy and the conduct of labor.

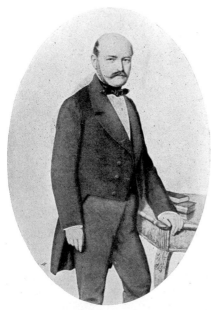

Semmelweis is thus the true pioneer of antisepsis in obstetrics, and while Holmes antedated him in some details by five years, the superiority of his work over that of his predecessor lies not only in the stiff fight he put up for his ideas, but in the all-important fact that he recognized puerperal fever as a blood-poisoning or septicemia (1847–49).[1] Like Holmes, he met with fierce opposition, and while Rokitansky, Hebra, Michaelis, and, to his lasting honor, Skoda stood by him, he was persecuted by Scanzoni, Carl Braun, and the orthodox obstetricians of the day. Disgusted, he suddenly left Vienna for Budapest, where he became in due course professor of obstetrics at the University (1855) and published his immortal treatise on "The Cause, Concept, and Prophylaxis of Puerperal Fever" (1861),[2] as well as his scathing "Open Letters to Sundry Professors of Obstetrics" (1861). But his sensitive nature was not equal to the strain of violent controversy, and brooding over

Ignaz Philipp Semmelweis (1818–65).

---

[1] Semmelweis' original communication is entitled "Höchst wichtige Erfahrungen über die Aetiologie der in Gebäranstalten epidemischen Puerperalfieber." Ztschr. d. k. k. Gesellsch. d. Aerzte in Wien, 1847–48, iv, pt. 2, 242; 1849, v, 64.

[2] Semmelweis: Die Aetiologie, der Begriff und die Prophylaxis des Kindbettfiebers, Budapest and Vienna, 1861.

his wrongs brought on insanity and death. He is one of medicine's martyrs and, in the future, will be one of its far-shining names, for every child-bearing woman owes something to him.

Medicine is also indebted to the New Vienna School for the introduction of **laryngoscopy and rhinoscopy.** On March 18, 1829,[1] a rude "glottiscope" was exhibited to the Hunterian Society of London by Benjamin Babington (1794–1866), of Guy's Hospital, and, in 1837, the Scotch surgeon, Robert Liston, described his mode of exploring the larynx.[2] These efforts passed unnoticed, however, and the modern laryngoscope came to be invented by Manuel **Garcia** (1805–1906), a Spanish singing teacher in London, who sent an account of his instrument to the Royal Society in 1855.[3] Three years later, his method of examining the throat was made a permanent part of laryngology by the Viennese neurologist, Ludwig **Türck** (1810–68), and his colleague, Johann Nepomuk **Czermak** (1828–73), of Bohemia, both publishing their initial communications in the same year (1858).[4] Separate treatises on laryngoscopy by the same writers appeared in 1860, and, about the same time, Czermak devised a method of exploring the nose and nasopharynx by means of small mirrors (1859–60).[5] Türck wrote an important treatise on diseases of the larynx, with atlas (1866),[6] and was an able neurologist, his studies on the sensible cutaneous areas of the separate spinal nerves (1856–68) being classic. He was also the first to note the correlation of retinal hemorrhage with tumors of the brain (1853).[7]

Other prominent members of the New Vienna School were Josef Hyrtl, the great anatomist, the physiologist Ernst von Brücke, the ophthalmologists Beer, Arlt, Stellwag von Carion, and Jaeger von Jaxtthal, Adam Politzer the otologist, the clinicians Bamberger, Winternitz, and Nothnagel, and the neurologists Meynert, Benedikt, and Ritter von Rittershain. Virchow was almost the only German spirit of his time who appreciated Bichat and Magendie, Bright and Addison, and it was largely due to the eminently practical tendency of these physicians of the New

---

[1] Babington: London Med. Gaz., 1829, iii, 555.

[2] Liston: Practical Surgery, London, 1837, p. 350.

[3] Garcia: Proc. Roy. Soc. London, 1854–55, vii, 399–410.

[4] Türck: Ztschr. d. k. k. Gesellsch. d. Aerzte zu Wien, 1858, xiv, 401; 1859, xv, 817. Czermak: Sitzungsb. d. k. Akad. d. Wissensch. Math.-naturw. Cl., Vienna, 1858, xxix, 557–584. Also Wien. med. Wochenschr., 1858, viii, 196; 1859, ix, 22; 145, et seq.

[5] Czermak: Wien. med. Wochenschr., 1859, ix, 518; 1860, x, 257.

[6] Türck: Klinik der Krankheiten des Kehlkopfes und der Luftröhre, Vienna, 1866.

[7] Türck: Ztschr. d. k. k. Gesellsch. d. Aerzte zu Wien, 1853, i, 214–218.

Vienna School—most of them Slavs—that German medicine finally crossed the Rubicon.

One other prominent feature of German medicine in the early part of the nineteenth century has yet to be mentioned, namely, the rise of **homeopathy,** which, in point of time, is really one of the many isolated theoretic systems of the preceding century. Its founder, Samuel Christian Friedrich Hahnemann (1755-1843), of Meissen, took his degree at Erlangen in 1779, and toward the end of the century, as the result of certain experiments, some of them made upon his own person, began to formulate those theories which characterize his system. These are, first, a revival of the old Paracelsian doctrine of signatures, namely, that diseases or symptoms of diseases are curable by those particular drugs which produce similar pathologic effects upon the body (*similia similibus curantur*); second, that the dynamic effect of drugs is heightened by giving them in infinitesimally small doses, which are to be obtained by carrying dilution or trituration to an extreme limit; third, the notion that most chronic diseases are only a manifestation of suppressed itch or "Psora." These doctrines were embodied in his "Organon der rationellen Heilkunde" (1810), and found wide acceptance, especially in the New World. The extreme popularity of Hahnemann's doctrines is probably due to the fact that they lessened the scale of dosage of drugs in practice. He was, in fact, the introducer of the small dose. Otherwise his system is but an offshoot of eighteenth century theorizing. He died a millionaire in Paris in 1843.

Of the earlier **American clinicians,** those who did the most original work were Otto, the Jacksons, North, the elder Mitchell, Ware, Gerhard, and Drake.

John Conrad **Otto** (1774-1844), born at Woodbridge, New Jersey, of German-American stock, took his medical degree at the University of Pennsylvania in 1796, succeeded Benjamin Rush at the Philadelphia Dispensary in 1813, and taught clinical medicine at the Pennsylvania Hospital for twenty-one years. He played an active part in the cholera epidemic of 1833, and is especially remembered by his paper on hemophilia (1803),[1] an investigation of a family of "bleeders," which was the first account of the condition in literature.

James Jackson (1777-1868), of Boston, a pupil of Louis, was the first physician to the Massachusetts General Hospital (1810), wrote an early text-book on practice (1825), and was widely read in his attractive "Letters to a Young Physician" (1855). He left one of the earliest accounts of alcoholic neuritis, which he

---

[1] J. C. Otto: Med. Respository, New York, 1803, vi, 1-4.

described as "arthrodynia à potu" (1822),[1] outlining the mental symptoms, and his report on typhoid fever (1838)[2] played a great part in putting the disease upon a definite basis in this country.

Jackson's son, James Jackson, jr. (1810–34), whose early death robbed American medicine of one of Louis' most promising pupils, left a valuable memoir on the cholera epidemic of 1832 and first described the prolonged expiratory sound as an important diagnostic sign of incipient phthisis (1833).[3]

Elisha **North** (1771–1843), of Goshen, Connecticut, was a pioneer in Jennerian vaccination (1800), established the first eye infirmary in the United

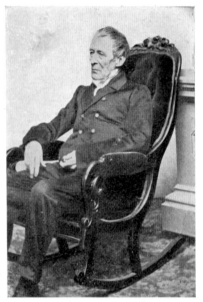

James Jackson (1777–1868).

States at New London (1817), and, in 1811, published the first book on cerebrospinal meningitis ("spotted fever"), in which he recommends the use of the clinical thermometer.

John Kearsley Mitchell (1793–1858), of Virginia, was educated in Scotland, graduated from the University of Pennsylvania in 1819, and after making three sea voyages as a ship's surgeon, commenced practice in Philadelphia, where he became eminent

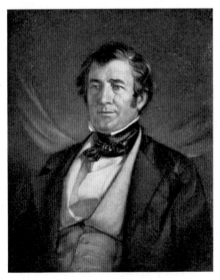

John Kearsley Mitchell (1793–1858).

[1] J. Jackson: New Engl. Jour. Med. and Surg., 1822, ii, 351.

[2] J. Jackson: Report founded on the cases of typhoid fever, Boston, 1838.

[3] Communicated to the Société médicale d'observation de Paris in 1833.

as an internist, neurologist, and teacher. The volume of monographs collected after his death by his distinguished son (1859)[1]
reveals an originality of mind far above the average, and, like the
latter, he was talented in poetry and fiction as well. He wrote
ably and suggestively on mesmerism, osmosis, liquefaction, and
solidification of carbonic acid gas, and ligature of limbs in spastic
conditions, and he was the first to describe the neurotic spinal ar-
thropathies (1831),[2] which have since been developed by Charcot,
Bechtereff, Strümpell, and Marie. His essay *On the Cryptogamous
Origin of Malarious and Epidemic Fevers* (1849) files the first brief
for the parasitic etiology of disease on *à priori* grounds—a rigorous,
logical argument which, as pure theory goes, ranks with Henle's
essay on miasms and contagia (1840).

John **Ware** (1795–1864), of Hingham, Massachusetts, a Harvard graduate, who was professor of practice at Harvard from 1832
to 1858, wrote an important monograph on croup (1842),[3] and his
exhaustive study of delirium tremens (1831)[4] is, in connection with
the earlier paper of Thomas Sutton (1813), the classic account
of this neurosis.

Jacob **Bigelow** (1787–1879), of Massachusetts, was one of the
greatest of American botanists, the three volumes of his "American
Medical Botany" (1817–20), illustrated with 60 plates and 6000
colored engravings, technically devised by himself, being a work
of international reputation, and, in America, only approached by
the writings of Barton, Raffinesque, Porcher, and Asa Gray.
Bigelow was visiting physician to the Massachusetts General
Hospital, professor of materia medica at Harvard, and a great
medical reformer. During the cholera epidemic of 1832 his wise
sanitary rulings limited the mortality in Boston to 100, as against
3000 in New York city. His discourse "On Self-limited Diseases"
(1835) exerted a powerful influence upon medical practice in the
United States, and, in the words of Dr. Holmes, did "more than
any other work or essay in our own language to rescue the practice
of medicine from the slavery to the drugging system which was a
part of the inheritance of the profession."

William Wood **Gerhard** (1809–72), born in Philadelphia, of
German extraction, was perhaps the most brilliant American pupil
of Louis. He was resident physician to the Pennsylvania Hospital
(1834–68), taught the institutes of medicine at the University of

---

[1] J. K. Mitchell: Five Essays, edited by S. Weir Mitchell, Philadelphia,
1859.
[2] Am. Jour. Med. Sc., Phila., 1831, viii, 55–64.
[3] Ware: "Contributions to the History and Diagnosis of Croup," Boston,
1842.
[4] Med. Communicat. Mass. Med. Soc., Boston, 1830–36, v, 136–194.

Pennsylvania (1838–72), and was much beloved in his native city for his geniality and kindliness. He investigated the endermic application of medicines (1830), described (with Pennock) the cholera epidemic at Paris in 1832, and wrote interesting papers on smallpox (1832)[1] and pneumonia (1834)[2] in children. His treatise on diseases of the chest (1842) was the most authoritative American work on the subject before the time of Flint. He left two contributions of enduring value, his monograph on tubercular meningitis in children (1833),[3] the first accurate clinical study of the disease, and his paper on differential diagnosis of typhus and typhoid fevers (1837),[4] which, in the United States at least, definitely settled the clinical and pathological status of the two affections. Isolated observers, like Willis in 1643,[5] Huxham in 1737,[6] or Hildenbrand in 1810,[7] had no doubt distinguished between the two diseases to their own satisfaction; but the subject remained upon a hazy basis until the time of Gerhard, for even Louis' masterpiece of 1829 took no cognizance of typhus fever, and British practitioners, with the possible exception of A. P. Stewart (1840)[8] or Perry of Glasgow, did not clearly separate typhus from typhoid until Sir William Jenner pointed the way in 1849.[9]

The greatest physician of the West, and one of the most picturesque figures in American medicine, was **Daniel Drake** (1785–1852), who was the first after Hippocrates and Sydenham to do much for medical geography, and has a unique position of his own in relation to the topography of disease. He was born in New Jersey in abject poverty, was reared in a log-cabin among the Kentucky pioneers, and the story of his struggles to gain an education, self-aided and single-handed, his rise to the height of his profession in the face of almost every obstacle, is a fine example of what honest ability can accomplish if persistent. A pupil of William Goforth, the pioneer of Jennerian vaccination in the West, his diploma, made out in the latter's handwriting, was the first to be issued west of the Alleghanies, although, in practice, Drake did not complete his medical education until 1815, when he received an academic degree at the University of Pennsylvania. He was one of Osler's "peripatetic physicians," constantly moving from

---

[1] Gerhard: Am. Jour. Med. Sc., Phila., 1832, xi, 368–408.

[2] *Ibid.*, 1834, xiv, 328; 1834–35, xv, 87.

[3] Gerhard: Am. Jour. Med. Sc., Phila., 1833, xiii, 313–359.

[4] Gerhard: *Ibid.*, 1837, xx, 289–322.

[5] Willis: De febribus, 1634, ch. xiv, xvii.

[6] Huxham: Essay on Fevers, 1755.

[7] J. V. von Hildenbrand: Ueber den ansteckenden Typhus, Vienna, 1810.

[8] Stewart: Edinb. Med. & Surg. Jour., 1840, 1 pl., liv, 289–369.

[9] Sir W. Jenner: Med. Chir. Tr., London, 1849–50, xxxiii, 23–42.

place to place in aid of the cause of medical education, "ever at war with man" (for his nature was combative), and apparently dissatisfied with every condition he met. He changed his locality as a teacher no less than seven times during his life, and two important medical faculties, the Medical College of Ohio (1821) and the Medical Department of Cincinnati College (1835), were founded by him. In the latter venture, he had as associates some of the best American teachers of his day, including Samuel D. Gross and Willard Parker. Drake was also the founder of the *"Western Journal of the Medical and Physical Sciences"* (1827–38), the

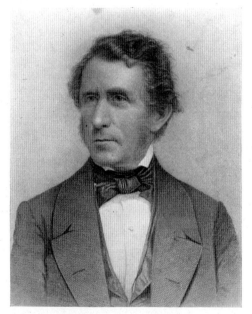

Daniel Drake (1785–1852).

most important medical periodical of the West in its time. It contains his celebrated essays on Medical Education, which were reprinted in 1832, and are, far and away, the most important contributions ever made to the subject in this country. They are written in a style which, for clarity and beauty, is, even today, a perfect model of what such writing should be. In 1841, Drake published one of the first accounts in literature on the local disorder known as "the trembles," or milk sickness.[1] He also described

---

[1] Early accounts were those of Thomas Barbee, in "Notices Concerning Cincinnati" (1809), and by Alexander Telford and Arthur Stewart in Med. Repository, New York, 1812, xv, 92–94.

epidemic cholera as it appeared in Cincinnati in 1832, and wrote a number of papers on the evils of city life (1831), mesmerism (1844), moral defects in medical students (1847), and an entertaining posthumous work on "Pioneer Life in Kentucky" (1870); but his crowning achievement was the great work on the *Diseases of the Interior Valley of North America* (1850–54), the result of thirty years' labor, based largely upon personal observation made during extensive travel. The first volume is a wonderful encyclopedia of the topography, hydrography, climate and meteorology, plants and animals, population (including diet, habitat and occupations), of the Mississippi Valley. The second volume, not published until after his death, treats of the autumnal malarial and other fevers, yellow fever, typhus fever, the exanthemata, and the unclassified "phlogistic fevers," in relation to topographic, meteorologic, and sociologic features. There was nothing like this book in literature, unless it might be Hippocrates on Airs, Waters, and Places, and even the latter made no attempt to map out or triangulate the geographical locale of disease. In its practical intention, Drake's book belongs in the class described by Billings as distinctively and peculiarly American, "in subject, mode of treatment, and style of composition."[1] When Alfred Stillé reported upon it to the American Medical Association in 1850, Drake was greeted with prolonged and thunderous demonstrations of enthusiasm and applause, such as had seldom been accorded to any physician before. "He covered his face with his hands and wept like a child." In connection with Drake's masterpiece, two of his earlier pamphlets should not be forgotten, for they are among the rarest of Americana. The first, a pamphlet on the Climate and Diseases of Cincinnati (1810), was the germ of the greater work; the second, his "Narrative of the Rise and Fall of the Medical College of Ohio" (1822), is one of the choicest bits of medical humor in existence. Drake, as described by Gross, was a tall, commanding figure, simple and dignified in manner. "He was always well dressed, and around his neck he had a long gold watch-chain, which rested loosely upon his vest." As a lecturer he had a splendid voice, and was possessed of fiery eloquence, causing him at times to sway to and fro like a tree in a storm. He was gentle, fond of children, hating coarseness, and had a genuine poetic side, writing very creditable verses.

---

[1] J. S. Billings, in "A Century of American Medicine," Philadelphia, 1876, p. 314. Dr. Billings was the first to emphasize the importance of Drake in American medicine. The latter has since been made the subject of an elaborate and excellent biography by Dr. Otto Juettner of Cincinnati (Daniel Drake and his Followers, Cincinnati, Harvey Publ. Co., 1909), which gives a detailed account of Western medicine in the early days, and should be read by all who wish to understand the conditions of the time.

Yet, although he practically created decent medical teaching in Cincinnati, he was subjected to many snubs and insults by snobs who affected to look down upon his origin and early chances. He assigned as a reason for not going to Europe that he did not wish to meet physicians who might plume themselves upon possessing greater advantages than himself, and said, with pathetic feeling, "I think too much of my country to place myself in so awkward a position."

Other prominent American physicians of the early period were George Bacon Wood (1797–1879) and Franklin Bache (1792–1864), of Philadelphia, who collaborated in the huge "Dispensatory of the United States" (1833), which ran through 17 editions; Alonzo Clark (1807–87), of New York, who introduced the opium treatment of peritonitis (1855)[1]; Elisha Bartlett (1804–55), of Rhode Island; John Y. Bassett (1805–81); Osler's "Alabama student," and Samuel Henry Dickson (1798–1872), of South Carolina, a trio of elegant and attractive medical stylists and litterateurs; that belligerent Celt, Charles Caldwell (1772–1853), of North Carolina, who founded two medical schools in the West, and whose "Autobiography" (1855) is a remarkable diatribe, surcharged with venom and rancor; Robley Dunglison (1798–1869), of Keswick, England, who compiled an excellent medical dictionary (1833) and wrote an amazing array of text-books on nearly every subject except surgery; David Hosack (1769–1835), in his day the best known practitioner in New York city, and editor of the "American Medical and Philosophical Register" (1810–14), in which work he was assisted by John Wakefield Francis (1789–1861), a German-American physician who came to enjoy something of Hosack's popularity in New York, was an attractive teacher and writer and something of a medical Mæcenas in the city; Nathaniel Chapman (1780–1853), of Virginia, a prominent teacher of clinical medicine at the University of Pennsylvania, who, in 1820, with Matthew Carey, founded the "Philadelphia Journal of the Medical and Physical Sciences," which, in 1827, under the guidance of Isaac Hays (1796–1879), became the "American Journal of the Medical Sciences" (Hay's Journal); Theodoric Romeyn Beck (1791–1855), of New York, whose "Elements of Medical Jurisprudence" (1823) was easily the best American work on the subject in its day, running through 10 editions and many translations; and Isaac Ray (1807–81), of Beverly, Massachusetts, who wrote the first treatise on the medical jurisprudence of insanity (1838), a solid, well-written book which is still of value.

Of isolated discoveries in internal medicine in the first half of the nineteenth century, we may mention the original description of "kondee," or sleeping sickness, in the African travels of Thomas Winterbottom (1803)[2]; the first accounts of cerebrospinal meningitis by Gaspard Vieusseux (1746–1814) at Geneva (1805),[3] and by L. Danielsson and E. Mann at Medfield, Massachusetts (1806)[4]; Charles Badham's little monograph on bronchitis, to which he gave the name (1808)[5]; Allan Burns on endocarditis (1809)[6]; William

---

[1] Clark: On the treatment of puerperal peritonitis by large doses of opium, 1855.

[2] Winterbottom: An Account of the Native Africans, London, 1803, vol. ii, pp. 29–31.

[3] Vieusseux: Jour. de méd., chir., pharm., etc., Paris, 1805, xi, 163–182.

[4] Danielsson and Mann: Med. & Agric. Register, Boston, 1806.

[5] Badham: Observations on the Inflammatory Affections of the Mucous Membrane of the Bronchiæ, London, 1808.

[6] Burns: Observations on Some of the Most Frequent and Important Diseases of the Heart, Edinburgh, 1809.

Charles Wells on rheumatism of the heart (1812)[1]; Romberg's thesis on achondroplasia (1817)[2]; John Clarke's account of laryngismus stridulus and tetany in children (1815);[3] John Bostock on hay-fever (1819)[4]; Louyer-Villermay's classic paper on appendicitis (1826)[5]; Kopp's description of "asthma thymicum" and "thymus-death" (1830)[6]; Lobstein's account of fragility of the bones, or osteopsathyrosis (1833)[7]; Carl Adolph Basedow's important paper on exophthalmic goiter, giving the three classic symptoms or "Merseburg triad" (1840)[8]; Mohr's case of tumor of the pituitary body with obesity (1840)[9]; Jakob Heine's monograph on infantile poliomyelitis (1840)[10]; Perrin on intermittent hydrarthrosis (1845)[11]; the independent accounts of leukemia by Virchow and John Hughes Bennett (1845)[12]; and Curling's note of the connection of absence of the thyroid with "symmetric swellings of fat tissue at the sides of the neck connected with defective cerebral development," or myxedema (1850).[13]

The neurological discoveries of the period will be considered later.

The earliest nineteenth century exponent of **anatomy** and of scientific medicine in France was Marie-François-Xavier **Bichat** (1771–1802), the creator of descriptive anatomy. The son of a physician, the favorite pupil, assistant, and household intimate of the surgeon Desault, and sometime an army surgeon in the French Revolution, Bichat soon developed from a light-hearted, rollicking, happy-go-lucky student into a successful surgeon and a master-worker in the science which sustained one of its gravest losses by his early death. His *Traité des membranes* (1799–1800), his five-volume "*Anatomie Descriptive*" (1801–03), and his work on general anatomy applied to physiology and medicine (1802) opened out an entirely new field for anatomists, that of a detailed description of the parts and tissues of the body in health and disease. Before Bichat's time, such text-books as those of the Monros were woefully rudimentary in spots and said next to nothing about

---

[1] Wells: Tr. Soc. Improve. Med. & Chir. Knowledge, 1804–10, London, 1812, iii, 373–412.

[2] M. H. Romberg: De rachitide congenita, Berlin, 1817.

[3] J. Clarke: Commentaries on some of the most important diseases of children, London, 1815, pp. 86–97.

[4] Bostock: Med.-Chir. Tr., London, 1819, x, 161–165.

[5] Louyer-Villermay: Arch. gén. de méd., Paris, 1824, v, 246–250.

[6] J. Kopp: Denkwürdigkeiten in der ärztlichen Praxis, Frankfurt a. M. 1830, i, 1; 368.

[7] Lobstein: Traité de l'anat. path., Paris, 1833, ii, 204–212.

[8] Basedow: Wchnschr. f. d. ges. Heilk., Berlin, 1840, vi, 197; 220.

[9] Mohr: Wchnschr. f. d. ges. Heilk., Berlin, 1840, 565–571.

[10] Heine: Beobachtungen über Lähmungszustände der untern Extremitäten und deren Behandlung, Stuttgart, 1840.

[11] Perrin: Jour. de méd., Paris, 1845, ii, 82. Union méd., Paris, 1878, 3, s. xxv, 821.

[12] Virchow: "Weisses Blut," in Neue Notizen a. d. Geb. d. Nat. u. Heilk., Weimar, 1845, xxv, 151–155. Bennett: Edinb. Med. & Surg. Jour., 1845, lxiv, 413–423.

[13] Curling: Med.-Chir. Tr., London, 1850, xxxiii, 303.

the detailed anatomy of the nerves and viscera; while teaching by dissection, as Robert Knox has recorded, was on the most rough and ready basis. Bichat was a forerunner of Henle and the histologists, dividing the tissues into 21 (non-microscopic) varieties, which he treated as indivisible parts, like the elements in chemistry, each tissue having its own particular kind of sensibility and contractility (*propriétés vitales*). Like Hunter, he regarded disease as an alteration of vital properties or principles. His error was to assign a specific vital property, a different mode of vitalism, to each tissue. This physiologic doctrine, now obsolete, is summed up in his famous and fallacious definition of life as "the sum of the forces that resist death,"[1] which, as has been often observed,[2] is only a

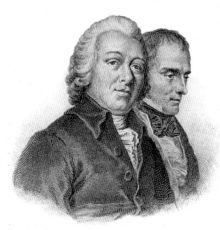

Desault (1744–95) and Bichat (1771–1802).

question-begging truism in the form of a reversible equation, in fact, a simple case of arguing in a circle.

In connection with Bichat's work may be mentioned the splendid atlas, "Anatomie de l'homme" (Paris, 1821–31), by Jules-Germain Cloquet (1790–1883), consisting of five volumes illustrated with 300 folio plates; and the discovery of the third corpuscles or blood-platelets by Alexandre Donné (1801–78) in 1842.[3]

Bichat's ideas were carried into pathology by Jean **Cruveilhier** (1791–1873), of Limoges, a pupil of Dupuytren's, who gave the first description (with plates) of disseminated sclerosis[4] and left an early description of progressive muscular atrophy of the Aran-

[1] Bichat: Recherches sur la vie et la mort, Paris, an viii (1800), p. 1.

[2] For example, in the inaugural dissertation of Dr. Abraham Jacobi (Cogitationes de vita rerum naturalium, Cologne, 1851, p. 24): "Prioribus iam temporibus Bichat alio modo vitam definire conatus est. Vitam igitur qualitatum et actionum materiæ *morte resistentium*, complexum nominat. Sed hæc num definitio est? num aliud est, quam circulus? Statim interrogandum erit *quidnam sit mors*, et quod solum respondere poteristis, id erit, mortem absentiam esse vitæ. Mors, constituta notione vitæ, vitæ negatione definienda est, non vice versa."

[3] Donné: Compt. rend. Acad. d. sc., Paris, 1842, xiv, 366–368.

[4] Cruveilhier: Anatomie pathologique, Paris, 1835–42, ii, livraison xxxviii, pl. 5.

Duchenne type (Cruveilhier's palsy), but, like Hunter before him, was led to the erroneous deduction that pyemia is the result of phlebitis, pushing his theory, indeed, to the extent of asserting that "Phlebitis dominates all pathology." Cruveilhier's atlases of pathology (1842) are among the most splendidly illustrated books on the subject. He did not use the microscope, and his errors were afterward corrected, as we shall see, by Virchow.

Sir Charles Bell (1774–1842), the leading British anatomist of the period, is now more celebrated as a physiologist and neurologist. The son of a Scotch Episcopal clergyman, he was a brother of John Bell, the well-known surgeon, who opened a private school

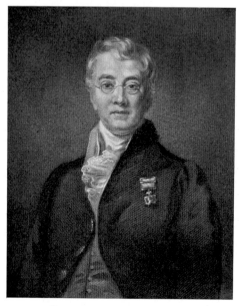

Sir Charles Bell (1774–1842).

of anatomy at Edinburgh in 1790. Both the Bells had an uncommon artistic gift, and Charles, in particular, illustrated his "System of Dissections" (1798), his "Engravings of the Brain and Nervous System" (1802), and his Bridgewater treatise on the hand (1833) with exquisite sketches. Coming up to London in 1804, he began teaching anatomy in his own house and later at Great Windmill Street. He also lectured to artists, his "Anatomy of Expression" (1806) being the result of these studies. Through his ardent devotion to private investigation, he never acquired the practice he had hoped for in London, and eventually accepted the chair of surgery at Edinburgh in 1836.   In 1811, Bell published "A New Idea of the Anatomy of the Brain and Nervous System," which contains the following sentence: "On laying bare the roots of the spinal nerves, I found that I could cut across the posterior fasciculus of nerves which took its origin from the posterior portion of the spinal marrow without convulsing the muscles of the back, but that, on touching the anterior fasciculus with the point of the knife, the muscles of the back were immediately convulsed." This is the first experimental reference to the functions of the spinal nerve-roots in literature, but Bell vitiated the effects of his discovery, to some extent, by holding fast to the old theory that all nerves are sensory, classifying them as "sensible and insensible," and, in reality, he demonstrated clearly the functions of the anterior roots only. An anatomist by training, his subsequent discoveries were all, in his own phrase, "deductions from anatomy," largely, no doubt, on account of his dislike of vivisection, and he failed to understand the true bearings of the experiment he had made or to interpret it correctly. The conclusive experimental proof that the anterior roots are motor, the posterior sensory, was made by Magendie upon a litter of eight puppies and published in 1822,[1] and confirmed by Johannes Müller in the frog in 1831.[2] In 1826, Bell himself (in a letter of January 9th) had acquired a clear idea of the difference between sensory and motor nerves. In 1829, he demonstrated that the fifth cranial nerve is sensory-motor discovered "Bell's nerve"; also the motor nerve of the face (portio dura of the seventh nerve) lesion of which causes facial paralysis (Bell's palsy). These discoveries are incorporated in his book on the nervous system (1830), which also contains early cases of pseudohypertrophic paralysis and "Thomsen's disease." Bell was a genial, unaffected, kind-hearted man, with a captivating twinkle behind his eye-glasses, a bit of a dandy in attire. He was much lionized during his London life, and in 1829 was knighted for his physiologic discoveries by the enthusiastic Lord Brougham. He was an able surgeon, and attended the wounded after Corunna and Waterloo, making interesting sketches of what he saw.

The ablest supporter of Bichat's ideas in Great Britain was the Scotch anatomist, Robert Knox (1791–1862), who was the first to teach general anatomy from the descriptive, histologic, and comparative angles, and attracted Edinburgh students in great numbers by his dramatic style of delivery and his showy appearance in the lecture-room. At this time, there were no public regulations

[1] Magendie: J. da physiol. expér., Paris, 1822, ii, 276–279.

[2] Müller: Froriep's Notiz a. d. Geb. d. Nat. u. Heilk., Weimar, 1831, xxx, 113; 129.   The experiment was further confirmed in fish by Wagner (1846) and Stannius (1849), and in birds by Panizza (1834) and Schiff (1858).

to supply dissecting material for teaching purposes, and the needs of the large anatomy classes were met by surreptitious methods. Body-snatching and even murder were rife. On the twenty-ninth of November, 1827, the dead body of an old man who owed £4 to his landlord, William Hare, was sold by Hare to Knox for £7 10s., to recoup the debt, and this stroke of business led Hare and his associate Burke to the idea of smothering their lodgers, or any other unfortunates who fell into their hands, as a money-making asset. The victim was first intoxicated, and then suffocated by closing the hands tightly over the nose and mouth ("Burking"). Sixteen bodies were secured in this way and sold before the crime was detected, and the last body was found in Knox's rooms. All Edinburgh went wild on the instant, and Knox was mobbed by the horrified populace, vituperated by press and pulpit, and threatened with hanging. The fact that "Daft Jamie," a harmless imbecile of the "Old Town," and the voluptuous figure of "a handsome Lais or Thais" had been among those victimized and dissected, added greater fuel to the flames. Knox, a man of powerful physique and self-possessed character, braved the clamor, made bold to outface his opponents, and eventually defended himself in writing, but he was never popular afterward and his only adherents were his faithful pupils.[1] This sensational and entirely discreditable episode led at least to one good reform, Lord Warburton's Anatomy Act of 1832 (2d and 3d William IV, cap. 75), which provided that all unclaimed bodies should, under proper conditions, go to the medical schools. Knox was an able and interesting writer on artistic anatomy and natural history, and his fragment on "The Races of Man" (1850), although full of eccentric views, is one of the most original and readable contributions ever made to anthropology. It was highly praised by Emerson.

An interesting work on artistic anatomy, which may be men-

---

[1] Of the odium which Knox incurred from the Burking incident, it may be said that, while he was technically guiltless, the aversion of his fellow-townsmen was not entirely without foundation, since they knew that the bodies of poor people were liable to be spirited away by "sham mourners" at funerals and other devices of the "Resurrectionists," while the showy, sensational methods of the lecturer himself were not strictly in accord with the best modern taste as to the dignity of medical teaching. Dissection and vivisection, to be respectable and scientific, should always be private and under proper legal restrictions. Even the public dissections depicted on the title-pages of Vesalius and Columbus reek a little too much of the Barnum's show-bill for modern taste, and a blood-pressure experiment demonstrated on a vivisected animal to a public audience, hardly any of whom understand its bearings, can best be judged in the light of the "Law" of Hippocrates: "Those things which are sacred are to be imparted only to sacred persons; and it is not lawful to impart them to the profane until they have been initiated into the mysteries of the science."

tioned in connection with Knox, is the "Anatomical Studies of the Bones and Muscles for the Use of Artists" (London, 1833), which were engraved from the posthumous drawings of John **Flaxman** (1755–1836) by Henry Landseer.

The leading **comparative anatomists** of the early nineteenth century were Lamarck, Cuvier, Owen, and Agassiz. Of these, Jean-Baptiste **Lamarck** (1744–1829), who gave up soldiering for medicine, medicine for botany, and botany for zoölogy, once famous for his Natural History of Invertebrates (1815–22), is now best remembered by his *Philosophie Zoölogique* (1809). In this he appears as a great pioneer of evolution, in his theory that variations are produced by the effects of use and disuse upon organs, by response to external stimuli, and by the direct inheritance of these acquired characters. Like Galen and Hunter, Lamarck believed that structure follows function (*La fonction fait l'organe*), and although this theory of the heredity of acquired characters is now hotly contested, he is still regarded as one of the greatest of philosophic biologists.

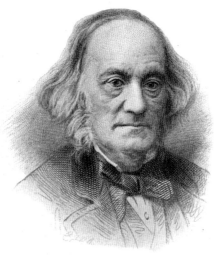

Georges **Cuvier** (1769–1832), whom Lamarck helped and who afterward turned against him, who once overshadowed him but is now regarded as his inferior, had, as Flourens said, "*l'esprit vaste.*" His great works on comparative anatomy (1801–05), on the fossil bones of Paris (1812), on the structure of fishes (1828), and on the animal kingdom (1836–49) are on the most extended scale. He was the founder of vertebrate paleontology, first stated the theory of morphologic types (vertebrate, molluscan, articulate, radiate), the doctrine of the structural correlation of parts of an organism, and the catastrophe theory of geologic forma-

Sir Richard Owen (1804–1892).

tions. But he believed in spontaneous generation, the fixity of species, and the preformation of the embryo.

Sir Richard **Owen** (1804–92), of Lancaster, England, a pupil of Abernethy's, and the associate and son-in-law of John Hunter's secretary, William Clift, edited Hunter's posthumous works, and began his studies in morphology with his great *Catalogue of the Physiological Series of Comparative Anatomy* (1833–40) in Hunter's collection. His *Anatomy and Physiology of the Vertebrates* (1866–68) was pronounced by Flower to rank next to Cuvier's Comparative Anatomy in scope. In 1840–45, he published the *Odontography*, a monumental treatise on the morphology of the teeth of living animals, illustrated with 150 plates. In paleontology, his monographs on British fossil mammals, birds, and reptiles (1846–84), extinct mammals of Australia (1877), and extinct wingless birds of New Zealand (1879), are of the highest importance. He described the Archæopteryx, the oldest known bird, the Apteryx, Notornis, and Dinornis, the latter class including the dodo and the giant moa. He was also the first to describe the Trichina spiralis (1835),[1] but he classified the sper-

---

[1] Owen: Tr. Zoöl. Soc. London, 1835, i, 315–324. *See, also*, Hilton: London, Med. Gaz., 1833, xi, 605.

matozoa as internal parasites under "Entozoa." Owen was one of the early workers with the microscope in England, a founder and charter member of the Royal Microscopic Society, and an accomplished violoncellist and chess-player. He was Hunterian professor at the Royal College of Surgeons (1836–56), and superintendent of the Natural History Department of the British Museum (1856–83). In 1843, he introduced the well-known distinction between serial homologies (organs of similar structure and development) and morphologic analogies (different organs of similar function). He followed Goethe and Oken in upholding the vertebrate theory of the skull,[1] and while admitting variation of species through an innate tendency to deviate from an ancestral archetype, was an opponent of Darwinism, but being worsted by Huxley in two important controversies, he eventually went over to it. After his death, Huxley wrote an appreciative study of his work.

Louis **Agassiz** (1807–73), of Mottier, Switzerland, settled in Cambridge, Mass., in 1846, and his Contributions to the Natural History of the United States (1857–62) is of especial interest to Americans. His Fossil Fishes (1833–44), describing over 1000 species, is his masterpiece, although his empirical classification by scales is now discarded. He was an opponent of Darwinism, and upheld the old Linnæan idea of the fixity of species; also the Recapitulation Theory, that "the history of the individual is but the epitomized history of the race."

The pioneers of American anatomy in the first half of the century were Wistar, Horner, Godman, and Morton.

Casper **Wistar** (1760–1818), born in Philadelphia of German extraction, taught anatomy at the University of Pennsylvania from 1791–1818, and his "System of Anatomy" (1811–14), now forgotten, was the earliest treatise on the subject published in this country. His description of the ethmoid bone was praised by Soemmerring, and his memory survives in the wisteria vine, which was named after him; in the "Wistar parties" of old time, weekly literary gatherings at which he was a cultured and amiable host, and in the present Wistar Institute of Anatomy and Biology in Philadelphia (1892).

William Edmonds **Horner** (1793–1853), of Warrenton, Virginia, studied medicine at Edinburgh and Philadelphia, and after serving as army surgeon in the war of 1812, settled in the latter city, where he became prosector to Wistar, Dorsey, and Physick, eventually succeeding the latter as professor of anatomy in the University of Pennsylvania in 1831, his successor being Joseph Leidy. Horner discovered the tensor tarsi muscle (Horner's muscle) supplying the lacrimal apparatus (1824),[2] and investigated the odoriferous axillary glands in the negro, the muscular tube of the rectum, and the membranes of the larynx. He performed and described important surgical operations, particularly on the eye, and published treatises on anatomy (1826) and pathol-

---

[1] Owen: On the Archetype and Homologies of the Vertebrate Skeleton, London, 1848.

[2] Horner: Phila. Jour. Med. and Phys. Sc., 1824, viii, 70.

25

ogy (1829). In 1834[1] he published an important paper showing that the rice-water discharges in Asiatic cholera consist of epithelium stripped from the small intestine.

John D. **Godman** (1794–1830), of Annapolis, Maryland, an anatomist of great talent, could not realize what was in himself because, as Gross puts it, "poverty literally pursued him from the cradle to the grave." Orphaned in infancy, friendless, cheated out of his inheritance by fraud, by turns a printer's apprentice and a sailor, he succeeded in gaining a medical education through

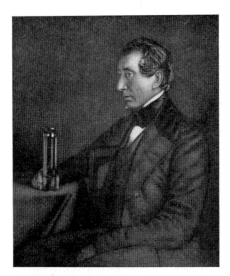

William Edmonds Horner (1793–1853).

a noble perseverance, attracted the kindly notice of Daniel Drake, who gave him a chair in surgery, and became editor of the short-lived "Western Quarterly Reporter of Medical, Surgical, and Natural Science" (1822–23), the first medical journal to be printed west of the Alleghenies. His life was one of grinding toil, his lectures were popular, but never remunerative, and he was an early victim of phthisis; but he produced three works of importance and originality—his treatise on the fascia (1824), his" Contributions to Physiological and Pathological Anatomy" (1825), and his "American Natural History" (1826).

Samuel George **Morton** (1799–1851), of Philadelphia, a graduate of the University of Edinburgh, published an elaborate treatise on general and microscopic anatomy in 1849, but he is now best remembered as craniologist, paleontologist, and phthisiographer. His "Crania Americana" (1839) and "Crania Ægyptiaca" (1844) are fine atlases, among the earliest of their kind, of permanent value and reputation. His book on organic remains (1834) is said to be the starting-point of all systematic study of American fossils. His "Illustrations of Pulmonary Consumption" (1834) is of great value as summing up the knowledge of his time. He believed that the races of mankind are of diverse origin, and his

---

[1] Horner: Am. J. Med. Sc., Phila., 1834, xv, 1545; 1835, xvi, 58; 277, 2 pl.

essay on hybridity (1847) demonstrated the fertility of hybrids, both which views made him a target for controversial abuse and theological hatred.

Among the earlier American works on zoölogy and morphology are Thomas Say's Crustacea of the United States (1817–18) and American Entomology (1824–28), Richard Harlan's Fauna Americana (1825), Godman's work on North American mammals (1826), Audubon's "Birds of America" (1827), Isaac Lea's Fresh Water Mussels (1829), Nuttall's Ornithology of the United States and Canada (1823–34), Holbrook's North American Herpetology (1836–40), De Kay's Zoölogy of New York (1846–9), and Audubon and Bachmann's Quadrupeds of North America (1846–54).

In Germany, the development of anatomy and physiology went hand in hand, and the ablest of the earlier morphologists and histologists—Müller, Schleiden, Schwann, Henle, Remak— were also, in the best sense of the term, physiologists. The founder of scientific medicine in Germany was, indeed, **Johannes Müller** (1801–58), of Coblenz, who was also the greatest German physiologist of his time, and, like Haller and John Hunter, one of the great all-round medical naturalists. He was equally eminent in biology, comparative morphology, physiological chemistry, psychology, and pathology, and through his best pupils—Schwann, Henle, Kölliker, Virchow, Du Bois Réymond, and Helmholtz, most of whom followed the same trend—we may trace the main currents of modern German medicine. Müller's "Handbuch der Physiologie des Menschen" (1834–40) resembles Haller's great treatise as a rich mine of novel facts and original ideas, and introduces two new elements into physiology—the comparative and the psychologic. His principal contributions to the science were his investigation of specific nerve energies (1826),[1] his explanation of the color sensations ("pressure-phosphenes") produced by pressure on the retina (1826),[2] his experimental proof (in the frog) of the Bell-Magendie law of the spinal nerve-roots (1831),[3] his discovery of the lymph-hearts in the frog (1832),[4] his law of the eccentric projection of sensations from the peripheral sense organs to other nerve-terminals (1833), his experiments on the vocal cords and the voice (1835–57),[5] his theory of color contrast (1837),[6] his isolation of chondrin and glutin (1837),[7] his demonstration of the function

---

[1] "Ueber die fantastische Gesichtserscheinungen," Coblenz, 1826; and Zur vergleichenden Physiologie des Gesichtssinnes, Leipzig, 1826.

[2] Zur vergleichenden Physiologie des Gesichtssinnes, p. 73.

[3] Notizen a. d. Gebiete d. Natur. u. Heilk., Weimar, 1831, xxx, 113; 129.

[4] Phil. Tr. London, 1833, pt. 1, 89–94.

[5] Handbuch d. Physiol., Coblenz, 1840, ii, 184–222.

[6] Handb. d. Physiol., 1840, ii, 372.

[7] Ann. d. Pharm., Heidelberg, 1837, xvi, 277–282.

of the bristle cells of the internal ear (1840),[1] and his examination
of the slimy secretions of the club-cells of the myxinoid fishes
(1845).[2] His broadest generalization, the Law of Specific Nerve-
energies,[3] which maintains that each sense organ, when stimulated,
gives rise to its own peculiar sensations and no other, has since
been extended far beyond its author's original intention, in the
idea that each nerve-fiber, as well as each organ or nerve, has its
specific sensations, differing in degree if not in kind under stimulation. As a morphologist, Müller made investigations of the

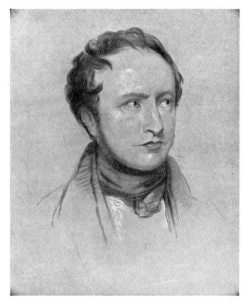

Johannes Müller (1801–58). (From a chalk drawing in the Surgeon General's
Library.)

first rank on the structural relations of the myxinoid and ganoid
fishes (1834–44), the Plagiostoma (with Jacob Henle in 1838–41),
and the echinoderms (1846–52). In embryology, his name is
associated with the discovery of the Müllerian duct (1825).[4]
As a histologist, he worked out the whole finer anatomy of the
glandular and cartilaginous tissues (1830)[5] and grouped the connective tissues. In pathology, as in histology, he was one of the

[1] Handb. d. Physiol., 1840, ii.
[2] Untersuchungen über die Eingeweide der Fische, Berlin, 1845, p. 11.
[3] Handb. d. Physiol., 1840, ii, 258.
[4] Nova acta Acad. Nat. Curios., Bonn, 1825, pt. ii, 565–672, 6 pl.
[5] De glandularum secernentium structura penitiori, Leipzig, 1830.

first to use the microscope, particularly in his monumental work on tumors (1838),[1] and he introduced the idea that fever is a nervous reflex (1840). In 1841, he described the parasitic disease now recognized as psorospermosis.[2] In 1834, he founded the journal everywhere known as *Müller's Archiv*, which was continued after his death by Reichert and Du Bois Réymond and, as containing a host of classical contributions, has exerted a profound influence upon the advancement of scientific medicine. Like every great investigator who has approached his subject from the broadest angle, Müller made a few mistakes. Following Hewson, Mascagni, and the Hunters, he maintained that absorption is the special and exclusive function of the lymphatics, although Magendie, in 1836, had shown that the blood-vessels also possess this power. As late as 1840, he held that respiration in the fetus is effected not (as John Mayow had shown in 1674) by the placenta, but by a special juice or plasma secreted in the maternal blood. In 1840, Müller stated that no one could ever hope to measure the velocity of a nervous impulse. Ten years later his pupil, Helmholtz, had done so. Temperamentally, he was a mystic, and, by the same token, a vitalist in theory. He believed that there is something in vital processes which does not admit of a mechanical or a material explanation, but he also believed that such explanation may be pushed to the limit "so long as we keep to the solid ground of observation and experiment." Strongly built, with broad shoulders and a massive Achillean head,—Virchow said it "seemed like that of some warrior of old,"—Müller was a striking, magnetic, impressive teacher, of rare personal charm, who influenced and inspired his pupils for good as only a great man can.

After Müller's time, the main trend of German anatomy was along histological and functional lines, and this new departure turned upon three important factors—the foundation of modern **embryology** by von Baer (1827–28), the improvement of the achromatic microscope by Joseph Jackson Lister in 1830, and the development of the cell theory by Schleiden and Schwann (1838–39).

Carl Ernst **von Baer** (1792–1876), the father of the new embryology, was a native of Esthland, in the Baltic Sea provinces of Russia, and was successively professor at Dorpat, Königsberg, and St. Petersburg. The special service of von Baer was that, where his predecessors had only studied the chick, he made embryology a comparative science, established the modern theory of the germ-layers, and the beginnings of histogenesis, organogenesis and

---

[1] Ueber den feinern Bau und die Formen der krankhaften Geschwülste, Berlin, 1838.

[2] Müller's Arch., Berlin, 1841, 477–496, 1 pl.

morphogenesis. Caspar Friedrich Wolff, in 1768, had already been close upon the germ-layer concept when he saw that the intestines are produced by the folding in and rolling together of "leaf-like" embryonic layers. In 1817,[1] Christian Pander (1793–1865), assisted by von Baer, in his observations upon the chick, extended the number of these layers to three. Von Baer, in his great work on the development of animals (1828–34),[2] showed, from comparative studies of all kinds, that these leaf-like layers are not true tissues of the developing organism, but the germs or germ-layers from which the alimentary canal, the nervous system and its other parts are unfolded, disappearing as the latter are completed. He recognized four layers in all, from the fact that the middle layer is made of two sheets; but this double layer was afterward shown to be a single structure by Robert Remak, who first defined the three categories, ectoderm, endoderm, and mesoderm (1845). The supreme merit of von Baer's work lies in the wonderful patience shown in working out, as Minot puts it, "almost as fully as was possible at this time, the genesis of all the principal organs from the germ-layers, instinctively getting at the truth as only a great genius could have done." This was in the trying early days of the modern microscope, and the clear and beautifully accurate results obtained, from sections cut without the aid of a microtome, have set the pace for all subsequent work, down to the recent phase of tracing the embryonic cell-lineage in minutest detail. Von Baer discovered the mammalian ovum in 1827,[3] and, at the same time, the chorda dorsalis or notochord. From his exhaustive studies in comparative embryology, he was led to classify animals into four groups, viz., Vertebrata, Articulata, Mollusca, and Radiata, which makes him, with Cuvier, the founder of modern morphology (Haeckel). Von Baer went to Russia in

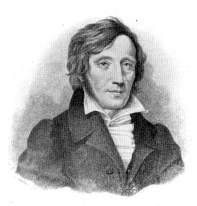

Carl Ernst von Baer (1792–1876). (From an engraving in the Surgeon General's Library.)

---

[1] Pander: Diss. sistens historiam metamorphoseos quam ovum incubatum prioribusque quinque diebus subit, Würzburg, 1817.

[2] Ueber Entwickelungsgeschichte der Thiere, Königsberg, 1828–34.

[3] De ovi mammalium et hominis genesi, Leipzig, 1827.

1834, and devoted the rest of his life to investigating the physical geography and anthropology of that country. In coöperation with Rudolf Wagner, he was instrumental in calling together the first Congress of Anthropologists in 1861. He was of a deeply religious nature, and his autobiography, privately printed in 1864, gives an interesting account of his experiences.

Contemporaneous with von Baer, was Purkinje's characterization of the formative substance ("protoplasm") of the embryo (1839), Schwann on respiration in the embryonic chick (1834), Reichert on the visceral arches in vertebrata (1837), Bischoff on the development of the rabbit (1848) and the guinea-pig (1852); but the latter-day embryology of von Kölliker, His, Haeckel, Balfour, Hertwig and Minot is part and parcel of the doctrine of the nucleated cell.

The development of the **cell-theory,** one of the fundamental principles of m o d e r n science, was almost entirely the work of botanists. In the seventeenth century, Robert Hooke (1665), Malpighi (1675), and Nehemiah Grew (1682) had noticed the cellular cavities in cork and green plants. In 1831, the cell-nucleus was discovered by the botanist Robert Brown (1773–1858), who also discovered the process of generation in plants by means of pollen. The cell nucleolus was discovered by Gabriel Valentin in 1836. The significance of the nucleus in vegetable histology was first emphasized by the Hamburg botanist, Matthias Jacob

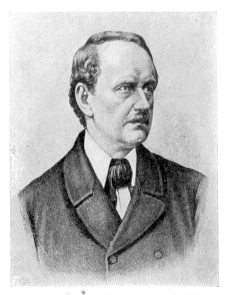

Matthias Joseph Schleiden (1804–1881).

Schleiden (1804–81), who, after studying law and medicine, became professor of botany at Jena, Dorpat, and Frankfort on the Main. In his important paper on *Phytogenesis* (1838)[1] Schleiden saw and proved that plant tissues are made up of and developed from groups of cells, of which he recognized the nucleus (or "cytoblast") as the important feature; but he held that young cells originate spontaneously from the cytoblast, which he thought to be encased

[1] "Beiträge zur Phytogenese," Müller's Arch., Berlin, 1838, 137–176, 2 pl.

in the solid cell-wall. He regarded the young cell as resting upon and expanding over the cytoblast like a watch-crystal over a watch, an idea which became known as the "watch-glass theory"(*Uhrglas-theorie*). Thus, he regarded cell reproduction as endogenous (free internal formation) instead of by division, and the cell-wall as a solid structure instead of a semi-permeable membrane. But Schleiden was a true physiological botanist withal, entertaining a lively contempt for the mere herbarium collector, and his "Grund-züge" (1842–43)[1] is perhaps the most important landmark in the modern history of the science. He was keen at controversy and, lawyer-like, did not hesitate to indulge in personalities to put his adversaries in a corner. A

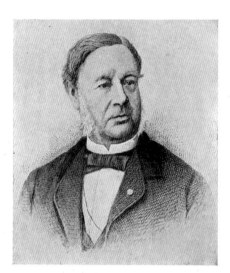

Theodor Schwann (1810–1882).

friendly after-dinner conversation between Schleiden and Schwann, who in the mean time, had discovered nucleated cells in the animal tissues, led the latter to look for cells in all the tissues he knew of and to formulate the most important generalization in the science of morphology, viz., the principle of structural similarity in animal and vegetable tissues: "There is one universal principle of development for the elementary parts of organisms, however different, and that principle is the formation of the cells."

To Schleiden's concept of the cytoblast, Schwann added the "cyto-blastema" or matrix of cell development, analogous to the mother liquor from which crystals spring. This, as Virchow pointed out, was a tacit acceptance of "spontaneous generation," the very thing which Schwann afterward did so much to overthrow.

Theodor **Schwann** (1810–82), born at Neuss near Düsseldorf, was a pupil of Müller's at Bonn and the latter's prosector at Berlin. After the publication of his classic on the cell theory in 1839,[2] he was called to the University at Louvain, and, in 1848, became

---

[1] Grundzüge der wissenschaftlicher Botanik, Leipzig, 1842–43.

[2] Mikroskopische Untersuchungen über die Uebereinstimmung in der Struktur und dem Wachsthum der Thiere und Pflanzen, Berlin, 1839.

professor of anatomy and physiology at Liège. A most careful
and accurate investigator, he discovered the sheath of the axis-
cylinder of nerves, which goes by his name (1838),[1] and the striped
muscle in the upper part of the esophagus (1837).[2] His inaugural
dissertation (1834)[3] showed that air is necessary for the development of the embryo; and, applying the same idea to the problem
of spontaneous generation, he was able to prove, in 1836,[4] that
putrefaction is produced by living bodies, which are themselves
destroyed if the surrounding air be heated or vitiated. In 1837,[5]
about the same time as Cagniard Latour, he discovered the organic
nature of yeast, and showed that the yeast-plant causes fermentation which can be suppressed by heating the culture-medium and
sterilizing the surrounding air by heat. As a physiologist, he
discovered pepsin in 1835,[6] showing its power to change non-
diffusible albumens into peptones; and, in 1841,[7] demonstrated,
by means of an artificial biliary fistula in a dog, that bile is absolutely essential to digestion. He was the first to investigate the
laws of muscular contraction by physical and mathematical
methods, in his classical experiment, demonstrating that the tension
of a contracting muscle varies with its length (1837).[8] In personality, Schwann was an amiable, unpretentious nature, somewhat
below the middle height, with an open, pleasant, genial countenance,
not unlike that of Claude Bernard. He is said to have visited
London twice without making himself known to any one. He was
a devout Catholic, submitting the manuscript of his work on the
cell theory to the Bishop of Maline for approval before publication,
but he did not hesitate to declare the Louise Lateau affair an
arrant imposture. During the last forty years of his academic
life, he seems to have done little scientific work, and Professor
Ray Lankester records that "to sit with him in front of a café in
the pleasant streets of Louvain and hear him discourse on the
progress of histology and the germ theory of disease" was "a
pleasure no less startling than that which could be conferred by
one risen from the dead."

---

[1] Froriep's Neue Notizen, Weimar, 1838, v, 228, and Schwann's book on
the cell-theory.

[2] Joh. Müller: Handbuch d. Physiologie, Coblenz, 1840, ii, 36.

[3] De necessitate aëris atmosphærici ad evolutionem pulli in ovo incubato,
Berlin, 1834.

[4] Ann. d. Physik u. Chemie Leipzig, 1837, xli, 184–193.

[5] Mitth. a. d. Verhandl. d. Gesellsch. naturf. Freunde zu Berlin, 1837, ii,
9–15.

[6] Müller's Archiv, Berlin, 1836, 90–114.

[7] Ibid., 1844, 127–159.

[8] Described in Müller's "Physiologie," 1840, ii, 59–62.

Following upon the researches of Schleiden and Schwann, cells were discovered which had not a cell-wall, but merely what physicists call a "surface of discontinuity" in relation to the surrounding medium; and it was found that the nucleus is contained, not in the cell-wall, as Schleiden had supposed, but in the ground-substance of the cell itself. From this time on, the nature and significance of this fundamental substance became the main object of investigation. In 1835, the French zoölogist Felix Dujardin (1801–60) had described and defined it in the protozoa as "sarcode."[1] Schleiden, in his paper of 1838, had noted it in plants and regarded it as a gum. Purkinje was the first to employ the term "protoplasm," applying it to the germinal ground-substance of the embryo (1839). In 1846–51, the botanist Hugo von Mohl (1805–72), of Stuttgart, described part of the contents of the vegetable cell (just under the cell-membrane) as "protoplasma,"[2] and the chemical nature of the same was investigated by a Swiss botanist, Carl Nägeli (1817–91), in 1862–63.[3] Ferdinand Cohn (1828–98), of Breslau, eminent for his work in bacteriology, declared, after a study of the protococcus, that animal and vegetable protoplasm are analogous, if not identical, substances (1850–53).[4] Heinrich Anton de Bary (1831–88), a Frankfurt botanist, showed this identity further in his work on the myxomycetes (1859).[5] In the mean time (1858), Virchow had already announced the continuity of cell development and its importance in pathology. Finally, Max Schultze, in 1861,[6] showed that the likeness between animal and vegetable protoplasm is not only structural and chemical, but also physiological. Thus the cell gradually came to be recognized as the structural and physiological unit in all living organisms, whether animals or plants, simple or complex, embryonic or adult, healthy or diseased, while, in our own time, the cell-nucleus is regarded as the chemical "center of oxidation" and the chromosome as the transmitter of inherited characters.

It was in this way that anatomic studies came to be more and more histologic or microscopic, and the "seats and causes" of disease itself to be referred to the cellular elements in the body and the unicellular organisms attacking them.

---

[1] Dujardin: Ann. d. sc. nat. (zool.), Paris, 1835, iv, 343–376.

[2] Von Mohl: Botan. Ztg., 1846, iv, 337; 353; 369; 385.

[3] Nägeli: Sitzungsb. d. k. bayer. Akad. d. Wissensch., München, 1862, ii, 280; 1863, i, 161; 483; 1863, ii, 119.

[4] Cohn: Zur Naturgeschichte des Protococcus pluvialis, Breslau, 1850, and Untersuchungen über die Entwicklungsgeschichte der mikroskopischen Algen und Pilzen, Bonn, 1853.

[5] de Bary: Die Mycetozoen, Leipzig, 1859.

[6] Schultze: Müller's Arch., Berlin, 1861, 1–27.

The importance of the cell theory is immediately sensed in the work of Jacob **Henle** (1809–85), the greatest German histologist of his time and one of the greatest anatomists of all time. Born of Jewish parents at Fürth, near Nuremberg, Henle was one of Johannes Müller's favorite pupils, one of his prosectors at Berlin, and later professor of anatomy at Zürich (1840), Heidelberg (1844), and Göttingen (1852–85). Henle did many important things for medical science. In his classic researches of 1836–37,[1] he was the founder of modern knowledge of the epithelial tissues of the body. He first described the epithelia of the skin and intestines, defined columnar and ciliated epithelium, and pointed out that this tissue constitutes the true lining membrane of all free surfaces of the body and the inner lining of its tubes and cavities. In 1840,[2] he demonstrated the presence of smooth muscle in the middle or endothelial coat of the smaller arteries, a discovery which was the starting-point of the present physiological theory of the vasomotor mechanism. He also discovered the external sphincter (striated muscle) of the bladder, the central chylous vessels, the internal root sheath of the hair, the Henle tubules in the kidney (1862),[3] and gave the first accurate account of the histology of the cornea and of the morphology and development of the larynx. He first pointed out many important structures in the brain, notably the relations of the hippocampus, and the vestigial character of the posterior lobe of the pituitary body. Altogether, the histological discoveries of Henle[4] take rank with the anatomical

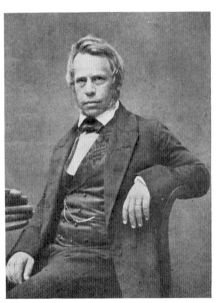

Jacob Henle (1809–1885).

---

[1] Symbolæ ad anatomiam villorum intestinalium imprimis eorum epithelii et vasorum lacteorum, Berlin, 1837.

[2] In his "Allgemeine Anatomie," Leipzig, 1841, pp. 510, 690.

[3] Contained in his "Handbuch der systematischen Anatomie," 1862, ii, 300–305.

[4] These discoveries are to be found in Henle's two treatises on anatomy.

discoveries of Vesalius. As a morphologist, he collaborated with Müller in his monograph on the plagiostomes (1838–41), and described the electric fish *Narcine*, and the annelid *Enchytræus*. In pathology he was, with his friend Pfeufer, the founder of the celebrated *Zeitschrift für rationelle Medizin* (1842–69), which exerted a powerful influence upon the advancement of German medicine and contains some of the best monographs of the period. His essay "On Miasms and Contagia" (1840)[1] contains the first clear statement of the idea of a *contagium animatum*. His essay on fevers[2] elaborates Müller's idea that fever is only a symptom, occasioned by disturbances in the central nervous system. In his "Hand Book of Rational Pathology" (1846–53)[3] he maintains that the physician's duty is to prevent and cure disease; that disease is a deviation from normal physiological processes; death the cessation of metabolism; and the hypothesis of a vital force, "just as good or as weak as that of electric attraction or gravitation." In practical medicine, he first connected the catarrhs and exanthemata with inflammation (1838), and pointed out the preponderance of left-sided varicocele and the relation of left-sided intercostal neuralgias to the hemiazygos vein. Of Henle's two books on anatomy, the earlier *Allgemeine Anatomie* (1841) was, in reality, the first treatise upon microscopic histology, and marks a great advance upon Bichat in that the tissues are considered in their developmental and functional, as well as their structural, relations. The classification of the tissues is the simplest and best ever made, and the book contains an admirable history of microscopy and histology, as also some of Henle's most important discoveries. The later "Hand Book of Systematic Anatomy" (1866–71)[4] is an exhaustive three-volume treatise of the highest scientific order. It contains the first logical account and nomenclature of the axes and planes of the body, the terminology is greatly simplified and the sections on the ligaments, the muscles, the viscera, and the vascular and nervous systems are of epoch-making importance. The illustrations of this work, made with Henle's own hand, are, as he puts it, architectural rather than diagrammatic, in that only so much of a structure is given in light and shade as is necessary for its comprehension, while the idea of plan and elevation is freely resorted to. As a lecturer, Henle was vivid and inspiring, making his own drawings with

---

[1] In his "Pathologische Untersuchungen," Berlin, 1840, pp. 1–82.

[2] *Ibid.*, 206–274.

[3] Handbuch der rationellen Pathologie, Braunschweig, 1846–53.

[4] Handbuch der systematischen Anatomie des Menschen, Braunschweig, 1866–71.

his crayon as he went along, and winning love and admiration by his sincerity and charm. He was not only a skillful artist, but something of a poet, and an accomplished musician, beginning with the violin and eventually learning to play both viola and violoncello, so that he might take any part at need in an impromptu string quartet. The experiences of his life, his peripatetic career as student and professor, the romantic circumstances of his first marriage, his friendships with such men as Humboldt, Gustav Magnus, and Felix Mendelssohn, make an interesting narrative.

Robert **Remak** (1815–65), of Posen, also of Jewish descent, was an assistant of Schönlein's at the Charité, and apart from his reputation as a microscopist, did a number of important things in other directions. In histology, he is memorable for his discovery of the non-medullated nerve-fibers (fibers of Remak) in 1838,[1] and of the ganglionic cells in the sinus venosus of the frog's heart (1848),[2] which some regard as the automatic centers causing the heart-beat. He was one of the first to point out that the proliferation of cells to form tissues is accomplished by cell-division (1852)[3] and not, as Schleiden and Schwann had supposed, by endogenous formation.

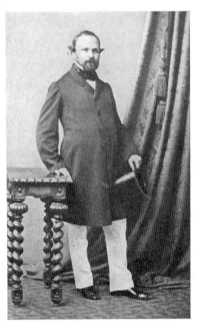

Robert Remak (1815–1865).

He simplified von Baer's classification of the germ-layers, as we have seen (1851).[4] In 1842, in Schönlein's clinic, he produced favus experimentally, *in propria persona*, separating the fungus from the genus Oïdium, and calling it Achorion Schönleini, after the master (1845).[5] He was the first to describe

[1] Remak: Observationes anatomicæ et microscopicæ de systematis nervosi structura, Berlin, 1838.

[2] Müller's Archiv, Berlin, 1848, 139.

[3] *Ibid.*, 1852, 47–57.

[4] Untersuchungen über die Entwickelung des Wirbelthiereies, Berlin, 1851.

[5] Remak: Diagnostische und pathogenetische Untersuchungen, Berlin, 1845, pp. 196; 205; 208.

ascending neuritis (1861), and he was, with Addison and Duchenne of Boulogne, one of the pioneers of electrotherapy, substituting the galvanic for the induced current (1856).[1]

Another important pioneer in the use of the microscope was Johannes Evangelista **Purkinje** (1787–1869), of Bohemia, who was also a physiologist of genius. He began life as a teacher, haviug previously taken orders, but graduated in medicine at Prague in 1819, his inaugural dissertation being an important work on subjective visual phenomena,[2] which won for him the friendship and protection of Goethe. It was perhaps through the latter's in-

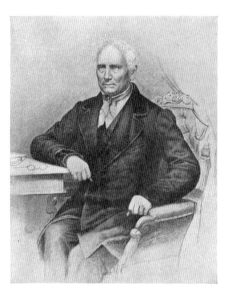

fluence that Purkinje was appointed professor of physiology and pathology at the University of Breslau in 1823. At Breslau, he was at first coldly received, on account of the current prejudice against Slavs, which he soon lived down, winning every one over by his superior knowledge and urbane demeanor. Purkinje remained at Breslau until 1850, when he was called to the chair of physiology at Prague. During his Breslau period he did some important work for the development of German science which is frequently overlooked. He was the founder of laboratory

Johannes Evangelista Purkinje (1787–1869).

training in connection with German university teaching. In 1824, he started a physiological laboratory in his own house, and the work done by the master and his pupils proved to be of such high character that the Prussian government finally erected a Physiological Institute for him at Breslau in 1842. As in the case of Carl Ludwig, many dissertations of Purkinje's pupils represent the ideas of the great physiologist himself. As a microscopist, Purkinje was the first to use the microtome, Canada balsam, glacial acetic acid, potassium bichromate, and the Drummond lime light (1839).

[1] Remak: Galvanotherapie der Nerven- und Muskelkrankheiten, Berlin, 1858.

[2] Beiträge zur Kenntniss des Sehens in subjectiver Hinsicht, Prague, 1819.

In 1825,[1] he described the germinal vesicle in the embryo, and he was the first histologist to employ the term protoplasm, which he applied to the embryonic ground-substance in 1839.[2] He discovered the sudoriferous glands of the skin with their excretory ducts (1833),[3] the pear-shaped ganglionic (Purkinje) cells in the cerebellum (1837),[4] the lumen of the axis-cylinder of nerves,[5] and the ganglionic bodies in the brain.[6] In 1834–35, he wrote (with Gabriel Valentin)[7] his famous essay on ciliary epithelial motion; described the "Purkinje fibers" of the cardiac muscle (1839)[8] and of the uterus (1840).[9] In 1837,[10] two years before Schwann, he pointed out the probable identity of structure in animal and plant cells and he also antedated the latter by two years in his work on artificial digestion (1838).[11] In 1823,[12] long before Francis Galton, he pointed out the importance of finger-prints, giving accurate figurations of the same, and he also noted that deaf-mutes can hear through the bones of the skull. He was an important pioneer in the description of most of the subjective visual figures (1819–23), notably those obtained by galvanic stimulation, the recurrent images, the entoptic appearances from the shadows of the retinal vessels, the dependence of brightness of color upon intensity of light, the choroidal figure, the rosettes of light produced by the use of digitalis, and the peculiar radiations following the instillation of belladonna. Purkinje was also the first to employ the terms "enchyma" for the basic substance of glands, "cambium" for the same thing in plants, and "protoplasm"

[1] Symbolæ ad ovi avium historiam ante incubationem, Breslau, 1825.

[2] Uebersicht d. Arb. u. Veränd. d. schles. Gesellsch. f. vaterl. Kultur, 1839, Breslau, 1840, p. 82. Also, De formatione granulosa in nervis aliisque partibus organismi animalis, student's dissertation by Joseph Rosenthal, Breslau, 1839.

[3] In student's dissertation "De epidermide humana," by Adolph Wendt, Breslau, 1833.

[4] Ber. ü. d. Versamml. deutsch. Naturf. u. Aerzte, 1837, Prague, 1838, xv, 180, plate, Fig. 18.

[5] Ibid., 177.

[6] Ibid., 178–179.

[7] Müller's Arch., Berlin, 1834, 391–400. Also "De phænomena generali et fundamentali motus vibratorii continui in membranis tum externis tum internis animalium plurimorum et superiorum et inferiorum ordinum obvii, Breslau, 1835.

[8] In student's dissertation by Bogislaus Palicki: De musculari cordis structura, Breslau, 1839.

[9] In student's dissertation by Wilhelm Kasper: De structura fibrosa uteri nongravidi, Breslau, 1840.

[10] Ber. d. Versamml. deutsch. Naturf. u. Aerzte, Prague, 1837, 175.

[11] Purkinje and Pappenheim: Ueber künstliche Verdauung, Müller's Arch., Berlin, 1838, 1–4.

[12] De examine physiologico organi visus et systematis cutanei, Breslau, 1823.

for the ground-substance of tissues. Altogether a physiologist of extraordinary range and keenness of perception, he was further distinguished as a pharmacologist, his experiments on the action of camphor, opium, belladonna, stramonium, and turpentine having been made upon himself (1829).[1] In relation to clinical medicine, Purkinje was the first to study the vertigo and rolling of the eyes produced by rotating the erect body in a vertical axis (1820-25),[2] and, although he did not connect the phenomenon with the semicircular canals, his description is the starting-point of modern work on vestibular and cerebellar nystagmus.

Albert von Kölliker (1817-1905).

After Henle's time, perhaps the most distinguished histologist of the early period was Albert von Kölliker (1817-1905), a Swiss who had heard Johannes Müller's lectures at Berlin, graduated at Heidelberg in 1842, and was Henle's prosector at Zürich in 1843. He became professor of anatomy at Zürich in 1846, and, the following year, received a call to Würzburg, where he remained for the rest of his active life. Kölliker was a follower of pure science and was equally remarkable in comparative embryology, histology, and morphology. In his monograph on the development of invertebrates (1843)[3] he was one of the first to apply Schwann's cell-theory to descriptive embryology, treating the ovum as a single cell and its segmentation as normal cell division only. In 1847, he first demonstrated the true development of the spermatozoa, showing that they are not extraneous bodies, but originate

---

[1] Neue Breslau, Samml. a. d. Geb. d. Heilk., Breslau, 1829, i, 423-444.

[2] "Beiträge zur Kenntnis des Schwindels aus heautognostischen Daten," Med. Jahrb., Vienna, 1820, vi, 79-125, and Rust's Mag. f. d. ges. Heilk., Berlin, 1825, xxiii, 284-310. See, also, the student's dissertation "De cerebri læsi ad motum voluntarium relatione, certaque vertiginis directione ex certis cerebri regionibus læsis pendente," by Heinrich Carl Krause, Breslau, 1824.

[3] Müller's Arch., Berlin, 1843, 68-141.

in the testicular cells and fertilize the ovum.[1] He was the author of the first work on comparative embryology (1861),[2] which embodies his important study of the relation of the vertebrate notochord to the adult spine and skull. In histology, he was the first to isolate smooth muscle (1846–48),[3] confirming Henle's discovery of the latter in the walls of blood-vessels; and he demonstrated the relation of the nerve-cell to medullated nerve-fiber (1889–94). He also confirmed Sharpey's theory of ossification and growth of bone (1860) and Corti's discoveries in the finer anatomy of the ear. His "Microscopic Anatomy" (1850–54)[4] and "Hand Book of Human Histology" (1852)[5] were the first formal text-books on the subject and the fifth edition of the latter was so enlarged by an added wealth of material as to be, in effect, a new book, the second volume literally creating the science of the comparative histology of the central nervous system in vertebrated animals. Minot says that "he knew more by direct personal observation of the microscopical structure of animals than any one else who has ever lived." In zoölogy, Kölliker's name will always be associated with the Cephalopoda, the Cœlenterata, the Gregarinidæ, Rhodope, Actinophrys, and other animals investigated by him. In 1849, he founded, with von Siebold, the "Zeitschrift für wissenschaftliche Zoölogie," the leading German organ of the science, which he edited for half a century. Kölliker was not only unrivalled in his notations of fact, but was also an able theorist and in advance of his time. Although ignorant of Mendel's work, he rejected the theory of natural selection in favor of saltatory or spontaneous variations (mutations); he regarded the cell nucleus as the transmitter of hereditary characters, and his theory of the mechanism of the male generative process (1863)[6] was confirmed by Eckhard. In 1862, he rediscovered the branched muscle plates in the heart which Leeuwenhoek had seen two hundred years before.[7] Personally, von Kölliker was a strong, grave, handsome, dignified figure, a veteran of pure science, whose prodigious industry was rewarded by a patent of nobility from the Bavarian government and the Prussian order "pour le mérite." Like his great predecessor, von Baer, he left an interesting autobiography (1899).

---

[1] Neue Denkschr. d. allg. schweiz. Gesellsch. f. d. ges. Naturwissensch., Zürich, 1847, viii.

[2] Entwicklungsgeschichte des Menschen und der Thiere, Leipzig, 1861.

[3] Mitth. d. naturf. Gesellsch. in Zürich, 1847, i, 18–28, and Ztschr. f. wissensch. Zoöl., Leipzig, 1848, i, 48–87, 4 pl.

[4] Mikroskopische Anatomie, Leipzig, 1850–54.

[5] Handbuch der Gewebelehre des Menschen, Leipzig, 1852.

[6] Würzb. naturw. Ztschr. (Sitzungsb., 1863), 1864, v, p. v.

[7] Proc. Roy. Soc. London, 1862–63, xii, 65–84.

26

The first and greatest teacher of topographic and regional anatomy in the nineteenth century was Josef **Hyrtl** (1810–94), of the New Vienna School, who was born at Eisenstadt, in Hungary. His father, a musician in Count Esterhazy's band, had played an oboe under Haydn, and Hyrtl, himself a chorister in his youth, had something the look of Haydn. As a student, he became Czermak's famulus at Vienna, made discoveries for which he was appointed prosector in 1833, and, at the age of twenty-six, became professor of anatomy at Prague. Appointed to the professorship of anatomy at Vienna in 1844, he was for thirty years the most

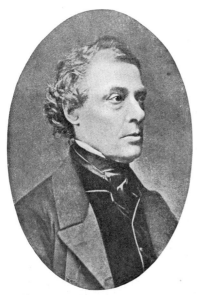

Josef Hyrtl (1810–1894). (Courtesy of Captain Henry J. Nichols, U. S. Army.)

fascinating and popular lecturer on the subject in Europe, his courses being followed by enthusiastic crowds of every race and class, even foreign nobles and consuls. His lectures were clear, concise, eloquent presentations of what he himself knew, interspersed to an extraordinary degree with witty epigrams, classical quotations, anecdotes, and veiled allusions of a questionable character. Hyrtl did not go in for merging his science into histology, like Henle, but kept up the straight Vesalian tradition of teaching gross or regional anatomy, and, for once, he succeeded, both as writer and lecturer, in making a dry subject piquant as well as interesting. Zuckerkandl said: "He spoke like Cicero and wrote like Heine." He made no great discoveries, and, as an independent investigator, he is not anywhere in Henle's class, but is to be regarded rather as the unapproachable teacher and technician and one of the greatest of medical philologists, a man to whom written and spoken Latin were as his mother tongue. His famous *Lehrbuch* (1846) passed through twenty-two editions, was translated into most languages, and has been pronounced by von Bardeleben to be the least soporific of all scientific treatises. Before reaching its twentieth edition (1889), it had no illustrations, the deficiency being largely supplied by Hyrtl's clear, beautiful, straightforward style, closing immediately with the subject in hand, and his wealth of historic and cultural allusions. Following the example of the French surgeons, Hyrtl published, in 1847,[1] the first topographic anatomy in the German language, which, despite its lack of illustrations, is doubly fascinating by reason of the same extraordinary display of historic and philologic knowledge. Hyrtl's manual of dissecting, published in 1860, is a classic of the same rank with Virchow's book on postmortem sections, and his *Corrosions Anatomie* (1873) is a permanent memento of his unique skill in making anatomical preparations. These, the wonder and admiration of Europe, included his unrivaled collection of fish skeletons, all prepared by himself; his models of the human and vertebrate ear; his microscopic slides and the corroded preparations (his own invention), consisting of injections of the blood supplies of the different organs and regions, with the adjacent parts eaten away by acids, to show the finest ramifications. His favorite fields of investigation were, in fact, the vascular and osseous systems. He discovered the portal vein of the suprarenal capsules, the branchial veins of fishes, the origin of the coronary arteries (1854), and made a collection of hearts devoid of blood-supply (*gefässlose Herzen*). Everything he did was stamped with originality and self-will. He once had the Laokoön represented as a life-sized skeletal group in support of his belief that bodily grace and poise depend, in the last analysis, upon bony structure. He opposed Brücke's theory of the autonomy of the heart with such harsh personalities that there came to be a Hyrtl faction and a Brücke faction in Vienna. Hyrtl had known the bitterness of poverty in his youth, but when he came into his own, and he was accounted wealthy as physicians go, his charity and humanity knew no bounds. Generous to a fault with his money, he endowed churches, orphanages, universities, with the same innate kindliness and liberality which prompted him to cheer his students at their work by his engaging presence and witty sallies. Nothing delighted him more than to lavish praise upon the work of a younger man, and in this unique regard he is like Müller and Ludwig, Virchow and Pasteur, those incomparable teachers of youth. Having filled his chair for thirty years, he resigned it voluntarily in 1874, in order to escape the (to him) humiliating experience of being pensioned off at seventy, retiring to a hermit-like existence at his country villa at Perchtoldsdorf. Here, in the society of his gentle, poetic wife, he produced his three masterpieces on Hebraic and Arabic elements in anatomy (1879),[2] on

---

[1] Hyrtl: Handbuch der topographischen Anatomie, Vienna, 1847.

[2] Hyrtl: Das Arabische und Hebräische in der Anatomie, Vienna, 1879.

anatomic terminology (1880),[1] and on old German anatomical expressions (1884).[2] Hyrtl ranks with Emile Littré as one of the greatest of modern medical scholars, and these books show him at his best in a field which was his very own. His declining years were clouded by a phase of pessimism that belied his cheerful, kindly nature.[3]

The group of investigators just considered includes a number of men who, under the influence of those great morphologists, John Hunter and Johannes Müller, approached physiological problems largely from the point of view of structure. Müller and his pupil Schwann employed both physical and chemical procedures in experimentation, but, after Müller's time, physiological investigation proceeded along two broadly divergent lines. The physical school, which aimed at purely mechanical modes of experimentation and interpretation, includes such names as Flourens, Poiseuille, Marshall Hall, the brothers Weber, Brücke, Carl Ludwig, du Bois Réymond, and Helmholtz. The chemical school, the followers of Liebig and Wöhler, was represented by Schwann, Beaumont, Tiedemann, Gmelin, Pettenkofer, and attained its highest development in the epoch-making work of Claude Bernard and Pasteur.

The pioneer of **experimental physiology** in France was François **Magendie** (1783–1855), of Bordeaux, who, like Müller, employed both physical and chemical procedure in his investigations, and was incidentally the modern founder of experimental pharmacology. Unlike Bichat, Magendie had not the slightest use for vitalistic or other theories, but regarded medicine as "a science in the making" (*une science à faire*) and sought to explain everything in terms of physics and chemistry. He compared himself to a rag-picker (*chiffonier*), who wanders through the domain of science collecting whatever he finds. This expressive phrase sums up the hard limitations which Magendie put upon himself or which existed in his own mind. He discovered only isolated facts, did not try to connect them with one another by any special hypotheses, and so arrived at no important generalizations. As the ardent protagonist of experimentation on living animals he is, of course, the particular aversion of the anti-vivisectionists, and there is no doubt that many of his experiments were without aim and needlessly cruel. But, before his time, physiology was made up of what Claude Bernard called *rêveries systématiques*, and it is the special distinc-

---

[1] Onomatologia anatomica, Vienna, 1880.

[2] Die alten deutschen Kunstworte der Anatomie, Vienna, 1884.

[3] See, "Ein Besuch bei Hyrtl," in Wien. med. Wochnschr., 1894, xliv, 1406. Contrast this with the jolly discourse of 1880 (*Las Culebras*) in Allg. Wien. med. Ztg., 1880, xxv, 521.

tion of Magendie to have headed the recent line of illustrious laboratory experimenters from Bernard himself to Pavloff, Loeb, and Ehrlich. Magendie was the founder of the first periodical devoted exclusively to physiology, the *Journal de physiologie expérimentale* (Paris, 1821–31). His greatest contribution to the science was his experimental proof (on a litter of puppies) of the truth of Bell's law, that the anterior roots of the spinal nerves are sensory, the posterior motor, in function (1822).[1] Through his bold vivisecting and lucid reasoning he arrived at a much clearer

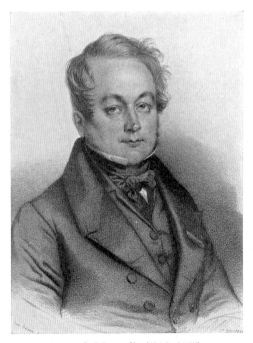

François Magendie (1783–1855).

conception of these functions than Bell; and, in adjusting the two claims, it seems proper to assign to Bell priority of discovery and demonstration in reference to the anterior roots, to Magendie priority of conclusive demonstration and interpretation of the functions of both motor and sensory roots. Magendie also made important investigations of the mechanism of deglutition and vomiting (1813);[2] of the effects of excision or section of the cere-

---

[1] Jour. de physiol. expér., Paris, 1822, ii, 276–279.

[2] Mémoire sur le vomissement, Paris, 1813.

bellum (1825),[1] and of the "circus movement" (*mouvement de manége*) obtained by lesion of the optic thalamus. He demonstrated that the pumping power of the heart is the main cause of the blood-flow in the veins, that chemical differences between the blood and the lymph will cause osmosis through the vessel-walls, and that the absorption of fluids and semisolids is a function of the blood-vessels as well as of the lymphatics (1821);[2] in other words, that absorption is not a specific vital property of the lymphatics, but only imbibition by vascular tissues. With Poiseuille, he was one of the first to notice that arterial blood-pressure rises with expiration, and his experiments on the circulation demonstrated the absurdity of the ancient idea of "points of election" in bloodletting, since the effects of venesection are the same at any site. Magendie's investigations in pharmacology introduced bromine, iodine, and such alkaloids as strychnine (showing its action on the spinal cord), morphine, veratrine, brucine, piperine, and emetine into medical practice (1821).[3] In experimental pathology, he induced Gaspard to repeat Haller's experiment of injecting putrid matter into the veins (1822).[4] His proof that secondary or subsequent injections of egg-albumen cause death in rabbits tolerant to an initial injection was the first experiment in anaphylaxis or supersensitization of the tissues (1839),[5] a phenomenon which Edward Jenner had already observed in variolous inoculations in 1798.

The most important French physiologists between Magendie and Claude Bernard are Legallois, Flourens, and Poiseuille.

Julien-Jean-César **Legallois** (1770–1814), a Breton who took part in the French Revolution, was some time in hiding for his political affiliations, and, after studying at the École de santé, received his medical degree in 1801. He was one of the earliest of the experimental physiologists, and his procedure was cruder and more brutal than Magendie's. He made such experiments as investigating the effect of submersion upon newly born animals or the temperature relations of brainless animals subjected to artificial respiration. In 1812,[6] he showed that bilateral section of the vagus nerve may produce fatal bronchopneumonia, and he greatly extended the observation of Robert Whytt (1750) that absolute integrity of the spinal cord is not necessary for the maintenance of

---

[1] Jour. de physiol. expér., 1825, v, 399.

[2] Jour. de physiol. expér., 1821, i, 1–31.

[3] Formulaire (etc.), Paris, 1821.

[4] Jour. de physiol. expér., Paris, 1822, ii, 1–45; 1824, iv, 1–69.

[5] In his "Lectures on the Blood," Phila., 1839, 244–249.

[6] Legallois: Expériences sur le principe de la vie, Paris, 1812.

the reflex functions.[1] His discovery that a lesion of a small circum-scribed area of the medulla inhibits breathing (1811)[2] was the first attempt to localize the center of respiration and was afterward com-pleted by the work of Flourens. Legallois is principally remem-bered today by his *Expériences sur le principe de la vie* (1812), in which he was the first, after Borelli, to revive the neurogenic theory of the heart's action. He maintained that the motor power of the heart is a principle or force contained throughout the spinal cord,

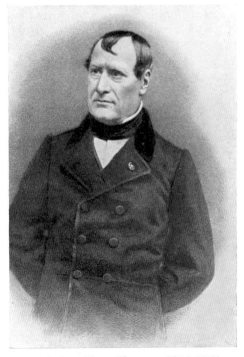

Marie-Jean-Pierre Flourens (1794–1867).

and transmitted to the heart by the branches of the sympathetic nerve. This was soon shown to be erroneous, but the neurogenic theory was further fortified by Robert Remak's discovery of in-trinsic nerve-ganglia in the heart (1844), and held its own until the revival of the myogenic theory by Gaskell and Engelmann.

Marie-Jean-Pierre **Flourens** (1794–1867) is memorable as the discoverer of the *nœud vital*, or "vital node," the bilateral center of

---

[1] Œuvres, Paris, 1830, i, p. 135.

[2] *Ibid.*, i, p. 248. Expériences (etc.), Paris, 1812 p. 37.

respiration in the medulla oblongata, a lesion of which causes asphyxia (1837).[1] Although the exact situation and extent of this vital spot have been in dispute down to the present time, the crucial feature of Flourens' experiment has never been set aside. In 1822–24,[2] he made his classical observations on the effects of removal of the cerebrum and cerebellum in pigeons, showing the absolute maintenance of reflexes with loss of cerebration and volition in the former case and the disturbance of equilibrium in the latter. These important experiments demonstrated that the brain is the organ of thought and of will power, while the cerebellum presides over the coördination of bodily movements, although Flourens denied the possibility of any cortical localization of functions. In 1828,[3] Flourens announced that a lesion of the semicircular canals in the internal ear will cause motor incoördination and loss of equilibrium, section of an individual canal producing rotatory motion around an axis at right angles to the plane of cleavage. From the analogy of these phenomena with the effects of a deep lesion in the cerebellum, Flourens inferred that both organs have to do with coördination of movement. Thus, where Purkinje had described only a presumable visual nystagmus, Flourens located the existence of a true cerebellar and labyrinthine vertigo. His results were confirmed physiologically by Vulpian, Goltz, Cyon, Ferrier; on the clinical side by Ménière; and have been ably elucidated, both surgically and clinically, by Robert Bárány as "vestibular nystagmus."

Jean-Léonard-Marie **Poiseuille** (1799–1869), of Paris, a medical graduate of 1828, was the first experimenter between Stephen Hales and Carl Ludwig to make any real advance in the physiology of the circulation. His name is permanently associated with the study of blood-pressure and the viscosity of the blood. Starting from Hales's original blood-pressure experiment of 1733, Poiseuille improved upon it by substituting a mercury manometer for the inconvenient long tube, connection with the artery being established by means of a hollow lead tip filled with potassium carbonate to prevent coagulation. This was Poiseuille's hemodynamometer (1828),[4] with which he showed that the blood-pressure rises and falls on expiration and inspiration, and measured the degree of arterial dilatation (about $\frac{1}{23}$ of the normal) at each

---

[1] Recherches expérimentales, Paris, éd. 2, 1842, p. 204. Compt.-rend. Acad. d. sc., Paris, 1858, xlvii, 803: 1859, xlviii, 1136.

[2] Arch. gén. de méd., Paris, 1823, ii, 344, 351; 1825, viii, 422–426; and Recherches expérimentales, Paris, 1824.

[3] Mém. Acad. d. sc., Paris, 1828, ix, 455–477.

[4] This instrument is described in Poiseuille's graduating dissertation: "Recherches sur la force du cœur aortique," Paris, 1828.

heart-beat. To this instrument Carl Ludwig, in 1847,[1] added a float, and, as Professor Stirling says, "had the genius to cause this float to write on a recording cylinder, and thus at one *coup* gave us the kymograph, or wave-writer, and the application of the graphic method to physiology." With these improvements, the science of blood-pressure (hemodynamics) became a definite part of recent medicine. Poiseuille's other great contribution to physiology was an investigation in mathematical physics, namely, on the flow and outflow of liquids in capillary tubes (1840).[2] He found that the average velocity of capillary flow varies directly with the sectional area of the tube, the grade of pressure, and the viscosity or stickiness of the moving fluid; also that the quantity of outflow is inversely as the length of the tube and directly proportional to the fourth power of its diameter, the pressure gradient, and the viscosity coefficient $\left(Q = \dfrac{D^4 PV}{L} \right)$, whence, for unit length, diameter, and pressure, the viscosity coefficient can be computed from the following formula: $V = \dfrac{QL}{D^4 P}$. This important equation is the mathematical expression of "Poiseuille's law," which, in recent times, has become fundamental in estimating the viscosity of the blood. The instrument used for the purpose (viscometer) was also invented by Poiseuille, and his name now stands, with those of Harvey, Hales, and Ludwig, as one of the founders of hemodynamics.

In applying the methods of laboratory physics to physiological problems, remarkable work was done by the brothers Weber, of Wittenberg. Of these, **Ernst Heinrich Weber** (1795–1878) was professor of anatomy and physiology at Leipzig (1821–66) up to the time of Carl Ludwig's advent, and afterward held the chair of anatomy there until 1871, when he was succeeded by Wilhelm His. He made an event in medical history by his discovery of the inhibitory power of the vagus nerve in 1845,[3] a find which threw much light upon such problems as the motion of the heart, the nature of fever, and the like. His original experiment, made with his brother, **Eduard Friedrich Weber** (1806–71), consisted in bringing the heart to a standstill by placing one pole of an electromag-

---

[1] Ludwig: Arch. f. Anat., Physiol. u. wissensch. Med., Berlin, 1847, 261.

[2] Poiseuille: Compt. rend. Acad. d. sc., Paris, 1840, xi, 961; 1041; 1841, xii, 12; 1843, xvi, 60.

[3] The discovery was communicated by the Webers to the Congress of Italian Scientists at Naples in 1845 ("Experimenta quibus probata nervos vagos rotatione machinæ galvano-magneticæ irritatos, motum cordis retardare et adeo intercipere," in Omodei's Ann. univ. de med., Milan, 1845, 3. s., xx, 227). It was afterward published at length in Wagner's Handwörterbuch der Physiologie, 1846, iii, 45–51.

netic apparatus in the nostril of a frog, the other on a cross-section of the cord at the level of the fourth vertebra. The field of inhibition was then localized to a region between the optic lobes and the calamus scriptorius, the vagi were found to be the channels of communication, and the results were extended to warm-blooded animals. Although the Webers at first thought that stimulation of both vagi was necessary for inhibition, and although Ludwig and Schmiedeberg afterward showed that the vagus contains accelerator as well as inhibitory fibers (1870–71), the original proof remains unshaken as one of the great monuments of physiologic

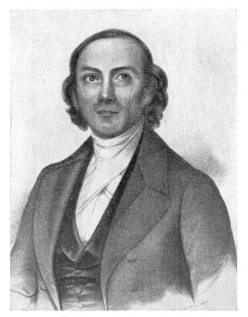

Ernst Heinrich Weber (1795–1878).

discovery. Ernst Heinrich Weber and Eduard Friedrich Weber also collaborated in the famous *Wellenlehre* or Hydrodynamics of Wave-Motion (1825), in which the velocity of the pulse-wave was measured for the first time and it was shown that it is delayed $\frac{1}{6}''$ to $\frac{1}{7}''$ in transmission, thus overthrowing Bichat's theory that the pulse is synchronous in all the arteries. In 1837, these two brothers again did clever work together in measuring and comparing the velocity of the blood and lymph corpuscles in the capillaries.[1] Ernst Heinrich Weber is again memorable for his model

---

[1] Müller's Arch., Berlin, 1837, 267–272.

to illustrate the hydrodynamics of the circulation (1850),[1] but the coping-stone of his single achievement is undoubtedly his great work on touch and temperature sense (Der Tastsinn und das Gemeingefühl, 1846), which was the starting-point of the experimental psychophysics of Fechner and Wundt. Johannes Müller, while assigning to each sense organ its proper, particular functions, did not admit the existence of any "common sensation" (such as pain or malaise) apart from the sense of touch. Weber was the first to show that this common sensation can be analyzed into its visceral and muscular components, and these separated from the tactile sensations. He boldly applied the idea of measurement to such phenomena as sensations of pain, heat, pressure, smell; noted that the threshold of painful sensation is also the threshold of nerve-injury, and stated the generalization known as Weber's law, viz., that intensity of sensation is not directly proportional to the degree of stimulus, but depends upon its mode of application. A given stimulus is less perceptible when added to a larger stimulus than to a smaller one; in other words, when the sensation increases in arithmetic progression, the stimulus must vary by geometric progression. Fechner afterward expressed this idea by saying that intensity of sensation varies with the logarithm of the stimulus (Weber-Fechner law), since the curve produced is a logarithmic curve.

A third brother of the Weber family was the celebrated electrician, **Wilhelm Eduard Weber** (1804–91), who was professor of physics at Göttingen all his active life (1831–91), constructed the first electromagnetic telegraph in 1833, made an atlas of the earth's magnetism (1840), and further distinguished himself by his important work in electric measurements. He collaborated with Eduard Friedrich Weber in the well-known classic on the mechanics of the human locomotor system (Mechanik der menschlichen Gehwerkzeuge, 1836), the most important study of the time on the physiology of motion and locomotion and the mechanism of the joints.

A remarkable all-round physiologist and anatomist was Ernst Wilhelm **von Brücke** (1819–92), of Berlin, who, in 1849, became professor of physiology at Vienna, where he was associated with the New Vienna School for the rest of his life. His investigation covered all branches of the subject, including the luminosity of the eye in animals (1845), phonetics (1856–62), the semilunar valves (1855), and artistic anatomy (1892), the latter one of the most attractive books ever written on the subject. He was the first to hold that normal urine may contain sugar (1858).

---

[1] Ber. ü. d. Verhandl. d. k. sächs. Gesellsch. d. Wissensch., Leipzig, 1850, 186.

The leading English exponent of physical experimentation in the early period was **Marshall Hall** (1790–1857), of Nottingham, whose Royal Society memoir on "The Reflex Function of the Medulla Oblongata and Medulla Spinalis" (1833)[1] established the difference between volitional action and unconscious reflexes. The idea that peripheral impulses can be reflected outwardly from the nerve centers connected with the brain, without relation to consciousness, had originally been suggested by Descartes in 1644 in his discussion of the batting of the eyes upon a threatened blow. Robert Boyle had noted that a viper, three days after decapitation, still wriggles upon being pricked. Johann Bohn had discussed the reflex movements of the decapitated frog as "a material phenomenon" (1686). Stephen Hales had shown that the movements of the decapitated frog are nullified when the spinal cord is destroyed. Robert Whytt, of Edinburgh, showed that destruction of the anterior optic lobe abolishes the contraction of the pupil to light (Whytt's reflex), and that a mere fragment of the spinal cord will suffice for the production of reflex movements. But most of these observers believed that reflex phenomena are bound up with sensation and ideation. The Bell-Magendie experiment (1811–22) was a great step forward and the discovery of the respiration center by Legallois (1826) and Flourens (1837) threw further light upon the problem. Independently of these last, and in apparent ignorance of the work of his predecessors, Marshall Hall showed that strychnine convulsions cease upon destruction of the spinal cord, that reflexes are more readily produced by stimulating the nerve-endings than the nerves themselves, and that there is a reflex contraction of sphincter muscles. It was Hall's work that gave "reflex action" a permanent place in physiology, although he did not realize, as Sherrington and others have pointed out, that volitional and reflex processes can pass from one to the other and that many nervous phenomena lie between the two extremes. He thought that the chief merit of his work lay in the discovery of special reflex paths dissociated from sensation and volition, an idea which was borne out by R. D. Grainger's discovery

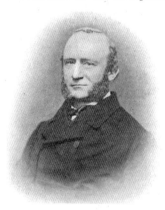

Ernst Wilhelm von Brücke
(1819–92).

---

[1] Hall: Phil. Tr., London, 1833, 635–665.

that the gray matter in the cord and its afferent roots is the true medium of reflex action (1837).

William **Sharpey** (1802–80), of Arbroath, Scotland, who was all his life a prominent teacher of physiology at University College, London (1836–74), is memorable for his papers on cilia and ciliary motion (1830–36),[1] and for his discovery of the "fibers of Sharpey" (1846).[2]

Sir William **Bowman** (1816–92), of Cheshire, England, an eminent ophthalmic surgeon, discovered and described striated muscle (1840–41),[3] basement m e m b r a n e s (1842), the ciliary region of the eyeball (1847), and, in 1842,[4] stated his theory of the urinary secretion that, as the tubes and their plexus of capillaries are probably the parts concerned in the secretion of the basic principles of the urine (the urea, lithic acid, etc.), the Malpighian bodies might be an apparatus destined to separate the watery portion from the blood.

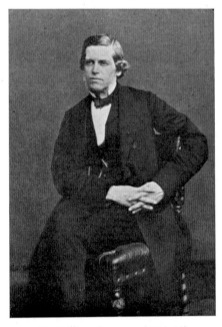

Sir William Bowman (1816–92).

The chemical tendency in modern experimental physiology, which led up to the magnificent work of Claude Bernard and Pasteur, was initiated by Liebig and Wöhler in Germany, and by Dumas and Chevreuil in France.

Justus **von Liebig** (1803–73), of Darmstadt, a pupil of Gay-Lussac, was the founder of agricultural chemistry, one of the prin-

---

[1] Sharpey: Edinb. Med. and Surg. Jour., 1830, xxxiv, 113–122, and Todd's Cyclopedia, London, 1835–36, i.

[2] Sharpey: in Jones Quain's anatomy, 5th ed., London, 1846, ii, pp. cxxxii–clxiii.

[3] Bowman: "On the Minute Structure and Movements of Voluntary Muscle," Phil. Tr., London, 1840, 457–501, 4 pl.; 1841, 69–73, the drawings by Bowman himself.

[4] Phil. Tr., London, 1842, pp. 67 et seq.

cipal founders of physiological chemistry and the chemistry of the carbon compounds, and the originator of laboratory teaching in chemical science. Liebig's laboratory, established at Giessen in 1826, was the first institution of the kind to be connected with university teaching and, bare and simple as its appointments, was soon thronged with enthusiastic, hard-working students. Here Liebig made his famous investigations of cyanides, cyanates, amides, aldehydes, benzoyls, benzoates, organic acids, and chemical fertilizers of soils, and here he founded Liebig's Annalen (1832–74), the leading literary organ of chemistry during his lifetime.

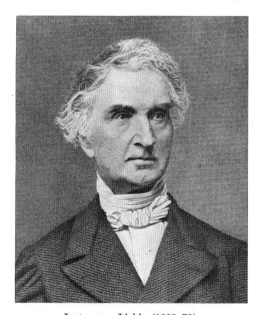

Justus von Liebig (1803–73).

Liebig's most important contributions to medicine were his discoveries of hippuric acid (Poggendorff's Ann., 1829), chloral and chloroform (1831),[1] his studies of uric acid compounds, his mode of estimating urea (1853),[2] and his important work on fats, blood, bile, and meat juice (Liebig's extract). His book on "Or-

---

[1] Ann. d. Pharm., Lemgo and Heidelberg, 1832, i, 182–230. Chloroform was discovered independently in the same year by Soubeiran (Ann. de chim., Paris, 1831, xlviii, 113–157), and by Samuel Guthrie, M.D. (1782–1848), of Bloomfield, Mass. (Am. J. Arts and Sc., 1831, xxi, 64; xxii, 105), at Jewettsville, near Sackett's Harbor, N. Y., where he hit upon the modern method of making chloroform by distilling alcohol with quicklime.

[2] Ann. d. Pharm., Lemgo and Heidelberg, 1853, lxxxv, 289–328.

ganic Chemistry in its Applications to Physiology and Pathology" (1842)[1] was the first formal treatise on the subject, introducing the term "metabolism" (*Stoffwechsel*); and his Familiar Letters on Chemistry (1844) did more than any other work to popularize that science. Liebig's investigations of fermentation and putrefaction were vitiated by his purely materialistic view of these phenomena, as based upon his theory of catalysis. He defined catalysis as the tuning-fork power of a system of molecules to set up sympathetic vibrations in another system, producing chemical change, and he affected only contempt or disbelief in regard to such vital agencies as bacteria or living ferments. He believed that fermentation and putrefaction are only physical disturbances of equilibrium which can be communicated by contact to other bodies. When, after long and bitter controversy, Liebig saw that his materialism had been refuted by Pasteur, he reluctantly stated that he had only attempted to assign a chemical cause for a chemical phenomenon. Yet Liebig was otherwise an uncompromising vitalist. Lord Kelvin relates that when he once asked the great chemist if he believed that a leaf or a flower could be formed or could be made to grow by chemical forces, Liebig replied: "I would more readily believe that a book on chemistry or on botany could grow out of dead matter by chemical processes."[2]

Friedrich **Wöhler** (1800–1882), of Eschersheim, Hesse-Nassau, was associated with Liebig in his investigations of uric acid, the cyanogen compounds, and the oil of bitter almonds, and himself made many important discoveries, two of which were epoch-making in the history of physiology. In 1828, Wöhler succeeded in effecting an artificial synthesis of urea[3] by heating ammonium cyanate, according to the equation: $NH_4CNO = CO(NH_2)_2$. This was the first time that an organic substance had ever been built up artificially from the constituents of an inorganic substance, without any intervention of vital processes, and it soon became clear that there is no essential difference between the structural chemistry of life and that of inanimate nature. This discovery led to a brilliant line of synthetic work, of which the highest point has so far been attained by Emil Fischer. In 1824, Wöhler made, and, in 1842, confirmed, a discovery which became the starting-point of the modern chemistry of metabolism, viz., that the benzoic

[1] Die organische Chemie in ihrer Anwendung auf Physiologie und Pathologie, Braunschweig, 1842.

[2] Lord Kelvin: Popular Lectures, London, 1894, ii, foot-note to p. 464.

[3] Wöhler: Ueber künstliche Bildung des Harnstoffs, Ann. d. Phys. u. Chem., Leipzig, 1828, xii, 253–256.

acid taken in with the food appears as hippuric acid in the urine.[1] This at once did away with the idea, current in Wöhler's time, that while plants can synthetize their complex materials, animals have to receive their constituent substances already synthetized from plants or other animals. Other modes of animal synthesis, such as those of uric acid from ammonium carbonate or of glycogen from glucose in the liver, were soon discovered and the problem of building up artificial foods from elementary materials had its inception here. Liebig and Wöhler were, in fact, the inaugurators of what von Noorden calls the qualitative period of metabolism experiments.

Among the earlier chemical investigations of importance to medicine were Sertürner's isolation of morphine (1806);[2] Wollaston's investigation of cystin calculi (1810);[3] Kirchhoff's conversion of starch into sugar (1811); Blackall and Wells on albumen in the urine (1812–14); the isolation of strychnine (1818),[4] brucine (1819), quinine,[5] and veratrine (1820) by Caventou and Pelletier; Alexander Marcet's investigation of black urine (1822);[6] Dutrochet's work on endosmosis and exosmosis (1827–35);[7] Geiger and Hesse's isolation of atropine (1833);[3] the investigations of Cagniard Latour[9] and Schwann on yeast cells and vinous fermentation (1837–38); Pettenkofer's test for bile (1844);[10] Hermann von Fehling's quantitative test for sugar in the urine (1848);[11] Henry Bence Jones's discovery of a special proteid (albumose) in the urine of patients with softening of the bones (myelopathic albumosuria, 1848);[12] Adolf Strecker's investigations of ox bile (1848–49);[13] Millon's discovery of a special reagent for proteids (1849);[14] and the invention of a ureometer for estimating the specific gravity of the urine (1849) by Florian Heller (1813–71), of the New Vienna School, his ring test for albumen[15] and his classic on urinary concretions (1860). Great impetus was given to chemical investigation in France by the work of Jean-Baptiste Dumas (1800–84), who isolated methyl alcohol, established the quantitative analysis of air and water, studied the chemical changes in the

---

[1] Ann. d. Phys. u. Chem., Leipzig, 1842, lvi, 638–641. One year before this, Alexander Ure, of Edinburgh, had pointed out that benzoic acid is changed to hippuric in the body (Provincial Med. and Surg. Jour., London, 1841, ii, 317). Wöhler's original experiment was given in Tiedemann's Ztschr. f. Physiol., 1824, i, 142, but his views were not definite until after Liebig's discovery of hippuric acid in 1829.

[2] Sertürner: J. d. Pharm., Leipzig, 1806, xiv, 47: 1811, xx, 99.

[3] Wollaston: Phil. Tr., London, 1810, 223–230.

[4] Caventou and Pelletier: J. d. pharm., Paris, 1819, v, 142–177.

[5] Ann. de chim. et phys., Paris, 1820, xv, 289; 337.

[6] Marcet: Med.-Chir. Tr., London, 1822–23, xii, 37–45.

[7] Dutrochet: Ann. de chim. et phys., Paris, v. 35, 37, 49, 52, 60.

[8] Geiger and Hesse: Ann. d. Pharm., Lemgo and Heidelberg, 1833, v, 43; vi, 44.

[9] Cagniard Latour: Ann. de chim. et phys., Paris, 1838, lxviii, 206–221.

[10] Pettenkofer: Ann. d. Chem. u. Pharm., Heidelberg, 1844, lii, 90–96.

[11] Fehling: Arch. f. d. physiol. Heilk., Stuttgart, 1848, vii, 64–73.

[12] Bence Jones: Phil. Tr., London, 1848, 55–62.

[13] Strecker: Ann. d. Chem. u. Pharm., Heidelberg, 1848, lxv, 1; lxvii, 1: 1849, lxx,149.

[14] Millon: Compt.-rend. Acad. d. sc., Paris, 1849, xxviii, 40–42.

[15] Heller's Arch. f. Physiol. u. path. Chem., Vienna, 1844, i, 192–199.

development of the chick, and (with Coindet) showed the value of iodine treatment in goiter (1820).[1] Michel-Eugene Chevreul (1787–1889) investigated the sugar in diabetic urine (1815),[2] and made an important study of animal fats (1823). In England, Thomas Graham (1805–69), of Glasgow, did work of capital importance in modern physiology by his discovery of the laws governing diffusion of gases (1829–31),[3] his investigation of osmotic force (1854),[4] and his method of separating animal and other fluids by dialysis, introducing the distinction between colloid and crystalloid substances (1861).[5] Graham's definition of osmosis as "the conversion of chemical affinity into mechanical power" still remains the most scientific ever made, as borne out by recent investigations of semi-permeable membranes.

The most important advance made by chemical investigation in the early period was in the physiology of digestion. The first work in this field, in order of time, is "An Experimental Inquiry into the Principles of Nutrition and the Digestive Process" (1803), by John R. Young, of Maryland, being his graduating thesis at the University of Pennsylvania. The labors of the earlier physiologists on digestion—Van Helmont, Sylvius, Borelli—were to a great extent impaired by their theories of innate heat and vital spirits, and, as William Hunter derisively remarked, they were fain to regard the stomach as a mill, a fermenting vat, or a stewpan. In the eighteenth century, Réaumur isolated the gastric juice and demonstrated its solvent effect upon foods (1752). Spallanzani confirmed the fact of its solvent and antiseptic character (1782), and thus did away with the various views of concoction, putrefaction, trituration, and fermentation in favor of a chemical theory of solution; but he failed to recognize that the solvent action of the gastric juice is due to its acidity. Young took up his work at this point and, by experiments made upon bull-frogs, snakes, and even *in propria persona*, showed that the solvent principle of the gastric juice is an acid, turning litmus paper red and softening bones into a pulp, and that this acid does not arise from any vinous or other fermentation in the stomach, but is part of the normal gastric secretion. He arrived at the important deduction, demonstrated in our own time by Pavloff, that the flow of gastric juice and of saliva are associated and synchronous, but he wrongly inferred that the acid principle of the stomach is phosphoric acid. In 1824, William Prout (1785–1850), an English chemist, was able to prove, by careful titration and distillation, that the acid of the gastric juice is free hydrochloric acid.[6] This result was soon confirmed by other

---

[1] Coindet: Ann. de chim. et phys., Paris, 1820, xv, 49–59.

[2] Chevreul: Ann. de chimie, Paris, 1815, xcv, 319.

[3] Graham: Quart. Jour. Sc., London, 1829, ii, 74–83; Phil. Mag., London, 1833, ii, 175–190.

[4] Phil. Tr., London, 1854, cxliv, 177–228.

[5] *Ibid.*, 1861, cli, 183–224.

[6] Prout: Phil. Tr., London, 1824, 45–49.
27

chemists, notably in the classical monograph on "Digestion, Experimentally Considered" (1826–27),[1] by Friedrich **Tiedemann** (1781–1861), of Cassel, and Leopold **Gmelin** (1788–1853), of Göttingen. In this work, Gmelin's nitric acid test for the bile-pigments is given, the limited quantity of the gastric secretion is pointed out, and it is shown that the saliva contains a sulphocyanate, and the pancreatic secretion a principle which turns red with chlorine water. This principle (tryptophan) was afterward shown by

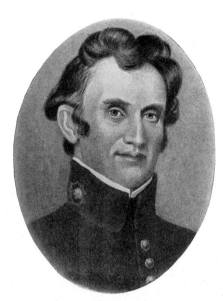

William Beaumont (1785–1853). (Courtesy of Dr. Jesse S. Myer, St. Louis. From his "Life and Letters of William Beaumont," 1912.)

Claude Bernard to be a by-product of pancreatic digestion and not a true constituent of the pancreatic juice.

In 1833, William **Beaumont** (1785–1853), of Connecticut, a surgeon in the United States Army, published his famous "Experiments and Observations" on an accidental gastric fistula in the Canadian half-breed, Alexis St. Martin, which threw so much light upon the nature of the gastric juice, the process of digestion in the stomach, and the early stages of gastritis. As far back as 1664, Regner De Graaf had published his account of artificial salivary and pancreatic juice in a dog, giving a picture of the dog; and there were earlier cases of gastric fistulæ; but Beaumont was the first to study digestion and the movements of the stomach *in situ* (1825).[2]   He began by carefully reviewing the work of his predecessors in a fair-minded spirit; gave an accurate description of the normal and pathological appearances of the gastric mucous membrane in life, and the movements of the stomach up to the completion of digestion; showed that the gastric juice is secreted only when food is present and that mechanical irritation of the mucous membrane produces congestion, but only a limited local secretion of gastric juice, thus fore-

    [1] Tiedemann and Gmelin: Die Verdauung nach Versuchen, Heidelberg and Leipzig, 1826–27.
    [2] Med. Recorder, Phila., 1825, viii, 14: 840: 1826, ix, 94.

shadowing the results of Pavloff, and overthrowing the doctrine of Magendie that the gastric secretion is continual. Beaumont's experiments on the effect of gastric juice upon different foods and the relative digestive values of the latter are the foundation of modern dietetic tables and scales; and his chemical examination of the gastric juice led him to the conclusion that it contains free hydrochloric acid plus some other active chemical substance, which Theodor Schwann, in 1835, proved to be pepsin. This was the most important work on the physiology of gastric digestion before the time of Pavloff, and the difficulties under which the experimenter completed his labors, first begun at an isolated military post in the primeval forests of Michigan, and completed only by dint of following up his patient, and bringing him nearly 2000 miles to Plattsburg Barracks, N. Y., make his experience one of the romantic episodes in the history of medicine. "Every physician who prescribes for digestive disorders," says Vaughan, "and every patient who is benefited by such a prescription, owes gratitude to the memory of William Beaumont, who, in 1825, on the island of Mackinaw, began his studies of digestion, which he pursued with labor and skill for the benefit of mankind." He was the true leader and pioneer of experimental physiology in our country.[1]

Early nineteenth century **surgery** was mainly a continuation of the surgery of the eighteenth century, with this difference, that the center of gravity had shifted from Paris to London, as a result of the mighty influence of Hunter's teaching and of the evil effects of the fanatical prohibitions of 1792–93, which abolished medical faculties and societies in France. Many bold operative feats were performed in this period, plastic surgery was revived, most of the larger arteries were successfully ligated, American and Russian surgery came into existence, but of general operating within the cranium, joints, abdomen, and female pelvis, or in isolated organs like the eye and ear, there was no sign until well after the year 1867.

The leading surgeons of the pre-Listerian period were the Bells, Cooper, Colles, Brodie, Liston, Syme, and Fergusson in Great Britain; Larrey, Dupuytren, Lisfranc, Delpech, Velpeau, Malgaigne, and Nélaton in France; the elder Langenbeck, Dieffenbach, the elder Graefe, and Stromeyer in Germany; Pirogoff in Russia; Physick, Post, Mott, the Warrens, and McDowell in America.

The brothers John and Charles Bell were leading figures among the London and Edinburgh surgeons of their day, but the fame of Sir Charles Bell now rests largely upon his discoveries in anatomy,

---

[1] For a very complete and interesting account of Beaumont and his work, see Dr. Jesse S. Myer's "Life and Letters of William Beaumont," with an introduction by Sir William Osler, St. Louis, C. V. Mosby Co., 1912.

physiology, and pathology. **John Bell** (1763–1820), of Edinburgh, belongs, in part, to an earlier period, but his great works upon surgical anatomy exerted a powerful influence upon the men of a later time, and he was, with Desault and John Hunter, a founder of the modern surgery of the vascular system. He himself had tied the common carotid and the posterior branch of the internal iliac successfully, and was the first to ligate the gluteal artery.[1] Like his brother Charles, John Bell was an artist of talent, one of the great medical men who have illustrated their own books. His "Anatomy of the Human Body" (1793–1803) was an important work in its time, afterward reissued with original plates drawn by Sir Charles Bell (1811); and his "Engravings," illustrating the different parts and organs of the body (1794–1804), the drawings and almost all the etchings and engravings being his own, is one of the milestones in the history of anatomical delineation. The third volume, dealing with the brain, nerves, sense organs and viscera (1804), is almost entirely the work of Sir Charles. John Bell's most enduring contributions to surgery are his "Discourses on the Nature and Cure of Wounds" (1795), the second of which is a valuable historical discussion of the surgery of the arteries; and his monumental "Principles of Surgery" (1801–1807), embellished with beautiful original engravings and full of unique historical and clinical matter relating to the ligation of the great vessels, fractures, trephining, tumors and lithotomy, of which he gives a detailed history, occupying 248 pages. The writings of John Bell are characterized by great sincerity and depth of feeling. He took his profession with a fine ethical seriousness, which, given his combative temperament, often involved him in hot and bitter controversy. He railed at the mistakes of Benjamin Bell and Monro *secundus*, which did not increase his popularity. He was kept out of practice in the Royal Infirmary through the machinations of James Gregory, who assailed him in a bulky volume under the now-forgotten pseudonym of "Jonathan Dawplucker." Toward the end of his life, broken in health by a fall from a horse, John Bell went to Italy to die, leaving an enduring memento of his visit in his posthumous "Observations on Italy" (1825), one of the best books of travel ever written by a physician. This work is again remarkable for beautiful original drawings, some of which exhibit a feeling for the details of Italian architecture akin to that of Piranesi.

Sir Astley Paston **Cooper** (1768–1841), of Norfolk, a pupil of John Hunter's, was the most popular surgeon in London during the first quarter of the century. A clergyman's son, he was some-

---

[1] See his "Principles of Surgery," 1801, vol. i, pp. 421–426.

thing like Hunter in his youthful pranks, and became demonstrator of anatomy of St. Thomas's Hospital at the age of twenty-one (1789), and surgeon at Guy's Hospital in 1800. He was one of the pioneers in the surgery of the vascular system, in experimental surgery and in the surgery of the ear. In 1808, he successfully ligated the common carotid and the external iliac arteries for aneurysms, making postmortem dissections of his cases in 1821[1] and 1826[2] respectively, and in 1817 came his celebrated feat of ligating the abdominal aorta.[3] Valentine Mott has left an inter-

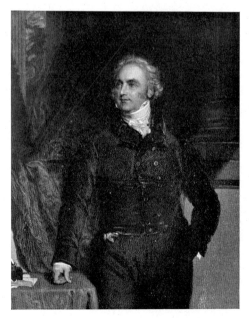

Sir Astley Paston Cooper, Bart. (1768–1841).

esting account of his attempt to tie the subclavian in 1809.[4] He also made experimental ligations of the arteries and nerves in dogs.[5] In 1824, he amputated at the hip-joint. His Royal Society memoir, on perforating the tympanic membrane for deafness resulting from obstruction of the Eustachian tube in 20 cases (1801),[6] gained

---

[1] Guy's Hosp. Rep., London, 1836, i, 53–58, 1 pl.

[2] *Ibid.*, 43–52, 2 pl.

[3] In Cooper and Travers's "Surgical Essays," London, 1818, pt. 1, 101–130, 2 pl.

[4] Med. Repository, N. Y., 1809–10, xiii, 331–334.

[5] Guy's Hosp. Rep., London, 1836, i, 457; 654.

[6] Phil. Tr., London, 1801, 435–450, 1 pl.

him the Copley Medal in 1802, and a slight operation performed on George IV, in 1820, was followed by his baronetcy. Cooper's professional life was thus one long trail of success, which can be sensed in the enormous number of engravings which were made of his likeness. "No surgeon, before or since," says Bettany, "has filled so large a space in the public eye." Although his early income was very small, his wife's fortune made his circumstances easy. Yet few medical men have ever worked so hard and so incessantly. He dissected every day of his life, even when traveling, paying large fees and liberal *douceurs* to the body-snatchers. With these, his experiences were such that he once stated before a House of Commons committee that "there was no person, whatever his worldly place, whom he could not dissect if he would." His daily course of life was to rise at six, dissect until eight, breakfast on two hot rolls and tea, see poor patients until nine, attend to his regular consulting practice until one, when he would drive rapidly to Guy's Hospital to visit the wards; at two, he lectured on anatomy at St. Thomas's Hospital, after which he went through the dissecting-rooms with the students and visited or operated on private patients until seven; he would then bolt his dinner, snatch forty winks of sleep and start out again for a possible clinical lecture, with another round of visits until midnight. He dictated whatever he wrote while in his carriage. He read little, but managed to absorb the best current knowledge, and his books on Hernia (1804–7), Injuries of the Joints (1822), Diseases of the Testis (1830), and the Anatomy of the Thymus Gland (1832) are still remembered, as also Cooper's fascia, Cooper's hernia and other eponyms. Cooper was one of the first surgical teachers to substitute practical demonstrations over an actual case for the old didactic theory-mongering of the past; and one of his best achievements was the large number of capable and spirited young surgeons he formed through contact with himself. In personality, he was no pedant or Philistine, but "courteous-eyed, erect and slim," the tall, handsome, engaging figure of Sir Thomas Lawrence's portrait, with a lively, expressive countenance, cheeks aglow with color, a clear voice and a chuckling laugh, and, in spite of his quick, imperious temper, idolized by the students, who followed his clinics in enthusiastic throngs. As an operator, he was unaffected, elegant, rapid but unhurried, thorough, masterful, "all ease, all kindness to the patients, and equally solicitous that nothing should be hidden from the observation of the pupils." He attributed his professional success to his uniform and unfailing courtesy to rich and poor alike, as well as to his zeal and industry, "but for this I take no credit, as it was given to me from above." Few men have so fully realized the truth of the poet's device, "We receive but what we give," in the possession of a cheerful, manly, and generous disposition.

Charles **Aston Key** (1793–1849), of Southwark, one of Cooper's juniors at Guy's, successfully ligated the external iliac artery for femoral aneurysm in 1822,[1] and the subclavian for axillary aneurysm in 1823.[2] He also tied the carotid in 1830 and introduced such improvements as the use of the straight staff in lithotomy (1824) and the principle of dividing the stricture outside the sac in strangulated hernia (1833). Like Cooper, he was a swift, neat operator and a popular teacher, smart in attire, but, unlike his chief, condescending, over-dictatorial and self-important in manner.

Benjamin **Travers** (1783–1858), of London, another of Cooper's pupils, collaborated with the latter in the valuable "Surgical Essays" (1818–19), to which he contributed a noteworthy paper on wounds of the veins. In 1809, he successfully ligated the common carotid artery in a case of aneurysm by anastomosis in the orbit.[3] He was one of those who followed Broussais in regarding constitutional irritation as a cause of disease, particularly in the nervous system (1824–34). His specialty was ophthalmology, in which field he introduced the use of mercury in non-specific iritis and wrote the best systematic treatise on diseases of the eye of his time (1820).

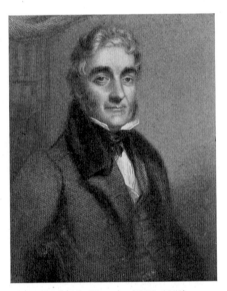

Benjamin Travers (1783–1858).

Abraham **Colles** (1773–1843), of Dublin, professor of surgery in that city for thirty-two years (1804–36), was the leading Irish surgeon of his day. He tied the subclavian artery twice (1811–15),[4] and was the first to tie it within the scaleni (1816). He is said to

---

[1] Key: Guy's Hosp. Rep., London, 1836, i, 68–70.
[2] Med.-Chir. Tr., London, 1823–7, xiii, 1–11.
[3] Travers: Med.-Chir. Tr., London, 1817, ii, 1–16.
[4] Colles: Edinb. Med. and Surg. Jour., 1815, xi, 1–25.

have been the first man in Europe to tie the innominate successfully.[1] He wrote treatises on surgical anatomy (1811) and on
surgery (1844–45), but his most important works are his original
description of fracture of the carpal end of the radius or "Colles'
fracture" (1814),[2] and his *Practical Observations on the Venereal
Disease* (1837), in which he states "Colles' law," relating to the
supposed immunity which a healthy mother acquires in bearing a
syphilitic child.

Robert **Liston** (1794–1847), of Scotland, was an Edinburgh
graduate who became professor of clinical surgery in University

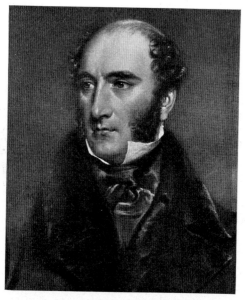

Robert Liston (1794–1847).

College, London, in 1834. Like the Bells and Astley Cooper, he
was a fine anatomist, keeping up his dissections all his life, and this
helped to make him one of the most brilliant and skilful operators
of his time, excelling in emergency cases which called for swiftness
of decision and originality of procedure. He introduced many
novelties, such as his popular mode of flap-amputation, his shoe
for club-foot and his devices for reducing dislocations, and crushing
and cutting for stone. He was especially successful in plastic opera-

---

[1] I have been unable to verify this statement, which is made in all biographies of Colles.

[2] Edinb. Med. and Surg. Jour., 1814, x, 182–186.

tions.   In 1836, he successfully excised the upper jaw, and, in 1837,[1] he described his method of laryngoscopy, in which he was one of the early pioneers.   His most important works were his "Elements of Surgery" (1831) and his *Practical Surgery* (1837), which passed through many editions and still contain things of permanent value.   Liston was often rough, abrupt and contentious in public relations, but kind and charitable to the poor, soft and gentle in the sick-room.   He was possessed of such Herculean strength that he could amputate a thigh with the aid of only one assistant, while compressing the artery with his left hand and doing all the sawing and cutting with his right.

James **Syme** (1799–1870), of Edinburgh, was a cousin of Liston's and taught anatomy with the latter in 1822.   Having quarreled with his partner, he could get no appointment in the Royal Infirmary until 1833, but when Liston went down to London in 1834, he succeeded to his very large Scotch practice.   The enemies were soon reconciled, and, after Liston's death in 1847, Syme succeeded him in London, but not liking the position, returned to Edinburgh.   Syme's most important contribution to surgery is his work on amputations and excisions.   In his *Excision of Diseased Joints* (1831) he was the first to show that excision is usually preferable to amputation, and the adoption of this new principle is due to him, although it was afterward developed *in extenso* by Fergusson.   He made his first three successful excisions of the elbow-joint in 1828–29.[2]   On September 8, 1842,[3] he performed his first successful case of amputation at the ankle-joint (Syme's amputation) of which he described eight cases in his "Contributions to the Pathology and Practice of Surgery" (1847).   In 1864, he published his work on "Excision of the Scapula" and, in the same year, successfully excised a large part of the tongue.   He treated aneurysm by tying the artery above and below and incising the tumor, performing this operation for carotid and iliac aneurysms in 1857, and, in 1862, he successfully treated an iliac aneurysm by ligation of the common, external and internal iliac arteries.[4]   Syme was a genial, happy, even-tempered man who "never wasted a word, nor a drop of ink, nor a drop of blood," yet a broad-minded, liberal spirit withal, welcoming all surgical innovations of value.   He was, with Pirogoff, perhaps the first European surgeon to adopt ether anesthesia (1847), and, in 1868, he was the first to welcome the

---

[1] In his "Practical Surgery," London, 1837, p. 350.

[2] Syme: Edinb. Med. and Surg. Jour., 1829, xxxi, 256–266.

[3] Lond. and Edinb. Month. Jour. Med. Sc., 1843, iii, 93–96.

[4] Proc. Roy. Med. and Chir. Soc., London, 1862, iv, 114–116.

antiseptic method of his best and greatest pupil, his son-in-law, Lord Lister.

Sir William **Fergusson** (1808–77), of Prestonpans, Scotland, was the founder of conservative surgery, that is, of the preservation of parts of the body which were needlessly sacrificed by earlier operators. Before Fergusson's time, denuded bones, diseased or painful (even neurotic) joints, were regarded as a sufficient reason for amputation. He held it to be "a grand thing when by prescience even the tip of a thumb can be saved." Fergusson was a pupil and prosector of Robert Knox, and soon became surgeon to the Edin-

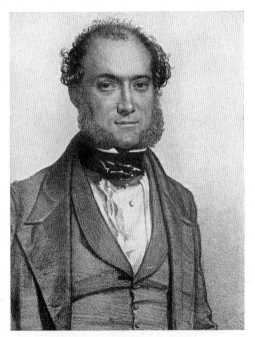

Sir William Fergusson (1808–77).

burgh Royal Dispensary (1831) and the Royal Infirmary (1839); but Syme's huge practice drove him to London where, after slow progress, he eventually attained the summit. He was one of the first in Scotland to tie the subclavian artery, and his progress in substituting excisions for amputation was rapid. He excised the head of the femur for incurable hip disease (1845), the scapula, in place of the interscapular-thoracic amputation (1847) and the knee-joint (1850). Between 1828 and 1864, he had operated 400 times for harelip, with only three failures, and 134 times for cleft-palate, with 129 successful cases. In lithotomy, he proceeded with such lightning speed and skill that some one advised a prospective visitor at his clinic to "look out sharp, for if you only wink, you'll miss the operation altogether." Yet he carefully planned every detail in advance, silently working out each step as he went along, even to the bandaging. He wrote a "System of Practical Surgery" (1842), and his "Progress of Anatomy and Surgery During the Present Century" (1867) is a historic work of permanent value. He was an indifferent lecturer and is said to have had a poor bed-side manner, but he fascinated his patients and was adored by the

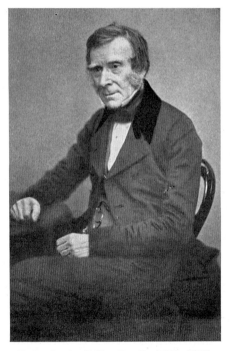

Sir Benjamin Collins Brodie (1783–1862).

children. He was highly accomplished, a good violinist, an inventor of many surgical instruments, so expert in carpentry and metal work that he could devise any necessary apparatus out of hand, an enthusiast at fly-fishing and in dancing Scotch reels. He was noted for his great generosity and hospitality to struggling authors, dramatists and medical students.

Sir Benjamin Collins **Brodie** (1783–1862) was the son of a Wilt-shire clergyman who was descended from a Jacobite exile in England. He was a pupil of Sir Everard Home, lectured at Great

Windmill Street (1805–12), and was subsequently assistant surgeon, and later full surgeon, at St. George's Hospital (1808–40).
Being profoundly influenced by Bichat, he at first devoted himself
to physiologic experimentation, producing four papers, important
in their day, on the influence of the brain on the action of the heart
(1810),[1] the effects of certain vegetable poisons (1811),[2] the influence of the nervous system on the production of animal heat
(1812),[3] and the influence of the pneumogastric on the secretions
of the stomach (1814).[4]   In these researches, the first two of which
gained him the Copley Medal (1811), he used the woorara poison
which had just been brought from Guiana.   In 1819, he published
his classic treatise "On the Pathology and Surgery of Diseases of
the Joints," his most important work, clearly describing the different articular diseases and differentiating the local lesions from
the hysterical and neuralgic forms.   He was a pioneer in subcutaneous surgery, performing his first operation on a case of varicose
veins in 1814, and made many improvements in surgical instruments and appliances.   He was the acknowledged head of the
medical profession in London for over thirty years, his income
often averaging £10,000 annually, and largely made up of guinea
fees at that.   He did not regard operative intervention as the
highest part of surgery, and "his vocation was more to heal limbs
than to remove them."   Brodie had been all his life assisted by
influential friends and family connections, but he held high places,
such as the presidency of the Royal College of Surgeons, with dignity, grace, and the kind of tactful self-effacement which aims to
stimulate and bring out the ideas of other men.   He seems to
have been "servile to none, deferential to none," standing on an
equal footing of friendliness and confidence with the poor in hospital or his titled intimates at Holland House or Windsor Castle.
"I hear you are ill," he once wrote to an almost unknown student;
"no one will take better care of you than I; come to my country
house till you are well," making the student remain with him two
months.
    Here may be mentioned two other surgeons of the Scotch group
—Lizars and Wardrop.
    John **Lizars** (1783–1860), of Edinburgh, a pupil of John Bell's,
was originally a naval surgeon, but became professor of surgery to
the College of Surgeons in his native city in 1831.   He was one of
the first to remove the lower jaw, but he is now best remembered as
the follower of McDowell (his fellow-pupil) in ovariotomy (1825),
and by his "System of Anatomical Plates" (1825), a superb series

---

[1] Brodie: Phil. Tr., 1811, 36–48.   [2] Ibid., 1811, 178–208: 1812, 205–227.
[3] Ibid., 1812, 373–393.   [4] Ibid., 1814, 102–106.

of 110 colored illustrations in folio, made largely from his own dissections.

James **Wardrop** (1782–1869), of Scotland, an Edinburgh graduate who settled in London in 1809, is now best remembered by his "Essays on the Morbid Anatomy of the Human Eye" (1808), a book of importance in its day, and by his method of treating aneurysm by ligating on the distal side of the tumor, which was first suggested by Brasdor in the eighteenth century. Wardrop performed this operation twice with success on the carotid artery (1809)[1] and once on the subclavian in a case of innomi-

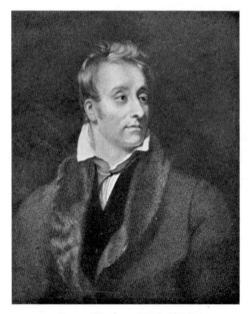

James Wardrop (1782–1869).

nate aneurysm (1827).[2] A curious side of Wardrop is that he stood in the way of his own success and estranged his colleagues through his acrimonious and abusive papers in the Lancet of 1826–27, and through the famous "Intercepted Letters," in the same journal for 1834, in which he foisted off more personal abuse by using the leading names of the London profession as stalking-horses.

---

[1] Med.-Chir. Tr., London, 1825, xiii, 217–226.
[2] Lancet, London, 1827, xii, 471; 601; 798: 1827–8, i, 408.

Other prominent English surgeons during the pre-antiseptic period were William Hey (1736–1819), of Leeds, who first described fungus hæmatodes and devised a useful saw for operating in fractures of the skull, and whose "Practical Observations on Surgery" (1803) passed through three editions; Allan Burns (1781–1813), of Glasgow, who wrote an important work on the Surgical Anatomy of the Head and Neck (1811), and first described the falciform process of the fascia lata in relation to femoral hernia; Samuel Cooper (1780–1848), whose "Surgical Dictionary" (1809) was the first thoroughgoing work of its kind to be published, passing through eight editions; Joseph Constantine Carpue (1764–1848), who was a pioneer in electrotherapy (1803),[1] revived the Hindu method of rhinoplasty (1816), and wrote a valuable "History of the High Operation for Stone" (1819); John Flint South (1797–1882), the historian of early British surgery, who translated Chelius, and whose posthumous manuscript of a "History of the Craft of Surgery in England" was edited and published by D'Arcy Power in 1886; O'Bryen Bellingham (1805–57), whose book on the treatment of aneurysm by compression (1847) preserves his name and fame in connection with the procedure; Thomas Pridgin Teale (1801–68), of Leeds, memorable for his treatise on abdominal hernia (1846), his method of amputation by a long and short rectangular flap (1858), and for his attempt to apply the Broussais doctrine of irritation to the nervous system (1829); Sir William Lawrence (1783–1867) and Sir William Bowman (1816–92), who did much to advance the surgery of the eye; Sir William Wilde (1815–76), of Castlerea, Ireland, one of the pioneers of aural surgery (1843–53) and cerebral surgery (Wilde's incision), who also discovered prehistoric lake dwellings on the Irish crannogs (1839) before Keller; William Henry Porter (1790–1861), who wrote an important work on the surgical pathology of the larynx and trachea (1826); and John Hieton (1804–78), of Guy's Hospital, whose "Rest and Pain" (1863) is one of the permanent classics of surgery.

Of isolated operations and operative procedures by English surgeons of the period we may mention the interscapular-thoracic amputation (excision of arm, scapula and clavicle) which was first performed by Ralph Cuming of the Royal Navy in 1808;[2] Anthony White's excision of the head of the femur for hip disease (1822);[3] the first English cases of gastrostomy (1858–59)[4] by John Cooper Forster (1824–96) of Guy's Hospital; Pridgin Teale's method of amputation by a long and a short rectangular flap (1858); Richard Carden's single flap amputation (1864);[5] and four successful cases of ligation of the external iliac artery by William Goodlad (1811),[6] William Stevens (1812),[7] John Smith Soden (1816),[8] and T. Cole (1817).[9] In Stevens' case, the patient lived ten years, the parts being dissected eight years later

[1] J. C. Carpue: An Introduction to Electricity and Galvanism, London, 1803.

[2] Cuming: Lond. Med. Gaz., 1829–30, v, 273.

[3] White: Lancet, London, 1849, i, 324.

[4] Forster: Guy's Hosp. Rep., London, 1858, 3. s., iv, 13: 1859, v, 1.

[5] Carden: Brit. M. J., 1864, i, 416–421.

[6] Goodlad: Edinb. Med. and Surg. Jour., 1812, viii, 32–39.

[7] Stevens: Med.-Chir. Tr., London, 1814, v, 422–434.

[8] Soden: *Ibid.*, 1816, vii, 536–540.

[9] Cole: London Med. Repository, 1820, xiii, 369–375.

(1830)[1] by Sir Richard Owen. The first successful ligation of the common carotid artery appears to have been performed by David Fleming, surgeon of H.M.S. Tonnant, in October, 1803.[2]

The leading English military surgeon of the time was George James **Guthrie** (1785–1856), of London, who had served in America and in the Napoleonic wars. At Waterloo, Guthrie successfully amputated the hip-joint[3] and ligated the peroneal artery (1815).[4] His most important work is his Treatise on Gunshot Wounds of the Extremities requiring Amputation (1815), which was epoch-

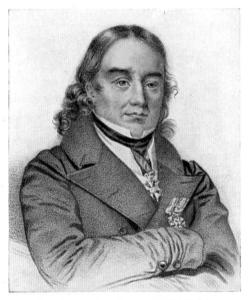

Dominique-Jean Larrey (1766–1842).

making and ran through six editions. Guthrie was also a skilled ophthalmic surgeon and left two important works on artificial pupil (1823) and the surgery of the eye (1812).

Dominique-Jean **Larrey** (1766–1842), the greatest French military surgeon of his time, also served in the Napoleonic wars. In his will, Napoleon left 100,000 francs to "Larrey, the most virtuous man I have ever known." Larrey was one of the first to amputate at

---

[1] Owen: Med.-Chir. Tr., London, 1830, xvi, 219–325.
[2] Fleming: Med.-Chir. Jour. and Rev., London, 1817, iii, 1–4.
[3] In his: Treatise on Gunshot Wounds, second ed., London, 1820, 332–340.
[4] Guthrie: Med.-Chir. Tr., London, 1816, vii, 330–337.

the hip-joint (1803),[1] performing the operation twice with success. He was surgeon-in-chief to the "Grande Armée," taking part in 60 battles and 400 engagements.   He was three times wounded, performed as many as 200 amputations in one day, was the inventor of the celebrated "flying ambulances," and sometime professor at the École de médicine militaire at Val-de-Grâce, which was founded in 1796.   Like Ambroïse Paré, he was adored by his comrades in arms for his good nature, courage, and humanity.   His most interesting work is contained in the four volumes of his "Memoirs of Military Medicine" (1812–17).   In a memoir published at Cairo in 1802, he was the first to point out the contagious nature of Egyptian ophthalmia or granular conjunctivitis.

The ablest and best trained French surgeon of his time was Guillaume **Dupuytren** (1777–1835), who was at once a shrewd diagnostician, an operator of unrivaled aplomb, a wonderful clinical teacher, and a good experimental physiologist and pathologist. Dupuytren rose from poverty and fought his way up, and his achievements are sometimes overlooked on account of the meanness of his character.   In 1808, he became one of the staff at the Hôtel Dieu, and by 1815 he was surgeon-in-chief.   Here his lectures and his extensive practice soon made him the leading surgeon of France, and he died a millionaire and a baron of the Empire.   His clinics drew crowds of students from all countries, and he turned out many brilliant pupils.   He was the first to excise the lower jaw (1812)[2] and to treat aneurysm successfully by compression (1818);[3] was the first to treat wry-neck by subcutaneous section of the sternomastoid muscle (1822),[4] and performed many feats in vascular surgery, such as the successful ligation of the external iliac (1815)[5] and two ligations of the subclavian (1819–29).[6]   He also devised an original method of treating artificial anus by means of a compressing enterotome of his invention (1828),[7] but his most enduring title to modern fame is in the field of surgical pathology.   His original descriptions of fracture of the lower end of the fibula (Dupuytren's fracture, 1819),[8] congenital

---

[1] Larrey: Mém. de chir. mil., Paris, 1812, ii, 180–195.

[2] Dupuytren: Leçons orales, Paris, 1839, ii, 421–453.

[3] Bull. Fac. de méd. de Paris, 1818, vi, 242.

[4] Described in Dupuytren: Leçons orales, Paris, 1839, iii, 455–461, and in Charles Averill's "Short Treatise on Operative Surgery," London, 1823, 61–64.

[5] Repert. gén. d'anat. et de physiol. path., Paris, 1826, ii, 230–250.

[6] Edinb. Med. and Surg. Jour., 1819, xv, 476, and Arch. gén. de méd., Paris, 1829, 7. s., xx, 566–573.

[7] Mém. Acad. de méd., Paris, 1828, i, 259–316, 3 pl.

[8] Annuaire méd.-chir. d. hôp. de Paris, 1819, i, 1–212.

dislocation of the hip-joint (1826),[1] and retraction of the fingers
from affection of the palmar aponeurosis, for which he devised
an operation (1832),[2] are his greatest works. His memoirs On
Injuries and Diseases of the Bones and on other phases of surgical
pathology were reprinted in translation by the Sydenham Society in
1847 and 1854. He also left a treatise on wounds in war (1834),
and his *Leçons orales* (1839) were often translated. In 1803, he
founded the Société anatomique de Paris, and he was also the
founder of the well-known Musée Dupuytren at Paris. Dupuytren was the type of man whom grinding poverty in youth has

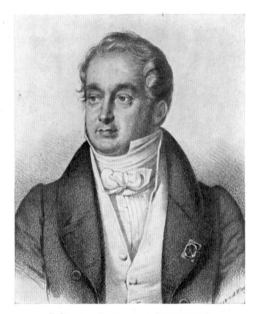

Guillaume Dupuytren (1777–1835).

made overambitious and overbearing. In Paris, he was regarded
as "nobody's friend," because he tolerated no rivals, and persecuted and intrigued against those who, like Velpeau, aspired to
that eminence, even pursuing them with vindictive hatred. He
was cold, hard, contemptuous, unscrupulous, and overbearing, and
more respected than beloved. Yet his fame was such that, when
he visited Italy he was treated *en prince.*

Jacques **Lisfranc** (1790–1847), surgeon at La Pitié, devised

---

[1] Repert. gén. d'anat. et de physiol. path., Paris, 1826, ii, 82–93.

[2] J. univ. et hebd. de méd. et de chir. prat., Paris, 1832, 2. s., v, 348–365.

28

many new operations, in particular his partial amputation of the foot at the tarsometatarsal articulation (Lisfranc's amputation, 1815),[1] his methods of disarticulating the shoulder-joint (1815), of excision of the rectum, of lithotomy in women, and of amputation of the cervix uteri.

Philibert-Joseph **Roux** (1780–1854), a pupil and friend of Bichat, was surgeon at the Charité in 1810, and succeeded Dupuytren at the Hôtel Dieu in 1835. He was the first French teacher to give a definite course of lectures (1812). He was a pioneer in plastic surgery, performing the first staphylorrhaphy in 1819

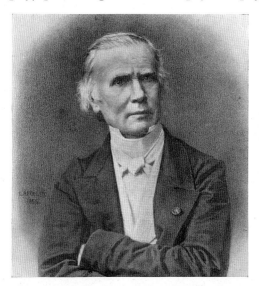

Alfred-Armand-Louis-Marie Velpeau (1795–1867).

(described in detail in his memoir of 1825),[2] and the first suture of the ruptured female perineum (1832).[3]

Jacques-Mathieu **Delpech** (1777–1832), of Toulouse, graduated in Montpellier (1801) and, in 1812, became professor of surgery there. He was the pioneer of orthopedic surgery in France, his principal work being "De l'orthomorphie" (1828). On May 9, 1816,[4] he performed, for the first time, a subcutaneous section of the tendo Achillis for club-foot, the object being to exclude the air and obtain union by first intention. This operation was twice

---

[1] Lisfranc: Nouvelle méthode opératoire [etc.], Paris, 1815.

[2] Roux: Arch. gén. de méd., Paris, 1825, vii, 516–538.

[3] Roux: Gaz. méd. de Paris, 1834, 2. s., ii, 17–22.

[4] In his: Clin. chir. de Montpellier, 1823, i, 147–231, pl. x.

repeated by Stromeyer in 1821–22. Delpech was also the first after Hippocrates to point out that Pott's disease (spinal caries) is tubercular in nature. He erected a large orthopedic institute at Montpellier, and, one morning, while on the way to it in his carriage, he and his coachman were shot and killed by a vindictive patient, who thought that an operation for varicocele had rendered him unfit for marriage.

Alfred-Armand-Louis-Marie **Velpeau** (1795–1867), a pupil of Bretonneau's, originally a blacksmith's son who had once been apprenticed to his father's trade, was surgeon to the Hôpital St.

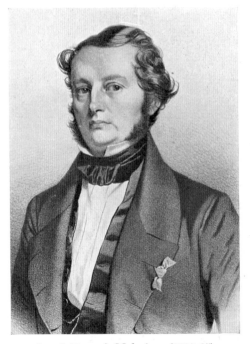

Joseph-François Malgaigne (1806–65).

Antoine (1828–30), La Pitié (1830–34), the Charité (1834–67), and professor of clinical surgery at the Paris Faculty (1834–67). He was not a scientific surgeon, but a strong, capable, hard-working teacher and operator, of whom Oliver Wendell Holmes said that "a good sound head over a pair of wooden shoes is a good deal better than a wooden head belonging to an owner who cases his feet in calf-skin." His principal works are his Treatise on Surgical Anatomy (1823), the first detailed work of its kind, his three-volume treatise on operative surgery, with atlas (1832), important for its historical data, and once edited in translation by Valentine Mott (1847), and his great treatise on Diseases of the Breast (1854),[1] the most important work on the subject in its time.

Joseph-François **Malgaigne** (1806–65), the son of a French health officer, is described by Billings as "the greatest surgical historian and critic whom the world has yet seen," and he is, with Petrequin, the most able writer on the surgery of the Hippocratic period. He wrote important works on operative surgery (1834), experimental surgery (1838), fractures and dislocations (1847–55), and edited the authentic modern edition of Ambroïse Paré, with

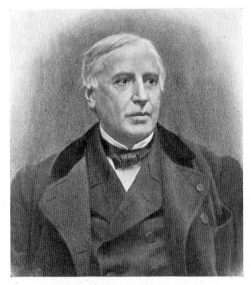

Auguste Nélaton (1807–73).

a fine biography of the latter (1840). In practical surgery his name is associated with the hooks of his invention used in treating fracture of the patella, but he is perhaps best remembered by the critical and historical discourses which Billings classes "among the most delightful reading in surgical literature."

Auguste **Nélaton** (1807–73), of Paris, who presided with Malgaigne at the Hôpital St. Louis, held the same unapproachable rank as an operator and teacher which Dupuytren had attained at an earlier period, but in personality he was the logical opposite of his self-seeking predecessor. He was modest, quiet, helpful, and friendly,

---

[1] Velpeau: Traité des maladies du sein, Paris, 1854.

generous to the unfortunate—in short, a gentleman. He invented a bullet-probe (first used in Garibaldi's case) and a valuable flexible rubber catheter (1860), and improved the treatment of nasopharyngeal tumors. In gynecology he is memorable as the first to describe pelvic (retro-uterine) hematocele (1851–52), and he did most to establish ovariotomy in France. His principal work is his *Éléments de pathologie chirurgicale* (1844–59).

Paul **Broca** (1824–80), who was, in succession, surgeon at St. Antoine, La Pitié, the Hôpital des Cliniques, and the Hôpital Necker, was the founder of the modern surgery of the brain and also of the modern French school of anthropology. In 1861,[1] he discovered that the third left frontal convolution of the brain is the center of articulate speech, a point which is now disputed, but which, in the first instance, undoubtedly led to mapping out the different centers of the brain for surgical operations. Broca was, in fact, the first to trephine for a cerebral abscess diagnosed by his theory of localization of function. In connection with his discovery, he introduced the term *aphemia* or "motor aphasia" (1861),[2] which is now undergoing destructive criticism at the hands of Pierre Marie. In anthropology, Broca is, with Topinard and Quatrefages, the greatest name of modern France. He originated the modern methods of determining the ratio of the dimensions of the brain to those of the skull (craniometry), and to this end devised the occipital crochet, a craniograph, and a goniometer, and did much to standardize the measurements of bones and the classification of colors of the hair and skin. He opposed the theory that the different races were originally developed from several separate pairs of

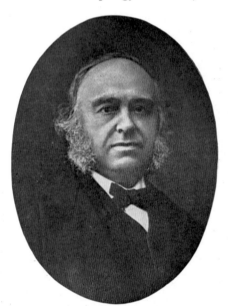

Paul Broca (1824–80).

[1] Broca: Bull. Soc. d'anthrop. de Paris, 1861, ii, 235–238, and Bull. Soc. anat. de Paris, 1861, xxxvi, 330; 398.

[2] *Ibid.*, 332.

species, in his law of "eugenesis," which maintains that the different varieties of the genus Homo are, and always have been, fertile with each other. This drove the "polygenists" to their last resort, diversity of language. Broca is also credited with the aphorism: "I would rather be a transformed ape than a degenerate son of Adam."

Among the isolated French contributions of importance are Richerand's resection of the fifth and sixth ribs (1818); the introduction of lithotrity by Leroy d'Étiolles (1822), Civiale (1824), and Heurteloup (1824–31); Béclard's excision of the parotid (1823);[1] Gensoul's excision of the upper jaw (1826); Lembert's method of enterorrhaphy (1826);[2] Maisonneuve's hair catheter (1845).[3] Sédillot's introduction of gastrostomy, which he performed for the first time on November 13, 1849;[4] Pravaz's hypodermic syringe (1851);[5] and Lallemant's method of autoplasty (1856).

Among the prominent German surgeons of the period were Vincenz von Kern (1760–1829), professor at Vienna (1805–24), who simplified wound-dressings by using bandages moistened with plain water (first proposed by Cesare Magati in 1616) as a substitute for the salves and plasters then in vogue; Christian Ludwig Mursinna (1744–1823), who was successively weaver, bath-keeper, barber's apprentice, and surgeon general of the Prussian Army (1787–1809); Conrad Johann Martin **Langenbeck** (1776–1851), professor of anatomy and surgery at Göttingen and surgeon general of the Hannoverian Army (1814), who devised the operation of iridocleisis for artificial pupil (1817), and attained such supreme swiftness in operating that he is said to have amputated a shoulder while a colleague present was taking a pinch of snuff; and Max Joseph von Chelius (1794–1876), whose "Handbuch der Chirurgie" (1822–23) was the standard text-book in Germany until the middle of the century, and who, according to Baas, was "the only professor in Heidelberg who kept a carriage." The most important German surgeons before 1850 were Dieffenbach, the elder von Graefe, the younger Stromeyer, Langenbeck, and Gustav Simon.

Carl Ferdinand von Graefe (1787–1840), of Warsaw, was one of the surgeon generals in the German struggle for independence (1813–15), having previously been professor of surgery at the University of Berlin in 1810, resuming this position after the war. He was the founder of modern plastic surgery, devising the

---

[1] Béclard: Arch. gén. de méd., Paris, 1824, iv, 60–66.

[2] Lembert: Repert. gén. d'anat. et physiol. path., Paris, 1826, ii, 100–107, 1 pl.

[3] Maisonneuve: Compt. rend. Acad. d. sc., Paris, 1845, xx, 70–72.

[4] Sédillot: Gaz. méd. de Strasbourg, 1849, ix, 366–377.

[5] Pravaz: Compt. rend. Acad. d. sc., Paris, 1853, xxxvi, 88–90.

operation for congenital cleft-palate in 1816.[1] In 1818, he introduced rhinoplasty (simultaneously with Bünger) and blepharo-
plasty (simultaneously with Dzondi). In the same year, he improved the technic of Cesarean section and excised the lower jaw
for the first time in Germany. He was also the first German surgeon to ligate the innominate artery (1822), his patient living
sixty-eight days.[2] His "Rhinoplastik" (1818) was the first handling of the theme of artificial nose-making after Tagliacozzi (1575)
and Carpue (1816).

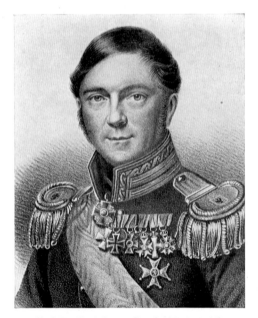

Carl Ferdinand von Graefe (1787–1840).

Johann Friedrich **Dieffenbach** (1792–1847), of Königsberg, also
fought (as a rifleman) in the German war for independence. His
doctor's dissertation at Würzburg (1822), on regeneration and
transplantation of tissues, already shows his leaning toward plastic
surgery.[3] He was surgeon at the Charité (Berlin) in 1829, and, in
1840, succeeded von Graefe as professor at the university. In
1829, following Stromeyer's proposal, he first treated strabismus

---

[1] von Graefe: Jour. f. Chir. u. Augenheilk., Berlin, 1820, i, 1–54, 2 pl.

[2] London Med. and Phys. Jour., 1823, xlix, 475.

[3] Dieffenbach: Nonnulla de regeneratione et transplantatione, Würzburg,
1822.

by severing the tendons of the eye muscles (with success).[1]   This
success perhaps led him to attempt the erroneous procedure of
subcutaneous division of the lingual muscles for stammering (1841),[2]
which produced many untoward results in his patients; but he
got wonderful results in tenotomy, skin-grafting, and orthopedic
surgery, and was a pioneer in transplantations and experimental
surgery on animals.   He wrote on treatment of urethral stricture
by incision (1826); transfusion of blood (1828), bandaging (1829),
nursing (1832), treatment of preternatural anus (1834) and urethral
fistula (1836), and a great treatise on operative surgery (1845–48).[3]

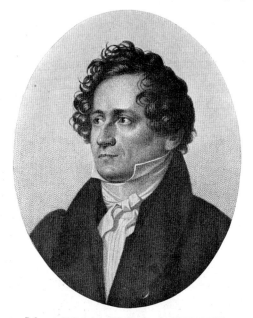

Johann Friedrich Dieffenbach (1792–1847).

He also made a brave attempt to treat vesicovaginal fistula by
every known method, and left a classical account of the sufferings
entailed by the condition (1845).   He was a genial, humane, attractive man, and an admirable teacher, upholding the highest
ideals of his profession.   He maintained that the surgeon should
be a many-sided Odysseus, full of native invention and resources
not to be found in books.   All great surgeons, he says, are, or
ought to be, clear thinkers, and therefore good writers.

---

[1] Ueber das Schielen, etc., Berlin, 1842.

[2] Die Heilung des Stotterns (etc.), Berlin, 1841.

[3] Die operative Chirurgie, Leipzig, 1845–8.

Georg Friedrich Louis **Stromeyer** (1804–76), of Hannover, professor at Erlangen, Munich, Freiburg, and Kiel, and successively surgeon general of the Schleswig-Holstein and Hannoverian armies, was the father of modern military surgery in Germany. He greatly extended the fields of conservative surgery of the joints and subcutaneous surgery. Stromeyer performed his first subcutaneous section of the tendo Achillis in 1831,[1] fifteen years after Delpech (1816), but if Delpech was the discoverer, Stromeyer was the *Mehrer des Reichs*. He practically created the modern surgery of the locomotor system by applying subcutaneous tenotomy to

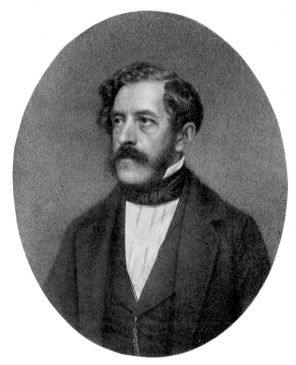

Bernhard von Langenbeck (1810–87).

all deformities of the body depending upon muscular defects. He is one of the founders of orthopedics in recent times, and his Maxims of War-Surgery (1855) made an epoch in German military medicine. He was a poet and wrote an attractive autobiography.

Bernhard von Langenbeck (1810–87), the nephew of Conrad, succeeded Dieffenbach at Berlin in 1847, and became the greatest

---

[1] Stromeyer: Mag. f. d. ges. Heilk., Berlin, 1833, xxxix, 195–218.

clinical surgeon and teacher of his day in Germany, having trained nearly every prominent operator up to the present time. In 1861, he started the *Archiv der klinischen Chirurgie* (known as Langenbeck's Archiv), and founded the German Society of Surgery, both of which have exerted a profound influence ever since. He has 21 operations credited to his name, of which the most important are his methods of excising the ankle, knee, hip, wrist, elbow, shoulder, and lower jaw, and of plastic surgery of the lip, palate, and nose.

Gustav **Simon** (1824–76), of Darmstadt, professor at Rostock (1861) and Heidelberg (1867), was a highly original operator and

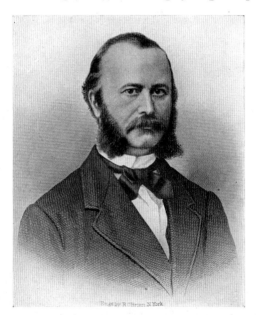

Gustav Simon (1824–76).

the author of admirable monographs on the treatment of vesico-vaginal fistula (1854), the excision of the spleen (1857),[1] on plastic surgery (1868)[2] and the surgery of the kidneys (1871–76).[3] He was the first in Europe to excise the kidney (1869).[4]

Albrecht Theodor **von Middeldorpf** (1824–68), of Breslau, performed the first operations for gastric fistula (1859) and eso-

---

[1] Simon: Die Exstirpation der Milz am Menschen, Giessen, 1857.

[2] Beiträge zur plastischen Chirurgie, Prague, 1868.

[3] Chirurgie der Nieren, Erlangen, 1871–6.

[4] Deutsche Klinik, Berlin, 1870, xxii, 137.

phageal tumor, was a pioneer in the use of the galvanocautery (1854), and made important contributions on fractures and dislocations. The greatest of Russian surgeons, and one of the greatest military surgeons of all time, was Nikolai Ivanovich **Pirogoff** (1810–81), who, like Paré and Hunter, had a remarkable career of self-development. Graduating in 1832, he studied for two years at Berlin and Göttingen, where he was disgusted with the small attention paid to anatomy. Langenbeck was, in his estimation, the only man who was well informed on the subject. Upon returning to Russia, he taught at Dorpat for five years, and, in 1840, was appointed professor of surgery at the Medico-Chirurgical Academy at St. Peters-

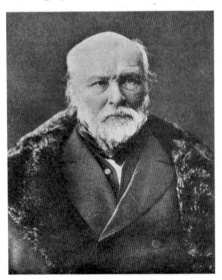

Nikolai Ivanovich Pirogoff (1810–81).

burg. In his forty-five years of service here, he introduced many important reforms, among others the teaching of applied topographical anatomy, for the first time in Russia, to which end he invited Hyrtl's pupil, Gruber, from Vienna. He made 11,000 postmortems, among them 800 of cholera victims in 1848. He saw a great deal of military surgery, serving in the field during the campaigns in the Caucasus (1847) and the Crimea (1854), and also reported upon the Franco-Prussian and Russo-Turkish campaigns. He served fourteen months in and around Sebastopol, and, in trenches and tents, witnessed all the horrors of pyemia, hospital gangrene, erysipelas, and purulent edema. Here he got himself into hot water with the governmental authorities by his sharp criticism of the bad management of the campaign, his attempts at segregation and other improvements, and was forced to resign his professorship. His experiences with sepsis led him to define war as a "traumatic epidemic." Through the aid of the Grand Duchess Helena Pavlovna, he introduced female nursing of the wounded in the Crimea, and, all his life, he was a warm advocate of freedom and higher education for women. In 1847, he was

already using ether anesthesia in his surgical practice.[1]   He devoted his latter days to advancing the cause of medical education
in his native country, in which he was again subjected to bitter
enmity and persecution at the hands of the official and military
tchinovniks.   Pirogoff is, in the esteem of cultivated Russians, the
most important figure in their medical history.   He is noted for
his method of complete osteoplastic amputation of the foot
(1854)[2]; for his great atlas of 220 plates (1851–54),[3] in which
frozen sections were first utilized on a grand scale in anatomic
illustration;[4] and for his treatise on military surgery (1864),[5] in
which he holds large hospitals responsible for the spread of epidemic diseases and recommends small, barrack-like pavilions,
such as were suggested by his Crimean experiences.   In speed,
dexterity, and strength of hand, Pirogoff, the operator, was
like those Slavic virtuosi of music whose execution is the astonishment of our times.   The usual portraits of the great surgeon
in his old age represent a broad-browed, serious face of venerable
aspect, strongly resembling two other great Russians, Glinka and
Turgenieff.   In relation to his country, we may apply to him the
exquisite tribute which Henry James paid to the latter: "His large
nature was filled with the love of justice but he was also of the stuff
of which glories are made."

American surgery in the pre-Listerian period was distinguished
principally by a great deal of bold operating on the vascular and
osseous systems, by the foundation of modern operative gynecology at the hands of McDowell and Sims, and by the permanent
introduction of surgical anesthesia.   Its leading representatives
in this period were Physick, the two Warrens, Post, Mott, Gibson,
the two Smiths, Willard Parker, McDowell, and Sims.

Philip Syng Physick (1768–1837), of Philadelphia, a pupil of
John Hunter's, and sometimes called the Father of American Surgery, was an Edinburgh graduate of 1792, surgeon to the Pennsylvania Hospital in 1794, and professor of surgery in the University
of Pennsylvania (1805–18).   He wrote nothing of consequence,—
all his teaching was preserved in the treatise on surgery of his
nephew, John Syng Dorsey,—and he is now remembered principally
by certain procedures of importance in their day, such as the in-

---

[1] Pirogoff: Recherches pratiques et physiologiques sur l'éthérisation, St.
Petersburg, 1847.

[2] Voyenno Med. Jour., St. Petersburg, 1854, lxiii, 2. sect., 83–100.

[3] Anatome topographica sectionibus per corpus humanum congelatum
triplice directione ductis illustrata, St. Petersburg, 1851–54.

[4] Frozen sections in anatomy were first used by Pieter de Riemer (1760–
1831) in his "Afbeeldingen" (The Hague, 1818).

[5] Pirogoff: Grundzüge der allgemeinen Kriegschirurgie, Leipzig, 1864.

troduction of absorbable kid and buckskin ligatures (1816),[1] the use of the seton in ununited fracture (1822),[2] an operation for artificial anus (1826),[3] the advocation of rest in hip-joint disease (1830),[4] and the invention of the tonsillotome (1828).[5] His modification of Desault's splint for fracture of the femur is still in use. He seems to have been the first to describe diverticula of the rectum (1836).[6]

John Warren (1753–1815), of Roxbury, Massachusetts, rendered distinguished army service in the Revolution and was founder

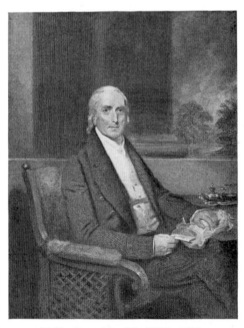

Philip Syng Physick (1768–1837).

and the first professor of anatomy and surgery of the Harvard Medical School (1783). He was first president of the Massachusetts Medical Society, an office which he held until his death (1804–15). He amputated at the shoulder-joint in 1781,[7] and excised the pa-

---

[1] Physick: Eclect. Repertory, Phila., 1816, vi, 389.
[2] Phila. Jour. Med. and Phys. Sc., 1822, v, 116–118.
[3] *Ibid.*, 1826, xiii, 199–202.
[4] Am. Jour. Med. Sc., Phila., 1830, vii, 299–308, 1 pl.
[5] *Ibid.*, 1828, ii, 116.
[6] Am. Cycl. Pract. Med. and Surg., Phila., 1836, ii, 123–126.
[7] Warren: Boston Med. and Surg. Jour., 1839, xx, 210.

rotid gland in 1804.[1] His son, **John Collins Warren** (1778–1856), of Boston, was a pupil of Astley Cooper and Dupuytren, and succeeded to his father's professorship in 1815. He was a pioneer in the excision of bones and joints, such as the hyoid (1804) and the elbow (1834), introduced the operation of staphylorrhaphy for fissure of the soft palate in 1828,[2] and was the first in this country to operate for strangulated hernia. He was the founder of the Massachusetts General Hospital (1811) and of the Warren Museum, and he practically introduced ether anesthesia in surgery (1847). His principal work is his "Surgical Observations on Tumors" (1837).

Wright Post (1766–1822), of Long Island, N. Y., was the first in America to ligate the femoral artery successfully (for popliteal aneurysm) according to John Hunter's method (1796),[3] and the second to ligate the external iliac successfully (1814),[4] having been preceded by Dorsey in 1811.[5] Post was also the first surgeon to tie the primitive carotid in its continuity with success (1813),[6] an operation which he successfully repeated in 1816;[7] and the subclavian artery was first successfully ligated outside the scaleni by him in 1817.[8]

Valentine Mott (1785–1865), of Long Island, was a pupil of Astley Cooper, and, like him, a great pioneer in vascular surgery. The innominate artery was ligated for the first time in the history of surgery by Mott in 1818,[9] the first successful operation being that of Smyth, of New Orleans, in 1864. In addition, Mott has to his credit the remarkable record of successfully ligating the common iliac at its origin (1827),[10] the carotid for subclavian aneurysm (1829),[11] the carotid for anastomosing aneurysm in a three-months' infant (1829),[12] the external iliac for femoral aneurysm (1831), the right subclavian within the scaleni (1833),[13] both carotids simultaneously (1833),[14] and the right internal iliac (1837).[15]

---

[1] In J. C. Warren: Surgical observations on tumors, Boston, 1837, p. 287.

[2] Am. Jour. Med. Sc., Phila., 1828, iii, 1–3, 1 pl.

[3] Post: Am. Med. and Phila. Register, New York, 1814, iv, 452.

[4] Post: *Ibid.*, 1813–14, iv, 443–453. Also in: Med. Repository, N. Y., 1815, n. s., ii, 196–199.

[5] Dorsey: Eclect. Repertory, Phila., 1811, ii, 111–115.

[6] Post: Am. Med. and Phila. Register, N. Y., 1814, iv, 366–377.

[7] Post: Med. Repository, New York, 1817, n. s., iii, 412.

[8] Post: Tr. Phys. Med. Soc. New York, 1817, i, 387–394.

[9] Mott: Med. and Surg. Register, New York, 1818, i, 9–54.

[10] Phila. Jour. Med. and Phys. Sc., 1827, xiv, 176–181.

[11] Am. Jour. Med. Sc., Phila., 1829, v, 297; 1830, vi, 532.

[12] Am. Jour. Med. Sc., Phila., 1829, v, 255; 1830, vii, 271.

[13] *Ibid.*, 1831, viii, 393–397.   [14] *Ibid.*, 1833, xii, 354.

[15] Am. Jour. Med. Sc., Phila., 1837, xx, 13–15.

Besides the innominate artery, says Billings, Mott "tied the sub-clavian 8 times, the primitive carotid 51 times, the carotid twice, the common iliac once, the external iliac 6 times, the internal iliac twice, the femoral 57 times, and the popliteal 10 times"—in all, 138 ligations of the great vessels for aneurysm. Mott was also a bold and successful operator on the bones and joints. He excised the

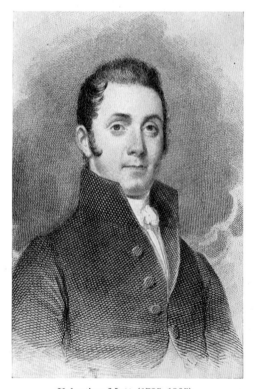

Valentine Mott (1785–1865).

right side of the lower jaw, after tying the carotid artery, in 1821;[1] successfully amputated at the hip-joint in 1824;[2] excised the left clavicle for osteosarcoma in 1828,[3] and removed a large fibrous growth from the nostril by dividing the nasal and maxillary bones (1841).[4]

---

[1] New York Med. and Phys. Jour., 1822, i, 385.
[2] Phila. Jour. Med. and Phys. Sc., 1827, xiv, 101–104.
[3] Mott: Am. Jour. Med. Sc., Phila., 1828, iii, 100–108.
[4] *Ibid.*, 1842, n. s., iii, 257; 1843, v, 87.

In connection with the work of Post and Mott, it is proper to mention here some other early operations by American surgeons in the same field. The primitive carotid artery was successfully ligated for primary hemorrhage by Mason Fitch Cogswell (1761–1830), of Connecticut, in 1803,[1] and, for secondary hemorrhage by Amos Twitchell (1781–1850), of New Hampshire, in 1807,[2] eight months prior to Sir Astley Cooper's case. Both primitive carotids were first successfully tied in continuity, within a month's interval, by George Macgill, of Maryland, in 1823,[3] to be followed by Reuben D. Mussey in 1827 and Mott in 1833. The primitive and internal carotids were first simultaneously tied by Gurdon Buck (1807–77), of New York city, in 1848[4]; and John Murray **Carnochan** (1817–87), of Savannah, Georgia, ligated the carotid on both sides for elephantiasis in 1867.[5] Carnochan was also the first to excise the superior maxillary nerve (including Meckel's ganglion) for facial neuralgia (1858).[6] John Kearny Rodgers (1793–1851), of New York city, a pupil of Wright Post, was the first to tie the left subclavian artery within the scaleni (1845),[7] but with fatal result, the first successful case being that of Professor W. S. Halsted, of Johns Hopkins, in 1892.[8] William Gibson (1788–1868), of Baltimore, Maryland, was the first American surgeon to tie the common iliac artery (1812).[9] In the preceding year, John Syng Dorsey (1783–1818) had successfully tied the external iliac,[10] to be followed by Post (1814), Horatio Gates Jameson (1821),[11] and Edward Peace (1841).[12] The internal iliac was successfully tied by S. Pomeroy White in 1827[13]; the femoral, by Henry M. Onderdonk (1813),[14] David L. Rogers (1824), and Carnochan (1851); the gluteal artery, by John B. Davidge, of Baltimore, and George McClellan, of Philadelphia; the aorta, for the first time after Sir Astley Cooper, by Hunter McGuire in 1868.[15] In addition, Gurdon Buck (1807–77), of New York, successfully ligated the femoral, profunda, external and common iliac arteries for femoral aneurysm in 1858[16]; Willard Parker (1800–84), of Francistown, N. Y., ligated the left subclavian inside the scalenus, together with the common carotid and vertebral arteries, for subclavian aneurysm in 1864,[17] the patient dying on the forty-second day; and Andrew Woods Smyth (1833–   ), of New Orleans, first successfully ligated the innominate artery, together with the common carotid, and subsequently the right vertebral, for subclavian aneurysm in 1864,[18] ex-

---

[1] Cogswell: New Engl. Jour. Med. and Surg., Boston, 1824, xiii, 357–360.

[2] Twitchell: New Engl. Quart. Jour. Med. and Surg., Boston, 1842–43, i, 188–193.

[3] Macgill: New York Med. and Phys. Jour., 1825, iv, 576.

[4] Buck: New York Med. Times, 1855–6, v, 37–42.

[5] Carnochan: Am. Jour. Med. Sc., Phila., 1867, n. s., liv, 109–115.

[6] Carnochan: Ibid., 1858, n. s., xxxv, 134–143.

[7] Rodgers: Am. Jour. Med. Sc., Phila., 1846, n. s., ix, 541.

[8] Halsted: Johns Hopkins Hosp. Bull., Balt., 1892, iii, 93.

[9] Gibson: Am. Med. Recorder, Phila., 1820, iii, 185–193, 2 pl.

[10] Dorsey: Eclect. Repertory, Phila., 1811, ii, 111–115.

[11] Jameson: Am. Med. Recorder, Phila., 1822, v, 118–124.

[12] Peace: Med. Exam., Phila., 1842, n. s., i, 225–228.

[13] White: Am. Jour. Med. Sc., Phila., 1827, i, 304–306.

[14] Onderdonk: Am. Med. and Phil. Register, Phila., 1814, iv, 176.

[15] McGuire: Am. Jour. Med. Sc., Phila., 1868, n. s., lvi, 415–419.

[16] Buck: New York Med. Jour., 1858, 3. s., v, 305–311.

[17] Parker: Am. Jour. Med. Sc., Phila., 1864, n. s., xlvii, 562.

[18] Smyth: Am. Jour. Med. Sc., Phila., 1866, n. s., lii, 280–282. (Exhibition of living patient.) New Orleans Jour. Med., 1869, xxii, 464–469. Repeated by J. Lewtas, of Murdan Hospital, Punjab (Brit. Med. Jour., London, 1889, ii, 312).

hibiting his patient alive in 1869, the specimen being now in the U. S. Army Medical Museum.

Of early American operations upon the bones and joints, we may mention the first amputation of the hip-joint in the United States, by Walter Brashear (1776–1860), of Maryland, in 1806[1]; the successful excision of part of the lower jaw, by William Henry Deadrick (1773–1858), of Winchester, Va., in 1810[2]; the first successful excision of the clavicle, by Charles McCreary (1785–1826), of Kentucky, in 1813[3]; the excision of the superior maxilla, by Horatio Gates Jameson (1788–1855), of York, Pa., in 1820[4]; the successful amputation at the elbow-joint, by James Mann, U. S. Army, in 1821[5]; an excision of the fifth and sixth ribs, with a portion of gangrenous lung, by Milton Antony (1789–1839), of Georgia (1821)[6]; excision of nearly the whole of both upper jaws, by David L. Rogers, of New York, in 1824[7]; amputation at the knee-joint, by Nathan Smith (1762–1869), of Massachusetts, in 1824[8]; osteotomy for ankylosis of the hip-joint, by John Rhea Barton (1794–1871), of Lancaster, Pa., in 1826[9]; successful wiring of an ununited fracture of the humerus (1827),[10] by J. K. Rodgers (1793–1851), of New York city; excision of the coccyx, by Josiah Clark Nott (1804–73), of Columbia, S. C., in 1832[11]; excision of the elbow-joint, by John Collins Warren (1778–1856), of Massachusetts, in 1834[12]; the interscapular-thoracic amputation, by Dixi Crosby (1801-73), of New Hampshire, in 1836[13]; and, in two stages, by Reuben Dimond Mussey (1818–82), of New Hampshire, in 1831–37[14]; excision of the olecranon process, by Gurdon Buck (1807–77), of New York city, in 1842[15]; the Fergusson operation for fissure of the hard and soft palates, by Jonathan Mason Warren (1811–67), of Boston, in 1842[16]; S. D. Gross's amputation at the ankle-joint in 1851[17]; Bigelow's excision of the hip-joint (1852)[18]; exsection of the ulna (1853),[19] the radius (1854),[20] and the os calcis (1857),[21] by John Murray Carnochan (1817–87), of Savannah, Ga., and Sayre's resection of the hip for ankylosis (1855).[22] In 1836, Paul Fitzsimmons Eve (1806–77), of Georgia, removed a large fibrous polyp from the base of the cranium,[23] and, in 1850, William Detmold (1808–94)

[1] Brashear: Tr. Kentucky M. Soc. 1852, Frankfort, 1853, ii, 265

[2] Deadrick: Am. Med. Recorder, Phila., 1823, vi, 516.

[3] McCreary: Tr. Kentucky Med. Soc., 1852, Frankfort, 1853, ii, 276.

[4] Jameson: Am. Med. Recorder, Phila., 1821, iv, 221–230, 1 pl.

[5] Mann: Med. Repository, New York, 1822, n. s., vii, pp. 17–19.

[6] Antony: Phila. Jour. Med. and Phys. Sc., 1823, vi, 108–117, 1 pl.

[7] Rogers: New York Med. and Phys. Jour., 1824, iii, 301–303.

[8] Smith: Am. Med. Rev. and Jour., Phila., 1825, ii, 370.

[9] Barton: North Amer. Med. and Surg. Jour., 1826, iii, 279–292; 400, 1 pl.

[10] Rodgers: New York Med. and Phys. Jour., 1827, vi, 521–523.

[11] Nott: New Orleans Med. Jour., 1844–45, i, 58–60.

[12] J. C. Warren: In Hodges's (J. M.) Excision of Joints, Boston, 1861, p. 69.

[13] Crosby: Med. Record, New York, 1875, x, 753–755. (Crosby was preceded by the English naval surgeon, Ralph Cuming, in 1808.)

[14] Mussey: Am. Jour. Med. Sc., Phila., 1837, xxi, 390–394.

[15] Buck: *Ibid.*, 1843, n. s., v, 297–301.

[16] J. M. Warren: New Engl. Quart. Jour. Med. and Surg., Boston, 1842–43, i, 538–547.

[17] Gross: cited on p. 457 of Am. Jour. Med. Sc., Phila., 1876, n. s., lxxi.

[18] Bigelow: Am. Jour. Med. Sc., Phila., 1852, xxiv, 90.

[19] Carnochan: Am. Med. Monthly, New York, 1854, i, 180–188.

[20] Carnochan: Am. Jour. Med. Sc., Phila., 1858, n. s., xxxv, 363–370.

[21] Carnochan: Am. Med. Gaz., New York, 1857, viii, 321–323.

[22] Sayre: New York Jour. Med., 1855, n. s., xiv, 70–82

[23] Eve: South. Med. and Surg. Jour., Augusta, 1836–37, i, 78–80.

29

opened the lateral sinus of the brain for abscess,[1] the report of which operation Virchow treated with scornful skepticism. Carnochan's three cases of excision of the fifth nerve for neuralgia (1858)[2] were followed by the ingenious and successful method of Joseph Pancoast (1805–82), of New Jersey, in 1872,[3] who was also the first to perform a successful plastic operation for exstrophy of the bladder in February, 1858.[4] This operation was repeated with success upon the female bladder by Daniel Ayres, of Brooklyn, N. Y., in November, 1858.[5] Cystotomy for inflammation and rupture of the bladder was first performed (1846–54)[6] by Willard Parker (1800–84), of Francistown, N. Y., who was also the first, after Hancock, of London (1848), to operate for appendicitis (1864),[7] and tied the subclavian artery five times. In lithotomy, Benjamin Winslow Dudley (1785–1870) was especially successful, having performed this operation 225 times with scarce a death. Next to Dudley, Physick is said to have cut for stone oftener than any other American surgeon, and his removal of over a thousand calculi from Chief Justice Marshall is a famous early case. The kidney was first excised (before Gustav Simon) by Erastus Bradley Wolcott (1804–80), of Benton, N. Y., in 1861.[8] John Stough Bobbs (1809–70), of Pennsylvania German descent, was the first to perform cholecystotomy for gall-stones (1868),[9] in which he was followed by Marion Sims (1878).[10] Among the special procedures introduced by American surgeons in this period are Nathan Smith's method of treating necrosis of bones with the trephine (1827),[11] Jonathan Wright's successful treatment of aneurysm by digital compression (1847),[12] the method of reducing dislocations by manipulation, without weights or pulleys, introduced by William W. Reid, of Rochester, New York, in his classical papers of 1851–55,[13] based upon dissections and experiments; the treatment of fractures of the femur by Nathan Ryno Smith's anterior splint (1860),[14] and by the weight and pulley apparatus of Gurdon Buck (Buck's extension, 1861).[15]

The Civil War in the United States (1861–65) brought forth the remarkable "Medical and Surgical History of the War of the Rebellion" (1870–88), by Joseph Janvier Woodward, Charles Smart, George A. Otis, and David L. Huntington, a remarkable collection of case histories and pathologic reports, embellished with fine plates, and, altogether, a work that is unique in the annals of military medicine. It was the subject of enthusiastic praise by Virchow.[16] Another important surgical work which came out of this war was the study of "Gunshot Wounds and Other Injuries of Nerves" (1864) by S. Weir Mitchell, George R. Morehouse, and William W. Keen, who were

---

[1] Detmold: Am. Jour. Med. Sc., Phila., 1850, xix, 86–95.

[2] Carnochan: Am. Jour. Med. Sc., Phila., 1858, n. s., xxxv, 134–143.

[3] Pancoast: Phila. Med. Times, 1871–72, ii, 285–287.

[4] Pancoast: North Am. Med.-Chir. Rev., Phila., 1859, iii, p. 710 (bracketed case, reported by S. D. Gross).

[5] Ayres: Am. Med. Gaz., New York, 1859, x, 81–89, 2 pl.

[6] Parker: New York Jour. Med., 1851, n. s., vii, 83–86. Also, Tr. Med. Soc. New York, 1867, 345–349.

[7] Parker: Med. Rec., New York, 1867, ii, 25–27.

[8] Wolcott: Med. and Surg. Reporter, Phila., 1861–62, vii, 126.

[9] Bobbs: Tr. Med. Soc. Indiana, 1868, 68–73.

[10] Sims: Richmond and Louisville Med. Jour., 1878, xxvi, 1–21.

[11] N. Smith: Phila. Month. Jour. Med., 1827, i, 11; 66.

[12] Wright: Boston Med. and Surg. Jour.. 1848, xxxviii.

[13] Reid: Buffalo Med. Jour., 1851–52, vii, 129–143.

[14] N. R. Smith: Maryland and Virginia Med. and Surg. Jour., 1860, xiv, 1; 177.

[15] Buck: Bull. New York Acad. Med., 1860–62, i, 181–188.

[16] Virchow: Die Fortschritte der Kriegsheilkunde, Berlin, 1874, p. 7.

then acting as army surgeons at the Turner's Lane Hospital in Philadelphia. This book was the first full-length study of the traumatic neuroses, introducing the use of massage in these cases, and was the starting-point of Mitchell's subsequent work on ascending neuritis, traumatic neurasthenia, and the psychic phenomena in those who have undergone amputation.[1]

The only successful amputation at the hip-joint during the Civil War was performed in a case of gunshot injury by Edward Shippen, of Philadelphia.[2]

The early history of the introduction of **ether anesthesia** in America has been the subject of rabid controversy, but the principal facts may be briefly stated as follows: In March, 1842, Dr. Crawford Williamson Long (1815–78), of Danielsville, Ga., a graduate of the University of Pennsylvania (1839), having previously noted some accidental anesthetic effects of ether, removed a small cystic tumor from the back of the neck of a patient under its influence, and subsequently used it in other cases (1842–43), which have been amply certified and vouched for by resident physicians of his locality.[3] But Long published no reports of his results, and, as Welch has admirably said, "we cannot assign to him any influence upon the historical development of our knowledge of surgical anesthesia or any share in its introduction to the world at large." Long had no one to take up and expand his work, as Lizars did for McDowell's. In 1800, Sir Humphry Davy (1788–1829), of Penzance, England, experimented upon himself with nitrous oxide, and stated that "it may probably be used with advantage in surgical operations in which no great effusion of blood takes place." In 1844, Horace Wells (1815–48), a dentist of Hartford, Connecticut, began to use nitrous oxide in dentistry, communicating his results to his friend and former partner, William Thomas Green Morton (1819–68), of Charlton, Massachusetts; but a fatal case caused Wells to withdraw from practice, and he eventually put an end to his life. Morton had, in the meantime, been studying medicine, having for his preceptor Dr. Charles T. Jackson, a chemist of ability, who pointed out to him the anesthetic effects of chloric ether, which he proceeded to apply in filling a tooth in July, 1844. Becoming interested, Morton pushed his inquiries further and subsequently learned from Jackson that sulphuric ether is also an anesthetic, whereupon he applied it at once in extracting a deeply rooted bicuspid tooth from one of his patients. Morton then visited Dr. John Collins Warren, of the Massachusetts General Hospital, and persuaded him to give

---

[1] Mitchell: Injuries to Nerves and their Consequences, Philadelphia, 1872.

[2] Surgeon General's Office : Circular No. 7, Washington, 1867.

[3] The original documents in support of Long's claim have been effectively brought together by Dr. H. H. Young in Bull. Johns Hopkins Hosp., Balt., 1896–97, viii, 174–184.

the new anesthetic a trial in surgical procedure, without, however, disclosing the name of the drug. The operation took place at the hospital on October 16, 1846, the case being a "congenital but superficial, vascular tumor, just below the jaw, on the left side of the neck." The tumor was dissected out by Warren in five minutes, and, as the patient came back to consciousness, he exclaimed, "Gentlemen, this is no humbug." The next day a large fatty tumor of the shoulder was removed by Hayward, with Morton as anesthetist, and again with success. On November 18, 1846, the discovery was announced to the world in a paper by Henry J. Bigelow, published in the Boston Medical and Surgical Journal.[1] It was largely due to the high character and repute of such men as Warren and Bigelow that ether anesthesia was taken up all over the world and became a permanent part of operative surgery, for Morton tried to patent the drug as "letheon" (1846),[2] squabbling with Jackson about their respective legal rights, and not announcing it as sulphuric ether until 1847.[3] In the meanwhile, Robert Liston had amputated a thigh under ether in December, 1846; Syme took it up in Edinburgh (1847), and Pirogoff wrote a little manual on etherization (1847), based upon his Crimean experiences. The terms "anesthesia" and "anesthetic" were proposed by Oliver Wendell Holmes. On January 19, 1847, Sir James Young Simpson (1811–70), professor of obstetrics at Edinburgh, used ether in midwifery practice for the first time in Great Britain, but on November 4, 1847, he was led to substitute chloroform, the discovery of Liebig, Guthrie, and Soubeiran, and was so much impressed with its advantages over ether in obstetric work that he published his results a week later.[4] The effect of these discoveries upon medicine and surgery was remarkable in many ways. First of all, the surgeon, who, in pre-anesthetic days, had to rush through an operation at lightning speed and under great disadvantages occasioned by the struggles and distress of the patient, could now take his time and therefore perform many new operations impossible under the old conditions.[5] The days of sleight-of-hand

---

[1] Boston Med. and Surg. Jour., 1846–47, xxxv, 309; 379.

[2] T. W. Morton: Circular, Morton's letheon, Boston, 1846.

[3] Morton: Remarks on the proper mode of administering sulphuric ether, etc., Boston, 1847.

[4] Sir J. Y. Simpson: Account of a new anesthetic agent, Edinburgh, 1847.

[5] "When I was a boy, surgeons operating upon the quick were pitted one against the other like runners on time. He was the best surgeon, both for patient and onlooker, who broke the three-minutes record in an amputation or a lithotomy. What place could there be in record-breaking operations for the fiddle-faddle of antiseptic precautions? The obvious boon of immunity from pain, precious as it was, when we look beyond the individual, was less than the boon of time. With anesthetics ended slapdash surgery; anesthesia gave time for the theories of Pasteur and Lister to be adopted in practice." Sir Clifford Allbutt, Johns Hopkins Hosp. Bull., Balt., 1898, ix, p. 281.

feats was over, and the prestidigitations of a Cheselden, a Langen-beck, a Fergusson, or a Pirogoff gave place to careful, deliberate procedure. Again, a few whiffs of chloroform enabled the lying-in woman to confront the fierce pangs of labor with greater ease and security, and the obstetrician was able to work under the same ad-vantages as the surgeon. Both surgeon and obstetrician special-ized at need, as operative gynecologists, while laboratory workers in physiology and other branches of experimental medicine could have no further misgivings about the sufferings of vivisected ani-mals. In these fields anesthesia was, in the memorable phrase of Weir Mitchell, the "Death of Pain."

Operative gynecology, which had no special existence before the beginning of the nineteenth century, was largely the creation of a number of surgeons from the Southern States, and, as has been suggested, had its origin in the attempt to repair the errors and omissions of backwoods obstetrics. In the eighteenth century, we find William Baynham (1749–1814), of Virginia, operating twice with success for extra-uterine pregnancy (1790–99),[1] and, in the early part of the nineteenth, John King (1819–93), of Edisto Island, South Carolina, performed a remarkable operation for abdominal pregnancy in 1816,[2] saving both mother and child by cutting through the walls of the vagina and applying the forceps, with abdominal pressure exerted upon the fetus from above. He afterward expanded his views on the subject in a volume of 176 pages, published at Norwich, England, in 1818, entitled "An Analysis of the Subject of Extra-uterine Fœtation, and of the Ret-roversion of the Gravid Uterus," the first book on the subject. The founders of operative gynecology were McDowell and Sims.

Ephraim **McDowell** (1771–1830), of Virginia, was a pupil of John Bell, of Edinburgh, in 1793–94, and, through Bell's eloquent teaching, was early impressed with the sad and hopeless fate of women afflicted with ovarian disease. In 1795, he settled in the village of Danville, Kentucky, then one of the outposts of civiliza-tion, and soon became known as a skilful and successful surgeon, especially in lithotomy, which he performed 22 times in succession without losing a case. In December, 1809, he performed his first ovariotomy upon Mrs. Crawford, a woman of forty-seven, who afterward lived to be seventy-eight. McDowell reported this case with two others in April, 1817,[3] following these with a report of

---

[1] Baynham: New York Med. and Phil. Rev., 1809, i, 160–170.

[2] King: Med. Repository, New York, 1817, n. s., iii, 388–394.

[3] McDowell: Eclect. Repertory and Analyt. Rev., Phila., 1817, viii, 242–244.

two more cases in 1819.[1] He performed the operation 13 times in his life, with a record of 8 recoveries. Although he may have been preceded by Weyer's swineherd of the sixteenth century, and by the partial operation (tapping of cyst) by Houstoun, of Edinburgh, in 1701, yet one swallow does not make a summer, and ovariotomy had no existence in surgical practice before McDowell produced his results and put it upon a permanent basis. He had sent a manuscript copy of his first paper to his old preceptor, John Bell, who was then ending his days in Italy and never saw it. It came, however, into the hands of Bell's pupil, John Lizars (1787–1860), of Edinburgh, who took up McDowell's work with interest, publishing his results in his "Observations on Extraction of Diseased Ovaria" (1825), the next important contribution to the subject. In the meantime, Dr. Nathan Smith had performed an ovariotomy at Norwich, Connecticut, in July, 1821,[2] in ignorance of McDowell's work, which was destined to receive its greatest impetus at the hands of the brothers, John L. and Washington L. Atlee, of Pennsylvania, the former of whom performed the operation 78 times, with 64 recoveries (1843–83), and the latter 387 times (1844–78). Ovariotomy was firmly established in English surgery through the admirable labors of Charles Clay (1801–93), of Manchester, and Sir Spencer Wells (1818–97), of London. The introduction of ovariotomy in France was due to Auguste Nélaton; to Jules Péan (1830–98), who performed the first successful operation in Paris (1864), and to the Alsatian surgeon Eugène Koeberlé (1828–   ), who was the first to perform the operation in present-day Germany.[3]

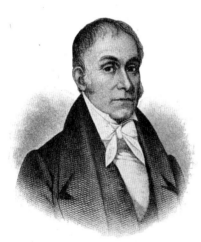

Ephraim McDowell (1771–1830).

Before the time of Sims, much important work of a scattered character was done in Europe and America, notably Ritgen's case of gastro-elytrotomy (1821),[4] Roux's operation for ruptured perineum (1834),[5] Récamier's invention

[1] McDowell: Eclect. Repert. (etc.), Phila. *Ibid.*, 1819, ix, 546–553.

[2] Smith: Am. Med. Recorder, Phila., 1822, v, 124–126.

[3] Koeberlé: Mém. Acad. de méd., Paris, 1862–63, xxvi, 371–472, 6 pl.

[4] Ritgen: Heidelberg klin. Ann., 1825, i, 263–277.

[5] Roux: Gaz. méd. de Paris, 1834, 2. s., ii, 17–22.

of the *speculum plein et brisé* (1842),[1] the simultaneous invention of special uterine sounds, in 1843, by Huguier, of Paris; Kiwisch, of Prague, and Sir James Young Simpson[2] (1811–70), of Edinburgh; Bennett's treatise on "Inflammation of the Uterus" (1845); Till on "Ovarian Inflammation" (1850); Nélaton's description of pelvic hematocele (1851–52);[3] Noeggerath's operation of epicystotomy (1853),[4] and Daniel Ayres's plastic operation for congenital exstrophy of the female bladder (1859).[5] In 1836, Michaëlis, of Kiel, reported the celebrated case of Frau Adametz, upon whom four Cesarean sections had been successively performed, his own operation being as successful as the rest[6]; and, in America, John Lambert Richmond performed the first Cesarean section at Newtown, Ohio, on April 22, 1827. Prevost, of Donaldsonville, Louisiana, performed the operation four times prior to 1830, with three successful cases; and William Gibson, of Baltimore, performed the Cesarean operation twice with success upon the same patient (1835–38),[7] who lived for fifty years after her first experience. Myomectomy for fibroid tumors of the uterus was performed twice with success by Washington L. Atlee in 1844,[8] and by Walter Burnham, of Lowell, Massachusetts, in 1853,[9] and, in the same year (1853),[10] Gilman Kimball (1804–92), of Lowell, Massachusetts, first performed this operation with deliberate intention.

Prior to the year 1852, the stumbling-block of gynecology was the relief of **vesicovaginal fistula.** Many surgeons, from the time of Paré onward, had attempted to operate for this condition, with no better result than to entail an additional amount of suffering and inconvenience upon their unfortunate patients. Roonhuyze (1672) and Fatio (1752) left admirable accounts of their operative methods, but no reports of successful cases. Dieffenbach left a classical account of the wretched plight of the women upon whom all his wonderful resources were tried in vain (1845). Jobert de Lamballe had written a whole treatise upon female fistulæ (1852),[11] but his autoplastic operation *par glissement* had only resulted in repeated failures and the death of many of his patients. Six successful operations for the condition had been reported in America by John Peter Mettauer (1787–1875), of Virginia[12] (1830–47);

---

[1] Récamier: Bull. Acad. de méd., Paris, 1842–43, viii, 661–668.

[2] Simpson: London and Edinb. Monthly Jour. Med. Sc., 1843, iii, 547; 701; 1009: 1844, iv, 208.

[3] Nélaton: Gaz. d. hôp., Paris, 1851, 3. s., iii, 573; 581: 1852, iv, 54; 66.

[4] Noeggerath: New York Med. Jour., 1853, 3. s., iv, 9–24.

[5] Ayres: Am. Med. Gaz., New York, 1859, x, 81–89, 2 pl.

[6] Michaelis: Mitth. a. d. Geb. d. Med. (etc.), Altona, 1836, iv, 7.–8. Hft., p. 60.

[7] Gibson: Am. Jour. Med. Sc., Phila., 1835, xvi, 351; xvii, 264: 1838, xxii, 13: 1885, n. s., xc, 422.

[8] Atlee: The Surgical Treatment of Certain Fibrous Tumors of the Uterus, New York, 1853.

[9] Burnham: Nelson's Am. Lancet, Plattsburgh, N. Y., 1853, vii, 147.

[10] Kimball: Boston Med. and Surg. Jour., 1855, lii, 249–255.

[11] A.-J. Jobert de Lamballe: Traité des fistules vésico-utérines, vésico-utéro-vaginales (etc.), Paris, 1852.

[12] Mettauer: Boston Med. and Surg. Jour., 1840, xxii, 154. Also, Am. Jour. Med. Sc., Phila., 1847, n. s., xiv, 117–121.

others by George Hayward (1791–1863), of Boston, in 1839[1]; by Joseph Pancoast, of Philadelphia, in 1847[2]; and, in France, by Maisonneuve (1848).[3]   The whole matter was changed, as Kelly says, "almost with a magic wand" by James Marion **Sims** (1813–83), of South Carolina.   A graduate of Jefferson Medical College, Philadelphia (1835), Sims settled in Alabama, where he soon became known as a capable and original surgeon, operating successfully for abscess of the liver in 1835, and removing both the upper and the lower jaw in 1837.   In 1845, he was called

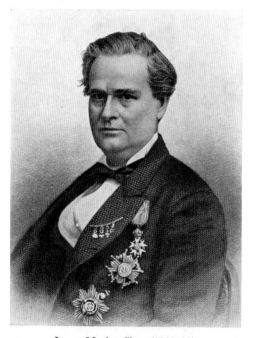

James Marion Sims (1813–83).

to see a country woman who had sustained a displacement of the uterus from a fall from a horse.   In making a digital examination to correct the displacement, he hit upon the peculiar lateral posture (Sims position), and was led to the invention of the special duck-bill speculum, which were to be the special factors of his success in operating for vesicovaginal fistula.   To the Sims position and

[1] Hayward: Am. Jour. Med. Sc., Phila., 1839, xxiv, 283–288.

[2] Pancoast: Med. Examiner, Phila., 1847, n. s., iii, 272–274; 1851, vii, 650–656.

[3] Maisonneuve: Clinique chirurgicale, Paris, 1848, vii, 660 et seq.

the Sims speculum, which enabled the operator to see the condition "as no man had ever seen it before," he added a special suture of silver wire, to avoid sepsis, and a catheter for emptying the bladder while the fistula was healing. With these four coefficients, Sims perfected his operation for repairing this almost irremediable condition, and published his paper in 1852.[1] It created a profound impression, and, in 1854,[2] was followed by a monograph of Gustav Simon, suggesting a method of uniting the edges of the fistula by means of double sutures. Sims removed to New York in 1853, and, in 1855, established the State Hospital for Women, which soon became the center of the best gynecological work of the time. Visiting Europe in 1861, Sims performed his fistula operation with great *éclat* before Nélaton, Velpeau, Larrey, and other surgical leaders, and was soon in request all over Europe as an operator in diseases of women. His "Clinical Notes on Uterine Surgery" (1866) was translated into German, and Robert Olshausen and August Martin have borne testimony to the high esteem in which Sims was held in that country.[3] Among his other important contributions were his methods of amputating the cervix uteri (1861),[4] his description of the condition "vaginismus" (1861),[5] his operation of cholecystotomy (1878),[6] and his great paper on "The careful aseptic invasion of the peritoneal cavity for the arrest of hemorrhage, the suture of intestinal wounds, and the cleansing of the peritoneal cavity, and for all intraperitoneal conditions" (1881).[7] Sims, a kind-hearted but impulsive man, was one of the most original and gifted of American surgeons. A statue, erected to his memory in 1894 by European and American admirers, is in Bryant Park, New York city.

In the Woman's Hospital in New York, Sims was assisted by Thomas Addis **Emmet** (1828–   ), a native of Virginia, who, under his training, became a great master of the plastic surgery of the perineum, the vagina, the cervix uteri, and the bladder. As Kelly says, he "caught Sims' idea at once, acquired his methods, and improved upon them and did more than any other surgeon to teach the members of the profession in this country how to do

---

[1] Sims: Am. Jour. Med. Sc., 1852, n. s., xxiii, 59–82.

[2] Simon: Ueber die Heilung der Blasen-Scheidenfisteln, Giessen, 1854.

[3] Olshausen: Ueber Marion Sims und seine Verdienste um die Chirurgie, Berlin, 1897. Martin: Ztschr. f. Geburtsh. u. Gynäk., Stuttgart, 1913, lxxiii, 946–948.

[4] Sims: Tr. Med. Soc. New York, Albany, 1861, 367–371.

[5] Sims: Tr. Obst. Soc. Lond., 1861, iii, 356–367.

[6] Sims: Richmond and Louisville Med. Jour., 1878, xxvi, 1–21.

[7] Sims: Brit. Med. Jour., London, 1881, ii, 925; 971; 1882, i, 184; 222; 260; 302.

these operations." Emmet's principal contributions are his papers on the treatment of dysmenorrhea and sterility resulting from anteflexion of the uterus (1865),[1] on the surgical treatment of lacerations of the cervix uteri (1869–74),[2] his monograph on vesicovaginal and rectovaginal fistula (1868),[3] and his papers on vaginal cystotomy (1872)[4] and the plastic surgery of the perineum (1882).[5]

Sims' work was further extended by Nathan **Bozeman** (1825–1905), of Alabama, who did many successful operations on vesical and fecal fistulæ in women, paying special attention to the complication of pyelitis, which he treated by catheterizing the ureter through a vesicovaginal opening (1887–88).[6]

In the group of Southern gynecologists may be included Prevost, of Donaldsonville, Louisiana, and William Gibson, of Maryland, both pioneers in Cesarean section, and Josiah Clark **Nott** (1804–73), of South Carolina, who, in 1844, described the condition which Sir James Y. Simpson, in 1861, called "coccygodynia."[7] Nott was also one of the first to suggest the "mosquito theory" in reference to the transmission of yellow fever (1848),[8] and wrote a number of works on ethnology.

Theodore **Gaillard Thomas** (1831–1903), of Edisto Island, South Carolina, like Marion Sims, practised in New York. In 1868, he published a treatise on diseases of women, which was esteemed the best that had yet appeared,[9] and was translated into French, German, Italian, Spanish, and Chinese. In 1870, Thomas revived Ritgen's operation of gastro-elytrotomy as a substitute for Cesarean section,[10] and in the same year was the first to perform vaginal ovariotomy.[11]

Robert **Battey** (1828–95), of Augusta, Georgia, a graduate of the Jefferson Medical College of Philadelphia, was the first to suggest the operation of oöphorectomy, or excision of the uterine appendages, for such non-ovarian conditions as painful menstruation and neuroses. This operation was first performed by him on August

---

[1] Emmet: New York Med. Jour., 1865, i, 205–219.

[2] Am. J. Obst., New York, 1868–69, i, 339–362; 1874–75, vii, 442–456.

[3] New York, 1868.

[4] Am. Pract., Louisville, 1872, v, 65–92.

[5] Tr. Am. Gynec. Soc., 1882, New York, 1884, viii, 198–216.

[6] Bozeman: Tr. Internat. Med. Cong., Wash., 1887, ii, 514–558; and Am. Jour. Med. Sc., Phila., 1888, n. s., xcv, 225; 368.

[7] Nott: New Orleans Med. Jour., 1844–45, i, 58–60. Simpson: Med. Times and Gaz., London, 1861, i, 317.

[8] Nott: New Orleans Med. Jour., 1848, iv, 563; 601.

[9] Thomas: A Practical Treatise on the Diseases of Women, Phila., 1868.

[10] Thomas: Am. Jour. Obst., New York, 1870, iii, 125–139.

[11] Thomas: Am. Jour. Med. Sc., Phila., 1870, n. s., lix, 387–390.

27, 1872.[1] "Battey's operation" was afterward applied to other pelvic conditions by Hegar in Germany, and Lawson Tait in England, and has more recently acquired a definite physiological significance in connection with modern work on the chemical correlation of the internal secretions.

The **advancement of scientific medicine in the second half of the nineteenth century** was characterized by the introduction of a biological or evolutionary view of morphology and physiology, out of which came the sciences of cellular pathology, bacteriology, and parasitology, new modes of seeing disease and its causes, which had in them the germ of novel methods of treatment by means of sera and vaccines. The discoveries of Pasteur led immediately to Listerian or antiseptic surgery, with its remarkable applications in such regions as the abdomen, the brain, the joints, the thorax, and special sense organs, and its great extension in operative gynecology. Great improvements in medical education, public hygiene, and military medicine followed upon these developments in due course, and were further helped out by the great increase in the number and quality of scientific periodicals and through the growth of rapid means of national

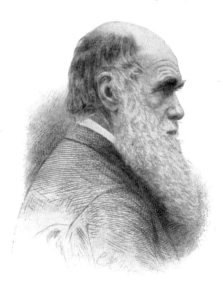

Charles Robert Darwin (1809–82).

and international communication by railway, steamship, telegraph, and cable. In this way, specialties like ophthalmology, otology, laryngology, orthopedics, dentistry, and veterinary medicine became something more than mere names.

The immense growth of general **biology** in our time was principally due to the evolutionary theories of Charles Robert **Darwin** (1809–82), of Shrewsbury, England, a Cambridge graduate, whose bent toward natural history was set by his boyhood interest in botany and his five years' cruise as naturalist on H.M.S. Beagle (1831–36), an experience which rendered him an expert geologist

---

[1] Battey: Atlanta Med. and Surg. Jour., 1872–73, x, 321–339.

and zoölogist. Although an invalid for the rest of his life, Darwin labored for twenty years before publishing his great work On the Origin of Species by Means of Natural Selection (1859), perhaps the most wonderful piece of synthesis in the history of science. This theory was arrived at independently by Alfred Russell Wallace (1822–1913) in 1858, although Darwin's priority dates back to 1838. Both Darwin and Wallace owed much to the Essay on the Principle of Population published by the English clergyman, Thomas Robert Malthus, in 1803. Darwin's extraordinary marshaling of facts, in evidence of the survival of the fittest by natural selection in the struggle for existence, had the same far-reaching influence upon biological speculation that the discoveries of Copernicus had upon astronomy. It dispensed with the ancient Linnæan concept of the fixity of species, that animals and plants were originally created as we find them today, and the ghostly metaphysical abstractions which were invoked to "explain" why this should be. It created the sciences of comparative physiology and pathology, by pointing to the close structural and functional relationship between human tissues and those of animals and plants. And though the idea of evolution was known to the Greeks and was more or less definitely outlined by Bacon, Buffon, Erasmus, Darwin, Goethe, Lamarck, Lyell, and Herbert Spencer, it became the salient fact of modern science through Darwin's work. The application of the idea of continuous development in "'The Descent of Man'" (1871) made an end of the anthropocentric theory that the universe was made for man. It began to be perceived that there is a rude and noble dignity in the story of man's painful evolution from the lower forms of life, even as Darwin's picture of the struggle for existence illuminated the true causes of human misery as never before. That there are flaws and gaps in Darwin's hypotheses; that he did not take sufficient account of those spontaneous accidental variations or mutations which, as Mendel and De Vries have indicated, may also originate species; that his theory of sexual selection is not borne out by the facts; that many specific characters in animals and plants are not true survival values, is all clear enough now. But it should not be forgotten that Darwin himself regarded natural selection "as the main, but not the exclusive, means of modification," and that a true specific character is a survival value only in regard to its possessor's essential environment, and not in respect of some accidental enemy. Darwin's essay on The Variation of Animals and Plants under Domestication (1868) is now mainly memorable for his attempt to explain the mechanism of inheritance by "pangenesis," or the transportation of gemmules from all parts of the organism to the ovum, to insure their reproduction, which has found an avatar in Starling's theory of the hormones. The great monograph on "The Expression of the Emotions in Man and Animals" (1873) ranks with the contemporaneous work of Duchenne, of Boulogne (1862), and the theory of evolution itself is the starting-point of comparative psychology. The investigations in botany and geology, the monographs on Climbing Plants (1875), Cross and Self-Fertilization (1876), Power of Movement in Plants (1880), Formation of Vegetable Mould (1881), Coral Reefs (1842), and Volcanic Islands (1844), can only be mentioned. Much harm has been done to Darwin's reputation among shallow-minded people through the attempt of the half-insane Nietzsche and his school to carry the idea of "war down the weak" into actual ethics. This contravenes the true intent of the Darwinian theory, which shows why nature is pitiless, but did not say that man should be. Over against these misinterpreters should be set the grave, self-possessed, entirely human figure of Darwin himself. Bearing in mind the magnificent sincerity of his work, his fame is safe enough from inexpensive caviling.

Darwin's work was popularized and extended in the philosophic writings of Herbert Spencer (1820–1903), whose "Principles of Biology" (1866–67), "Principles of Psychology" (1871), and "Descriptive Sociology" (1873–81) are all of a high order of merit; by Alfred Russel Wallace, whose "Geographical Distribution of Animals" (1876) is his best work; and by Huxley and Haeckel.

Thomas Henry **Huxley** (1825–95), of Ealing, England, was a medical graduate of the London University (1845) who became a surgeon in the Royal Navy. As with Darwin, his interest in biology was awakened by a sea voyage, a five years' cruise on H.M.S. Rattlesnake (1846–50). Prior to this experience he had already discovered the layer of cells in the root-sheath of hair which goes by his name (1845),[1] and upon his return he made many important contributions to marine zoölogy, in recognition of which he became Fellow and gold-medallist of the Royal Society (1851–52). Resigning from the navy, he became lecturer on natural history at the Royal School of Mines, and introduced the idea of teaching morphology by means of a series of typical animals, as norms of their species, which afterward became the feature of Huxley and Martin's "Elementary Biology" (1875). He applied evolution to paleontology, in his extended studies of fossil fishes, crocodiles, and other vertebrata, and in his work on the ancestry of the horse. His Croonian Lectures on the theory of the vertebrate skull (1858) overthrew Owen's concept of an archetype in favor of a morphologic type, an assemblage of

---

[1] Lond. Med. Gaz., 1845, n. s., i, 1340.

features common to all its class, as in a composite photograph. With this may be bracketed Huxley's important lectures
on the craniology of birds (1867). In 1861,[1] he demonstrated
the inaccuracy of another contention of Owen's, relating to the
supposed backward projection of the cavities of the brain into the
posterior horn and the hippocampus minor, as a specific character in man. The essays on the Comparative Anatomy of Man
and the Higher Apes (1859–62), and On Evidence as to Man's
Place in Nature (1863), reveal the follower of Darwin, of whose
ideas Huxley was indeed the ablest modern interpreter. A master

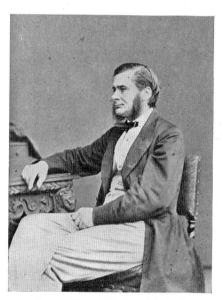

Thomas Henry Huxley (1825–95).

of vigorous English, he
wrote several volumes of
essays, which are among
the most delightful of
modern contributions to
popular science; and his
text-books on physiology
(1866), which passed
through 30 editions, on
vertebrate and inverte-
brate anatomy (1871–77)
and on physiography
(1877) are little master-
pieces of their kind. Huxley defined himself as one
who cared more for free-
dom of thought than for
the mere advancement of
science, and this is the interest of his personality.
Vigorous and resolute in
form and features, a stalwart, masculine-minded
man who ruined his health by sedentary labors, he was, in the circumstances of his marriage, as in his championship of Darwinism
or his Napoleonic warfare on theologians, a romantic, like Vesalius.
No man ever fought more bravely and openly for truth and honesty,
for the right of people to think and express their own thoughts. No
man ever admitted his own errors more readily or was more generous
to a fallen adversary. His conviction that "there is no alleviation
for the sufferings of mankind except veracity of thought and action
and the resolute facing of the world as it is, when the garment of

[1] Nat. Hist. Rev., London, 1861, 67–84. Proc. Zoöl. Soc., London, 1861, 247–260.

make-believe by which pious hands have hidden its uglier features is stripped off," is the final justification of Darwinism and sounds the keynote of the social medicine of the future.

Ernst **Haeckel** (1834–   ), of Jena, a great morphologist, carried Darwinism into Germany, where the opposition of Virchow created the necessity for such a defender.   Haeckel's greatest work is his *Generelle Morphologie* (1866), in which organisms and the forms of organic structures are considered and classified in relation to serial homology, heredity, and evolution.   In 1868, appeared his "Natural History of Creation"; in 1874, the *Anthropogenie*, a great treatise on human embryology; and, in 1884, his monograph on the Gastræa Theory, which regards the two-layered gastrula as the ancestral form of all multicellular animals. These were all contributions of the most effective kind, the result of years of patient investigation. Haeckel's popular writings include his delightful letters of East Indian travel and such uncritical works as The Riddle of the Universe.   In the latter, he combines an ironclad materialism, like that of the French   Encyclopædists, with the notion that aggregations of molecules have souls (*Plastidul Seelen*), which was ridiculed by Virchow.   At the present time Haeckel, the sage of Jena, is highly revered among scientific men, and looked up to as one of the greatest of fighters for freedom in thought and teaching.   His Phyletic Museum at Jena is said to be the most wonderful collection of serial illustrations of evolution and development in the world.

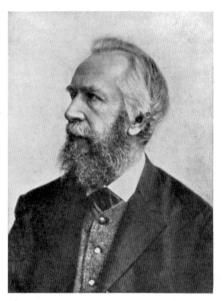

Ernst Haeckel (1834–   ).

The problem of **heredity** was attacked in four different ways by Mendel, Hering, Galton, and Weissmann.

Gregor **Mendel** (1822–84), abbot of the Augustinian monastery at Brünn, Austria, discovered the mathematical law governing the dominant and recessive characters in hybrids (1866–67), the application of which belongs to the twentieth century.

Ewald **Hering** (1834–   ), a Saxon professor, is the author of the psycho-physical theory (1870) that facultative memory, the automatic power of protoplasm to do what it has done before, is the distinctive property of all living matter. The transmission and reproduction of parental characters are supposed to be the result of the organism's unconscious memory of the past, the mechanism being, in Hering's view, the persistence of wave motions of molecules. This idea was also advanced by Haeckel (Perigenesis of Plastidules) and by Samuel Butler (1835–1902), of Langar, England, who translated Hering's essay and applied the doctrine in his polemics against Darwinism.

Sir Francis **Galton** (1822–1911), a cousin of Darwin's, began to investigate heredity experimentally in 1871. His observations upon the inheritance of transfused blood in rabbits, of tricolored spots on the coat of Bassett hounds, of stature and other characters in human families, led him to reject the Lamarckian theory of the inheritance of acquired characters as well as the Darwinian Pangenesis. In his book on "Natural Inheritance" (1889), he proceeds, by statistical induction, to the Law of Filial Regression, which asserts that the offspring of parents unusual in height, talent, etc., regress to the average of the stock; also to the Law of Ancestral Inheritance, in virtue of which each parent contributes one-fourth $[(\frac{1}{2})^2]$ of the total inheritance, each of the four grandparents one-sixteenth $[(\frac{1}{2})^4]$, each of the eight great-grandparents $\frac{1}{128} = (\frac{1}{2})^6$, while, in general, the ancestors in degrees removed contribute $(\frac{1}{2})^{2n}$ each. The latter theorem has been confirmed, with slight mathematical changes, by the biometric methods of Karl Pearson. Galton's work on Finger-prints (1892) is the first contribution of importance after Purkinje. He introduced the doctrine of eugenics (a term of his coinage), founded the Eugenics Laboratory in London (1904), and, with Pearson and Weldon, founded "Biometrika" (1901), a journal for the study of biologic problems by advanced statistical methods.

An important extension of evolutionary theory is the idea of the unbroken continuity or immortality of the germ-plasm, which was elaborated by August **Weissmann** (1834–   ), of Frankfort on the Main, between 1893 and 1904. The general idea of continuity of growth and development by direct cell-lineage was already inherent in Virchow's cell-theory. Owen, in his paper on Parthenogenesis (1849), distinguished betweeen cells forming the body and germ-cells. Haeckel emphasized the idea of continuous descent all through his Generelle Morphologie (1866). Jaeger coined the phrase "continuity of the germ protoplasma" in 1878, and the capacity of the latter for transmitting hereditary qualities was clearly stated by Nussbaum in 1875. Weissmann insisted on the continuity of descent in unicellular organisms, and, in tracing the gradual evolution of multicellular organisms from these, pointed out that the complex organism, made up of body-cells, is only the vehicle of the germ-cells. The germ-plasm, a complex structure contained in the nuclei of these reproductive cells, is the parent of the germ-cells of the succeeding generation, securing a relative immortality for the species, although individuals die out. The union of the two germs is "amphimixis." Weissmann maintained that variation is produced by sexual selection, and latterly by a nutritional selection among the components of the germ-plasm (germinal selection). Another feature of Weissmann's theory is his experimental proof that acquired characters are not directly transmitted. This apparent overthrow of the Lamarckian theory has caused much controversy, but the balance of experimental evidence seems in favor of Weissmann. If true, the Weissmann theory is of far reaching social significance, since it seems probable that moral qualities cannot be transmitted to children, but have to be acquired, in each case, by intensive early training.

Another outgrowth of biologic and evolutionary thinking was the nineteenth-century science of **anthropology,** which was built up by the labors of such men as Darwin, Huxley, Lyell, Spencer, Prichard, and Tylor in England; in France, by Broca, who invented some 27 craniometric and cranioscopic instruments; in Germany, by Virchow, who was an expert in craniology, and took the whole field of anthropology for his province; in Italy, by Cesare Lombroso, who developed the study of the criminal and the morbid side of the man of genius.

Anthropological societies were founded in Paris (by Broca) in 1859, in London in 1863, in Madrid in 1865, in Berlin in 1868, in Vienna in 1870, in Italy in 1871, and in Washington, D. C., in 1879. Physical anthropology was developed through the craniological investigations of Broca and Virchow, the treatises of Paul Topinard, Quatrefages' studies of fossil and savage men (1861) and pygmies (1887), Virchow's statistics on the physical anthropology of the Germans (1876), Lombroso's book on criminal man (*L'uomo delinquente*, 1876), Alphonse Bertillon's method of identifying criminals by selected measurements (*Bertillonage*, 1886), and Francis Galton's mode of identification by finger-prints (1892). Ethnological societies had been founded in Paris in 1839, New York (1842), and London (1844), and the principal monuments of the science are the monographs of Prichard (1813), Pickering (1848), Knox (1850), Latham (1850–59), Nott and Gliddon (1857), Waitz (1859–72), Herbert Spencer (1873–81), Friedrich Müller (1873), Peschel (1873), Ratzel (1885–88), Haddon (1894–1909), Achelis (1896), and Ripley (1900). In the field of ethnic craniology, we may mention Morton's albums of American and Egyptian skulls (1839–44), the "Crania ethnica" of de Quatrefages and Hamy (1872–82), Rütimeyer and His on Swiss skulls (1864), Retzius' albums of Finnish and Swedish skulls (1878–1900), and Virchow's "Crania ethnica Americana" (1892). The subject was carried into a pedantic excess of detail in Sergi's polysyllabic subdivisions of racial types of skulls, and in Aurel von Török's "Systematic Craniometry" (1890), with its 5000 proposed measurements of a single skull. Ethnic psychology was developed by Andrew Lang (1884–1901), Adolf Bastian (1886–90), Alfred Fouillée (1903), Wilhelm Wundt (1904), and in such monographs as those of the Torres Straits Expedition (1898). Other phases of comparative ethnology are the studies of Pitt-Rivers on technology (1860–75), Sir Henry Maine on Ancient Law (1861), J. J. Bachofen on the Matriarchate (*Das Mutterrecht*, 1861), Jnt. MacLennan on Primitive Marriage (1865), E. B. Tylor on Primitive Culture (1871), L. H. Morgan on Systems of Consanguinity (1871), Herbert Spencer on Descriptive Sociology (1873–81), William Black (1883) and Max Bartels (1893) on medical folk-lore, J. G. Frazer on Totemism (1887), Totemism and Exogamy (1910), and Taboo (*The Golden Bough*, 1890), Westermarck on Human Marriage (1891), Alfred C. Haddon on Evolution in Art (1895), Edwin Sydney Hartland on Primitive Paternity (1910), and W. I. Thomas on Social Origins (1909). The excavations of bones and flint implements by M. Boucher de Perthes at Abbeville, during 1805–47; the later unearthing of similar finds in the Devonshire caves; the exploration of lake-dwelling remains in the Irish crannogs by Sir William Wilde (1839), and of the Swiss *Pfahlbauten* by Ferdinand Keller (1853–54), led to extensive and intensive study of these prehistoric objects all over the world. The results were systematized in Gabriel de Mortillet's classic, Le *Préhistorique* (1883), and carried forward by Sir John Evans in England, Virchow in Germany, Piette in France, and Holmes in America. The discovery of the prehistoric skull and skeletal remains at Neanderthal in 1856, which Virchow pronounced diseased, Broca normal, and Huxley human but ape-like, led Huxley to his famous assignment of man's place in nature as "more nearly allied to the higher apes than the latter are to the lower" (1860). The subsequent cranial finds at Spy (1886), Krapina (1889), Heidelberg (1907), Le Moustier (1908), La Chapelle aux Saints (1909), and Sussex (1912), and Eugène Dubois' discovery, in Java, of the teeth, calvarium, and femur of the Pithecanthropus erectus (1891), which he regarded as a sort of "missing link" between the anthropoid apes and man, only added fuel to the ensuing controversy which is bound up with the question of the single or diverse origin of the human species. In general, man is now classed, where Linnæus left him in 1735, with the Simiidæ. The unity of the human species has been maintained by Linnæus, Buffon, Prichard, Sir William Lawrence, Broca, the English anthropologists and the followers of Haeckel, while the multiple or polygenist theory has been favored largely by those Germans who have followed the somewhat official leadership of Virchow.

After the labors of such masters as Bichat, Bell, Henle, and Hyrtl, there was little to be added to the subject of descriptive

30

HISTORY OF MEDICINE

human **anatomy** and most investigation in this field became merged into morphology and histology. Splendid atlases of gross or macroscopic anatomy were published, such as those of the Bells, Cloquet (1821–31), Sir William MacEwen's Atlas of Head Sections (1893), and the albums of the younger Retzius (1896) and Carl Wernicke (1897–1904) on the brain. Frozen sections, introduced by Pieter de Riemer (1760–1831) in 1818, were utilized in Pirogoff's epoch-making "Anatome topographica" (1852–59) and in the atlases of the pregnant uterus (1872) and of normal topographic anatomy (1872) by Christian Wilhelm Braune (1831–92). Artistic anatomy was ably treated by John Flaxman (1833), Robert Knox (1852), Matthias Duval (1881), the physiologists, Paul Richer (1890) and Ernst Wilhelm Brücke (1891); and, by direct photography from the nude, in the different works of Carl Heinrich Stratz, the motion pictures of Eadweard Muybridge (1901), and the splendid treatise of Julius Kollmann (1886). Treatises on gross anatomy were published by Sappey (1850–64), Gray (1859), Gegenbaur (1883), Testut (1889–91), and Bardeleben (1896). The history of anatomy was taken up by Hyrtl, Knox, Robert von Töply (1898), the history of anatomic methods by William W. Keen (1852), and Ludwig Choulant's History of Anatomical Illustration (1852) is a monograph of permanent value. There were isolated discoveries in plenty, such as the island of Reil (1809), Clarke's columns (1851), Broca's convolution (1861), Auerbach's plexus (1862), Bigelow's demonstration of the Y-ligament (1869), or Waldeyer's ring (1884). Perhaps the most important of these was the description of the parathyroid glands by the Swedish anatomist, Ivar Sandström, in 1879.

The leading German anatomist of recent times was Wilhelm **Waldeyer** (1836–1906), of Hehlen, Brunswick, professor at Berlin (1883), who made important researches on the development of cancer (1867–72), retroperitoneal hernia (1868), ovary and ovum (1870), and the neuron theory (1891), to which he gave the name. He first described the open ring of lymphoid tissue[1] formed by the faucial, lingual, and pharyngeal tonsils (1884), which is now regarded as a prominent portal of infection.

Joseph **Leidy** (1823–91), of Philadelphia, who succeeded Horner as professor of anatomy at the University of Pennsylvania, was the leading American anatomist of his time, and a biologist of the type of Hunter and Müller, doing important work in botany, zoölogy, mineralogy, and paleontology, as well as in comparative and human anatomy. His "Fresh Water Rhizopods of North America" (1879) is one of our biological classics. He made valuable re-

---

[1] Waldeyer: Deutsche med. Wochenschr., Leipzig and Berlin, 1884, x, 313.

searches on the comparative anatomy of the liver (1848), the bones, trichinosis in hogs, etc., and his Elementary Treatise on Human Anatomy (1889) has a special interest in that it was illustrated by himself. Minot records that he discovered the bacterial flora of the intestines (1849)[1] and made the first experiment in transplanting malignant tumors (1851).[2] Like Gerhard and Gross, Leidy was a fine type of the German-American physician, as modest and unassuming as he was learned and versatile.

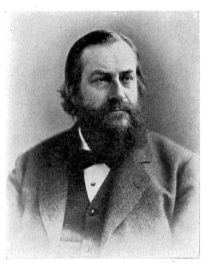

Oliver Wendell **Holmes** (1809–94), of Boston, whose work on puerperal fever has been mentioned, was Parkman professor of anatomy at the Harvard Medical School (1847–82), and resembled Hyrtl in his skill in making a dry subject interesting through his liveliness and wit. He made no discoveries of importance, but he wrote many clever medical poems, and his "Medical Essays"

Joseph Leidy (1823–91).

(1883) was easily the most important American book dealing with medical history in its day.

Prominent among the **comparative anatomists** of the transition period were Gegenbaur and Wiedersheim. Carl **Gegenbaur** (1826–1903), a native of Würzburg and a fellow-student of Haeckel's, established the point that comparative morphology, and not embryology, is the true criterion for determining the relation of homologies or pedigrees of organs (phylogeny), thus bringing the matter of the genealogy of organs back to Owen's original concept. In recent times, a large number of facts in corroboration of Owen's theory were produced, but many others which showed that similar structures may arise in different ways. At present, embryology is studied as a phase of morphology. Gegenbaur also gave the *coup de grâce* to the vertebrate theory of the skull (Goethe-Owen), by showing that, in the embryo, there are a large number of head segments corresponding to the branchial clefts and the cranial nerves; that, in the lowest order of fishes, the head, instead of being composed of vertebræ, is unsegmented, while, in the higher, many cranial bones arise from the skin. In 1861, Gegenbaur demonstrated that the ovum of every vertebrate is a single cell. His principal works are his Comparative Anatomy of Vertebrates (1864–72), his Elements of Comparative Anatomy (1870), and his Text-book of Human Anatomy (1883). He was editor of the *Morpholog-*

---

[1] Leidy: Proc. Acad. Nat. Sc., Phila., 1848–9, iv, 225–233.

[2] *Ibid.*, 1851, 212.

isches Jahrbuch (1875–1902), and professor of anatomy at Heidelberg, where he had many American pupils.

Robert **Wiedersheim** (1848–   ), professor of anatomy at Freiburg, was the author of important works on the Comparative Anatomy of Vertebrates (1882–83) and The Structure of Man as an Evidence of his Past (1887).

After the time of Schleiden, Schwann, and Henle, the study of the finer or **microscopic anatomy** of the tissues became the word of ambition. Histological investigation was rapidly improved by the introduction of new staining methods, microtomy, and other technical procedures. Purkinje, as we have seen, had a microtome and used Canada balsam, glacial acetic acid, and potassium bichromate, but these things were not generally known, and the common procedure was to examine the tissues in the fresh state, sliced by a razor between layers of vegetable pith. Hardening of the tissues in alcohol came long after. In 1847, Joseph von Gerlach, Sr. (1820–1896), of Mayence, began to inject capillaries with a transparent mixture of carmine, ammonia and gelatine; and, by 1855, he was employing carmine as a nuclear stain for the tissues. Virchow did practically all his work with carmine. Gerlach was also a pioneer in the use of aniline and gold chloride and, after his time, differential staining became rapidly specialized.

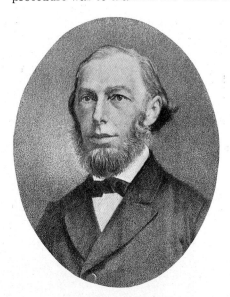

Max Schultze (1825–74).

The microtome was definitely introduced by Wilhelm His in 1866, but was not perfected until about 1875, after which it became an important labor-saving device.

The master worker in histology was Max **Schultze** (1825–74), of Freiburg, who was professor of anatomy at Halle (1854–59), and, succeeding Helmholtz at Bonn in 1859, became director of the Anatomical Institute there in 1872. Schultze introduced the dilute chromic acid solution, the osmic acid stain, iodated serum as a preservative, and invented the heatable object-stand. An important contributor to marine zoölogy, in his studies of the Turbellaria (1848–51), the Polythalamia (1854–6), and the

embryology of Petromyzon (1856), he made an epoch in histology
by his great monographs on the nerve-endings of the sense organs,
in particular, the internal ear (1858),[1] the nose (1863),[2] and the
retina (1866).[3]

In 1865, he founded the *Archiv für mikroskopische Anatomie*,
which he edited until his death. Schultze had a lasting influence
upon the cell theory through his essay of 1861,[4] in which, contem-
poraneously with Brücke, he defined the true cell as a clump of
nucleated protoplasm, thus emphasizing the point which Leydig
had made in 1856, that the cell membrane, even in the ovum, is a
secondary physico-chemical formation, probably due to surface-
tension condensation of the cell contents. In his memoir on the
protoplasm of rhizopods and plant cells (1863),[5] Schultze definitely introduced the term protoplasm, and showed that it is
practically identical in all living cells. In 1863, he gave the most
accurate contemporary account of the furrowing and segmentation
of the frog's egg.[6] Schultze was a striking, keen-eyed investigator, an accomplished draftsman, and a friend of music, devoting his leisure hours to the violin.

The next most important step in the cell doctrine was taken by
Walther **Flemming** (1843–1905), of Schwerin, professor at Prague
(1873–76) and Kiel (1876–1905), whose important monograph,
Zellsubstanz, Kern- und Zelltheilung (1882), gives the classic
account of cell division and karyokinesis. Some phases of the
latter process had been observed by Virchow and Schneider, and
Heitzmann had noted (1873) that all protoplasm is a continuous
network, the granular appearance of which is only optical.
Flemming's memoir put the whole matter in a new light. He
worked out the phenomena of nuclear division, as crystallized in
his aphorism "*Omnis nucleus e nucleo*"; and showed that protoplasm is a complex structure, made up of an active, contractile,
net-like material, and an inert, semifluid, inter-reticular substance,
which, from their behavior toward various stains, he called chromatin and achromatin, respectively. Histologists hold this to be
the most important work on the cell after Schwann's and Virchow's.

Many important discoveries and innovations in histology were made in
this period, such as Corti's investigations of the mammalian cochlea (rods of
Corti, 1851),[7] Virchow's discovery of the neuroglia (1854),[8] Wilhelm His' in-

---

[1] Schultze: Müller's Arch., Berlin, 1858, 343–381.

[2] Abhandl. d. naturf. Gesellsch. zu Halle, 1863, vii, 1–100.

[3] Zur Anatomie und Physiologie der Retina, Bonn, 1866.

[4] Arch. f. Anat., Physiol. u. wissensch. Med., Leipzig, 1861, 1–27.

[5] Das Protoplasma der Rhizopoden und der Pflanzenzellen, Leipzig, 1863.

[6] De ovorum ranarum segmentatione, Bonn, 1863.

[7] Corti: Ztschr. f. wissensch. Zoöl., Leipzig, 1851, iii, 109–169.

[8] Virchow: Arch. f. path. Anat., Berlin, 1854, vii, 135–138.

vestigations of the structure of the lymphatic glands (Leipzig, 1861) and
lymphatic vessels (1863), Willy Kühne's memoir on the peripheral end-organs
of the motor nerves (Leipzig, 1862), Deiters' memoir on the brain and spinal
cord in man and mammals (Brunswick, 1865), the islands of Langerhans (1869),[1]
Ranvier's investigations on the histology of the nervous system (nodes of
Ranvier, 1878), Ehrlich's investigations of the leukocytes (1880),[2] and his
intravital (methylene-blue) stain for nerve substance (1886),[3] and Camillo
Golgi's epoch-making work on the nervous system (1873–86).[4]   The third
elements of the blood, the so-called blood plaques or platelets, were first
noticed by Alexander Donné (1801–78)[5] in 1842, afterward by Max
Schultze, and more fully described by Sir William Osler (1873)[6] and Giulio
Bizzozero (1883).[7]

Toward the close of the nineteenth century, the storm center of histologic controversy was the **neuron theory,** the doctrine of the physiologic
autonomy of the nerve-cell and its branches.   The cell theory seemed adequate
to account for this as far as the nerve-cell itself was concerned, but the great
stumbling-block was the origin and true significance of the far more abundant
nerve-fibers, which had always been described as detached formations, separate
from the cells.   In 1850, Augustus Volney **Waller** (1816–70), of Faversham,
England, showed that if the glossopharyngeal and hypoglossal nerves be severed, the outer segment, containing the axis-cylinders cut off from the cells, will
undergo degeneration, while the central stump will remain relatively intact for
a long period of time.[8]   This "law of Wallerian degeneration" indicated that
the nerve-fibers are simply prolongations of the cells from which, as Waller
maintained, they receive their nourishment.   The classical researches of Deiters (1865)[9] showed that each nerve-cell has an axis-cylinder or nerve-fiber process growing from it, and a number of protoplasmic processes or dendrons, which
branch into dendrites, forming arborizations.   The material continuity of the
nerve-fibers with the terminal arborizations was demonstrated by Gerlach's
gold chloride stain in 1871, and later the use of carmine with Weigert's mordant
showed the continuity of the nerve-body with the axis-cylinder.   In 1883[10] Camillo **Golgi** (1844–   ), of Pavia, applied his silver nitrate stain of 1873[11] to the
central nervous system, and strikingly demonstrated the existence of multi-
polar nerve-cells, having long and short axis-cylinder processes (Golgi cells)
with the arborization of dendrites.   In 1886,[12] Wilhelm **His** showed how the
nerve-cell develops from a columnar epiblastic cell into a neuroblast by thrusting out a pseudopodium, which becomes the axis-cylinder, the polar pseudo-
podia remaining protoplasmic and becoming the dendrites.   Progress was now
rapid.   Forel, in 1887, confirmed the work of His on the pathologic side by
studying experimental degenerations.   A host of investigations by von Kölliker
(Switzerland), von Lenhossék (Hungary), the younger Retzius (Sweden), Van

---

[1] Paul Langerhans: Berlin dissertation, 1869.

[2] Ehrlich: Ztschr. f. klin. Med., Berlin, 1879–80, i, 553–560.

[3] Ehrlich: Deutsche med. Wochenschr., Leipzig and Berlin, 1886, xii, 49–52.

[4] Golgi: Sulla fina anatomia degli organi centrali del sistemo nervoso,
Milan, 1886.

[5] Donné: Compt. rend. Acad. d. sc., Paris, 1842, xiv, 366–368.

[6] Osler: Proc. Roy. Soc., London, 1873–74, xxii, 391–398

[7] Bizzozero: Di un nuovo elemento morfologico del sangue, Milan, 1883.

[8] Waller: Phil. Tr., London, 1850, 423–430.

[9] Otto F. C. Deiters: Untersuchungen über Gehirn und Rückenmark
(etc.), Brunswick, 1865.

[10] Golgi: Riv. sper. di freniat., Reggio-Emilia, 1882, viii, 165; 361: 1883,
ix, 1; 161; 385: 1885, xi, 72; 193.

[11] Golgi: Gazz. med. ital. lombard, Milano, 1873, 6. s., vi, 244–246, 1 pl.

[12] His: Abhandl. d. math.-phys. Kl. d. k. sächs. Akad. d. Wissensch., Leipzig, 1887, xiii, 477–513, 1 pl.

Gehuchten (Belgium), and the eminent Spanish histologist, Santiago **Ramon y Cajal** (1852–) greatly extended the knowledge of those terminal arborizations in the brain and cord, which Obersteiner likened to an espalier growth and Ramon y Cajal to the network of lianas and mosses in a tropical forest. Many new staining methods were introduced, in particular, that of Bethe, who made Ehrlich's intravital (methylene-blue) stain a permanent one by adding ammonium molybdate, and thus clearly demonstrated the continuity of the cell-body and axis-cylinder (1875).[1] The neurofibrillæ, which Max Schultze had seen in the electric lobe of the torpedo in 1872, were beautifully brought out in violet by the gold chloride stain of the Hungarian, S. Apáthy (1897),[2] who thought he saw them extending from one neuron into another. This was, however, confuted by the remarkable staining methods of Ramon y Cajal (1903), Bielschowsky (1903), and Donaggio (1905). Meanwhile the whole doctrine had been brought to a focus in the celebrated essay of Wilhelm **Waldeyer** (1891),[3] which affirmed that the nervous system is made up of epiblastic cells or neurons, each consisting of a cell-body with two sets of processes, an axon (axis-cylinder) having efferent (cellulifugal) functions and one or more dendrites with afferent (cellulipetal) functions. Upon these countless neurons the functional activity of the nervous system depends, the nerve-fibers being nowise independent, but axonic and dendritic outgrowths. In America, the whole subject was ably and critically expounded in the treatise of Lewellys F. Barker (1899),[4] who has dealt particularly with the controversies which raged down to the year 1904. Implicit in the neuron doctrine itself is the basic idea of the autonomy of its units, viz., that the branches of the neurons are contiguous, but not continuous, transmitting sensations and impulses by contact alone. But Gerlach believed that the *sensorium commune* is made up of a continuous network (*rete mirabile*); Apáthy, Held, and Bethe upheld the notion of a continuum of neurofibrillæ, Henson, the concept of a system of intercellular bridges, Nissl, the theory that the gray matter (*nervöse Grau*)[5] is the conducting medium, Held and Bethe that nerve-fibers can be formed by a fusion of certain cells (pluricellular doctrine). In battling over these views, many able investigators wandered away from actual facts into journalistic pettifogging. The conclusion of the whole matter was reached in a series of beautiful and convincing experiments by Ross Granville **Harrison** (1870–), who eventually demonstrated the ameboid outgrowth of the nerve-fibers from the cell in an extravital culture (1910).[6] Thus, by purely physical and chemical methods, the whole nervous system was finally brought under the cell doctrine of Schwann and Virchow.

By the close of the nineteenth century, **embryology** had become a highly complex science, its main developments being along such paths as the investigation of the origin of tissues, the morphology and pathology of the embryo as a whole, the significance of maturation and fertilization of the ovum, the tracing of cell lineage (cytogenesis), the study of embryology in the light of evolution (Recapitulation Theory), the structural relations of the placenta, and the beginnings of experimental embryology.

Highest among contemporary names, perhaps, stands that of

---

[1] Albrecht Bethe: Arch. f. mikr. Anat., Bonn, 1894–95, xliv, 579–622.

[2] Apáthy: Mitth. a. d. zoöl. Station zu Neapel, 1897, xii, 495–748.

[3] Waldeyer: Deutsche med. Wochenschr., Leipzig and Berlin, 1891, xvii, 1244; 1267; 1287; 1331; 1352.

[4] Barker: The Nervous System and its Constituent Neurons, New York, 1899.

[5] Franz Nissl: München. med. Wochenschr., 1898, xlv, 988; 1023; 1060.

[6] Harrison: J. Exper. Zoöl., Phila., 1910, ix, 784–846, 3 pl.

Wilhelm **His** (1831–1904), of Basel, Switzerland, who did the best work of his time on the origin of tissues and the serial and morphological study of the embryonic and adult organism. As Bichat dealt with the coarser aspects of tissues, Henle and Kölliker with their microscopic appearances in health, Virchow with the same in disease, so the name of His will always be associated with the science of their origins (histogenesis). His came of a distinguished Basel family, and apart from the advantages derived from his parentage, his education was of the very best, his teachers being Johannes Müller, Robert Remak, Virchow, and Kölliker. Professor of anatomy at Basel from 1857 to 1872, he was, through the influence

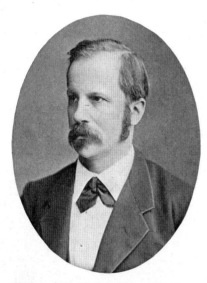

of Carl Ludwig, appointed in the latter year, to the same chair at Leipzig where he remained for the rest of his life. His earlier studies were on such themes as the normal and pathological histology of the cornea (1853–56), the structure of the thymus gland (1859–61), the histology of the lymphatic glands (1861) and the lymphatic vessels (1862–63), the latter illustrated with unrivaled plates. In 1865, he published his great academic program "On the Tissue-layers and Spaces of the Body,"[1] introducing a new classification of tissues as a guide in embryological research. It contains a sympathetic appreciation of Bichat, a defense of his classification as being related to the germ-layers, and points out that all the serous spaces arise in the mesoderm and are lined with the special membrane which His called endothelial. His monograph on the embryology of the chick appeared in 1868, and during 1880–85 his famous *Anatomie menschlicher Embryonen*, in which, from carefully selected specimens, the human embryo was studied as a whole for the first time. In 1886, His established, by embryological investigation, the fact that the axis-cylinder is a process of the nerve-cell. In 1900, he introduced his concepts of the lecithoblast and angioblast (the *Anlage* of the blood and capillaries). In the mean

Wilhelm His (1831–1904). (Courtesy of Miss Davina Waterson.)

---

[1] His: Die Häute und Höhlen des Körpers, Basel, 1865.

time, he had been approaching his subject from a larger angle. A beautiful draughtsman and a skilful photographer from boyhood up, his aim in teaching was to visualize everything to his pupils by means of microphotography, lantern-slides, models and his own unrivaled drawings, and he was able to utilize the advantages given him at Leipzig in a most remarkable way. In 1866, he invented a microtome which he gradually improved, and, from the serial sections so obtained, he conceived the idea of a graphic reconstruction of the embryo in two and three dimensions (1868), the former process being attained by means of the "embryo-graph" (his invention), the latter by the models of his assistant F. J. Steger, and afterward, by the device, invented by Born, of drawing the sections upon wax plates and setting them in juxta-position. These serial sections, all from the same embryo, soon obviated the errors made by comparing chance sections of embryos of different sizes and ages. The His-Steger models, now seen in all anatomical museums, are permanent memorials of his success in demonstrating morphological relations in three-dimensional space. This is especially true of his *Präparate zum Situs viscerum* (1878), which included models of the female pelvic viscera. In 1874, he published *Unsere Körperform*, which argues that the form of an organism is due to such mechanical effects as the migrations of cells, tissues and organs, although a mechanical causation of cell growth is denied. While not the same thing as developmental mechanics, this idea may be said to have led up to it. His was one of the founders of the Anatomische Gesellschaft and in 1895, he drew up its report on the revision of anatomical nomen-clature (B. N. A.) which, it is said, reduced current anatomical terms by about eighty per cent. This was presented in English dress by Lewellys F. Barker in 1907. In 1876, His founded the *Zeitschrift für Anatomie und Entwicklungsgeschichte*, which, in 1877, became merged into the old Müller-du Bois Reymond *Ar-chiv*, His and Braune editing the *Anatomische Abteilung* (1877–1903). The great Anatomisches Institut at Leipzig was constructed under the direction of His, and opened April 26, 1875. He was also one of the founders of the *Archiv für Anthropologie* (1876), and his interest in the subject is evidenced in the monograph on Swiss crania which he made with Rütimeyer in 1864, his studies of the Rhætian population (1864), of the skeletons belonging to Vesa-lius and Plater (1879), of the development of human and animal physiognomies (1892), and his identification of the remains of Johann Sebastian Bach (1895). The latter were found in a coffin in the yard of the old Johanniskirche and, by comparative measure-ments and averages taken from other cadavers, His enabled the sculptor Seffner to construct a bust in clay which was at once recognized as a counterfeit presentment of the great seventeenth century composer. Unlike his colleague Ludwig, His founded no school, believing that it is best for the student to go his own way and follow his own bent. His work on the anatomy of the human embryo has been carried forward to a unique conclusion by his pupils, Franz Keibel and Franklin P. Mall (1910–12).

The problem of the dynamics of the maturation, fertilization, and segmentation of the ovum, which had remained insoluble since Harvey's time, was worked out in the following way: In 1826[1], Prévost and Dumas first described the segmentation of the frog's egg. The mammalian ovum was discovered by von Baer in 1827, and was shown to be unicellular in every vertebrate by Gegenbaur in 1861. The spermatozoa, discovered by Hamen in 1677, were shown, in a filtration experiment of Spallanzani's, to be essential to fertilization (1786), and their cellular origin was demonstrated by Kölliker in 1841. In 1865, Schweigger-Seidel and La Valette St. George proved that the spermatozoön is a cell possessing a nucleus and cytoplasm.[2] Its union with the ovum was first observed (in the rabbit) by Martin Barry in 1843. Virchow clearly stated that the ovum is derived, in continuous line of descent, from preëxisting fertilized ova (1853). In 1875, Oscar **Hertwig** demonstrated that the spermatozoön enters the ovum and that fertilization is accomplished by the union of the male and female pronuclei so formed.[3] Huxley conceived that, "regarded as a mass of molecules, the entire organism may be compared to a web of which the warp is derived from the female and the woof from the male" (1878). The polar bodies, given off by the ripe ovum, were shown to be formed by division of its nucleus by Bütschli in 1875, and by Fol in 1876. In 1883, the splitting of chromosomes in the cell-nucleus (karyokinesis) was discovered by Flemming (1880); and in 1883, Van Beneden discovered that the associated male and female pronuclei in the fertilized egg each contain half as many chromosomes as the normal body cells in the same species. Weissmann believed that the object of this was to keep the number of chromosomes constant in the given species. In 1875, Flemming discovered a minute body in the ovum of the Anodon, usually lying outside the nucleus and often paired. This was discovered independently by Van Beneden in 1876, and was termed the centrosome by Boveri in 1888. The centrosome was soon found to be common to many other cells of the body and to unicellular organisms, and came to be regarded as the special organ of cell division, the "dynamic center" of the cell. Boveri supposed it to be the specific organ of fertilization in the spermatozoön, initiating mitosis by its own division, or, as Wilson once put it, "the web is to be sought in the chromatic substance of the nuclei," while "the centrosome is the weaver at the loom." While the latter point has not been entirely substantiated, the study of the reduction of the chromosomes has led to an exact comprehension of oögenesis and spermatogenesis (Oscar Hertwig, 1890), and latterly to the elucidation of the part they play in heredity and the determination of sex by McClung, Morgan, Wilson, Miss Stevens, and others.

The science of the germ-layers was founded by von Baer (1828–34) and Robert Remak (1845). In 1849, Huxley showed that the embryonic epiblast (ectoderm) and hypoblast (endoderm) can be assimilated to the two layers of cells which make up the body of the adult Hydra. This was regarded as a great advance at the time, but later investigation has shown that the developments from the germ-layers in different animals are by no means constant; that the mesoderm may originate from either ectoderm or endoderm, and that many organs can be traced back to certain predestined cells, rather than to cell-layers. Cell lineage or cytogenesis has therefore become a subject of ardent investiga-

---

[1] Prévost and Dumas: Ann. d. sc. nat., Paris, 1827, xii, 415–443.

[2] F. Schweigger-Seidel: Arch. f. mikr. Anat., Bonn, 1865, i, 309–335.

[3] O. Hertwig: Morph. Jahrb., Leipzig, 1875–6, i, 347–434, 4 pl.

tion, and, since the initial labors of Blochmann (1882), most of this work has been done in America. In such finely illustrated monographs as those of Charles Otis Whitman on the embryology of Clepsine (1878), Edmund B. Wilson on Nereis (1892), C. A. Kofoid on Limax (1895), Frank R. Lillie on the Unionidæ (1895), H. S. Jennings on Asplanchna (1896), W. E. Castle on Ciona (1896), and E. G. Conklin on Crepidula (1897), the germ layers have been traced out, cell by cell, from the beginning of segmentation, and it has been shown that there is nothing constant about the development of the mesoderm and its derivatives.

The net result of the vast amount of embryological investigation, up to the year 1881, was summed up in the master-work of Francis Maitland **Balfour** (1851–82), of Edinburgh, whose tragic death robbed science of one of its brightest, most attractive and most promising spirits. At Cambridge, Balfour came under the influence of Michael Foster, and from that master he acquired his interest in embryology, collaborating with him in the well-known Elements (1874) which was the standard text-book of its time in English and American schools. In 1873, Balfour went to study under Anton Dohrn at the Naples Zoölogical Station, and here he made an important research upon the embryology of Elasmobranch fishes,[1] which was particularly strong in regard to the early stages of the ovum and embryo, the development of the kidneys, and the origin of the spinal nerves. In the meantime, Balfour had been appointed fellow and lecturer on animal morphology at Cambridge, and was soon attracting large classes of enthusiastic pupils. In 1880–81, appeared his great *Treatise on Comparative Embryology*, which is not only indispensable as a digest of all that was known up to that time, but, as embodying the work of himself and pupils, is the most compact and lucid exposition of the science which has yet appeared. Foster describes it as brushing away many cobwebs and mooted points "with a firm but courteous sweep." In acknowledgment of the value of this work, Balfour was made professor of animal morphology at Cambridge in 1882, but he was not to enjoy the fruits of his labors. Taking up Alpine climbing to improve his health, he attempted, in July, 1882, to make an ascension of a virgin peak and was never seen alive again. His body and that of his guide were found at the bottom of a chasm a day later. Balfour was described by Foster as a keen, quick observer and logician, a high-minded, fascinating, and very able man. Had he lived, he would undoubtedly have been one of the topmost figures of modern science. Locy says that "the speculations contained in the papers of the rank and file of embryological workers for more than two decades, and often fondly believed to be novel, were for the most part anticipated by Balfour, and were also better expressed, with better qualifications."

---

[1] Balfour: Jour. Anat. and Physiol., London, 1876–78, *passim*.

The close resemblance between the early stages of the embryo in different animals had been noticed by Meckel and Oken. Von Baer is said to have admitted that he could not distinguish between three unlabeled embryos of a bird, a reptile and a mammal before him. Agassiz, in his "Essay on Classification" (1859), stated that the developmental phases of all living animals correspond to the morphological changes in their fossil successors throughout geological time. Fritz Müller, in 1863, showed that the larval stages of crustaceans can be interpreted as a recapitulation of the evolution of the race. Kovalevsky, in 1866, showed that the early stages of Amphioxus (the lowest vertebrate), and of the invertebrate order of Tunicata are identical. He also demonstrated that all animals pass through the so-called gastrula stage, which led Haeckel to his Gastræa Theory (1884), viz., that the two-layered gastrula is the analogue of the hypothetic ancestral form of all multicellular animals (gastræa). Haeckel's biogenetic law asserts that the developmental history of the individual (ontogeny) tends to recapitulate the developmental history of the racial type (phylogeny). The most critical and conservative statements of the Recapitulation Theory are those of von Baer and Balfour. Von Baer's "laws" assert that the resemblance of early embryonic stages in different vertebrates is limited to a certain short period at which the embryo in question not only differs, in special class features, from all other embryos, but has already begun to put on generic and specific characters of its own. Balfour pointed out that the recurrence of certain ancestral characters, such as the fish-like branchial clefts and the two-chambered heart in the frog, indicate that these "were functional in the larva of the creature after they ceased to have any importance in the adult." The De Vries theory, that species can originate by sudden jumps or mutations, has created a great spirit of antagonism to the old Darwinian idea of the slow gradual evolution of species through accidental variations, although it is perfectly possible that both processes may coexist in the scheme of nature. In any case, the recapitulation doctrine is now regarded as a mere literary analogy or formal interpretation, as something read into the facts of comparative embryology by human prepossessions. Concerning the hypothetical family tree of the vertebrata through the Amphioxus, the Annelida, the worms of Sagitta type, the spiders, Limulus and the Echinoderms, Driesch quotes the scathing remark of du Bois Reymond that "phylogeny of this sort is of about as much scientific value as are the pedigrees of the heroes of Homer."

Among the important embryological researches of the century may be mentioned Wilhelm Waldeyer's studies on the ovary and ovum, including his discovery of the germinal epithelium (1870), Édouard Van Beneden on the early development of the mammalian ovum (1875) and the history of the germinal vesicle and embryonic nucleus (1876), the work of Alexander Agassiz (1835–1910) on the Echinoderms (1872–83) and the Ctenophora; the discovery of the atrio-ventricular bundle of the heart by Wilhelm His, Jr. (1893), Johannes Sobotta on the formation of the corpus luteum (1896), and Alfred Schaper on the earliest phases of differentiation in the central nervous system (1897).

Of Americans, William Keith **Brooks** (1848–1908), of Cleveland, Ohio, professor at the Johns Hopkins University (1876–1908), is memorable for his monographs on the oyster (1891), the genus Salpa (1893), which corrected the earlier views entertained as to its "alternation of generations," the Stomatopoda of the Challenger expedition, the genera Lucifer and Macrura, and his books on Pangenesis (1877), Heredity (1883) and The Foundations of Zoölogy (1899). He founded the Chesapeake Zoölogical Laboratory (1878), and was a fascinating, inspiring teacher, especially through his unusually beautiful drawings.

Charles Otis **Whitman** (1842–1910), of Woodstock, Maine, professor of zoölogy in the University of Chicago (1892), founded the *Journal of Morphology* (1887) and the *Biological Bulletin* (1899), and is memorable for his papers on the embryology of Clepsine (1878) and the inadequacy of the cell theory of development (1895).

Franklin Paine **Mall** (1862–   ), of Belle Plaine, Iowa, professor of anatomy at the Johns Hopkins University, a pupil of His and Carl Ludwig, did good work on the physiology of the circulation under the latter, and is known for his important investigations on monsters, the pathology of early human embryos (1899–1908), and the structural unit of the liver (1905). He collaborated with Franz Keibel in the valuable *Manual of Human Embryology* (1910–12), the best modern work of its kind.

Charles Sedgwick **Minot** (1852–   ), of West Roxbury, Massachusetts, professor of embryology and comparative anatomy at Harvard University, is the author of an important treatise on Human Embryology (1892), which introduced many novel theories, also of a Bibliography of Vertebrate Embryology (1893), and a Laboratory Text-book of Embryology (1903). He invented two different kinds of automatic microtomes, and is widely known for his original investigations, particularly those on the origin and structure of the placenta (1891). His "Age, Growth, and Death" (1908) states the "law of cytomorphosis," in virtue of which these processes result from the steady change of protoplasm into more highly differentiated forms.

Experimental embryology is a branch of experimental morphology or developmental mechanics (*Entwicklungsmechanik*), a phrase introduced by Wilhelm **Roux** (1850–   ) of Halle, who may be regarded as the founder of the science. Roux was a pupil of Virchow and Haeckel, and his bent was already shown in his graduating dissertation (Jena, 1878), which dealt with the hydrodynamic conditions governing the formation of the lumina of branching blood-vessels. In 1894, he founded the *Archiv für Entwicklungsmechanik*, the principal organ of his science to date. Most of the early work in experimental embryology was done upon the frog's egg, as being the easiest to obtain. The first step was taken by the physiologist Eduard **Pflüger** (1829–1910), who, in 1882–83, made a number of experiments on cross-fertilization with different species of the frog. In 1883, Pflüger made a series of still more important experiments upon the effect of gravity upon the development of the egg, showing that the initial planes of cleavage will be vertical and the development normal, no matter how the egg is placed. In 1884, Born showed that gravity brings about a slow rearrangement of the contents of a rotated egg, according to their specific gravity. In the same year, Roux demonstrated that eggs whirled in a centrifugal machine do not differ in development from the normal controls. Pflüger, in 1884, showed that compression of the unsegmented egg between two planes of glass modifies the planes of cleavage according to the direction of pressure. Later, in 1892, Hans **Driesch** (1867–   ) showed that continued pressure applied to an Echinus egg can produce a flat plate of 16 or 32 cells, which will proceed to normal development in three dimensions, directly the pressure is removed. In 1888, Roux published his celebrated experiment of killing one of the two initial blastomeres with a hot needle, producing a typical half-embryo. This led to the Roux-Weissmann hypothesis of mosaic or qualitative development, which assumes that the center of formative changes is the complex structure of the nucleus, the sifting of the differential characters in the daughter cells being purely qualitative. Driesch, however, found, in 1891, that if the two blastomeres could be separated and set free by shaking, the segmentation in each would go on unilaterally up to the blastula stage, after which the open side of the latter would close over, resulting in a fully developed but small-sized embryo. Thomas Hunt **Morgan** (1866–   ), by rotating the surviving blastomere in Roux's hot-needle experiment, so that the white pole was turned upward, produced a whole embryo of half size (1894), showing that the completed development was due to a rearrangement of the contents; and Schultze, in 1894, produced double monsters by inverting a fertilized frog's egg between two glass plates, so that the dark pole of the egg came uppermost. In 1895, Driesch and Morgan, by cutting off a piece of the protoplasm of a ctenophore egg, prior to segmentation, without damaging the nucleus, produced the same half-embryo which ordinarily results from isolating the blastomeres of this egg. In 1889, Boveri had succeeded in fertilizing a non-nucleated piece of sea-urchin egg with the sperm of another species. All this indicated that the protoplasm, rather than the nucleus, is the principal agent in the production and regulation of form (morphogenesis). Herbst pointed out (1894–1901) that the formative and directive stimuli are usually external in plants and internal in animals. From a number of facts of this order, including the many novel experiments upon regeneration in adult marine hydroids by Loeb, Morgan, Miss Bickford, and others, Driesch was led to formulate his quantitative theory of cell-division, viz., that the "prospective value" of any embryonic cell is simply a function of its location; and that protoplasm is a "polar bilateral structure," capable of regulating its development symmetrically in any of the three dimensions of space, also a "harmonious equipotential system," having the same potency for development in all its parts. From the totipotency of protoplasm, Driesch argued that its functions can never be explained mechanically, since a machine, the smallest part of which is identical in structure and functional capacity with the whole machine itself, is unthinkable. The same sharp distinction which is made in mechanics and patent law between a "tool" and a "machine" is, therefore, to be observed between a machine and a living organism or substance, since the former is always a clumsy imitation of the latter, and never *vice versâ*. If this point were constantly observed by biologists, the superfine vitalism of Driesch would soon dwindle into a truism, for the eminent morphologist has latterly invoked, as a substitute for the medieval vital principles, the old Aristotelian "entelechies," which is again, only a *petitio principii*. Driesch has given up experimentation to philosophize in the Cloud-Cuckoo-Land of "harmonious equipotential systems," but his quantitative theory of the development of the ovum had the advantage of being identical with the "epigenesis" of Wolff and von Baer, while Roux's "mosaic theory" is only a modified form of the old "preformation" hypothesis of Bonnet and Haller. Roux, having become enmeshed in these difficulties, devoted a great deal of labor to the task of extricating himself by means of "sage provisos, sub-intents and saving clauses." Thus, two of the ablest experimental morphologists of recent times have lapsed into scientific inactivity through the effect of their own theories.

The masters of **physiology** in the second half of the nineteenth century were Helmholtz, Claude Bernard, and Carl Ludwig. In the second rank come du Bois Reymond, Brücke, Goltz, Pflüger, Brown-Séquard, and, among the physiological chemists, Willy Kühne, Hoppe-Seyler, and Kossel. About the middle of the century, the physical principles of the Conservation, Transformation, and Dissipation of Energy came into prominence, and we may begin with the great mathematician and physician who made these an essential part of physiological theory.

Hermann **von Helmholtz** (1821–94), of Potsdam, was of mingled German, English, and French extraction, and was educated as a surgeon for the Prussian army. At the University of Berlin, he came under Johannes Müller and Gustav Magnus, and met such younger men as Virchow, du Bois Reymond, Brücke, Kirchhoff and Clausius. His inaugural dissertation dealt with the origin of nerve-fibers from cells in the ganglia of leeches and crabs, which he had observed with a rudimentary compound microscope (1842). During his barrack life at Potsdam he published his essay, *Ueber die Erhaltung der Kraft* (1847), which established his reputation, although, at first, appreciated only by the mathematician Jacobi. In 1849, Helmholtz was appointed professor of physiology and pathology at Königsberg, subsequently occupying the chairs of anatomy and physiology at Bonn (1855–58), physiology at Heidelberg (1858–71), and physics at Berlin (1871–94).

The essay on the Conservation of Energy established the first law of thermodynamics, viz., that all modes of energy, as heat, light, electricity and all chemical phenomena, are capable of transformation from one to the other but otherwise indestructible and impossible of creation. This had actually been demonstrated for physiological processes by the Heilbronn physician, Robert Mayer, and, for physical phenomena, by James Prescot Joule, in 1842, but Helmholtz gave it universal application. During the years 1850–52, Clausius and Lord Kelvin established the second law of thermodynamics, which asserts that energy, in all its modes, is continually flowing or tending to flow from states of concentration to phases of dissipation and never otherwise. This was applied to all physical and chemical phenomena by one of Helmholtz's pupils, the Yale professor, Willard Gibbs (1872–78), of whose work Helmholtz wrote an appreciative study in 1882. That the muscles are the main source of animal heat was demonstrated by Helmholtz in isolated preparations in 1848,[1] and, in 1850–52,[2] he measured the velocity of the nervous impulse with the pendulum-myograph of his invention. His invention of the ophthalmoscope, in

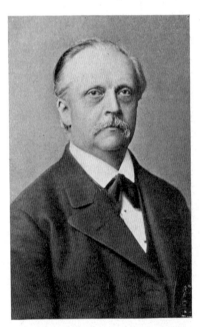

1851,[3] made ophthalmology an exact science, and it was followed by his phakoscope and ophthalmometer (1852). With the latter, he was able to determine the optical constants and explain the mechanism of accommodation (1854), particularly the part played by the lens. His great Handbook of Physiological Optics (1856–67) is a permanent classic, containing his revival of the Young theory of color vision, which he regarded as a special case of Müller's law of specific nerve energies. The *Tonempfindungen* (1863) shows the same wonderful sweep and mastery, revealing, at the same time, the accomplished musician. Never has the subject of acoustics been so exhaustively dealt with, except, perhaps, in Lord Rayleigh's treatise. Among other things which cannot be recorded here, Helmholtz also made an important study of the mechanism of the tympanum and ossicles of the middle ear (1869), which did much to elucidate the phenomenon of audition. After assuming the chair of physics at Berlin and becoming director of the Physico-Technical Institute at Charlottenburg in 1887, he devoted the rest of his life to the field in which his true genius lay and in which he was

Hermann von Helmholtz (1821–94).

only equaled, in modern times, by such men as Clerk Maxwell and Lord Kelvin. In mathematical physics, Helmholtz made contributions of the first rank to the principles of dynamics, hydrodynamics, thermodynamics, and electrodynamics. He investigated the spin or vortex motion of an ideal, frictionless fluid (1858–73), he introduced the idea of the convection of electricity by moving material systems and, in his Faraday lecture of 1881, stated his belief that the chemical atoms are, in their ultimate nature, electric. Independently of Gibbs, he defined the "free (available) energy" of a chemical system as the difference between its total

---

[1] Arch. f. Anat., Physiol. u. wissensch. Med., Berlin, 1848, 144–164.

[2] *Ibid.*, 1850, 71; 276: 1852, 199.

[3] Beschreibung eines Augen-Spiegels zur Untersuchung der Netzhaut im lebenden Auge, Berlin, 1851.

(intrinsic) energy and its molecular (unavailable) energy; and he was the first to introduce the idea that the "hidden motions" of material bodies are those of cyclic systems with reversible circular motions (as in the gyroscope or the governor of a steam-engine), in other words, rotational stresses in the ether or "whirls of energy." The Gibbs-Helmholtz equation, which asserts that the electromotive force of a galvanic cell (the actual work it can do) is equal to its free energy per electro-chemical equivalent of decomposition, is now one of the basic principles of physical and physiological chemistry, containing, as Nernst says, "all that the laws of thermodynamics can teach concerning chemical processes." It was in Helmholtz's laboratory that Rowland investigated the properties of a moving body charged with electricity, so important in colloidal chemistry, and that Hertz discovered the electric (Hertzian) waves, which led to wireless telegraphy.

Yet, although he stood at the summit of the highest department of human thought, Helmholtz never forgot that he was a physician. "Medicine," he said, with pride, "was once the intellectual home in which I grew up; and even the emigrant best understands and is best understood by his native land." He even made a little contribution to medical practice, the application of quinine sulphate to the nasal mucous membrane in hay-fever (1869).[1] As a lecturer on "popular science," Helmholtz was approached only by Huxley, Tyndall, and Ernst Mach. His writings in this field have an elevation and dignity, a genial command of vast resources which is peculiarly his own. In them one senses the personal nobility of the scientific gentleman. Helmholtz was of middle height, a man of extremely serious, dignified manner, his head of Goethean proportions, with fine, earnest eyes. With the sincere, he was absolutely sincere and helpful. With shallow or trivial persons, he was apt to invest himself with "the subtle ether of potential disapprobation," which, as some have testified, made them feel as if they were dealing with the fourth dimension of space. He had the northern tendency toward the impersonal, and this was manifested even in his attitude toward religion. As to his ultimate views of the great questions of life, death, and immortality, Helmholtz was inscrutable and gave no sign. And, in this regard, his impersonal contributions to mathematical and physiological science are a true expression of his strong and dignified character.

Emil **du Bois Reymond** (1818–96), of Berlin, the founder of modern **electrophysiology,** was of French extraction, and he wrote in German with the clarity and precision commonly associated with the French language and literature. Like Helmholtz, he was one of Johannes Müller's pupils, and succeeded the latter as professor of physiology at Berlin in 1858, holding the chair for the rest of his life. Here he added a new luster to the Berlin Faculty, turning out many fine pupils, and supervising the construction of the palatial Physiological Institute (opened November 6, 1877), the best equipped laboratory of its kind in the world. The studies of

---

[1] Ueber das Heufieber, Arch. f. path. Anat., Berlin, 1869, xlvi, 100–102.

du Bois Reymond relate almost entirely to the physiology of those muscle-nerve preparations which he did so much to introduce into laboratory experimentation, and his numerous investigations were twice printed in collective form, in 1848–60 and 1883. After the discovery of muscular electricity by Galvani, and of physiological tetanus by Volta, in 1792, there was little done in electrophysiology beyond the introduction of the astatic galvanometer by Leopoldo Nobili (1784–1834), of Florence (1825); and the brief investigations of Carlo Matteucci (1811–68), who introduced the word "tetanize" (1838), and of Stefano Marianini (1790–1866). Du Bois Reymond introduced faradic stimulation by means of the interrupted (make-and-break) current from the special induction coil which is called after him (1849), made a thoroughgoing investigation of physiological tetanus, and was the first to describe and define electrotonus (1843), representing both conditions graphically by means of algebraic curves.

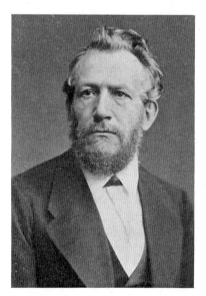

In 1843, he discovered that there is a difference of potential between the cut end of an excised muscle or nerve and the uninjured end, producing a current which can be demonstrated with a galvanometer, by closing the circuit. He wrongly inferred that this difference of potential exists in normal uncut muscle, but Hermann has since shown that it is due to chemical changes in an injured end. Since du Bois Reymond's time, a tetanic condition of injured or uninjured muscle has been regarded as the summation of individual responses evoked by rapidly succeeding stimuli. He showed that tetanized muscle yields an acid, resting muscle a neutral, reaction; that stimulation with a constant current has no effect upon nerve, and stated the "law of stimulation," in virtue of which the excitation of nerve depends, not upon the intensity of the current, but upon the rapidity of its variation or upon maximum variations in unit time. He believed that the "currents of rest" and other electric phenomena which he found in muscle, nerve and the glands, were due to electromotive molecules of prismatic form, arranged in series end to end, unbroken circuits being maintained by the fact that these tissues are all moist conductors. He applied the same reasoning to the organs of electric fishes, which he was the first to study in detail, and he summed up his view by stating that electrophysiological stimulation is merely a phase of electrolysis.

Emil du Bois Reymond (1818–96).

During his long life, du Bois Reymond wrote many fascinating essays and many fine biographical memoirs, in particular, his scien-

31

tific studies of the French materialists, Voltaire, La Mettrie, Diderot, Maupertuis; and of Johannes Müller and Helmholtz, the latter being the standard sources of information in regard to their achievements. These lectures are written with great verve and *esprit*, displaying wide culture, but are more loaded with erudition than those of Helmholtz. Two have attracted especial attention— those on the Limits of Natural Science (1872) and the "Seven World-Riddles" (1880), in which their author professes a rigid denial of final causes in regard to such problems as the nature of force and matter, the origin of motion, the origin of life, the purposeful character of natural phenomena, the origin of sensation, thought and speech, and the freedom of the will, summing up his view in the oft-quoted phrases, *Ignorabimus, Dubitemus*. In person, du Bois Reymond was a man of middle height, of ruddy countenance and energetic features, strong and athletic, with fiery glance and lively gestures. He left two sons, both of whom became well-known physicians.

The example of Helmholtz and du Bois Reymond gave an added interest to the study of the **physiology of muscle and nerve,** and the special advance that was made was in the introduction of new instrumental procedures. Many of these, such as the cosine lever, the myotonograph, and the improved thermopile, were introduced by Adolf **Fick** (1829–1901), of Cassel, a pupil of Ludwig's, who wrote two important works on medical physics (1856)[1] and on mechanical work and heat-production during muscular activity (1882).[2] The method of obtaining myograms, introduced by Helmholtz, was vastly improved by Étienne-Jules **Marey** (1830–1904), of Paris, who showed that, in order to avoid the errors from inertia and other causes, it is best to have a very light writing style for the tambour. Investigation was also materially aided by such instruments as d'Arsonval's galvanometer, Lippmann's capillary electrometer, Bernstein's differential rheotome (1890), and Mosso's ergograph (1890),[3] for the study of voluntary muscular contractions in man. Photography was effectively employed by Sir John **Burdon Sanderson** (1828–1905) and by Julius **Bernstein** (1839–   ) in measuring the time relations of the period of latent stimulation of muscle, which they reduced from the figures Helmholtz gave to about 0.0035".[4] Bernstein, one of du Bois Reymond's best pupils, has also done important work upon the thermodynamics of muscular contraction (1902–08). Willy Kühne proved that muscle plasma is coagulable (1859) and fluid within the living fiber (1863). Ludimar Hermann investigated muscular metabolism (1867), showing that there is increased elimination of CO_2 upon contraction. Angelo **Mosso** (1846–   ), of Turin, investigated muscular fatigue with the ergograph (1890–91),[5] and, by injection experiments with the blood of a fatigued animal, indicated that fatigue is due to a toxic product of muscular contraction (1890).[6] Auguste **Chauveau** (1827–   ) investigated the heat and

---

[1] Fick: Die medizinische Physik, Braunschweig, 1856.

[2] Fick: Mechanische Arbeit und Wärmeentwicklung bei der Muskelthätigkeit, Leipzig, 1882.

[3] Mosso: Arch. ital. de biol., Turin, 1890, xiii, 124–141.

[4] Sanderson: Jour. Physiol., London, 1895, xviii, 146. Bernstein: Arch. f. d. ges Physiol., Bonn, 1897, lxvii, 207.

[5] Mosso: La fatica, Milan, 1891.

[6] Tr. Internat. Med. Cong., 1890, Berlin, 1891, ii, 2. Abth., 13.

energy relations of muscular work (1891), and Theodor Wilhelm **Engelmann** (1843–   ), the mechanics and thermodynamics of muscular contraction, illustrating his theory by an artificial muscle made of a violin-string. Some of the best work on muscle was done in Carl Ludwig's laboratory, in particular, H. P. Bowditch's demonstration of the staircase phenomenon (*Treppe*) in smooth (heart) muscle (1871),[1] von Kries upon the effect of tension upon the response of muscle to stimuli (1880), and the work of Kronecker.

Hugo **Kronecker** (1839–   ), of Liegnitz, Silesia, a pupil of Helmholtz, Wundt, Kühne, Traube and Ludwig, and professor of physiology at Bern (1885), has especially distinguished himself by his work on fatigue and recovery of striped muscle (1871),[2] his proof that heart muscle cannot be tetanized (1874),[3] his investigation of the mechanism of deglutition (with S. J. Meltzer, 1883), his inventions of the phrenograph, the thermo-esthesiometer and a perfusion-cannula, his studies of reflex action, animal heat, innervation of respiration, and many other things of importance. The classic experiments of Bowditch and Kronecker on heart-muscle have led to the principle that the heart's motto is "all or none," *i. e.*, no matter what the stimulus, it will either contract to the fullest extent possible or not at all.

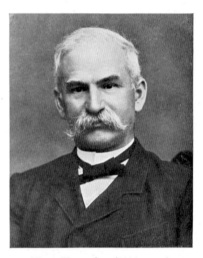

Hugo Kronecker (1839–   ).

The **mechanics of locomotion** was first investigated by the Weber brothers (1836), later by Samuel Haughton (1873), and along rigid mathematical lines by Christian Wilhelm Braune and Otto Fischer (1891–95). The idea of investigating locomotion by serial (cinematographic) pictures was first suggested by the astronomer Janssen, who observed the transit of Venus in this way (1878). The method was perfected and utilized by E. A. Marey (*Le mouvement*, 1894), and by Eadweard Muybridge in his atlases of animals and of the nude human figure in motion (1899–1901).

After du Bois Reymond, the most interesting investigations upon the **physiology of nerve** were the discovery of the inhibitory power of the vagus nerve by the Weber brothers (1845); Helmholtz's measurement of the velocity of the nerve current (1850–52), which was avowedly suggested by du Bois Reymond's work; Eduard Pflüger's monograph on electrotonus (1859), in which he first stated the famous laws governing the make and break stimulation of

---

[1] Bowditch: Ber. d. k. Sächs. Gesellsch. d. Wissensch., Leipzig, 1871, xxiii, 652–689.

[2] Kronecker: Arb. a. d. physiol. Anst. zu Leipzig, 1871, 177–266.

[3] Kronecker: Ludwig Festschrift, Leipzig, 1874, pt. 1, pp. clxxiii–cciv.

nerve with the galvanic current; the Ritter-Rollet phenomenon (1876); the studies of mechanical irritation of nerve by Rudolf Heidenhain (1858), Robert Tigerstedt (1880), and von Uexküll ("nerve-shaker," 1895); Paul Grützner on the effect of chemical stimulation (1893); the investigations of Magnus Blix upon the specific energies of the cutaneous nerves (1884–85), of Alfred Goldscheider upon the temperature nerves (1884–85), and of Henry Head upon the effects of injury and section of peripheral nerves (1905–08).

One of the most important experiments was the demonstration of the indefatigability of nerve (1890)[1] by Henry Pickering **Bowditch** (1840–1911), of Boston, Massachusetts, who founded the first physiological laboratory in the United States (1871), made the first investigation of the *Treppe* in heart muscle (1871) and did important work upon reënforcement of the knee-jerk

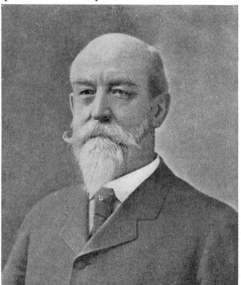

Henry Pickering Bowditch (1840–1911).

(1890). Bowditch's proof that nerve cannot be tired out was accomplished by paralyzing the motor nerve-endings in the muscle, to eliminate the latter, and stimulating the nerve at intervals, under artificial respiration, until the effect of the drug wore off, when it was seen, from the muscular twitchings, that, in spite of the prolonged excitation, the nerve had responded and still responded to the stimulus. Bernstein (1877) and Wedensky (1884) varied the experiment by blocking off the nerve from the muscle by means of a galvanic current (Wedensky effect),[2] and

---

[1] Bowditch: Arch. f. Physiol., Leipzig, 1890, 505–508.

[2] Wedensky: Centralbl. f. d. med. Wissensch., Berlin, 1884, xxii, 65–68.

Maschek, in 1887, blocked the nerve by local application of ether vapor to a part between the stimulated region and the muscle, the nerve still responding after twelve hours' excitation. Thus the initial experiment of Bowditch led in time to the idea of anesthetic blocking of the nerve-trunks by Crile and Cushing, which is one of the fundamental principles of recent surgery.

The whole subject of muscle-nerve preparations was exhaustively treated in the *Electrophysiologie* (1895) of Wilhelm Biedermann (1854–   ), and du Bois Reymond's studies upon electrical fishes were continued by Gustav Theodor Fritsch (1887–90), Karl Schönlein, and the late Francis Gotch (1887–95). The chemical side of nervous activity has been investigated by William D. Halliburton (London, 1901), A. B. Macallum, and Menten (1906).

The starting-point of the neuron theory was the epoch-making experiment of Augustus Volney **Waller** (1816–70), of Elverton Farm, Kent. He showed that when a nerve is cut, the distal stump (the axis-cylinders, severed from the nerve-cells) will soon degenerate, while the proximal stump remains relatively intact (1850), from which he inferred that the nerve-cells nourish the nerve-fibers. By the same method, Waller showed that, if an anterior spinal nerve-root is severed, the degenerative changes indicate that the nutritive centers of the motor fibers must lie in the spinal cord, while, in the case of section of the posterior (sensory) roots, they are seen to lie in the posterior root ganglia. These experiments won for Waller the Montyon Prize of the French Academy of Sciences (2000 francs) in 1856, and they have been repeatedly confirmed by the observations of the histologists who worked on the neuron theory. Some important observations on old amputations, made by the late William Howship Dickinson (1832–1913), of Brighton, England, in 1865, demonstrated that the proximal stump of a severed nerve eventually undergoes atrophy.[1]

The theory that the functions of the brain can be localized in the cerebral cortex was introduced in somewhat fantastic form by Franz Joseph **Gall** (1757–1828) as organology or cranioscopy, and by his pupil, Johann Caspar **Spurzheim** (1776–1832), as phrenology, their joint researches appearing as a four-volume treatise, with atlas, in 1810–19.[2] This contained many really important additions to cerebral anatomy and also the theory that the brain is a bundle of some twenty-seven (later 37) separate "organs," presiding over the different moral, sexual and intellectual traits of the individual, their size being proportional to the preponderance of these traits and manifested on the surface of the skull as protuberances. Gall's theory drove him out of Vienna, but two medals were struck off in his honor in Berlin, and, like Hahnemann, he died rich in Paris. Spurzheim's propagandism led to the formation of secret phrenological societies and phrenological journals in Great Britain and the United States. The theory attracted the favorable notice of Goethe, who shrewdly

---

[1] Dickinson: Jour. Anat. & Physiol., London, 1869, iii, 88–96, 1 pl.

[2] Gall and Spurzheim: Anatomie et physiologie du système nerveux, Paris, 1810–19.

pointed out that the secret of its hold upon the popular mind lay in the fact that it dealt with particulars rather than general propositions; in other words, the folk-mind, even in fashionable people, was not unnaturally preoccupied with the various cranial "bumps" which located the specific amativeness, combativeness, philoprogenitiveness, etc., of the person in question. Exploited by quacks and charlatans, phrenology soon became an object of derision among scientific men.

The first real advance, after the experiments of Flourens and Legallois, was also the most important one, viz., the work of Gustav **Fritsch** (1838–91) and Eduard **Hitzig** (1838–　　), establishing the electric excitability of the brain (1870),[1] which had been doubted since the time of Flourens. Motor aphasia from injuries or lesions in the region of the third left frontal (Broca's) convolution had, indeed, been established by Bouillaud (1825) and Broca (1861), and localized, epileptiform spasms from definite cerebral lesions had been described by Richard Bright (1836) and Hughlings Jackson (1875); but the experiments of Fritsch and Hitzig upon the dog's brain were the first to show that local bodily movements and convulsions can be produced by stimulation of definite areas in the brain, always identical in different animals of the same species, and that, *per contra*, removal of these areas will produce paralysis or loss of function of the corresponding parts of the body. These observations were verified and greatly extended by the work of Sir David **Ferrier** (1843–　　), upon mammals, birds, frogs, fishes, and other creatures (1872–76)[2]; and the later observations of Horsley and Schäfer (1884–88) and Beevor and Horsley (1887–94) have tended to confirm Ferrier's inference that the motor area of the cerebral cortex is around the central sulcus of Rolando. The special motor and sensory, as well as the "silent" or inexcitable, areas were mapped out by the labors of Flechsig (1876), Munk (1877–89), Bechtereff (1887), François Franck (1887), Gudden (collected in 1889), Henschen (1890–94), and Monakow (1891–92), while the subject was most carefully considered on the clinical and pathologic side by Charcot and Pitres (1895).

The subject of the total functions of the cerebral hemispheres and the spinal cord will always be associated with the name of Friedrich Leopold **Goltz** (1834–1902), of Posen, one of Helmholtz's pupils, who became professor of physiology at Halle (1870–72) and Strassburg (1872–1902). Goltz did important work upon cardiac pressure and the mechanism of shock (*Klopfversuch*, 1862),[3] and the functions of the semicircular canals (1870), but his most

---

[1] Fritsch and Hitzig: Arch. f. Anat., Physiol. u. wissensch. Med., Berlin, 1870, 300–332.

[2] Ferrier: West Riding Lun. Asyl. Rep., London, 1872, iii. Functions of the Brain, London, 1876.

[3] Goltz: Königsb. med. Jahrb., 1862, iii, 271–274.

telling experiments were those upon the effect of excision of the brain and spinal cord in the frog (1869–72)[1] and the dog (1874–96).[2] He showed how the decerebrated or "spinal" frog will hop, swim, jump out of boiling water, croak like the frogs in Aristophanes, and adjust itself mechanically to every stimulation, but will otherwise sit like a mummy and, though surrounded with food, die of starvation, because it is a spinal machine, devoid of volition, memory, or intelligence; how, if the optic thalami remain intact, the animal will show some intelligence in regard to its own nutrition and sexual instinct, and how ablation of the cerebral hemispheres in the dog is followed by restless movements, unintelligent response to stimuli, and inability to feed itself or to swallow. Similar experiments had already been made upon fish, pigeons, and smaller mammals by Rolando, Flourens, Longet, and Vulpian, but no one ever described the phenomena so carefully and graphically as Goltz, who brought out the important fact that the effects of decerebration are the more profound, the higher the animal, as evidenced by amentia in man. The other experiment (excising the spinal cord) had to be performed with the greatest delicacy and care if the animal was to live;

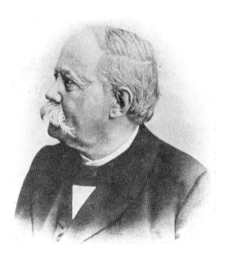

Friedrich Leopold Goltz (1834–1902).

and Goltz's data showed that, under these conditions, the muscles supplied by spinal nerves are totally paralyzed, with a complete loss of sensation in the corresponding parts, the viscera and blood-vessels lose their tone, the power of adaptability to temperature and other environmental changes is lessened, and perspiration abolished, although pregnancy, labor, and lactation can occur. Goltz's exposition of the "spinal" animal as a brainless mechanism which, in Bernard Shaw's phrase, "blunders into death," and of the animal deprived of its spinal cord as a conscious intelligence

---

[1] Goltz: Beiträge zur Lehre von den Functionen der Nervencentren des Frosches, Berlin, 1869; and Arch. f. d. ges. Physiol., Bonn, 1872, v, 53.

[2] Goltz: *Ibid.*, 1874, viii, 460; 1892, li, 460; 1896, lxiii, 362.

with lessened power of coördination and adaptation, initiated much of the work of recent times upon the complex reflexes of the body.

While du Verney had successfully excised the cerebrum and cerebellum (1697), the earliest investigation of the cerebellar functions was Rolando's *Saggio* of 1809. This was followed by Flourens' classical experiments on the pigeon (1822) and those of Luciani upon the dog (1882–91), which brought out the ataxic incoördination. Experimental excisions of fractional parts were made by a host of observers, from Rolando and Magendie on. Rolando likened the cerebellum to the Voltaic pile, in that it augments and reënforces the voluntary movements initiated by the cerebrum, a view which was reiterated and emphasized by Weir Mitchell (1869). Flourens introduced the idea of nervous coördination, which was again emphasized by John Call Dalton (1861). Hughlings Jackson regarded the cerebellum as the center for continuous movements, the cerebrum as the center for changing movements. The effect of excision of the medulla oblongata and pons Varolii was investigated by Schrader (1887). Robert Whytt found that removal of the anterior part of the corpora quadrigemina abolishes reflex contraction of the pupil to light (1768), Ivan Michailovich Setchenoff thought it contained an inhibitory center for the spinal reflexes (1863), and Charles S. Sherrington showed that a condition of "decerebrate rigidity" obtains upon complete transection (1896–97). The relation of the optic thalamus to opposite-sided sensation, especially in the eye, was noted simultaneously by Panizza and Joseph Swan (1856), and brought out, on the clinical and pathologic side, in an important postmortem by Hughlings Jackson (1875).[1] The sympathetic system was investigated by Friedrich Wilhelm Bidder (1810–94) and Alfred Wilhelm Volkmann (1800–77), who showed that it is largely made up of small, medullated fibers originating from the sympathetic and spinal ganglia (1842)[2]; by Claude Bernard, Brown-Séquard, Waller, and Budge, who demonstrated the effect of section and stimulation of the cervical sympathetic (1852–53); by Kölliker (1889) and other modern histologists, who studied the structure of sympathetic cells by improved staining methods; by W. H. Gaskell, who studied visceral and vascular innervation (1886); by J. N. Langley, who studied reflexes from sympathetic ganglia (1894)[3] and defined the "autonomic system" (1900); and latterly by Henry Head. Of special nerves, the vagus was investigated by the Webers (1845), Schmiedeberg (1871) and Gaskell (1882), the nerves of the heart and chorda tympani by Carl Ludwig, the vasoconstrictors and vasodilators by Claude Bernard (1858), the dilator nerves of the peripheral vessels by Carl Ludwig (1866), the intestinal plexuses by Auerbach and Meissner (1862), the secretory and trophic nerves of glands by Heidenhain (1878), the temperature nerves (1884) and nerves of cutaneous sensation (1885) by Alfred Goldscheider, the distributory fibers of the cranial nerve by Vulpian (1885), the erector mechanism by Eckhard (1863) and Gaskell (1887), the end-organ of the eighth nerve by Julius Ewald (1892), the pilomotor nerves by J. N. Langley (1893), and the nerve-endings for painful sensations by Max von Frey (1896).

The modern concept of **reflex action** was an outgrowth of the cell theory, with its most important corollary, the neuron theory; for it was through the labors of the different histologists and experimenters who worked on the latter, from Deiters to Harrison, that the complex paths for transmitting impulses from nerve-cell to nerve-cell were traced out and their morphological continuity demonstrated. The initial data were the Bell-Magendie law of the

---

[1] Jackson: London Hosp. Rep., 1875, viii.

[2] Bidder and Volkmann: Die Selbstständigkeit des Nervensystems, Leipzig, 1842.

[3] J. N. Langley: Jour. Physiol., London, 1894, xvi, 410–440.

spinal nerve-roots, the law of Wallerian degeneration of nerve-fibers after section, and Goltz's work on the effects of the excision of large segments of the central nervous system. Türck's investigations of the cutaneous distribution of the separate pairs of spinal nerves (1858–68) were of capital importance, as also the discovery of the cerebral inhibition of spinal reflexes by Setchenoff (1863),[1] and the investigation of such localized reflexes as the knee-jerk or the mechanism of deglutition. Under the neuron theory, the simple reflex mechanism of external stimulus, afferent path, nerve-center, and efferent path became converted into a "reflex arc," requiring a sensory neuron centered in the ganglia of the posterior spinal roots or the cranial nerves and a motor neuron in the anterior horn of the cord or in the motor nucleus of a cranial nerve. Even this complex was soon perceived to be only an abstraction, since an isolated system of nerve-cells, functionating apart, is unthinkable. It became clear that most reflexes are compounded or coördinated, and that the nervous system functionates as a whole. This idea was specially developed by Charles Scott **Sherrington,** who did a large amount of experimental work on all phases of the subject. Sherrington was the first to investigate the phenomena of "decerebrate rigidity" produced by transection between the corpora quadrigemina and the thalamus opticus (1896–98),[2] and of "reciprocal innervation" and reciprocal inhibition, in virtue of which antagonistic muscles, e. g., flexors and extensors, when under reflex stimulation, are so related that excitation of one center is simultaneous with inhibition of the other (1893–98).[3] Sherrington expanded the theoretical concept of the "synapse," the separating surface which Foster postulated to exist between two neurons or their terminations, to complete the circuit in the reflex arc; and he did much to develop the knowledge of reënforcement and antagonism in simple and compound reflexes and of coördination in successive (chain) reflexes. The whole trend of his teaching is to the effect that a reflex action is seldom an isolated phenomenon, but one in which several reflex arcs are concerned, so that the true function of the nervous system is to integrate the organism, in the sense of giving it an individuality which is not possessed by a mere collection of cells or organs.[4] No one has handled this abstruse subject with more ability than Sherring-

---

[1] I. M. Setchenoff: Physiologische Studien über die Hemmungsmechanismen für die Reflexthätigkeit des Rückenmarks im Gehirn des Frosches, Berlin, 1863.

[2] C. S. Sherrington: Proc. Roy. Soc., London, 1896, lx, 415; and Jour. Physiol., London, 1898, xxii, 379.

[3] Proc. Roy. Soc. London, 1892–3, lii, 556, et seq.

[4] Sherrington: The Integrative Action of the Nervous System, New York, 1906.

ton, and, in connection with his work, it is proper to mention the important experiments of Erb and Westphal (1875), Jendrassik (1885), Weir Mitchell and Morris J. Lewis (1886), Lombard (1889), Bowditch and Warren (1890), on reënforcement and inhibition of the knee-jerk, of Sigmund Exner on reënforcement (*Bahnung*) of reflexes (1882), and of Jacques Loeb on "chain-reflexes" (1899).

Experimental **psychology** began in Ernst Heinrich Weber's laboratory, and its modern phases are principally the work of Lotze, Fechner, and Wundt. Rudolph Heinrich **Lotze** (1817–81), of Bautzen, a medical graduate who went over to metaphysics and philosophy, was the author of many important works on analytic psychology, in particular his *Medicinische Psychologie*, or Psychology of the Soul (1852). He was a pioneer in the investigation of space perception and in the scientific exploration of subconscious states. The elaborate analytics of Jung and the Freudian school are foreshadowed in such works as J. C. A. Heinroth's treatise on lying (1834), in which the concept of "pathological lying" was, in effect, introduced, and Kussmaul's investigations of the psychic life of the new-born child (1859).

Gustav Theodor **Fechner** (1801–87), professor of physics at Leipzig (1839–75), who did much experimental and editorial work in physics and chemistry, was perhaps the first after Weber to apply mathematical physics to the physiology of sensation, and wrote the first treatise on psychophysics (1860).[1] He made extended experimental studies of cutaneous sensation and muscular sense, for example, his record of 24,576 separate judgments of weights; he pointed out the personal or egotistic nature of painful sensation, he followed Weber in his investigations of the threshold limits of sensation, and stated Weber's law in its modern form. In 1838, he first investigated the color phenomena produced by rotating disks with black and white sectors, and mention can only be made of such optical novelties as his "side-window experiment" and his "paradoxical experiment."

Wilhelm **Wundt** (1832–   ), of Neckarau, Baden, was professor of physiology at Heidelberg (1864), Zürich (1874), and Leipzig (1875) and founded the Institute for Experimental Psychology in the latter city (1878). He wrote a text-book of physiology (1865), and three enduring memoirs on muscular motion (1858),[2] sensory perception (1862),[3] and the mechanics of the nerves and nerve-centers (1871–76),[4] which were the foundation of his future work. The first of these is memorable for the famous "isotonic curves" produced by muscle under continuous and constant (amounting to continual) excitation, which, as Burdon Sanderson says, have been copied into every text-book. It also contains valuable researches on muscular action under drugs and after transection of the nerves and spinal cord. The book on the nervous mechanism deals with such matters as reaction time and reflex time through the spinal cord and ganglia, and muscle sense. Wundt's contributions to psychology proper are a long list, and include his Elements of Physiological Psychology (1874),[5] Logic (1880–83), Ethics (1886), and Comparative Psychology (1904–10).[6] In 1883 he founded the *Philosophische Studien*, a serial devoted to experimental psychology and epistemology.

Other noteworthy contributions to psychology are the measurement of

---

[1] Fechner: Elemente der Psychophysik, Leipzig, 1860.

[2] Wundt: Die Lehre von der Muskelbewegung, Brunswick, 1858.

[3] Beiträge zur Theorie von der Sinneswahrnehmung, Leipzig, 1862.

[4] Untersuchungen zur Mechanik der Nerven und Nervencentren, Erlangen, 1871–76.

[5] Grundzüge der physiologischen Psychologie, Leipzig, 1873–74.

[6] Völkerpsychologie, Leipzig, 1904–10.

the velocity of the psychic impulse by Donders (1868),[1] the monographs of Duchenne (1862) and Darwin (1873) on the expression of the passions and emotions, Stanley Hall's study of Laura Bridgman (1879),[2] the work of Romanes, Jacques Loeb, Lloyd Morgan, Jennings, and others on comparative psychology, and of Krafft-Ebing, Havelock Ellis, and Freud on morbid sexual psychology.

Much of our knowledge of the digestive and vasomotor systems was developed by **Claude Bernard** (1813–78), the greatest physiologist of modern France, who was born in the village of Saint-Julien (Rhône), where his father was one of the many vine-growers and wine-makers of this region. A chorister and pupil of the Jesuits of the college at Villefranche, young Bernard was

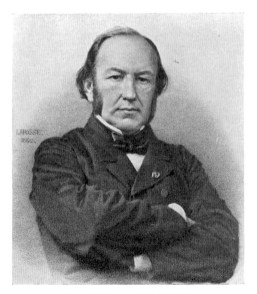

Claude Bernard (1813–78).

driven by straitened family circumstances to become a pharmacist's assistant at Lyons. Sharing the romantic aspirations of the youth of his time, he turned his attention to literature and wrote "La Rose du Rhône," a vaudeville comedy which was produced with some success, and "Arthur de Bretagne," a five-act tragedy which was long afterward handsomely printed (1886). With the latter in hand, he went up to Paris to consult the critic Saint-Marc Girardin, who saw the merits of his work as a dramatic poet, but shrewdly advised him to study medicine as a surer means of

---

[1] Donders: Arch. f. Anat., Physiol. u. wissensch. Med., Leipzig, 1868, 657–681.

[2] Hall: Mind, London, 1879, iv, 149–172.

gaining a livelihood. This advice was the turning-point in Bernard's career, for it brought him into close contact with Magendie, who directed his genius into its proper channels. Magendie, after three or four demonstrations of Bernard's superb talents, announced, with characteristic generosity, "You are a better man than I." As compared with Magendie, who often experimented at haphazard, like one groping in the dark, Bernard's attitude toward scientific investigation is best summed up in his own words:

"Put off your imagination, as you take off your overcoat, when you enter the laboratory; but put it on again, as you do your overcoat, when you leave the laboratory. Before the experiment and between whiles, let your imagination wrap you round; put it right away from you during the experiment itself lest it hinder your observing power."

All of Bernard's greatest discoveries were based upon accidentally discovered facts, which he used as clues to larger results through his wonderful power of thinking physiologically. It came to be said of him that he was no mere physiologic experimenter, but "physiology itself." Like Magendie and Johannes Müller, he made his bow to "vitalism," but he gave it the widest possible berth. Where Magendie had left medicine "une science à faire," Bernard boldly advanced to the position that the chief aim of physiologic experimentation is to throw light upon morbid conditions. He is the founder of experimental medicine, or the artificial production of disease by means of chemical and physical manipulation.

In 1843, he discovered that cane-sugar, when injected into the veins, appears in the urine, but not if treated with gastric juice prior to the injection. This was the starting-point of his investigation of the **glycogenic function of the liver.** He arrived at this by the accidental discovery of sugar in the hepatic vein of a dog fed upon sugar, whence he proceeded to experiment with a dog[1] fed upon meat, with the same results, and published his papers in 1848–50. By 1857, he had, through a number of ingenious experiments, established the glycogenic function of the liver upon a permanent basis, and had succeeded in isolating glycogen.[2] The fact that this substance could be obtained, seen as such and experimented with was more potent even than Wöhler's work in establishing the fact that the animal body can build up chemical substances as well as break them down. Furthermore, Bernard made it clear that the glycogenic function of the liver is in the nature of an "internal secretion," a term which he first introduced. "This," says Foster, "at one blow, destroyed the then dominant conception that the animal body was to be regarded as a bundle of organs, each with its appropriate functions." In 1849, Bernard made his celebrated discovery that a puncture (*piqûre*) of the fourth ventricle of the brain in dogs produces temporary diabetes.[3] Equally important for the physiology of the digestive system was his work on the **pancreatic**

---

[1] Bernard: Compt. rend. Acad. d. sc., Paris, 1848, xxvii, 249; 253; 514; 1850, xxxi, 571: 1855, xli, 461.

[2] *Ibid.*, 1857, xliv, 578; 1325.

[3] Compt. rend. Soc. de biol., 1849, Paris, 1850, i, 60.

juice (1849–56).[1] Up to the time of Bernard, gastric digestion was the whole of digestive physiology. Eberle, in 1834, suggested that the pancreatic juice emulsifies fats, and Valentin, in 1844, showed that it acts upon starch, but this was all that had been done and even this was not generally known. Bernard cleared up the whole subject. He showed that "gastric digestion is only a preparatory act," that the pancreatic juice emulsifies the fatty foods passing through the intestines, splitting them up into fatty acids and glycerin; and he demonstrated its power of converting starch into sugar and its solvent action upon the proteids undissolved by the stomach. Bernard put the experimental pancreatic fistula upon a working basis. His third great achievement was his exposition of the **vasomotor mechanism** (1851–53).[2] In 1840, Henle, as we have seen, demonstrated the existence of smooth muscle in the endothelium of the smaller arteries; and, in 1846, Kölliker showed that such involuntary muscles are made up of small, spindle-shaped cells. The term "vasomotor" was first employed by Benedict Stilling, in 1840, as a hypothetic designation of the nerve filaments supplying the blood-vessels. Bernard started out with the idea that the nervous system sets up chemical changes producing animal heat. On dividing a rabbit's cervical sympathetic nerve (1851), he found, instead of the expected fall in temperature, a sensible rise (4°–6° C.) and a marked increase in vascularity of the ear, but he left it an open question whether the congestion was the cause or the effect of the increased temperature. In August, 1852,[3] Brown-Séquard, then residing in America, showed that galvanism applied to the superior part of the divided sympathetic really causes contraction of the blood-vessels and a fall of the temperature on that side, whence he inferred that the effect of section of the sympathetic was to paralyze and dilate the blood-vessels. Bernard performed the same experiment independently, in November, 1852, and similar results were obtained by Waller and Budge, in 1853. In 1853, Bernard shut off the circulation in the ear by ligating two of its veins and, finding the same rise of temperature upon section of the sympathetic, argued that the latter controls the temperature relations, a view which he held to the end of his life. In 1858, he demonstrated that the sympathetic is the constrictor nerve and the chorda tympani the dilator of the blood-vessels. This discovery of vasodilator and vasoconstrictor nerves[4] completes his work on the circulation. Among his lesser achievements are his experiments with curare (1850–56),[5] in which, by paralyzing the nerve, he demonstrated the independent excitability of muscle, thus giving the classical proof of Haller's doctrine of specific irritability; his investigations of carbon monoxide poison (1853–58),[6] showing that it displaces the oxygen in the red blood-corpuscles; and his studies of the "paralytic secretions" occasioned by section of glandular nerves (1864).[7]

During the later years of his life Bernard expounded and extended his doctrines by means of courses of lectures at the Collège de France and the Sorbonne, in particular those on experimental physiology (1855), the effect of poisonous substances and drugs (1857), the physiology and pathology of the nervous system (1858), the liquids of the organism (1859), experimental pathology (1872),

---

[1] Arch. gén. de méd., Paris, 1849, i, 60–61. Compt. rend. Acad. d. sc., Paris, 1856; suppl., 379–563, 9 pl.

[2] Compt. rend. Soc. de biol., Paris, 1851, xxxiii, 163; 1852, xxxiv, 472; xxxv, 168; 1853, xxxvi, 378.

[3] Brown-Séquard: Med. Exam., Phila., 1852, viii, 481–504.

[4] Compt. rend. Acad. d. sc., Paris, 1858, xlviii, 245; 393.

[5] Compt. rend. Acad. d. sc., Paris, 1850, xxxi, 533; 1856, xliii, 825.

[6] Compt. rend. Acad. d. sc., 1858, xlvii, 393.

[7] J. de l'anat. et physiol., Paris, 1864, i, 507–513.

anesthetics and asphyxia (1875), and operative physiology (1879). The later of these reveal the unapproachable master in the technique of experimental procedure, and all of them the accomplished man of letters, who began his career as a poet and dramatist. Scattered through his writings are many luminous aphorisms which are to medicine what the "Pensées" of Vauvenargues and Joubert are to literature, in that they deal, as never before, with the high calling, the honorable aims and aspirations of the scientific physician. In the early days, Bernard was looked upon askance as a mere vivisector of animals, and he relates that he owed much immunity from persecution to an accidental friendship with a police-commissioner, in whose district he was afterward careful to pitch his tent. For the same reason, he was not happy in his married life, even his daughters becoming estranged from him through his wife, who had no sympathy with his genius, and was soured by the fact that he did not become a successful practitioner. But honors came in due course. A special chair of general physiology was created for him at the Sorbonne during Magendie's lifetime; and, in 1855, he succeeded the latter as full professor of physiology at the Collège de France, and was admitted to the Académie Française in 1868. Napoleon III was so fascinated with his personality that he gave him two fine laboratories at the Sorbonne and the Muséum d'Histoire Naturelle, and made him a senator in 1869. Among his friends were Duruy, Gambetta, Pasteur, Rayer, Davaine, St. Claire Deville, Berthelot and Renan, who succeeded to his *fauteuil* in the French Academy. Claude Bernard was tall and imposing in presence, with a noble brow and a countenance expressing depth of thought and kindliness of feeling. "As he walked the streets, passers-by might be heard to say, 'I wonder who that is? He must be some distinguished man.'"

Of Bernard's pupils, Willy **Kühne** (1837–1900), of Hamburg, professor of physiology at Amsterdam (1868–71) and Heidelberg (1871–1900), is memorable for his investigation of the peripheral end-organs of the motor nerves (1862), of hemoglobin (1865), of the digestion of proteids by the pancreatic juice (1867),[1] of the proteolytic enzyme in the pancreas, which he called trypsin (1876),[2] of the cleavage of the albumens in gastric and tryptic digestion (1877),[3] of rhodopsin, or "visual purple," and the "chromophanes" of the retina (1877)[4]; of the electrical storms in a muscle stimulated under pressure, and its power to excite

[1] Kühne: Virchow's Arch., Berlin, 1867, xxxix, 130–174.
[2] Verhandl. d. naturh.-med. Ver. zu Heidelb., 1874–77, n. F., i, 194; 233.
[3] *Ibid.*, 236.
[4] Untersuch. a. d. physiol. Inst., Heidelberg, 1877, i, 15; 105; 109; 119; 455.

another muscle compressed with it (1888),[1] and particularly the remarkable series of chemical studies of the intermediate products of peptic and intestinal digestion which he carried on with his pupil, Russell Henry **Chittenden** (1856–   ), of New Haven, Connecticut, many new substances being isolated and named for the first time by these investigators (1883–88).[2] Kühne was a man of infinite resource in experimentation, notably in his "opto-grams," or photographs made directly on an excised retina, and his use of pancreatic ferments as a reagent in histology.

Paul **Bert** (1830–86), of Auxerre, Bernard's favorite pupil and his successor at the Sorbonne (1868), spoiled a brilliant scientific career by mixing in politics. He was fiercely radical and anticlerical, and, being sent by Gambetta as consul general to Tonkin in 1886, died there of dysentery shortly after. He discovered an unanalyzed substance in the mammary gland (1879), but his best work was *La Pression Barometrique* (1878), a bundle of scattered essays dealing with the gases of the blood, caisson disease, and particularly with the toxic effects of oxygen at high pressure. In prosecuting these experiments, Bert induced three balloonists to make a high ascension, armed with bags of oxygen, and only one survived the attempt. The theory of the glycogenic function was formally opposed by Frederick William Pavy (1829–1911), whose work will be considered in relation to internal medicine.

In connection with the work of Bernard, we may follow the modern developments of the **physiology of digestion,** of metabolism, and of the ductless glands.

The classical description of the mechanism of the act of deglutition was given by Magendie (1817),[3] who described the three stages in the passage of food through the mouth, pharynx, and esophagus. He thought that the principal coefficients of the motor power were the constrictor muscles of the pharynx, but it was afterward shown by Hugo Kronecker (1839–   ), of Bern, and Samuel James Meltzer (1851–   ) that the swallowing reflex is a complex coördinated mechanism, depending mainly upon the mylohyoid and hyoglossal muscles (1880–83).[4] The essential reflex character of the act was demonstrated in 1876 by Angelo Mosso (1846–   ), of Turin, who showed that, even after section or ligation of the esophagus, the peristaltic wave from the pharynx will, in time, be taken up on the lower side of the gap by means of the nerve-supply and pass to the stomach, while section of the nerves will abolish the reflex completely.[5] The movements of the stomach were first studied *in situ* by William Beaumont, and more accurately by Walter Bradford Cannon[6] (1871–   ), of Wisconsin, who studied them with the Röntgen rays, after ingestion of bismuth (1898). That the stomach is, like the heart, an automatic motor mechanism, independently of the nervous mechanism which adjusts its function, was shown by the observations of Hofmeister and Schütz upon the

---

[1] Ztschr. f. Biol., Munich, 1888, xxiv, 383–422.

[2] Kühne and Chittenden: Zeitschr. f. Biol., Munich, 1883, xix, 160; 1884, xx, 11; 1886, xxii, 409; 423; 1888, xxv, 358.

[3] Magendie: Précis élémentaire de physiologie, Paris, 1817, ii, 58–67.

[4] Kronecker and Meltzer: Arch. f. Physiol., Leipzig, 1880, 299; 446; 1883, Suppl.-Bd., 328.

[5] Mosso, in Moleschott's Untersuch. z. Naturlehre (etc.), Frankfort, 1876; xi, 331–349.

[6] Cannon: Am. Jour. Physiol., Boston, 1898, i, 359–382.

movements of an excised stomach kept warm (1886), by Rud. Heidenhain; by W. B. Cannon, at Harvard (1906), who proved that the gastric movements and secretions continue unabated after section of the extrinsic fibers of the vagus and splanchnic nerves; and latterly in the "visceral organism" which Alexis Carrel has kept alive in an extravital culture-medium (1912). The mechanism of vomiting was first described by Magendie (1813), who thought that the sole agent was the contraction of the abdominal muscles. Later investigations have shown that he was only half right, the act being a complicated reflex in which the walls of the stomach play an equal part. After the time of Prout and Beaumont, it was contended by Claude Bernard and Barreswil, Lehmann, and others, that the free acid of the gastric juice was, in reality, lactic acid, but this was finally set at rest by the laborious analyses of Bidder and Schmidt (1852), which proved that normally the gastric juice always contains hydrochloric acid in excess. Brücke (1872) and others had shown, however, that during carbohydrate digestion, starch can be converted directly into lactic acid in the stomach, probably through the action of the lactic acid bacillus. The hydrochloric acid in the stomach was shown by Voit (1869) and Cahn (1886) to be derived from the chlorides in the blood-plasma. In regard to the mechanism of its formation, the different theories advanced by Maly, Gamgee, and others are still *sub judice*. The histologic changes in the gastric glands during secretion were studied by Heidenhain (1878), and intravitally by J. N. Langley (1880). The stages of conversion of proteids into peptones in the stomach were first described by Meissner (1859–62), and more exhaustively and finally by Willy Kühne (1877).

The movements of the intestines were studied by Carl Ludwig (1861),[1] who described the swaying motions (*Pendelbewegungen*) between the intervals of peristalsis; by W. B. Cannon, who observed the latter by means of the Röntgen rays (1902),[2] and by Bayliss and Starling, who described peristalsis as a reflex through the intrinsic ganglia (1899).[3] That the peristaltic wave is in one direction and due to some definite arrangement in the intestinal walls was proved by Franklin P. Mall, who cut out a piece of the gut and reversed it *in situ*, producing intestinal obstruction from accumulation of food above the section (1896).[4] The intrinsic nerve plexuses were described by Auerbach and Meissner. Pflüger, in 1857,[5] showed that stimulation of the splanchnic nerves inhibits the intestinal movements. The net result of investigation goes to show that the intestines, like the stomach, are an automatic mechanism which is regulated by, but not dependent upon, the extrinsic nerves. Similar conclusions in regard to the rectal functions have been reached through the experiments of Goltz upon dogs deprived of the spinal cord (1874), and the skiagraphic observations of Hertz (1907). In 1895, it was shown, by G. H. F. Nuttall and H. Thierfelder, that healthy animal life and perfect digestion are possible without the presence of bacteria in the alimentary canal. Harvey Cushing showed that, above and below the ileum, the intestines are relatively free from bacteria, and that the intestinal tract can be sterilized by fasting (Welch-Festschrift, 1900). Our knowledge of the chemistry and histology of intestinal absorption is largely due to the work of Kühne (1877), Heidenhain (1888–94), and Pavloff and his pupils (1897). What we know of the functions of the liver and pancreas will always be associated with the great name of Claude Bernard. His pupil, Willy Kühne, as we have seen, worked out the cleavage changes of the proteins in the stomach and intestines, but, before him, Purkinje and Pappenheim had noticed the proteolytic power of pancreatic extracts (1836), and Lucien Corvisart, in a long series of re-

---

[1] Ludwig: Lehrbuch der Physiologie, 2. Aufl., 1861, ii, 615.

[2] Cannon: Am. Jour. Physiol., Boston, 1901–2, vi, 251–277.

[3] W. M. Bayliss and E. H. Starling: Jour. Physiol., London, 1899, xxiv, 99.

[4] Mall: Johns Hopkins Hosp. Rep., Baltimore, 1896, i, 93.

[5] Pflüger: Ueber 'den 'Hemmungsnervensystem für die peristaltischen Bewegungen der Gedärme, Berlin, 1857.

searches (1857–63),[1] had shown that proteids are converted by the pancreatic juice into the ordinary digestive products, at the temperature of the body, and in alkaline, acid, or neutral media. This corrected the error of Claude Bernard, who supposed that pancreatic proteolysis cannot take place without the previous action of bile. The sugar-forming ferments of the salivary glands and pancreas were investigated by the pathologist, Julius Cohnheim (1863).[2] Ptyalin was isolated by Mialhe (1845),[3] trypsin by Kühne (1876).[4] The derivatives of bile were studied by Thénard (1809), Gmelin (1826), Plattner, who first obtained "crystallized bile" (1844), and particularly by Adolf Strecker (1822–71), who showed that Plattner's crystals were a mixture of the sodium salts of glycocholic and taurocholic acids, which, treated with acids, yield the amido-acids, glycocoll, and taurine, with cholic acid as a common product (1848–49).[5] Bilirubin was first isolated by Heintz (1851); biliverdin, by Berzelius (1840), who confused it with chlorophyll, and by Valentiner, who first obtained it in crystalline form (1859). Urobilin was discovered in the urine by Max Jaffé in 1868. Austin Flint, Jr., in 1862, claimed that cholesterin is removed from the blood by the liver and discharged from the body as stercorin, but Naunyn and his pupils have assumed it to be a product of the gall-bladder and ducts, and not of the liver-cells (1892). The common bile-tests were introduced by Gmelin (1826), Pettenkofer (1844), and Paul Ehrlich (1883).

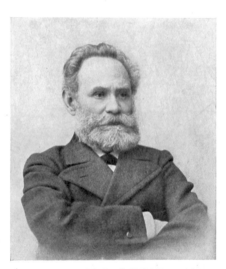

Ivan Petrovich Pavloff (1849–   ).

Recent knowledge of the relation of the nervous system to the salivary, gastric, and pancreatic secretions is mainly due to the work of the physiologists of the Russian school, in particular Ivan Petrovich **Pavloff** (1849–   ), of the Ryazan Government, who, in 1904, was awarded the Nobel prize for his investigations.[6] The success of Pavloff's experiments was mainly due to certain improvements which he and his pupils made in the operative production of gastric and pancreatic fistulæ.

---

[1] L. Corvisart: Collection de mémoires sur une fonction seu connue du pancreas, Paris, 1857–63.

[2] Cohnheim: Arch. f. path. Anat., Berlin, 1863, xxviii, 241–253.

[3] Mialhe: Compt. rend. Acad. d. sc., Paris, 1845, xx, 654; 1483.

[4] Kühne: Verhandl. d. naturh.-med. Ver. zu Heidelberg, 1876, n. F., i, 190.

[5] Strecker: Ann. d. Chem. u. Pharm., Heidelberg, 1848, lxv, 1; lxvii, 1: 1849, lxx, 149.

[6] Collected in his "Le travail des glandes digestives" (Russian text, St. Petersburg, 1897. French translation, Paris, 1901).

32

As early as 1852, Bidder and Schmidt had reported that the sight of food will produce a copious flow of gastric juice in a gastrostomized dog, and Richet, in 1878, had obtained a similar effect in a patient who had to be fed through a gastric fistula, on account of a strictured esophagus.   Heidenhain failed to obtain this result in a fistulized dog, whence it was inferred that he had in some way damaged the nerve connections in preparing his fistula (1880). Pavloff improved the Heidenhain fistula by keeping the nerve-supply intact, and so standardized it for modern procedure.[1] In addition, he severed the dog's esophagus in such wise that swallowed food might be discharged at the upper opening, and unswallowed food ingested into the stomach at the lower. Three sets of experiments were then possible: The dog might be allowed merely to see or smell the food, a Barmecide feast which Pavloff called "psychical feeding"; or, the animal might chew the food which passed through the esophageal opening, constituting a sham meal (Scheinfütterung); or; a true feeding might be obtained by introducing the food through the lower stoma of the esophagus.   In the first two instances, the effect of smell, sight, taste, chewing, and swallowing was such that a copious and continual gastric secretion—as much as 700 c.c. in five or six hours—was. obtained without the introduction of any food into the stomach. Pavloff called this effect a "psychical secretion."   He next showed that severing the splanchnic nerves does not affect the phenomenon, but section of both vagi will abolish the reflex secretion, and direct stimulation of the peripheral ends of the cut vagi will, after a short interval, produce it again. This proved that the gastric secretion is regulated by the vagus. Under the third condition set by Pavloff, mere mechanical stimulation of the stomach by the introduction of food through the esophageal opening, while the dog is asleep or inattentive, does not necessarily stimulate secretion, contrary to received opinion. Chischin, Pavloff's pupil, found that, when the psychical stimuli are shut off in this way, the amount of secretion varies with the kind of food, being positive for meats and peptones generally, and negative for other substances, which, when eaten, might cause a psychical secretion (1894). By means of a special pancreatic fistula, Pavloff was able to indicate that the secretory fibers of the pancreas are in the vagus nerve. In 1895, Dolinsky found that the introduction of acids into the duodenum causes a flow of pancreatic juice, from which it is inferred that the acid in the gastric juice sets up this secretion, probably through the production of the hormone which Bayliss and Starling call secretin (1902). Chepovalnikoff, another Pavloff pupil, discovered that pancreatic juice from a fistula acquires a powerful solvent action on proteids from contact with the duodenal membrane or its extract, and the latter Pavloff assumed to contain a special enzyme, "enterokinase," which activates the pancreatic juice (1899).[2] Like Purkinje and Carl Ludwig, Pavloff has developed many of his ideas through the medium of his pupils.

The scientific study of **metabolism** has been divided by von Noorden into three stages: First, the qualitative period, inaugurated by Liebig and Wöhler, in which the end-products of animal metabolism and the conditions of their formation were determined. Second, the quantitative period of von Voit and von Pettenkofer, in which food values were carefully studied in dietetic tables and the balance of nutrition determined, after which the thermodynamic relations of metabolic processes were calculated in terms of heat and energy units. Third, the recent era of the study of the intermediate products of metabolism, which is again qualitative, but already in process of becoming quantitative. Curiously

---

[1] Described in Chischin's St. Petersburg dissertation, 1894.
[2] N. P. Chepovalnikoff: St. Petersburg dissertation, 1899.

enough, the initial experiments in metabolism were quantitative, viz., Sanctorius' efforts to measure his own "insensible perspiration" on the steelyard, and the attempt of Lavoisier and Laplace to establish an equation between the quantity of heat formed in the body of a mammal and that formed in a burning candle, assuming the quantities of carbon dioxide formed to be identical in both cases. The latter has been signalized by Jacques Loeb as the foundation of scientific biology.[1] All of Lavoisier's work on the exchange of gases in the lungs belongs, in fact, to the subject of metabolism, in the strict modern sense.

During the early period, Magendie was the first to emphasize the importance of the nitrogenous substances in the organism. Prout divided food-stuffs into the saccharine, oily, and albuminous, from the fact that milk, nature's ready-made perfect food, is made up of these ingredients. Next came the work of Liebig and Wöhler on urea and uric-acid compounds, in particular Wöhler's syntheses of urea (1828) and hippuric acid (1842). Liebig was the first to classify the organic food-stuffs and the processes of nutrition (1842). He held that oxygen is the principal chemical coefficient in living processes, that muscular work is done at the expense of albumen, that fat can be formed in the body from albumen or sugar, and, like Claude Bernard, he believed that food-stuffs have to be changed into physiologic albumen before they can be utilized in the body. The embryologist Theodor Ludwig Wilhelm Bischoff (1807–1882), of Hannover, was the first to demonstrate the presence of free CO_2 and oxygen in the blood (1837), studied the urea as a measure of metabolism (1842), and (with Voit) the laws of nutrition and inanition in carnivora (1860). The Alsatian chemist, Boussingault, first attempted to tabulate the metabolic intake and output in different animals (1835–40), and (with Dumas) defined an animal as an oxidizing, a plant as a reducing, apparatus (1844). Bischoff's assistant, Carl von Voit (1831–1908), of Amberg, made many interesting studies on dietetics, particularly in his Handbook of the Physiology of Metabolism in Nutrition (1881), which introduced new methods of determining the intake and outgo in the balance of nutrition and the amount of proteid necessary in foods. In collaboration with the Bavarian hygienist, Max von Pettenkofer (1818–1901), Voit first estimated the amounts of proteins, fat, or carbohydrates broken down in the body (from the total nitrogen and CO_2 eliminated) by means of a special respiration apparatus, constructed at the expense of King Maximilian of Bavaria (1861), which was further elaborated and improved by Voit himself. These two investigators also demonstrated that fats are formed from the food proteids (1862–81), but, later, this view was not exclusively held to, even by Voit (1886), and was absolutely denied by Pflüger (1892). Voit distinguished between organized or tissue-proteids and unorganized or circulating proteids (1881), and held that the food carbohydrates and proteids are directly consumed in the body (1881), in opposition to the Liebig-Bernard-Pflüger hypothesis, that they have first to be changed into body-substance. Pettenkofer introduced the well-known test for bile (1844), and a new method of estimating the CO_2 in the air. The estimate of the nitrogen content in metabolism was rendered relatively easy by the method introduced by J. Kjeldahl in 1883. Max Rubner (1854–   ), of Munich, was one of the first to investigate metabolic changes in terms of heat and energy units by means of the calorimeter, or by using the animal body as a calorimeter (1891). The heat relations of the body were first investigated by Lavoisier and Laplace (1780), Crawford (1788), and Scharling (1849), who used ice, water, and air calorimeters respectively. Since the time of Voit and Pettenkofer, these investigations have been improved by such instruments as

---

[1] J. Loeb: The Mechanistic Conception of Life, Chicago, 1912, pp. 4, 5.

d'Arsonval's differential air calorimeter (1886), and the respiration calorimeters of Atwater and Rosa (1899) and Atwater and Benedict (1905). The value of quantitative work by improved means has been especially shown in such researches as those of Nathan Zuntz on the blood gases and respiratory metabolism, Pavy and Moleschott on dietetics, Atwater and Langworthy on the balance of nutrition, R. H. Chittenden on the minimum nutritive requirements of the body in relation to its capacity for work and nitrogenous equilibrium (1904), and F. G. Benedict on the influence of inanition on metabolism (1907). Much of recent effort has been concentrated on the diathetic diseases, diabetes, gout and rheumatism, obesity and the disorders of the ductless glands, and most of this has been concerned with the discovery and significance of novel chemical compounds. The pathology and treatment of diabetes has been rendered a purely chemical problem through such advances as Petters' discovery of acetone in diabetic urine (1857); the work of Kussmaul on acetonemia (1874); of Stadelmann (1883), Külz (1884–87), Minkowski (1884), and Magnus-Levy (1899–1909) on β-oxybutyric acid in relation to diabetic coma, von Mering's experimental production of diabetes by exhibition of phlorizin (1886); and the dietetic studies of Carl von Noorden (1895–1911), in particular his oatmeal diet. The true metabolic relations of uric acid, first isolated from the urine by Scheele (1776) and found in gouty and urinary concretions by Wollaston (1797), have been a matter of keen controversy. Important landmarks in its history are Marcet's discovery of xanthin (1819); Strecker's demonstration of the same in the urine (1857); Kossel's proof that xanthin bases are derivatives of the urine (1879); the discovery of nuclein in pus-cells and spermatozoa by Miescher (1874); Kossel's and Hoppe-Seyler's classifications of the nucleins; Horbaczewski's synthesis of uric acid *in vitro* (1882), and his proof that it is derivable from nuclein (1889); Minkowski's discovery that a diet of xanthin bases will increase uric-acid excretion (1886), and that, in birds, the latter is synthetized in the liver through the influence of lactic acid (1886); and Emil Fischer's family tree of gout, based upon the idea that uric acid and the xanthin bases have a common purin-nucleus (1895). The relation of the liver to metabolism was studied to advantage through a method introduced by the Russian physiologist, Nikolai Vladimirovich **Eck** (1847–   ) in 1877. This consisted in establishing a permanent communication between the portal vein and the inferior vena cava (Eck's fistula), abolishing the portal circulation by ligation of the portal vein, so that ligation of the hepatic artery under these conditions is equivalent to excising or excluding the liver.

The name of Rudolph **Heidenhain** (1834–97), professor of physiology at Breslau (1859–   ), is intimately associated with the interpretation of all secretory phenomena as intracellular, rather than mechanical, processes. He investigated the histologic changes in the cells concerned in the secretion of saliva, milk, the gastric and intestinal juices, and the pancreatic ferments, and opposed Ludwig's filtration theory of the formation of lymph and urine on the same grounds, describing lymph as a secretion from the cells forming the walls of the capillaries, and urine as a product of the renal glomeruli, so far as water and inorganic salts are concerned, urea and uric acid being regarded as secretions of the epithelial cells in the convoluted tubes. Most of these theories are contained in his memoir on secretions in Hermann's Handbuch der Physiologie (1880, v). He also investigated the action of poisons on the nerves of the submaxillary gland (1872), the trophic and secretory fibers of the secretory nerves (1878), and the phenomena of intestinal absorption (1888–94). Under du Bois Réymond, he began his studies of the mechanics, metabolism, and heat-production of muscular activity (1864), leading to the construction of a "tetanomotor." With Bürger, he made some experimental investigations in hypnotism, but his most striking work was undoubtedly his method of staining the kidney-cells by the injection of indigo-carmin into the blood, which, whatever his hypotheses, shows him to have been an investigator of great power.

The beginnings of the theory of **ductless glands and internal secretions,** especially in relation to metabolism, were Claude Bernard's work on glycogen (1848–57), the pancreatic functions (1849–56), his fourth ventricle *piqûre*, Addison's description of the suprarenal syndrome (1849–56), and the experiments of Brown-Séquard and Schiff.

Charles-Edouard **Brown-Séquard** (1817–94), a native of Mauritius, was the son of an American father and a French mother, but his life-work was mainly associated with French medicine. He led a roving existence, posting from one country to another at intervals, and, whether in London, Paris, or New York, he could have attained almost any eminence by continuous effort. He succeeded Claude Bernard as professor of experimental medicine in the Collège de France in 1878, and he was successively a professor in the Harvard and Paris medical faculties. In 1852, he confirmed Bernard's work on the sympathetic. Previous to this he had made his mark by his experimental transections and hemisections of the spinal cord (1849); his description of hemiplegia with crossed anesthesia (1850)[1] of which he gave an incorrect physiological explanation; his investigations of the associated pains of visceral disease (1857); the effect of tropical heat on the temperature of the body (1859); the "tremospasm" feature of the knee-jerk (1858); the experimental production of epilepsy (1869–70); the experimental production of vasomotor changes in the pulmonary circulation (1872); and the vasodilator effect produced by heat stimulation of the cerebral cortex (1887). He is, with Claude Bernard, the principal founder of the doctrine of the internal secretions, through his experimental production of an exaggerated Addison's disease in animals by excision of the suprarenal capsules (1856–58),[2] his use of the testicular and other organic juices as remedies (1889–91),[3] his theory that the kidney has an internal secretion (1892),[4] and his treatment of acromegaly by animal extracts (1893).[5] He was founder and editor of the *Journal de la physiologie de l'homme et des animaux* (1858–63), and, with Charcot and Vulpian, of the *Archives de physiologie normale et pathologique* (1868–94).

Moritz **Schiff** (1823–96), of Frankfort on the Main, a pupil of Magendie and Longet, was professor of comparative anatomy at Bern (1854–63), and of physiology at Florence, Italy (1863–76), and Geneva (1876–96). He was a zoölogist by training, attaining particular eminence in ornithology, and there are few aspects of physiology which he did not investigate. Schiff's work was characterized by great originality in the minutiæ of experimental procedure, displaying an almost prophetic insight into many things of present moment. He liked to cross swords with contemporary theorists, and the fact that he sometimes abandoned his own theories, or that some of them have been abandoned by others, has tended to obscure his very solid merits. Thus, in 1849, he took the somewhat arbitrary standpoint that the vagus is the motor, rather than the inhibitory, nerve of the heart, from his results on stimulation of the terminal motor fibers, which anticipated the discovery of the accelerator vagus fibers by Ludwig and Schmiedeberg in 1870. He noticed that the ventricle of a dying heart sometimes beats more slowly than the auricle, which overthrew the old Haller idea of a peristaltic, muscular wave passing from the great veins through the heart to the aorta, and all but afforded a vista into the phenomenon of heart-block. He believed that the localized "idiopathic" muscular contractions at the outset of rigor mortis are due to a special chemical stimulus (hormone) formed at death. In 1856, he made experiments which foreshad-

---

[1] Brown-Séquard: Compt. rend. Soc. de biol., 1850, Paris, 1851, ii, 70–73.

[2] Compt. rend. Acad. d. sc., Paris, 1856, xliii, pt. 2, 422; 542. Jour. de la physiol. de l'homme, Paris, 1858, i, 160–173.

[3] Arch. de physiol. norm. et path., Paris, 1889, 5. s., i, 739; 1890, ii, 201; 443; 646; 1891, iii, 746.

[4] Arch. de physiol. norm. et path., Paris, 1892, 5. s., v, 778–786.

[5] Compt. rend. Soc. de biol., Paris, 1893, xlv, 527.

owed the existence of the vasodilator nerves discovered by Bernard in 1858. In 1867, in anticipation of Pavloff's pupils, he noted that the reflex flow of saliva in a dog with a parotid fistula varies with the methods and substances employed in stimulation. He was one of the earliest to study the effects of removal of the cerebellum, hemisection of the cord, and transection of the cerebral peduncles and spinal nerve-roots (1858); he was the first to notice the effect of excitation of the cerebral cortex upon the circulation; first described the vasoconstrictor function of the great auricular nerve and the inhibitory effect of section of the small superficial petrosal upon reflex salivary secretion; and first regarded the Rolandic area as sensory, although he later abandoned this view. His epoch-making experiments on the effects of excision of the thyroid in dogs, their prevention by thyroid grafts and by the injection or ingestion of thyroid juices (1856–84),[1] which will be described under twentieth century medicine, make him a pioneer of the doctrine of internal secretions and a prophet of thyroid therapy. To this field belong also his experiments on artificial diabetes (1856) and the relation of the nervous system to its production (1859).

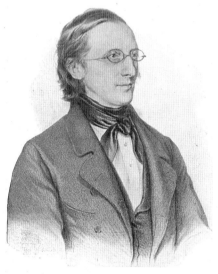

Carl Ludwig (1816–95).

"More than to any one else since the time of Harvey," says Sir Lauder Brunton, "do we owe our present knowledge of the **circulation** to Carl Ludwig . . . Like the great architects of the Middle Ages, who built the wonderful cathedrals which we all admire, and whose builder's name no man knows, Ludwig has been content to sink his own name in his anxiety for the progress of his work, and in his desire to aid his pupils." **Carl Ludwig** (1816–95) was a native of Witzenhausen, Hesse, a Marburg graduate (1840), professor of anatomy at the latter university (1846–49), professor of anatomy and physiology at Zürich (1849–55), professor of physiology and zoölogy in the Josephinum at Vienna (1855–64), and finally professor of physiology at Leipzig (1865–95), where he founded the Physiological Institute in which so much of his work was done. Ludwig was perhaps the greatest teacher of physiology who ever lived. He had over 200 pupils of all nationalities, and most of the younger generation of investigators in his science were

---

[1] Schiff: Untersuchungen über die Zuckerbildung in der Leber, Würzburg, 1859, pp. 61–63. Rev. méd. de la Suisse Rom., Geneva, 1884, iv, 65–75.

trained by him. Beyond a text-book of physiology (1852–56), two inaugural addresses on the mechanism of urinary secretion (1843) and on blood-pressure (1865), and a few minor essays, he did but little independent writing. Most of his important discoveries were published under the names of his pupils, some of whom, von Kries tells us, merely sat on the window-sill, while Ludwig and his faithful assistant, Salvenmoser, did all the work. He had a wonderful capacity for selecting themes which would make the pupil find himself. His object was to form capable investigators, while carrying out his own ideas, and, to this end, he always mapped out the experimental problem himself, including its technical details, and usually wrote out the final draft of the paper also.[1]

His principal contributions to physiology are the introduction of the graphic method (1847), with new instruments, like the kymograph, blood-pump, and Stromuhr; perfusion of excised organs (1865–67), his theories of the mechanism of urinary secretion and lymph-formation, his discovery of the innervation of the salivary glands, and his many excursions into the physiology of the circulation. Nearly all these things were done before he came to Leipzig.

To the Marburg period belongs the mechanical theory of the secretion of urine by osmosis. In 1842,[2] Sir William Bowman, in describing the capsule around the glomeruli and the urinary tubules, advanced the theory that the proximal principles of the urine are secreted in solid form from the epithelium of the venous tubules, solution being effected by water discharged from the glomerulus. Ludwig's theory (1843–44)[3] starts with the idea that the secretion of urine depends upon the beating of the heart, the blood-pressure causing the urinary constituents to pass from the blood through the capillary walls as a dilute liquid, which becomes concentrated, as it passes through the tubules, by osmosis of water to the more concentrated lymph outside. Bowman and Heidenhain treated the glomerular epithelium as a secreting gland. Ludwig regarded it as a passive filter. Ludwig's theory has been accepted by most physiologists, although strong objections to it have been made by Heidenhain[4] and others. In 1869–70, as Brunton points out,[5] Ludwig himself, in collaboration with his pupil, Ustimovitch, performed an experiment which forced him to modify his views somewhat.[6] This consisted in dividing the medulla in the neck of a dog, causing the blood-pressure to fall, and stopping the urinary secretion. Sub-

---

[1] These monographs were published simultaneously, under the pupils' names, in the "Berichte" of the Saxon Academy of Sciences, and in the famous *Arbeiten aus der physiologischen Anstalt zu Leipzig* (1866–77), but, after 1877, in du Bois Reymond's Archiv. They cover every aspect of the subject except the physiology of the brain, and reveal, at every turn, the master experimenter, the man of infinite resource in investigation.

[2] Bowman: Phil. Tr., London, 1842, 57–80.

[3] Ludwig: Beiträge zur Lehre vom Mechanismus der Harnsecretion, Marburg, 1843, and Wagner's Handwörterb. d. Physiol., 1844, ii, 637.

[4] Heidenhain: Arch. f. path. Anat., Berlin, 1866, xxxv, 158.

[5] Brunton: Proc. Roy. Soc. Med., London, 1912, v, Therap. Sect., 139–151.

[6] C. Ustimovitch: Arb. a. d. physiol. Anst. zu Leipzig, 1870, v, 217.

sequent injection of urea into the veins caused a renewal of the urinary secretion and forced Ludwig to conclude that the effect of pressure was dependent upon the chemical constituents in the blood; in other words, upon osmosis through a selective, semipermeable membrane. In 1847, Ludwig changed Poiseuille's mercury manometer into the kymograph.[1] In 1848 he discovered the ganglionic cells in the interauricular septum.[2] During the Zürich period, he stated, through his pupil, F.W.Noll, the theory that lymph is formed by the diffusion of fluids from the blood through the vessel-walls into the surrounding tissues, the motor power being the capillary blood-pressure (1850).[3] In 1851, Ludwig, (with Becher and Rahn) discovered the innervation of the submaxillary glands,[4] and, in 1856, he showed that the stimulation of the sympathetic nerve will cause secretion by the submaxillary gland.[5] During the Viennese period, his pupil, Lothar Meyer, investigated the gases of the blood (1857–58); Cloetta discovered inosite, taurin, leucin, and uric acid in the animal body (1855); and Ludwig himself collaborated with the physicist Stephan in a hydrodynamic investigation of the pressure exerted by flowing water in a plane perpendicular to its direction (1858). In 1864, he studied, with Thiry, the effect of the spinal cord upon the blood current,[6] and his Leipzig inaugural address (1865) introduced the idea of keeping excised portions of an organism (*überlebende Organe*) active by an artificial circulation or "perfusion." During the Leipzig period, research was varied, but the main object of study was the heart and the circulation. Thus, in 1866, we find him, with Elie von Cyon, investigating the effect of temperature on heartbeat, and in the same year he discovered the depressor nerve of the heart, and the "nervi erigentes" of the peripheral vessels (1866).[7] With Dogiel, he invented the *Stromuhr* for measuring the amount of blood passing in unit time (1867)[8]; in 1868, with the same pupil, he found, upon auscultating the heart after ligation of the vena cava, pulmonary artery and vein, and aorta, that the first (systolic) sound is not of valvular origin entirely, but is partly produced by the cardiac muscle.[9] In 1869–70, Lauder Brunton and O. Schmiedeberg began to study the effects of drugs upon the circulation; and in 1871, Schmiedeberg traced the accelerator fibers of the vagus nerve in the dog.[10] In 1871, H. P. Bowditch, experimenting with an excised heart and a frog manometer, showed that the heart muscle always gives a maximal contraction or none at all ("all or nothing"); and Kronecker, investigating fatigue and recovery of muscle, showed that heart muscle cannot be tetanized. In 1871–73, Ludwig, with Dittmar, was the first to localize a vasomotor center (in the medulla oblongata).[11] With Mosso, he made plethysmographic studies on the blood-vessels of the excised kidney (1874); with von Kries, he measured the blood-pressure in the capillaries (1875);[12] with Schmidt-Mülheim, he began to experiment with the injection of peptones into the blood (1880);[13] in 1883, Wooldridge made his important studies on the chemistry of coagulation of the blood, and in 1884, Conrad Gompertz investigated the

---

[1] Ludwig: Arch. f. Anat., Physiol. u. wissensch. Med., Berlin, 1847, 241–302.

[2] Ludwig: Müller's Arch., Berlin, 1848, 139–143, 1 pl.

[3] Ludwig and Noll: Zeitschr. f. rat. Med., Heidelberg, 1850, ix, 52.

[4] Ludwig, Becher and Rahn: *Ibid.*, 1851, n. F., i, 225–292.

[5] According to his pupil, Czermak.

[6] Ludwig and Thiry: Sitzungsb. d. k. Akad. d. Wissensch. Med.-naturw. Cl., Vienna, 1864, xlix, 2. Abth., 421–454.

[7] Ludwig's Arbeiten (1866), Leipzig, 1867, i, 128–149.

[8] *Ibid.*, ii, 196–271.

[9] Ber. d. k. sächs. Gesellsch. d. Wissensch., Leipzig, 1868, xx, 89.

[10] Ludwig and Schmiedeberg: *Ibid.*, 1871, xxiii, 148–170.

[11] Ludwig and Dittmar: Ber. d. k. sächs. Gesellsch. d. Wissensch., Leipzig, 1871, 135; 1873, 460.

[12] Von Kries: *Ibid.*, 1875, 148.   [13] Arch. f. Physiol., 1880, 33.

arrangement of muscular fibers in the heart. Other important investigations from Ludwig's laboratory were his monograph on the lymphatics (with Schweig-ger-Seidel, 1872–74);[1] introducing the puncture method of injection in his-tology; Flechsig's investigations of medullated nerve-fibers (1876); Ludwig's study of the digestion of proteids after excision or exclusion of the stomach (with Ogata, 1883),[2] and Bowditch's proof of the non-fatigability of nerve (1890).

The titles listed give but a faint idea of the immense amount of valuable work done in the Leipzig laboratory, where not a few stu-dents, as Burdon Sanderson tells us, "for the first time in their lives came into personal relation with a man who was utterly free from selfish aims and vain ambitions, who was scrupulously con-

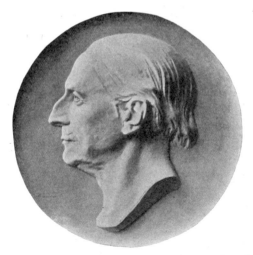

Carl Ludwig (medallion). (Courtesy of Professor William Stirling, Man-chester, England.)

scientious in all that he said and did, who was what he seemed to be and seemed what he was, and who had no other aim than the advancement of his science." All who met Ludwig, says Kron-ecker, "came under the influence of his enchanting personality." He lived with his pupils in a "*schöne Gemeinsamkeit,*" and was, indeed, in some respects, the personification of Browning's hawk-nosed, high-cheek-boned, blue-eyed German professor, absolutely sincere and unpretentious, and, however rigorous and exact in method, captivating every one by his warmth of heart, his genial sympathy, and the simplicity of his life and aims. Ludwig was a splendid draftsman, and his mind was of the purely plastic kind,

---

[1] Die Lymphgefässe der Fascien und Sehnen, Leipzig, 1872.

[2] Ludwig and Ogata: Arch. f. Anat. u. Physiol., Leipzig, 1883, 89.

which visualizes everything as a material phenomenon. For this reason, he had little use for mathematics, psychology, or any of the sciences which repose upon a metaphysical basis. He was devoted to music, however, a great patron of the *Gewandhaus* concerts, and he often had chamber music at his house. The charm of his personality has been admirably conveyed in the reminiscences of his old pupils, Kronecker, von Kries, Burdon Sanderson, and William Stirling.

The innervation of the heart was investigated by Henle (1841); by Friedrich **Bidder,** who discovered the ganglionic cells at the junction of the auricles and ventricles (1852)[1]; by Albert **von Bezold,** who demonstrated the accelerator nerves of the heart and their origin in the spinal cord (1862); and by Walter Holbrook **Gaskell,** who showed that the innervation of the heart is the same in cold-blooded and warm-blooded animals, and that the vagus nerve weakens the heart as, well as slows it (1882–4).   A striking experiment upon the heart-beat was made by Hermann **Stannius** (1808–83), of Hamburg, who, by placing a ligature at the junction of the auricle and the sinus venosus, brought the heart to a standstill, while a second ligature, applied to the auriculo-ventricular groove, caused the ventricle to beat again (1852).[2] In the early days of the neurogenic theory of the heart's action, the effect of the Stannius ligatures was supposed to be due to inhibition of the ganglia of Bidder and Remak, but the subject took on a new light with the discovery of the auriculo-ventricular bundle of His. The pulse was specially studied by Étienne-Jules **Marey** (1830–1904), who invented the sphygmograph, although the graphic method in pulse-examination had already been introduced by Karl Vierordt (1855). Other studies of the pulse were made by Landois, von Kries, and von Frey. Blood-pressure was especially investigated in Alfred Wilhelm Volkmann's *Die Hæmodynamik nach Versuchen* (1850), by Ludwig Traube (1818–76), who first described the rhythmic variations in the tone of the vasoconstrictor center (Traube-Hering waves) in 1865, and by Roy and Adami (1892).

Coagulation of the blood was investigated by Andrew Buchanan, who extracted the fibrin ferment (1845); and by Alexander Schmidt (1831–94), who gave it its name, but supposed that coagulation was due to the combination of fibrinogen and serum-globulin. This error was corrected by Olof Hammarsten (1841–   ), who showed that coagulation is accomplished by splitting up of the fibrinogen into fibrin and other substances (1875). Henry Newell **Martin** (1848–96), of Newry, Ireland, professor of biology at the Johns Hopkins University (1876–93), studied the effect of variations of blood-pressure and temperature upon the rate of beat of the mammalian heart (1882–83), His pupil and successor, William Henry **Howell** (1860–   ), of Baltimore. Maryland, has investigated such problems as the accelerating effect of increased venous pressure on the heart (1881), the life-history of the blood-corpuscles (1890), blood-serum deprived of proteids as an improvement on Ringer's solution (1893), and the rôle of the "hormones," antithrombin and thromboplastin, in the coagulation of the blood (1911). The art of keeping animal tissues active extravitally was introduced by Carl Ludwig in his perfusion experiments, and was perfected by **Sydney Ringer** (1835–1910), of Norwich, England, who showed that a frog's heart can be kept beating for long periods of time in a mixture of the chlorides of sodium, potassium, and calcium. This was afterward shown to be equally true of the mammalian heart.[3] Ringer's work showed the importance of the calcium salts in maintaining tissue activity, and "Ringer's solution," so widely used in physiological experiments, was the culture-medium in which Carrel latterly grew his "visceral organism."

---

[1] Stannius: Müller's Arch., Berlin, 1852, 163–177.   [2] *Ibid.*, 85–100.
[3] Ringer: Jour. Physiol., London, 1880–87, iii–vii, *passim.*

The most important work on **respiration** was done by Eduard F. W. **Pflüger** (1829–1910), of Hanau-am-Main, a pupil of Johannes Müller and du Bois Reymond, who succeeded Helmholtz as professor of physiology at Bonn in 1859, and held the chair the rest of his life. Under Pflüger, the new Institute of Physiology at Bonn was opened in 1878, and in 1868 he founded the famous *Archiv für die gesamte Physiologie* (Pflüger's Archiv), which ran through 130 volumes under his direction, and became the most popular journal of physiology in Germany.

Pflüger early made his mark as a master investigator by his monograph on electrotonus (1859).[1] By his experiments in crossing species (1883) he became the founder of experimental embryology. In his work on metabolism, he opposed the view of Voit that organized (tissue) proteid, in order to undergo metabolism, must first be converted into unorganized (circulating) proteid, maintaining just the opposite view, viz., that proteids can never undergo metabolism or assimilation except in the organized or stationary form; in other words, that proteid metabolism cannot take place until the material is built up into protoplasm. He adopted as a criterion for a proteid the capacity to maintain life and to enter into the composition of protoplasm, which would, of course, exclude the polypeptides, proteoses, protamins, and the poisonous proteids. Pflüger also made laborious researches to prove that glycogen does not originate from protein material, and, like Pavy, he was forced to surrender his position toward the end of his life. The most effective work of Pflüger and his pupils is the proof that the essential seat of respiration is not in the blood, but in the tissues. This was accomplished in his important memoirs on the gasometry of the blood (1866),[2] on the cause of dyspnea, apnea, and the mechanism of respiration (1868),[3] on the origin and rationale of the oxidative process in the animal organism (1872),[4] and on the heat-production and oxidation of living matter (1878).[5] He proved his thesis by showing that frogs, the blood of which had been entirely replaced by normal salt solution, gave off just as much carbon dioxide and took in just as much oxygen as normal control animals.[6] He invented new physiological instruments, such as the improved mercurial gas-pump (1865), the lung catheter (1872), the aërotonometer (1872), and the pneumonometer (1882).

Pflüger was of a combative disposition, fond of arguing for the sake of argument, and actually believing that science is advanced by vigorous controversy. This has been held to explain his somewhat unseasonable and ill-advised attacks on the neuron theory and on the work of Emil Fischer. He seems to have led the uneventful life of a man devoted exclusively to scientific research, and it is said that he spent his last days in bed, correcting the proof-sheets of papers sent to his Archiv.

Lavoisier, as we have seen, showed that **respiration** and combustion are analogous, and that both are essentially an oxidation with water and carbon dioxide as by-products (1771–80). Hassenfratz showed that the oxygen of the

---

[1] Untersuchungen über die Physiologie des Electrotonus, Berlin, 1859.

[2] Centralbl. f. d. med. Wissensch., Berlin, 1866, iv, 305–308.

[3] Arch. f. d. ges. Physiol., Bonn, 1868, i, 61–106.

[4] *Ibid.*, 1872, vi, 43; 190.

[5] *Ibid.*, 1878, xviii, 247–380.   [6] *Ibid.*, 1875, x, 251–367.

inspired air, being dissolved in the blood, takes up carbon and hydrogen from the tissues. The fact of tissue respiration was demonstrated by Gustav Magnus in 1837, who extracted oxygen and carbon dioxide from both arterial and venous |blood by means of a mercurial pump, from which he inferred that these gases are simply dissolved in the blood. Lothar Meyer, working in Ludwig's laboratory in 1857, obtained these results by the more refined method of heating the blood to extract the gases, and arrived at similar conclusions. Liebig, however, had pointed out, in 1851, that the blood gases were probably in loose combination with some unknown substance, and this substance Hoppe-Seyler subsequently obtained in crystalline form as hemoglobin (1862–64). The discovery of Sir George Gabriel Stokes that oxygen can be removed from hemoglobin by reducing agents proved that the latter is the agent of combination (1864). The combining agency of the carbon dioxide is still obscure. The extraction of gases from the blood has been further refined by means of the improved mercurial gas-pumps of Ludwig and Setchenoff (1859), Pflüger (1865), Grehant, and Leonard Hill (1895). The other gas of the blood, nitrogen, was shown to be in a state of simple solution by Lothar Meyer (1857), Pflüger (1864–68), and Paul Bert (1878). The difficult subject of the metabolism in respiration was investigated by Pettenkofer and Voit (1863), Zuntz (1880), Atwater and Rosa (1899), and Atwater and Benedict (1905).

The action of the intercostal muscles in respiration was first investigated by Haller, and, in geometric manner, by G. E. Hamberger (1748). The latter's view was confirmed experimentally by Henry Newell Martin and Edward M. Hartwell at the Johns Hopkins University (1879). The action of the vagus on respiration was first investigated by Isidor Rosenthal (1864), who showed that section of both vagi is always followed by deeper, slower breathing, while the amount of air taken in in unit time is the same as before. He held that the vagus contains two sets of fibers—one to contract the diaphragm, the other to relax it. In 1868, Hering and Breuer showed, by alternate closure of the trachea at the end of inspiration and expiration, that the mechanism of breathing is automatic and self-regulative, the distention and contraction of the lungs being, in themselves, a normal stimulus of the vagi, the effect which Rosenthal had obtained by stimulation of the divided nerve.

In 1889,[1] Henry **Head,** of London, working in Hering's laboratory at Prague, carried these experiments much further by such novel means as freezing the nerve or etherizing it inside a rubber tube, and the sum of his investigations is that the vagus acts like the governor of a steam engine in economizing the energies of respiration, preventing the center in the medulla from wearing itself out. This was shown by section of the vagi, which produced a condition of "spendthrift activity" in the respiratory center.

Normally, each inspiration stimulates the fibers which eventually inhibit it, and, at each expiration, the collapse of the lungs stimulates the inspiratory fibers, thus keeping up a steady automatic rate of respiration, which is largely due to the inhibitory fibers in the vagus. Head, the present editor of "Brain," has also done most important work on the cutaneous distribution of pain and tenderness in visceral disease (1893–96),[2] showing that the segmentation of the cutaneous areas affected by the different viscera (Head's zones) corresponds strikingly with those belonging to the root ganglia of the spinal nerves. With A. W. Campbell, he showed that herpes zoster is a hemorrhagic inflammation of the posterior nerve-roots and the homologous cranial ganglia (1900).[3]

---

[1] Head: J. Physiol., London, 1889, x, 1; 279.

[2] Brain: London, 1893, xvi, 1: 1894, xvii, 339: 1896, xix, 153.

[3] *Ibid.*, 1900, xxiii, 353–523, 17 pl.

In April, 1903,[1] he submitted to the unique experiment of division of his own left radial and external cutaneous nerves, in order to study the loss and restoration of sensation, which led to a new classification of the sensory paths.

Even before Pflüger, respiration of the tissues had been carefully investigated by Felix **Hoppe-Seyler** (1825–95), of Freiburg (Saxony), who is the greatest physiological chemist between Liebig and Emil Fischer. Hoppe-Seyler studied under the three Webers, Skoda, and Virchow, was Virchow's assistant in the Pathological Institute at Berlin (1856–64), professor of applied chemistry at Tübingen (1864–72), and professor of physiological chemistry at Strassburg (1872–95). He was founder of the *Zeitschrift für physiologische Chemie* (1877–95); also the author of a handbook of chemical analysis applied to physiology and pathology (1858), and an epoch-making treatise on physiological chemistry (1877–81).

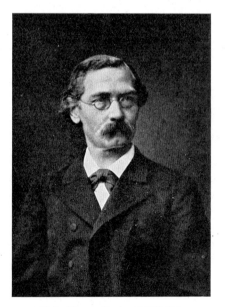

Felix Hoppe-Seyler (1825–95).

In 1854, he made investigations of the physics of percussion and auscultation, correcting certain errors of Skoda, and he also did some important work in inorganic chemistry and mineralogy. He is particularly remembered by his studies on the blood (1857–91), of which he made analyses for over thirty years. He first obtained hemoglobin in crystalline form, described the spectrum of oxyhemoglobin (1862), first ascertained the formulas of hemin, hematin, and hematoporphyrin (1863), discovered hemochromogen and methemoglobin (1864), and showed that hemoglobin is loosely combined with oxygen, but cannot be separated from carbon dioxide. He also made studies in metabolism, and constructed an apparatus for measuring gaseous interchanges. He was the first to observe the appearance of gas in the blood following a sharp and sudden fall of the atmospheric pressure. His investigations of pus and of pathological transudates led to the discovery of nuclein by his pupil Miescher, and of paranuclein by Lubavin. He first obtained lecithin in the pure state, and introduced the term "proteids." He investigated the chemistry of cartilage, and, in his laboratory, glycosamin was discovered by Ledderhose (1876) and chitosan by himself. He made important analyses of milk, bile, and urine, investigated the chemical products of fermentation, especially in yeast, and his study of chlorophyll was the starting-point of Ehrlich's work on the dynamics of the cell periphery. Personally, he seems to have been an attractive man, of happy, genial disposition.

---

[1] *Ibid.*, 1908, xxxi, 323–450.

Of his many pupils, Albrecht **Kossel** (1853–   ), of Rostock, professor of physiology at Marburg (1895–1901) and at Heidelberg (1901–   ), is to be remembered for his important work on the chemistry of the cell and its nucleus (1882–96), on nucleinic acid (1893), on albuminoids (1898), for the discovery of adenin, thymin, thymic acid, histidin, and agamatin, for his classification of the proteids, his studies of the fundamental units (*Bausteine*) of the protein molecule, and of the substitution products of albuminoids. He made important investigations in the chemistry of metabolism, and received the Nobel prize for medicine in 1910.

The **physiological chemistry** of the nineteenth century was rich in the discovery of new compounds, notably in the analysis and formulation of the decomposition products of proteids at the hands of Paul Schützenberger and others. After Kirchhoff had effected the hydrolysis of starch by diastase in 1815, Braconnot, in 1820, first hydrolyzed proteins by acids and discovered glycin, the simplest form of proteid.

Of the amino-acid constituents of proteins (Kossel's *Bausteine*), cystin was found in calculi by Wollaston (1810), tyrosin was discovered by Liebig (1846), glycocoll (1848) and alanin (1849) by Strecker, serin by Cramer (1865), phenylalanin by Schulze (1879), histidin by Kossel (1896), while tryptophan was named as a hypothetical product by Neumeister (1890), and isolated by Gowland Hopkins (1902). Leucin was discovered in putrefying cheese by Proust (1818), and named by Braconnot (1820). Both leucin and tyrosin were found in the pancreas after death by Virchow (1853), and in the living body by the clinician Frerichs (1855). Glutamic acid was obtained by Ritthausen and Kreutzer (1871), aspartic acid by Radziejewski and Salkowski (1873), ornithin by Jaffé (1877), argimin by Schulze and Steiger (1886), lysin by Drechsel (1889), prolin by Willstätter (1900) and Emil Fischer (1901), diaminobutyric acid and oxyprolin by Emil Fischer (1901–02).

The effect of animal enzymes on proteids was studied by Willy Kühne, Kossel, Drechsel, and others, and Schulze studied the effect of vegetable enzymes. Drechsel discovered that the protein molecule contains di- as well as mono-amino acids, and these were investigated by Kossel, Kutscher, and Emil Fischer. The nucleins were investigated by Worm Müller (1873) and Miescher (1874); the nucleic acids by Kossel (1893), Altmann (1889), Abderhalden, and Schittenhelm (1906); the albuminoids by Kossel (1898), Drechsel (1891), and Alberhalden (1905). β-oxybutyric acid was isolated by Eduard Külz (1884–87), and investigated in relation to diabetes by Ernst Stadelmann (1883) and Adolf Magnus-Levy (1899–1909). Acetone was discovered in diabetic urine by Wilhelm Petters (1857), and investigated by Carl Gerhardt (1865), Rudolf von Jaksch (1885), and, in the blood, by Adolf Kussmaul (1874). Max Jaffé discovered urobilin in the intestinal contents (1871) and indican in the urine (1877). Ehrlich introduced his diazo-reaction in 1882, and cryoscopy of the urine was introduced by Sandor Korányi in 1894. Myelopathic albumosuria (proteinuria) was described by Henry Bence Jones in 1848; acetonuria and diaceturia by von Jaksch (1885), and pentosuria by Ernst Salkowski (1895). The ptomains were investigated by Selmi, Gautier, Brieger, Vaughan, and Novy. The theory of the open carbon chain and the closed benzene ring was stated by August Kekulé in 1865, developed by van't Hoff and LeBel, and brilliantly applied to the structural theory of chlorophyll by Hoppe-Seyler, and to the "side-chain" theory of immunity by Paul Ehrlich.

Physical chemistry was made available for physiology through the labors of Sadi Carnot (1824), Robert Mayer (1842), Lord Kelvin (1848–52), Helmholtz (1847), Clausius (1850), Willard Gibbs (1872–78), van't Hoff (1887), Arrhenius (1887), Ostwald, and the chemists of the Dutch school. Its laws were applied to the physiology of muscles by Julius Bernstein (1902–08), to the question of surface tension by Isidor Traube (1910–11) and Macallum (1910–11), and to various biological problems by Jacques Loeb. The theory of osmosis and of semi-permeable membranes was investigated by Dutrochet (1827–35), Graham (1854–61), Moritz Traube (1867), Willard Gibbs (1876), van't Hoff and Arrhenius (1887), and H. J. Hamburger (1902–04), and colloids were studied by Graham, Siedentopf, and Zsigmondy.

Almost every great teacher of the subject has written a treatise on physiology. To the early period belong those of Magendie (1816–17), H. Mayo (1827), Joh. Müller (1834–40), Rudolf Wagner (1838–42), W. B. Carpenter (1842), G. Valentin (1844, 1846), Senhouse Kirkes (1848), F. C. Donders (1850), F. A. Longet (1850), and Wagner's *Handwörterbuch* (1842–53). In the second half of the century, we have those of Carl Ludwig (1852–56), J. C. Dalton (1859), W. Wundt (1865), T. H. Huxley (1866), Austin Flint, Jr. (1866–74), Sir Michael Foster (1877), L. Landois (1879–80), W. Stirling (1888), A. D. Waller (1891), E. H. Starling (1892), Max Verworn (1895), Robert Tigerstedt (1898), L. Luciani (1898–1903), W. H. Howell (1905), M. Duval and E. Gley (1906), H. Zwaardemaker (1910), and M. von Frey (1911). Foster's book is a masterpiece. The "Text-book" edited by Sir Edward A. Schäfer on the coöperative plan (London, 1898), is remarkable for its wonderful assemblage of historical data, in respect of which it has been likened to Haller's great "Elementa" of 1757–66. Of American treatises, that of William H. Howell (1905) is incomparably the best, on account of its clean-cut, lucid presentation of what is known.

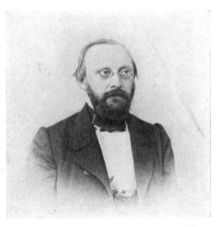

Rudolf Virchow (1821–1902). (From a carte de visite photograph in the Surgeon General's Library.)

The rise of modern medical science, German or other, is inseparably connected with the name of Rudolf **Virchow** (1821–1902), the founder of **cellular pathology.** A native of Schievelbein in Pomerania, Virchow graduated at Berlin in 1843, became Froriep's prosector at the Charité in 1845, full prosector in 1846, and, in 1847, founded the *Archiv für pathologische Anatomie*, known everywhere as Virchow's Archiv. His first paper in this periodical advanced the idea that an unproved hypothesis of any kind is a very leaky bottom for practical medicine to sail or trade upon, and scouted the notion that any one man is infallible in respect of judgment or knowledge. It is one of the strongest manifestos of the modern spirit in recent medicine. In 1848, Virchow was sent by the Prussian government to investigate the epidemic of typhus or "famine" fever then raging among the weavers of Upper Sile-

sia.   His exhaustive account of what he saw reminds us of the
piling up of horrors in Gerhart Hauptmann's social drama of
"Die Weber," and his recommendations included not only hygienic measures and a large charity for these unfortunates, but
filled an actual brief for democracy and freedom ("*volle und un-
umschränkte Demokratie . . . Bildung mit ihren Töchtern, Frei-
heit und Wohlstand*"). This bold pronouncement, along with
the tendencies of his semipolitical periodical, *Die medizinische
Reform* (1848–9), soon got Virchow into trouble with the governmental authorities, and, in 1849, he was deprived of his pro-
sectorship, obtaining, at the same time, through the offices of
the obstetrician Scanzoni, the chair of pathologic anatomy at
Würzburg.   Seven years later, after making a brilliant record
as lecturer and teacher, he was asked to come back to Berlin
upon honorable terms, and, in 1856, was duly installed as professor
of pathology at that University, at the same time assuming the
directorship of the Pathological Institute, which had been erected
for him.   Here he entered upon a career of almost unparalleled
activity in many directions.   He was a man of wide culture and
deepest human interests, and he soon became known everywhere
as anatomist and pathologist, epidemiologist and sanitarian, anthropologist and archeologist, editor and teacher, social reformer
and "old parliamentary hand."   He joined the Prussian Lower
House in 1862, and from 1880 until 1893 he served in the Reichstag
as a faithful and reliable representative of the rights of the people.
During the Franco-Prussian War, he organized the Prussian Am-
bulance Corps and superintended the erection of the army hospital
on the Tempelhof.   He had much to do with securing a good
sewage system for Berlin, and, as president of many different societies, he became easily the most influential medical personality
in the Prussian capital.   As he grew older, honors came to him from
all quarters, and, in 1899, he dedicated the Pathological Museum,
to which he gave his private collection of 23,066 preparations, each
of which had been prepared, labeled, and placed upon the shelves
by his own hand.   On his eightieth birthday, he received a purse
of 50,000 marks from his German colleagues, in aid of the Virchow
Institute, with a unique gold medal from the Emperor, and shortly
before his death he saw the completion of the splendid municipal
hospital in Berlin (January 15, 1902) which is now called by his
name.

    Virchow derived the inspiration for his life-work from Johannes
Müller, and what he accomplished was in every way worthy of his
great teacher.   In pathology, he had only Morgagni as a possible
competitor before him and no one after him.   His *Cellular-Pathol-
ogie* (1858) set in motion a new way of looking at the body as "a

cell-state in which every cell is a citizen," disease being "merely a conflict of citizens in this state, brought about by the action of external forces." Virchow's aphorism, "Omnis cellula e cellula," means that cell development is not discontinuous (as Schleiden and Schwann had supposed), and that there are no specific cells in disease, but only modifications of physiologic types. In other words, "A new growth of cells presupposes already existing cells." This morphologic view is the basis of his work on tumors (1863–67),[1] which treats of these formations as physiologically independent new-growths of either histioid or cellular structure. The two most prominent errors in the cellular pathology were the theories that the cell-contents are the controlling feature of the whole organism, and that there can be no diapedesis of blood-cells, which was afterward disproved by Cohnheim.

Virchow was the first to observe and define leukocytosis, and in 1845, simultaneously with the clinical record of John Hughes Bennett, he described leukemia as "white blood."[2] In 1846, he separated pyemia from septicemia, and between the years 1846 and 1856 created the doctrine of embolism,[3] his greatest single achievement in pathology, and one which is, in every sense, his very own. Before Virchow, as we have seen, both John Hunter and Cruveilhier saw thrombosis as a sequel of phlebitis, with the latter as the prime factor in pyemia also. Virchow revolutionized existing knowledge by showing that a thrombus is the primary essential condition in phlebitis. His studies of embolism were based upon experiment, and he was the first to recognize the cerebral and pulmonary varieties. In 1856, he demonstrated the embolic nature of the arterial plugs in malignant endocarditis, and attributed the condition to parasites. As a parasitologist, he also did good work on trichinosis (1859–70), and discovered the sarcinic and aspergillic forms of mycosis in the lungs and bronchial tubes. He also pointed out the true relationship between lupus and tuberculosis, introduced new pathological concepts like agenesia, heterotopia, ochronosis, and first described leontiasis ossea, hematoma of the dura mater, and the aortic hypoplasia with contracted heart in chlorotic maidens (1872). In 1861, he gave the name "arthritis deformans" to rheumatic gout. In histology, he made two important discoveries—the neuroglia (1846)[4] and the special lymphatic sheaths of the cerebral arteries (1851). He made hundreds of contributions to anthropology (his special hobby), from the great atlas of "Crania Ethnica Americana," prepared "in memory of Columbus and the Discovery of America" (1892), to well-known papers upon racial characters and abnormities, anthropometry, physical anthropology of the Germans, prehistoric finds, prehistoric syphilis, tattooing, and relics of the Trojan War. To medical history he contributed valuable monographs on the leprosoria and other hospitals in the Middle Ages, biographical studies of Morgagni, Johannes Müller, and Schönlein, and he was the first to write upon medicine in relation to the fine arts (1861).[5]

Personally, Virchow was a small, elastic, professorial figure,

---

[1] Virchow: Die krankhaften Geschwülste, Berlin, 1863–67.

[2] Froriep's Neue Notizen a. d. Geb. d. Nat. u. Heilk., Weimar, 1845, xxv, 151–155.

[3] Beitr. z. exper. Path. (Traube), Berlin, 1846, ii, 227–380, and Virchow: Ges. Abhandl., Frankfurt a. M., 1856, 219–732.

[4] Arch. f. path. Anat., Berlin, 1854, vi, 135–138.

[5] Virchow's Arch., Berlin, 1861, xxii, 190–192.

with snappy, black eyes, quick in mind and body, with a touch of the Slav, something of a martinet in the morgue or lecture-room, often transfixing inattention or incompetence with a flash of sarcasm. Yet he was generous, whole-souled, and broad-minded withal, and none who "made good" were ever lost from sight or memory. In extreme old age, Virchow, always "liberal in politics," became "reactionary in science"; but love of truth, generosity in word and deed, were the essence of his youth and mature manhood. All his life, he had been keen and ardent in controversy. He began his career by giving Rokitansky's theory of "crases" a wholesale slashing, with the result that the Viennese pathologist withdrew all reference to the matter from the second edition of his book and never afterward referred to it again. Yet there is no finer tribute in literature to the best features of Rokitansky's work than Virchow's. Then came his disputes with Hughes Bennett about leukemia, and his destruction of the Cruveilhier dogma that phlebitis is the whole of pathology. At the same time, he was cheerfully encouraging Cohnheim to combat the Virchow hypothesis of the non-migration of blood-cells. Believing that the nervous system is not the center of life and does not control the nutrition of peripheral parts, Virchow declined to see anything in Charcot's ataxic joint symptoms but a simple local lesion. He believed in the duality of tuberculosis. He opposed the Darwinian theory; and the new views of Koch and Behring about toxins and antitoxins were hardly acceptable to one who had obliterated the humoral pathology. The peculiarities of the Neanderthal skull were wrongly attributed by Virchow to the effects of disease. An accidental shelling of the Muséum d'histoire naturelle in Paris, during the war of 1870–71, led Quatrefages to write a sentimental pamphlet claiming that the Prussians were not a Germanic, but a barbaric, destructive Mongol race. This stirred Virchow's patriotism to the extent of instigating a colossal public census of the color of the hair and eyes in 6,000,000 German school-children, the solemn official character of which frightened some of the children out of their wits. The sight of a copy of Grimmelshausen's "Simplicissimus" is said to have caused him the same indignation that Wordsworth experienced when he heard the first line of Keats's "Ode to a Grecian Urn." These vagaries may be set off by the generosity of his touching defense of Pasteur, his discriminating tribute to the American Army Medical Department, or the laurel-wreaths of praise which he has laid upon the tombs of so many of his predecessors and contemporaries. Above all, he was, in respect of civic courage, an ideal modern man. He did not believe in a characterless, stock-jobbing bourgeoisie, but warmly espoused the cause of those who labor for the common good of all. His lifelong championship of the rights of industrial humanity, valiantly upheld in the very stronghold of the Prussian military government, shows the kind of fiber he was made of.

Of Virchow's pupils, the most eminent was Julius **Cohnheim** (1839–84), of Demmin, Pomerania, who, after serving as a Prussian army surgeon in the Austrian war (1864–65), became an assistant in the Pathological Institute, and was subsequently professor of pathology at Kiel (1868–72), Breslau (1872–78), and Leipzig (1878–84). Under Willy Kühne, Cohnheim made an important investigation on the sugar-forming ferments (1863),[1] but his inaugural dissertation on the inflammation of serous membranes (1861) marks his bent as a pioneer in experimental histology and pathology. He introduced the method of freezing fresh preparations in microscopical work, investigated the nerve-endings in muscle by means of silver salts (1863–65), discovered the mosaic fields in cross-sections of muscle which bear his name (1865), and first used gold salts, with brilliant results, in his studies of the sensory nerve-endings in the cornea (1867). His monographs on inflammation and suppuration (1867–73)[2] revolutionized pathology, showing, in direct opposition to the teaching of Virchow, that the essential feature of in-

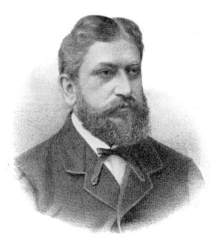

Julius Cohnheim (1839–84).

flammation is the passage of white blood-cells through the walls of the capillaries, and that pus and pus-cells are formed in this way from the blood. Diapedesis had already been noticed by Addison, but Cohnheim's experiments traced the direct migration of the stained leukocytes to a center of inflammation in the cornea. Valuable papers on venous stasis (1867) and on the relation of the terminal arteries to embolic processes (1872) followed, but the summit of Cohnheim's experimental achievement was his successful inoculation of tuberculosis

---

[1] Arch. f. path. Anat. (etc.), Berlin, 1863, xxvii, 241–253.
[2] Neue Untersuchungen über die Entzündung, Berlin, 1873.

in the anterior chamber of the eye of the rabbit (1877),[1] which
Weigert wittily described as a demonstration *"in oculo ad oculos."*
Two years before, Robert Koch had demonstrated his cultures
of anthrax bacillus, and Cohnheim made the prophetic statement that Koch would surpass all others in this field. The last
years of Cohnheim's life were clouded by severe complications of
gout, an old enemy, and his brilliant career was cut short at the
early age of forty-five. He is described as a man of robust,
cheerful, energetic disposition, swift and sure of speech, with great
powers of wit and sarcasm. Among his pupils were Heidenhain,
Litten, Lichtheim, Welch, Ehrlich, Neisser, and Weigert at Breslau, and, at Leipzig, Roy and Councilman.

Carl **Weigert** (1845–1904), of Münsterberg, Silesia, is memorable for his investigations of the pathological anatomy of smallpox (1874–75)[2] and Bright's disease (1879),[3] and by the fact that
he was the first to stain bacteria (1871),[4] in which he later had
great success with anilin colors (1875).[5] He introduced many
improvements in the differential staining of the nervous system,
notably with acid fuchsin (1882). He also made investigations
of the neuroglia (1890–95), and of coagulation-necrosis (1880),
described tuberculosis of the veins (1882), and stated the well-
known quantitative "law" that the amount of repair in an injured
tissue is always in excess of what is needed.

Among the special pathological studies of the period were those of Ludwig
Traube (1855), Hermann Senator (1873), Carl von Liebermeister (1875), and
Ernst von Leyden (1870–79) on the pathology of fever, Peter Ludwig Panum
(1820–85) on the experimental pathology of embolism (1863–64), Thomas
Bevill Peacock on malformations of the human heart (1866), Carl Thiersch on
phosphoric necrosis of bones (1867), Wilhelm Waldeyer on the development
of cancer (1867–72), F. D. von Recklinghausen on neurofibroma (1882)
Paul Grawitz on the origin of renal tumors from suprarenal tissues (1884),
Julius Wolff on the law of transformation in bones (1892), Paul Ehrlich and
Adolf Lazarus on anemia (1898). Among Americans, William Pepper (1843–
98) described the changes in the bone-marrow in pernicious anemia (1875),
William Henry Welch (1850–   ) investigated acute edema of the lungs
(1877) and embolism and thrombosis (1899), Reginald Heber Fitz (1843–1913)
gave conclusive demonstrations of the pathology of perforating inflammation
of the vermiform appendix (1886), hemorrhagic pancreatitis with fat necrosis
(1889), and described intrapleural lipoma of the mediastinum. Ludvig
Hektoen (1863–   ), of Westby, Wisconsin, has done good work in the
experimental pathology of hepatic cirrhosis (1901), measles (1911), and the
isolation of antibodies.

Following the eighteenth-century works of Astruc (1743), Gaub (1758),

---

[1] Die Tuberkulose vom Standpunkt der Infectionslehre, Leipzig, 1880.

[2] Weigert: Anatomische Beiträge zur Lehre von den Pocken, Breslau,
1874–75.

[3] Samml. klin. Vorträge, Leipzig, 1879, No. 162, 163 (Innere Med., No. 55),
1411–1460).

[4] Centralbl. f. d. med. Wissensch., Berlin, 1871, ix, 609–611.

[5] Jahresb. d. schles. Gesellsch. f. vaterl. Cultur, 1875, Breslau, 1876, liii,
229.

Morgagni (1761), Matthew Baillie (1791), and Kurt Sprengel (1795–97), pathology was the subject of special treatises by Carl Friedrich Burdach (1808), J. W. H. Conradi (1811), A.-F. Chomel (1817), E. D. A. Bartels (1819), J. C. C. F. M. Lobstein (1829–33), Herbert Mayo (1836), and Thomas Hodgkin (1836–40). The first exhaustive treatise on pathology in English was that of Samuel David Gross (Boston, 1839), which was followed by the treatises of Rokitansky (1842–46), Jacob Henle (1846–51), Alfred Stillé (1848), Salvatore De Renzi (1856), Virchow (1858), Samuel Wilks (1859), P. Uhle and E. Wagner (1862), Eduard Rindfleisch (1867–69), Victor Cornil and L. Ranvier (1869–76), F. V. Birch-Hirschfeld (1876), Cohnheim (1877–80), Ernst Ziegler (1881), Sims Woodhead (1883), Henri Hallopeau (1884), Francis Delafield and T. Mitchell Prudden (1885), Edwin Klebs (1887), D. J. Hamilton (1889–94), V. V. Podwyssotsky (1891–94), Anton Weichselbaum (1892), Otto Bollinger (1896–97), Alfred Stengel (1898), Ludvig Hektoen and David Riesman (1901–02), Guido Banti (1905–07), and John George Adami (1908–12). Noteworthy atlases of pathological illustration are those of Johann Friedrich Meckel (1817–26), Jean Cruveilhier (1829–42), Alexander Auvert (1856), F. A. Thierfelder (1872–81), The Sydenham Society (1877–1906), Alfred Kast and Theodor Rumpel (1892–97), and Paul Grawitz (1893). Important works on experimental pathology are those of Ludwig Traube (1871–78), Claude Bernard (1872), Salomon Stricker (1877), Victor Paschutin (1885), and Paul Ehrlich (1909); and the monographs of August Hirsch (1860–64), Andrew Davidson (1892), and Frank G. Clemow (1903) on geographical pathology, John William Ballantyne on fetal pathology (1902–4), F. B. Mallory and J. H. Wright on pathological technic (1897), deserve mention.

The founders of **bacteriology** were Louis Pasteur and Robert Koch, the former being also the pioneer of the modern theory of preventive inoculation against disease, while to the latter we owe the development of the correct theory of specific infectious diseases.

Before the time of Pasteur, Leeuwenhoek had seen protozoa (1675) and bacteria (1687) under the microscope. A. Bassi showed that silkworm disease is due to the presence of microörganisms (1836), John Goodsir described sarcinæ in the stomach (1842), Casimir Davaine the microörganisms of anthrax (1865), and Ferdinand Cohn the morphological and botanical characters of bacteria (1870). Before the time of Koch, Kircher (1658), Plenciz (1762), and Henle (1840) had announced the theory of a contagium animatum, Hermann Klencke had shown that tuberculosis may be transmitted by cow's milk (1846), Jean-Antoine Villemin (1827–92) had demonstrated that the tubercular virus is specific and inoculable, in a series of masterly experiments (1868) which were confirmed by the further investigations of Edwin Klebs (1873), L.-A. Thaon and J.-J. Grancher (1873), and Julius Cohnheim (1880).

Louis **Pasteur** (1822–95) was born at Dôle (Jura), where his father, one of Napoleon's old soldiers, was a local tanner. As a youth, Pasteur was remarkably good at portrait sketching, but was otherwise only a harmless, enthusiastic fisherman. Awakening to the call of duty, he went to study at Besançon, where he acquired his interest in chemistry, and graduated at the École normale at Paris in 1847. After this he was successively professor of physics at the Lyceum at Dijon (1848), professor of chemistry (1852–54) at the University of Strassburg, dean and professor of chemistry in the Faculty of Sciences at Lille (1854–57), director of scientific studies at the École normale at Paris (1857–63), professor of geology and chemistry at the École des beaux-arts (1863–67), professor of chemistry at the Sorbonne (1867–89), and director of the Institut Pasteur (1889–95). As set forth in the inscriptions on the arches over his tomb, Pasteur is memorable for his work on molecular dyssymmetry (1848), fermentation (1857), spontaneous generation (1862), diseases of wine (1863), diseases of silkworms (1865), microörganisms in beer (1871), virulent diseases (anthrax, chicken cholera, 1877), and preventive vaccinations (1880), particularly of hydrophobia (1885).

The first of these, his classic investigations of the conversion of dextro-tartaric acid into the inactive forms (racemic and mesotartaric acids), and

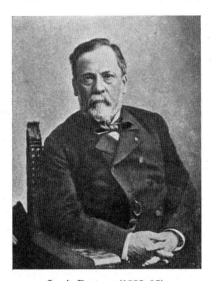

Louis Pasteur (1822–95).

his discovery of the splitting up of racemic acid into right- and left-handed tartaric acid by means of optically active substances, gained him the Rumford medal of the Royal Society (1856), and undoubtedly led to the work of van't Hoff and Le Bel on stereochemistry or chemistry in space. They also led Pasteur to the study of ferments and microörganisms through his initial experiment of inducing fermentation in racemic acid by means of albumen, causing the destruction of the dextro-rotatory product by fermentative microörganisms. From this he proceeded to those studies of beer yeasts and lactic-acid fermentation which resulted in the discovery of lactic-acid bacteria, and confuted the errors which Liebig and even Helmholtz had made in regard to the significance of fermentation. He next discovered the anaërobic character of the bacteria of butyric fermentation, introducing the concepts of aërobism and anaërobism. A comparison of flasks of yeast in nutrient media, one of which had been sterilized, demonstrated the rôle of microörganisms in changing atmospheric oxygen into carbon dioxide (1861). His dispute with Pouchet about spontaneous generation was obscured by the fact that Pouchet's hay infusion was more difficult to sterilize than the yeast infusion employed by Pasteur, but the latter prevailed in his contention,[1] winning a prize and membership in the Academy of Sciences. About this time, he discovered that the pellicle so necessary to the formation of vinegar from wine consists of minute, rod-like microörganisms (*Mycoderma aceti*). The investigation of acetic fermentation[2] confuted Liebig's mechanical theory of the latter process, and led Pasteur to study the causes detrimental to the three great industries of his country, those of wine, silk, and wool. In 1867, the wine industry of

---

[1] Compt. rend. Acad. d. sc., Paris, 1860, l, 303; 849; li, 348; 675: 1864, lviii, 21: 1865, lxi, 1091.

[2] Études sur la vin, Paris, 1866.

France was worth 500,000,000 francs to the nation, and this gain was due to Pasteur's discovery that the ageing of wine by microörganisms can be prevented by partial heat sterilization (Pasteurization) at a temperature of 55° to 60° C., without any alteration of the taste or bouquet of the vintage (1863–65). This process is now applied to all perishable foods, and is of inestimable importance in the nutrition of infants. In 1849, the silkworm industry of France began to be crippled by the disease *pébrine.* By 1861, the annual revenue from this source had sunk from 130,000,000 to 8,000,000 francs, and enormous sums were spent in importing healthy silkworm eggs from Spain, Italy, and Japan. The mulberry plantations in the Cevennes were abandoned, and the state was petitioned, in 1865, to remedy the evil. In a little house near Alais Pasteur and his assistants worked for five years on an apparently insoluble problem, and even after he had discovered the cause and prevention of pébrine there came his burst of despair: " *Il y a deux maladies!* " The second disease, *flâcherie*, was conquered in time,[1] but at a terrible cost, the death of one of his daughters and the worry incident to harsh criticism of his failures bringing on a severe attack of paralysis. Even his pleasure in such tokens of recognition as a degree of M.D. from Bonn, a prize from the Austrian government, membership in the Royal Society, and a nomination as senator, was spoiled by the outbreak of the Franco-Prussian War. He returned the Bonn diploma and took up the study of the spoiling of beer by microörganisms, again showing the advantages of Pasteurization.[2] About this time, his definition of a ferment as "a living form which originates from a germ" was contested in a posthumous essay of Claude Bernard's,[3] but, in 1874, Lister had sent him the celebrated letter acknowledging the value of his work in relation to antiseptic surgery. Thus Pasteur was gradually transformed from a chemist to a medical man, particularly in his mode of attacking the problem of infectious diseases. In his studies on anthrax, he was preceded by Davaine, who discovered the bacillus and showed that the virulence of the disease was in proportion to the number of bacteria present (1850–65); by Klebs, who indicated that anthrax virus is non-filterable, since the filtrate will not produce the disease (1871), and by Koch, who first cultivated pure cultures of anthrax bacilli, described their full life-history and their relation to the disease (1877). Pasteur confirmed Koch's results, and disposed of the controversial question of a separate virus by carrying the bacilli through a hundred generations and producing anthrax from the term of the series.[4] At the same time, he discovered, with Joubert and Chamberland, the bacillus of malignant edema (*vibrion septique*), the first find of an anaërobic microörganism of a pathogenic character; and he showed the relation of animal heat to bacterial virulence. As he cared nothing for the morphological aspects of bacteriology, it is sometimes forgotten that he discovered the Staphylococcus pyogenes in boils as "*microbe en amas de grains*," and the Streptococcus pyogenes in puerperal septicemia as "*microbe en chapelet de grains*" (1878–9).[5] His discovery of preventive inoculation was due to the accidental fact that virulent cultures of chicken cholera virus, during a vacation from the laboratory, became sterile or inactive, and, when injected, were found to act as preventive vaccines against a subsequent injection of a virulent character. The attenuated virus could be carried through several generations and still maintain its immunizing property. In 1881, he succeeded in producing a vaccine against anthrax, injection of which lowered the mortality-rate to 1 per cent. in sheep and to 0.34 per cent. in horned cattle. Experiments with the viruses of anthrax, chicken cholera, and swine measles (*rouget des porcs*) brought out the principle that the pathogenic properties of a virus can be attenuated or heightened by successive passages through the bodies of appropriate animals, and led to one of the most luminous thoughts in the history of science—that the origin

---

[1] Études sur les maladies des vers à soie, Paris, 1870.

[2] Études sur la bière, Paris, 1876.

[3] Bernard: Rev. scient., Paris, 1879, xv, 49–56.

[4] Compt. rend. Acad. d. sc., Paris, 1880, xci, 86; 455; 697: 1881, xcii, 209.

[5] *Ibid.*, 1880, xc, 1033–1044.

or extinction of infectious disease in the past (syphilis, for instance) may be simply due to the strengthening or weakening of its virus by external conditions, or in some such way as the above. This principle was applied with success against anthrax at the sheep-folds near Chartres, and in preventive vaccinations against hydrophobia, the culture-medium being the spinal marrow of the infected animal.[1] Pasteur's first patient was Joseph Meister, an Alsatian boy, bitten all over by a rabid dog, who was treated with success in July, 1885. Shortly afterward, the Pasteur Institute was opened, and special institutes for hydrophobia inoculations were founded all over the world. Here Pasteur labored almost to the end of his life, with such brilliant pupils as Metchnikoff, Roux, Yersin, Calmette, Chamberland, and Pottevin. With Ch. Chamberland, he devised the celebrated filter which is called after him, while Émile Roux did epoch-making work on the diphtheria antitoxin, Metchnikoff on phagocytosis and the lactic-acid bacillus, Alexandre Yersin on the plague bacillus, Albert Calmette on preventive inoculations against snake-bites.

Pasteur's last years were crowded with honors from all parts of the world, and, after his death, an appropriate mausoleum for his remains, copied from the tomb of Galla Placidia at Ravenna, was built in the Pasteur Institute by his family. Deeply religious, intensely serious, endowed with a mind the quality of which Roux has compared to the action of a blow-pipe flame, Pasteur was a *sensitif*, who suffered unduly, in his life, from the captious cavillings of lesser men.His return of the diploma from the genial Rhineland University of Bonn can be excused only by his child-like, high-strung devotion to his native land. Literary snobbery has descanted sufficiently upon his "peasant origin," but the man himself was a gentleman of the type described by Wordsworth and Cardinal Newman, one who never inflicts wanton or needless pain upon others. His sympathy with the sufferings of dumb animals was of a kind which, said Roux, might have seemed comic had it not been touching. We have the testimony of his pupils as to his power of establishing an immediate sympathetic relation between himself and any one sincerely interested in his work, and his sympathies extended, circle-wise, as in Emerson's parable, from the intimate group of his family and pupils, to embrace the people (even the animals) of his native land and the entire human race.[2] His humanity was of that rare and noble kind which, in Emerson's words, "approves itself no mortal, but a native of the deeps of absolute and inextinguishable being."

Robert **Koch** (1843–1910), of Klausthal, Hannover, was educated in the gymnasium of his native town, and took his medical degree at Göttingen (1866), where he was profoundly influenced by the teachings of Jacob Henle, whose theory of contagion (1840)

---

[1] Compt. rend. Acad. d. sc., Paris, 1885, ci, 765: 1886, cii, 459; 835; ciii, 777.

[2] The writer once had the privilege of hearing an account of Pasteur in which these qualities were very strikingly set forth by one of his pupils.

may have started Koch upon his life-work in science. After serving in the Franco-Prussian War, he became district physician (*Kreisphysicus*) at Wollstein, where he varied the monotony of long journeyings over rough country roads by private microscopic studies. He began with anthrax, and, in April, 1876, wrote to the eminent botanist Ferdinand Cohn at Breslau to the effect that he had worked out the complete life-history and sporulation of the anthrax bacillus. About a week later, at Cohn's invitation, he gave a three-day demonstration of his culture methods and results at the Botanical Institute (Breslau), in the presence of Cohn, Weigert, Auerbach, Traube, Cohnheim, and others. The latter declared that Koch's was the greatest bacteriological discovery yet made, and Cohn immediately published his paper in his Beiträge (July, 1876).[1] This memoir demonstrated that the anthrax bacillus is the cause of the disease, and that pure cultures grown through several generations outside the body can produce it in various animals. Koch's results were violently opposed by Paul Bert, but completely confirmed by Pasteur. In November, 1877, Koch published his methods of fixing and drying bacterial films on cover-slips, of staining them with Wei-gert's anilin dyes, of staining flagellæ, and of photo-

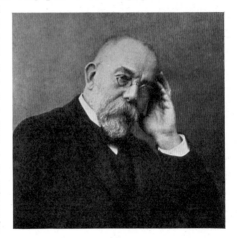

Robert Koch (1843–1910). (Courtesy of Captain Henry J. Nichols, U. S. Army.)

graphing bacteria for identification and comparison.[2] In 1878, appeared his great memoir on the etiology of traumatic infectious diseases,[3] in which the bacteria of six different kinds of surgical infection are described, with the pathological findings, each microörganism breeding true through many generations *in vitro* or in animals. These three memoirs elevated Koch to the front rank in medical science, and, through Cohnheim's influence, he was appointed to a vacancy in the Imperial Health Department (*Kaiserliches Gesund-*

---

[1] Cohn's Beitr. z. Morphol. d. Pflanzen, Breslau, 1876–7, ii, 277–310, 1 pl.

[2] *Ibid.*, 399–434, 3 pl.

[3] Untersuchungen über die Aetiologie der Wundinfektionskrankheiten Berlin, 1878.

heitsamt), with Löffler and Gaffky as assistants, in 1880. Here, in 1881, he produced his important paper upon the method of obtaining pure cultures of organisms by spreading liquid gelatin with meat infusion upon glass plates, forming a solid coagulum.[1]   When Koch demonstrated his plate cultures at the International Medical Congress in London, Pasteur is said to have rushed forward with the exclamation: *C'est un grand progrès!* and so it proved.   The year 1882 was marked by the discovery of the tubercle bacillus by special culture and staining methods.   This paper[2] contains the first statement of "Koch's postulates," establishing the pathogenic character of a given microörganism.   About the same time, he and his assistants had introduced steam sterilization by dry heat. In 1883, Koch, at the head of the German Cholera Commission, visited Egypt and India, discovered the cholera vibrio,[3] its transmission by drinking-water, food, and clothing, and incidentally found the microörganisms of Egyptian ophthalmia or infectious conjunctivitis (Koch-Weeks bacillus, 1883),[4] for which results he received a donation of 100,000 marks from the Prussian State. In 1885, he was appointed professor of hygiene and bacteriology at the University of Berlin, where his laboratories were crowded with bright pupils from all over the world, among whom were Gaffky, Löffler, Pfeiffer, Welch and Kitasato.

At the tenth International Medical Congress at Berlin, in 1890, Koch announced his belief that he had found a remedy for tuberculosis. The introduction of tuberculin,[5] his one mistake, in that it was prematurely considered, was hailed all over the world as an event of the greatest scientific moment, and honors and felicitations of all kinds were showered upon its discoverer.   Although he himself had limited his claims to the possible cure of early cases of phthisis, the great hopes which had been entertained of the remedy were not realized in time, and the number of failures and fatal cases impaired the confidence of the profession, but abated little of Koch's great reputation, especially after the discovery that tuberculin is the most reliable means of diagnosis.   In 1891, the Institute for Infectious Diseases was founded in Berlin, and remained under his direction until he resigned in 1904, in favor of his pupil Gaffky.   In 1892, his ideas were applied in fighting the cholera epidemic at Hamburg, and in 1893 he wrote an important paper on water-borne epidemics, showing how they may be largely prevented by proper filtration.[6]   In 1896, he investigated Rinderpest in South Africa at the request of the English government, devised a method of preventive inoculation, and

---

[1] Mitth. a. d. kaiserl. Gesundheitsamte, Berlin, 1881, i, 1–48, 14 pl.

[2] Berl. klin. Wochenschr., 1882, xxi, 221–230.   The bacillus was probably seen, though not positively identified in a causal relation, by Aufrecht (1881) and Baumgarten (1882).

[3] Deutsche med. Wochenschr., Berlin, 1884, x, 725–728.

[4] Wien. med. Wochenschr., 1883, xxxiii, 1550; also described by John E. Weeks, in Arch. Ophth., New York, 1886, xv, 441–451.

[5] Deutsche med. Wochenschr., Leipzig u. Berlin, 1890, xvi, 1029: 1891, xvii, 101; 1189.

[6] Ztschr. f. Hyg. u. Infektionskr., Leipzig, 1893, xiv, 393–426.

made valuable studies of Texas fever, blackwater fever, tropical malaria, surra, and plague.[1] In 1897, he produced his new tuberculin (T. R.), and in 1898 he investigated malarial fever in Italy. At the London Tuberculosis Congress (1900) he announced his view that the bacilli of bovine and human tuberculosis, which had been separated and studied by Theobald Smith in 1898, are not identical, claiming that there is little danger of transmission of the bovine type to man. These views were reiterated at the Washington Congress of 1908, and on both occasions aroused violent controversy, the general trend of opinion at present being provisionally in favor of Koch. In 1902, he studied Rhodesian red-water fever (*Küstenfieber*), horse-sickness, trypanosomiasis, and recurrent fever in German East Africa, and, in the same year, established methods of controlling typhoid which have been adopted almost everywhere.

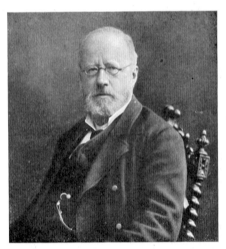

Koch received the Nobel Prize in 1905, and, in 1906, visited Africa again, at the head of the Sleeping Sickness Commission, introducing atoxyl for the treatment of the disease. Although he was honored by a membership in the Prussian Academy of Sciences and the title of *Excellenz*, he was not happy in the later years of his life. Certain changes in his domestic arrangements estranged many of

Edwin Klebs (1834–1913). (Courtesy of Dr. Arnold C. Klebs, Lausanne, Switzerland.)

his friends, and subjected him to harsh criticism, which he bore with stoicism and dignity, but which told upon him in the end. He died of heart-failure on May 27, 1910, at the age of sixty-seven. His body was cremated at his own request, and his ashes deposited in the Institute which he had founded. In appearance, Koch was the typical German savant of the Prussian type, in character dignified, modest, and fair-minded, altogether one of the greatest men of science that his country has produced.

Edwin **Klebs** (1834–1913), of Königsberg, Prussia, one of the earlier assistants of Virchow at Berlin (1861–66), who became professor of pathology at Bern (1866), Würzburg (1871), Prague (1873), Zürich (1882), and Chicago (Rush Medical College, 1896), is, with Pasteur, perhaps the most important precursor in the bacterial theory of infection; indeed, did most to win the pathologists over to this view. He saw the typhoid bacillus before Eberth

---

[1] Reiseberichte über Rinderpest (etc.), Berlin, 1898.

(1881),[1] the diphtheria bacillus before Löffler (1883),[2] made solid cultures of bacteria, and investigated the pathology of traumatic infections before Koch (1871),[3] inoculated monkeys with syphilis before Metchnikoff (1878),[4] and, in his experiments on anthrax (1871)[5] and other diseases, he was one of the first to experiment with the filtrates of bacterial cultures.   He wrote two text-books on pathology (1869–76, 1887–89), monographs on bacteriology in relation to gunshot wounds, based upon his experiences in the Franco-Prussian war (1872), on tumors (1877) and gigantism (1884), made many investigations on tuberculosis, and he was, with Gerlach, the first to produce bovine infection of *Perlsucht* by feeding with milk (1873).[6]   He investigated the genesis of endocarditis (1878), and his studies of malarial fever (with Tommasi Crudeli, 1879) were translated for the Sydenham Society. He experimented with various products for the treatment of tuberculosis, and was the first to experiment with the therapeutic possibilities of the tubercle bacilli of cold-blooded animals (1900). The original discoveries of Klebs, "so often (as Osler says) a pioneer," had great heuristic value in their day, and undoubtedly stimulated Koch and others in their work.

Friedrich **Löffler** (1852–   ), of Frankfort on the Oder, was for many years a Prussian army surgeon, and eventually became professor of hygiene at Greifswald (1888).   He discovered the bacteria of erysipelas in swine (1882–83),[7] and glanders (1882)[8]; established the causal relation of the diphtheria bacillus (1884),[9] differentiating it from the organisms causing the disease in doves and calves; eradicated the field-mouse plague in Thessaly by means of the Bacillus typhi murium (1892); and, in his investigations of the foot and mouth disease (1898),[10] he was able to prove experimentally that the latter is caused by a filterable virus, thus establishing this concept and introducing a preventive inoculation against the disease (1899).   He wrote an admirable history of bacteriology (1887), still unfinished.

George **Gaffky** (1850   ), of Hannover, also a Prussian army

---

[1] Klebs: Arch. f. exper. Path. u. Pharmakol., Leipzig, 1880, xii, 231: 1881, xiii, 381, 3 pl.

[2] Verhandl. d. Cong. f. innere Med., Wiesbaden, 1883, 139–174.

[3] Cor.-Bl. f. schweiz. Aerzte, Bern, 1871, i, 241–246.

[4] Arch. f. exper. Path. u. Pharmakol., Leipzig, 1878–79, x, 161–221, 4 col. pl.

[5] Cor.-Bl. f. schweiz. Aerzte, Bern, 1871, i, 279 (Nachschrift).

[6] Arch. f. exper. Path. u. Pharmakol., Leipzig, 1873, i, 163–180.

[7] Löffler: Arb. a. d. k. Gesundheitsamte, Berlin, 1885, i, 46–55.

[8] Deutsche med. Wochenschr., Leipzig u. Berlin, 1882, viii, 407.

[9] Mitth. a. d. k. Gesundheitsamte, Berlin, 1884, ii, 451–499.

[10] Centralbl. f. Bakteriol., 1. Abt., Jena, 1898, xxiii, 371–391.

surgeon, became associated with Koch in Berlin, and, after filling the chair of hygiene at Giessen (1888) for several years, succeeded Koch as director of the Hygienic Institute. He made important studies of experimental septicemia (1881), cholera, and anthrax, and is a well-recognized modern authority on infectious diseases and public hygiene.

The work of these men led to a wonderful output of epoch-making discoveries in bacteriology and parasitology, which constitute one of the chief glories of nineteenth century medicine. These are the establishment of the causal relations of the bacteria of leprosy by Armauer Hansen (1871–74), of gonorrhea by Albert Neisser (1879), of typhoid fever by Carl Joseph Eberth (1880), of lobar pneumonia by Pasteur (1880–81), George Miller Sternberg (1880–81), Albert Fränkel (1884), and Carl Friedländer (1883), of glanders by Friedrich Löffler (1882–86), of erysipelas by Friedrich Fehleisen (1883), of swine erysipelas by Löffler (1882–86), of diphtheria by Edwin Klebs (1883) and Friedrich Löffler (1883–84), of cholera nostras by Dittmar Finkler and J. Prior (1884), of tetanus by Arthur Nicolaier (1884), of Bacillus coli infection by Theodor Escherich (1886), of Malta fever by Sir David Bruce (1887), of cerebrospinal meningitis by Anton Weichselbaum (1887), of fibrinous pneumonia by Nicolaus Gamaleia (1888), of influenza by Richard Pfeiffer (1892), of Bacillus aërogenes infection by William Henry Welch and George H. F. Nuttall (1892), of bubonic plague by Shibamiro Kitasato and A. Yersin (1894), of dysentery by Isagiyoi Shiga (1897), of bovine peripneumonia by Edmond Nocard and Émile Roux (1898), and of whooping-cough by Jules Bordet and Octave Gengou (1906).[1] The microörganisms of the surgical and puerperal infections were discovered and investigated by Pasteur (1878–9), Koch (1878), Gaffky (1881), and Welch (1892). Toxins were first isolated and named (typhotoxine and tetanine) by Ludwig Brieger in 1888. The bactericidal effect of blood-serum was discovered by Hans Buchner (1889), bacteriolysis by Richard Pfeiffer (1894), bacterial hemolysis by Jules Bordet (1898). L. Landois, in 1875, made the important discovery that animal serum will hemolyze human blood. The subsequent discoveries of Maragliano (1892), Landsteiner (1901), and Eisenberg (1901), that the sera of diseased, and even of normal, donors, will hemolyze alien blood, have revolutionized the whole subject of transfusion. Anaphylaxis was discovered by Edward Jenner (1798) and François Magendie (1839), and investigated by C. Richet (1903), Rosenau and Anderson (1906), and von Pirquet (1907). Bacterial agglutination was discovered by Max Gruber and Ferdinand Widal (1896). **Parasitology** was greatly advanced by such monumental treatises as those of K. A. Rudolphi on entozoa (1808–10), G. F. H. Küchenmeister on cestodes (1853) and parasites in man (1855), Carl Theodor von Siebold on teniæ and hydatids (1854), Casimir Davaine on entozoa in man and animals (1860), Thomas Spencer Cobbold on entozoa (1864), Rudolf Leuckart on human parasites (1867), and Raphael Blanchard on medical zoölogy (1886–90). Of parasites producing disease, that of favus was discovered by Schönlein (1839), of psorospermosis by Johannes Müller (1841), of tinea favosa (alopecia) by David Grüby (1841–44), of anchylostomiasis by Angelo Dubini (1843), of recurrent fever by Otto Obermeier (1873), of malarial fever by Alphonse Laveran (1880), of parasitic hemoptysis (paragonomiasis) by Erwin Baelz (1880), of Texas fever (piroplasmosis) by Theobald Smith (1889).[2] The parasite of aspergillosis was discovered and described by Bennett in 1842, that of actinomycosis in man by von Langenbeck (1848) and James Israel (1878), that in cattle by Otto Bollinger (1876), the identity of both being established by Ponfick (1880), that of Nocardiosis by Edmond Nocard

---

[1] For bibliographical references to these discoveries see Index Catalogue, Surgeon General's Library, 1912, 2. series, xvii, pp. 135–137.

[2] *Ibid.*, pp. 138, 139.

(1888–93), that of blastomycosis by Thomas Casper Gilchrist (1896), and that of sporotrichosis by Benjamin R. Schenck (1898). The two latter discoveries were made in the Johns Hopkins Hospital.

The theory that mosquitos can transmit malarial fever was indicated even in the Sanskrit Susruta,[1] and the same theory was advanced for yellow fever by Josiah Clark Nott, of South Carolina (1848),[2] and Louis Daniel Beauperthuy (1854),[3] while the hypothesis was |more definitely stated for yellow fever by Carlos Finlay (1833–   ), of Cuba (1881),[4] and for malarial fever by Albert F. A. King (1883).[5]   In the mean time Sir Patrick Manson (1844–   ) had proved that the mosquito is a vector of Filaria sanguinis hominis (1879),[6] and the plasmodium of malarial fever had been discovered by Alphonse Laveran (1845–   ), a French army surgeon, in 1880.[7] These hemocytozoa were accurately described by Ettore Marchiafava and Angelo Celli (1885), and it was shown by Camillo Golgi, the histologist, that malarial paroxysms are coincident with sporulation of parasites (1886), and that the parasite of quartan fever differs from that of tertian (1889).   In 1889, Marchiafava and Celli showed that the organisms of the pernicious and the tertian and quartan forms are different; B. Grassi and R. Feletti studied the parasites in birds (1891), D. L. Romanovsky devised a special stain for them (1890), and Ronald Ross, in India, demonstrated the infection of birds by means of the mosquito (1897–98). W. G. McCallum and E. L. Opie demonstrated sexual conjugation in the flagellated forms (1897–98), and Grassi and A. Bignami showed that the parasites develop only in the Anopheles mosquito (1899).   Intracorpuscular conjugation in the parasite as a cause of latency and relapse was demonstrated by Charles F. Craig (1907), also the possibility of malaria carriers.

About 1890, Pasteur's theory of attenuated viruses was extended to the science of toxins and antitoxins by Emil von Behring (1854–   ), a Prussian army surgeon who became professor of hygiene at Halle (1894) and Marburg (1895).   In his studies on chicken cholera, Pasteur had already noticed the pathogenic effects of a clear filtrate of the specific organism, and, in 1888, his pupils, Roux and Yersin, got the same results from diphtheria filtrates.[8]   Hans Buchner, in 1889, had established the bactericidal effect of blood-serum.[9]   While working in Koch's Institute with Kitasato, Behring demonstrated that the serum of animals immunized against attenuated diphtheria toxins can be used as a preventive or therapeutic inoculation against diphtheria in other animals, through a specific neutralization of the toxin of the disease (1890–93).[10]   After trying out the remedy in man, Behring began to produce it upon a grand scale (1894), and it soon became rec-

---

[1] Sir H. A. Blake: J. Ceylon Branch, Brit. Med. Ass., Colombo, 1905, ii, 9.

[2] Nott: New Orleans M. & S. J., 1848, iv, 563; 601.

[3] Gaz. offic. de Cumana, 1854, No. 57.

[4] Finlay: An. r. Acad. de cien. med. . . . de la Habana, 1881–2, xviii, 147–169.

[5] King: Pop. Sc. Month., New York, 1883.

[6] Manson: J. Linnæan Soc., London, 1879, xiv, 304–311.

[7] Laveran: Compt. rend. Acad. d. Sc., Paris, 1880, xciii, 627.

[8] Ann. de l'Inst. Pasteur, Paris, 1888, ii, 629; 1889, iii, 273.

[9] Buchner: Centralbl. f. Bakteriol., Jena, 1889, v, 817; vi, 1.

[10] Behring: Deutsche med. Wochenschr., Leipzig and Berlin, 1890, xvi, 1113; 1145; 1893, xix, 389; 415.

ognized as the specific treatment for diphtheria. The success of diphtheria antitoxin led to many attempts to treat other specific infections by immune sera, but, except in the case of tetanus and serpent-poisoning, these have not been uniformly successful. Meanwhile the subject of immunity was developed on the solidist or cellular side by Elie **Metchnikoff** (1845–   ), the eminent Russian biologist, who, in his studies of inflammation (1884), showed how the white blood-corpuscles destroy bacteria by absorbing them (phagocytosis). This theory, in the hands of Sir Almwroth Wright and others, led to vaccinotherapy. Metchnikoff also demonstrated that Pfeiffer's phenomenon (bacteriolysis) can take place in vitro (1895);[1] with Roux, he showed that the higher apes can be inoculated with syphilis (1903–04),[2] and his

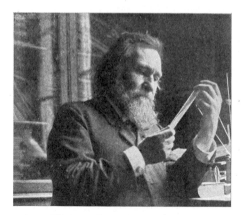

Elie Metchnikoff (1845–   ).

theories of the effect of lactic acid on bacteria in counteracting the intestinal poisons and prolonging life (1906), have attracted much attention. He received the Nobel prize in 1908.

Bacteriology and pathology have been specially advanced in America by William Henry **Welch** (1850–   ), of Norfolk, Connecticut, a pupil of Cohnheim's, who became professor of pathology at the Bellevue Hospital Medical College (1879–84) and at the Johns Hopkins University (1884), where he has turned out a long line of worthy pupils. Welch investigated acute edema of the lungs in Cohnheim's laboratory (1877), discovered the Staphylococcus epidermidis albus and its relation to wound infection (1892),[3]

---

[1] Ann. de l'Inst. Pasteur, Paris, 1895, ix, 433–461, 1 pl.

[2] *Ibid.*, 1903, xvii, 809; 1904, xviii, 1.

[3] Welch: Tr. Cong. Am. Phys. & Surg., New Haven, 1892, ii, 1–28.

also the Bacillus aërogenes capsulatus (1892),[1] grouping the diseases caused by it (1900).[2]   He also made important studies of embolism and thrombosis, and, with Flexner, demonstrated the pathological changes produced by experimental injection of the toxins of diphtheria (1891–92)[3] simultaneously with von Behring.

Simon **Flexner** (1863–   ), of Lexington, Kentucky, now director of the Rockefeller Institute for Experimental Research (1903), has distinguished himself by his work on terminal infections, his experimental work on venoms (1901), and the etiology and therapy of cerebrospinal meningitis (1909) and infantile poliomyelitis (1910–13).

George H. F. **Nuttall** (1862–   ), of San Francisco, professor of biology at the University of Cambridge (1906), editor and founder of the *Journal of Hygiene* (1901) and of *Parasitology* (1908), first summarized the rôle of insects, arachnids, and myriapods as transmitters of bacterial and parasitic diseases (1899), and his monograph on "Blood Immunity and Blood Relationship" (1904) establishes the identification of different kinds of blood by the precipitin test.

Theobald Smith (1859–   ), of Albany, New York, professor of comparative pathology in Harvard University (1896), has been one of the pioneers in the theory of infectious diseases.   In 1886, working with D. E. Salmon, he demonstrated that immunity from hog cholera can be secured by injection of the filtered products of the specific organisms. This was the first experiment in immunization, and was soon followed by the work of Behring, Roux, and others. Smith's demonstration of the parasite of Texas fever (*Pirosoma bigeminum*) (1889),[4] and his work (with F. L. Kilborne) in tracing its transmission by the cattle tick (Boöphilus bovis), was a great advance in the science of protozoan disease (1893). He also demonstrated anaphylaxis from the bacterial products of diphtheria prior to 1903, a discovery which Ehrlich called the "Theobald Smith phenomenon."   He made the first clear differentiation between the bovine and human types of tubercle bacilli (1898),[5] his work having been substantiated by Koch, Spengler, and others, and has [made many other discoveries in bacteriology, notably the first observation of pleomorphism in bacteria.

While Pasteur was investigating fermentation and putrefaction, the foundations of the most important application of his work were

---

[1] Johns Hopkins Hosp. Bull., Baltimore, 1892, iii, 81–91 (with G. H. F. Nuttall).

[2] *Ibid.*, 1900, xi, 185–204.   [3] *Ibid.*, 1891, ii, 107; 1892, iii, 17.

[4] Smith: Med. News, Phila., 1889, lv, 689–693.

[5] J. Exper. Med., New York, 1898, iii, 451–511.

being laid by Joseph Lister, a young English surgeon who was destined to make his art a science in the same sense in which the mathematician Cayley defined bookkeeping as a perfect science. **Lord Lister** (1827–1912), the last and greatest of the interesting line of English Quaker physicians, was born at Upton, Essex (April 5th). His father, Joseph Jackson Lister, a London wine merchant, who devoted his leisure hours to the study of optics, was, in a sense, the founder of modern microscopy through his epoch-making improvements in the achromatic lenses of the instrument (1830), and his special bent was not without its influence upon his son. After graduating in medicine from the University of London in 1852, Joseph Lister produced a number of papers on the histology of muscle illustrated by drawings which are rare and delicate examples of the talent which so many great physicians have displayed in illustrating their own works. Two of Lister's teachers, William Sharpey and Thomas Graham, were Scots, and it was upon their advice that he went up to Edinburgh to follow surgery under Syme, who made him his house surgeon in 1854, and whose eldest daughter afterward became his wife. In 1860,

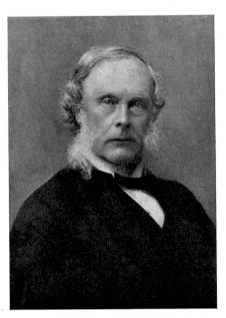

Lord Lister (1827–1912).

Lister became professor of surgery in the University of Glasgow, and it was during the latter years of his residence there that his greatest contribution to the science was made. Meanwhile, he had verified Kölliker's observation that the contractile tissues of the iris consist of smooth muscle (1852);[1] he had overthrown the current theory that coagulation of the blood is due to liberation of ammonia, showing that, in the blood-vessels, it depends upon their injury (1859–63);[2] and he had made his mark in surgery by

---

[1] Lister: Quart. Jour. Micr. Sc., London, 1853, i, p. 8 *et seq.*

[2] Edinb. Med. Jour., Dec., 1859; and Croonian lecture, Proc. Roy. Soc., London, 1863.

34

530   HISTORY OF MEDICINE

his classical paper on excision of the wrist for caries (1865).[1] Early
in his hospital experience, Lister had been deeply impressed with
the high mortality from such surgical pests as septicemia, pyemia,
erysipelas, tetanus, and hospital gangrene. In his own statistics
of amputation (1864–66), he found 45 per cent. of fatal cases, although he had constantly employed Syme's methods of keeping
the wound clean by silver wire sutures, drainage, frequent change of
dressings, and scrupulous cleanliness. These were the days of
"laudable pus," yet Lister had already begun to think of the old
Hippocratic healing by first intention as the surgeon's ideal. Notic-
ing that the latter, when attainable, was always dissociated from
putrefaction, his attention was accidentally drawn to Pasteur's
work, and, immediately grasping its tendency, he set out definitely
to prevent the development of microörganisms in wounds. Per-
ceiving that Pasteur's heat sterilizations would avail nothing here,
he turned to chemical antiseptics, and, after trying out chloride of
zinc and the sulphites, he hit, by lucky chance, upon carbolic acid,
which had been employed, a short while before, in the disinfection
of sewage at Carlisle.[2] On August 12, 1865, he employed it in a
case of compound fracture with complete success, and, in 1867,
published the results of two years' work in two papers,[3] the second
of which bears the significant title, "On the Antiseptic Principle
in the Practice of Surgery." The criticisms which were heaped
upon this paper turned upon such non-essentials as the question of
priority in the use of carbolic acid, or the character of Lister's
dressings, which, complex at the start, were only accidental features of the great surgical principle with which they were confused.
Undisturbed by these attacks, Lister proceeded to develop his
thesis in the broadest and most scientific manner by original investigation of lactic-acid fermentation, of the relation of bacteria
to inflammation, and of the antiseptic healing of wounds. All his
life, he labored constantly to improve his dressings, from the
earlier devices of putty, block tin, layers of oiled silk or gauze,
and the carbolic acid spray, to his later experiments with the double
cyanides of mercury and zinc and his great innovation of catgut
ligatures in the surgery of the vascular system (1880).[4] He boldly
applied the antiseptic principle to such conditions as abscesses
in the spine and the joints, excision of the knee-joint (1878),
operations on the breast (1881), fracture of the patella (1883),

[1] Lancet: London, 1865, i, 308; 335; 362.
[2] This substance had already been recommended by François-Jules
Lemaire, a French chemist, in 1860, but Lister had heard of neither Lemaire
nor Semmelweis.
[3] Lancet, London, 1867, ii, 95; 353, 668.
[4] Tr. Clin. Soc., London, 1880–81, xiv, pp. xliii–lxiii.

and all manner of operations on the locomotor system, doing as much to extend the domain of surgery as any man of his time. Modern surgery, it is true, has become almost entirely aseptic, in the sense of discarding strong antiseptics in the dressing of wounds, but in both, the Listerian ideal of avoiding sepsis remains the same. In 1869, Lister succeeded Syme at Edinburgh, and, in 1877, accepted the chair of surgery at Kings College, London, retiring from practice in 1896, before which time his fame had become international. He was president of the Royal Society during 1895–1900, received his baronetcy in 1883, and was the first medical man to be raised to the peerage (1897). In France, his ideas were defended by Lucas-Championnière, who pointed out that asepsis, the Listerian ideal, must always be preceded by antisepsis, and even heat sterilization is, in the truest sense, anti-septic. This was the weak point of Lawson Tait's argument against Listerism, for the Birmingham gynecologist, who denied that bacteria are pathogenic, could not admit that his own marvelous success in ovariotomy was due to those housewifely antiseptics, soap and hot water.[1] The military applications of antisepsis, which Lister suggested in 1870,[2] were not taken up until late in the Franco-Prussian War, but his methods were soon grasped by von Volkmann, Thiersch, Mikulicz, and others, and his tour through Germany, in 1875, was in the nature of a triumphal progress. Upon hearing of Semmelweis, in 1883, Lister generously declared him to be his forerunner; and, in the obstetrician's hands, Listerism is now the main safeguard of the woman in childbed. To Listerism are due all modern developments of the surgery of the hollow cavities of the body, including the cranium, chest, abdomen, the joints, and the male and female pelvic viscera. At Pasteur's jubilee, in 1892, Lister paid a feeling tribute to the man whose work he had been first to appreciate. As an operator, Lister was not brilliant, but deliberate and careful, aiming, like Kocher today, to make the recovery of his patient a mathematical certainty. His Quaker sobriety, his severe and austere ideals, were not the traits that make for rapid and showy success. His progress was slow; he left no school; but, before he died, the entire guild of surgeons "lived in his mild and magnificent eye." When his body was laid at rest in Westminster, England had buried her greatest surgeon.

The character of Lister was one of rare nobility. As the Quaker is the Puritan transposed into a softer and more grateful key, so his nature had those elements of sweetness which proverbially can

---

[1] The cavillings of von Bruns ("*Fort mit dem Spray!*"), Tait, and Bantock have, in the end, proved to be of little moment, so far as the generic idea of surgical cleanliness is concerned.

[2] Brit. Med. Jour., London, 1870, ii, 243.

come only out of strength, and no praise of him is more touching
than that of one of the Scottish clergymen after his death:

"Of Joseph Lister's winsome personality, those speak most warmly who
knew him best. It was his gentleness, above all, that made him greater. His
very presence was a spiritual force. Clear-eyed and pure of soul, he cherished
from earliest days that love of truth which guided him to the end. His noble
passion for humanity extinguished all thoughts of self and personal fame, im-
pelling him along that path which he steadfastly pursued till he found the
secret of his search, and bestowed on the world probably the greatest boon
which science has been able to win for the physical life of mankind. Yet
greater than his greatest achievement was the man himself, and the final
secret of his greatness was that serene simplicity which was his most distinguished characteristic . . . . His was the grave and thoughtful courtesy
which bespoke the Christian
gentleman and the earnest
lover of his kind. Hence we
are not surprised to learn how
he stirred enthusiasm and
moved men to reverence, how
he gained such love and affection as rarely falls to a scientific teacher. Behind his acknowledged mastery of his
science, his grave and noble
face, marked by soft lines of
tranquil thought, revealed a
soul of singular beauty and
sweetness, of high integrity
and stainless honour. That
such a man, dowered with
God's gift of genius, should rise
to lofty heights and achieve
great things was inevitable."—
(*Rev. Wallace Williamson*:
Memorial Discourse, Edin-
burgh, February, 1912.)

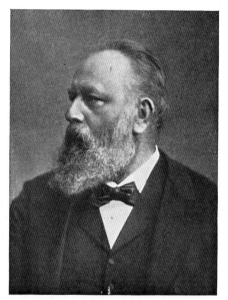

Theodor Billroth (1829–94).

Of the surgeons of
Lister's time, who devel-
oped his ideas in new
fields, perhaps the first
place belongs to Theodor
Billroth (1829–94), the
pioneer of **visceral surgery**. Born on the island of Rügen, a
Berlin graduate of 1852, Billroth became an assistant in Langenbeck's clinic, and subsequently professor of surgery at Zürich
(1860–67) and Vienna (1867–94). Billroth was early interested
in wound infections, and, in his "coccobacteria septica," he had
undoubtedly grasped the causal idea, but regarded one generic
group of bacteria as the cause of a whole family of affections. He
wrote an admirable volume of lectures on surgical pathology and
therapeutics (1863),[1] which was translated into almost every

[1] Billroth: Die allgemeine chirurgische Pathologie und Therapie, Berlin,
1863.

modern language, but he is especially remembered as the surgeon of the alimentary tract. In 1872, he made the first resection of the esophagus,[1] and, in 1881, the first resection of the pylorus for cancer, which was successful.[2] He also made the first complete excision of the larynx (1873),[3] is said to have been the first to perform the "interilio-abdominal amputation" (1891),[4] and did a large number of intestinal resections and enterorrhaphies (1878–83).[5] All these operations upon the gastro-intestinal tract did much to elucidate the pathology of those regions, as being, in Naunyn's phrase, "autopsies *in vivo*." Billroth was a man of charming, genial personality, with a strong artistic bent, delicately revealed in the few specimens of verse and music which he left, and in his delightful *Briefe*, in some sort, a memorial of his life-long friendship with the great North German composer, Johannes Brahms.

Billroth's most prominent pupils were Mikulicz, Czerny, Wölfler, and Gersuny, all Slavs, and von Eiselsberg, an Austrian.

Johann **von Mikulicz-Radecki** (1850–1905), of Czernowitz, Poland, who was Billroth's assistant up to 1881, and professor of surgery at Königsberg (1887) and Breslau (1890), did much to improve antiseptic methods, introduced the present modes of exploring the esophagus and the stomach (1881),[6] first treated cancer of the esophagus by resection and plastic transplantation (1886),[7] introduced lateral pharyngotomy in excising malignant tumors of the tonsillar region (1886),[8] described symmetrical inflammation of the lacrimal and salivary glands (Mikulicz's disease (1892),[9] greatly extended the operative surgery of the stomach and the joints, and collaborated in an atlas (1892) and a treatise (1898) on diseases of the mouth. He was one of the first to wear gloves in operative work, but the cotton gloves he used were soon superseded by those of rubber, introduced by Halsted in Baltimore (1890), and, shortly afterward, by W. Zoege-Manteuffel.

Vincenz **Czerny** (1842–   ), of Trautenau, Bohemia, professor of surgery at Freiburg (1871) and Heidelberg (1887), in-

---

[1] Arch. f. klin. Chir., Berlin, 1872, xiii, 65–69, 1 pl

[2] Wien. med. Wochenschr., 1881, xxxi, 162–165.

[3] Arch. f. klin. Chir., Berlin, 1874, xvii, 343–356, 1 pl.

[4] Billroth did not report upon an unsuccessful operation, said to have been performed about 1891, so that, by the law of priority, credit is given to Mathieu Jaboulay, who published the first paper in Lyon méd., 1894, lxxv, 507–510.

[5] Zeitschr. f. Heilk., Prague, 1884, v, 83–108.

[6] Mikulicz: Wien. med. Presse, 1881, xxii, 1405, *et seq.*

[7] Prag. med. Wochenschr., 1886, ix, 93.

[8] Przegl. lek., Krakow, 1886, xxv, 173.

[9] Billroth Festschrift (Beiträge zur Chirurgie), Stuttgart, 1892, 610–630, 1 pl.

534 HISTORY OF MEDICINE

troduced the enucleation of subperitoneal uterine fibroids by the vaginal route (1881),[1] and extended Billroth's work on the excision of the larynx, the esophagus, the kidneys, and general visceral surgery. He introduced the concept, "exudative diathesis" (1907).

Anton **Wölfler** (1850–   ), of Kopezen, Bohemia, professor of surgery at Graz (1886) and Prague (1895), introduced gastro-enterostomy (1881),[2] and devoted special attention to the surgical treatment of goiter (1887–91).

Robert **Gersuny** (1844–   ), of Teplitz, Bohemia, who succeeded Billroth as director of the Rudolfinerhaus (1894), is now best remembered for the introduction of prothetic paraffin injections (1900).

Karl **Thiersch** (1822–95), of Munich, one of Stromeyer's pupils, who became professor of surgery at Erlangen (1854) and Leipzig (1887), was a great pioneer of Listerism, and through his studies of epithelial cancer (1865),[3] phosphoric necrosis of the jaws (1867),[4] the healing of wounds (1867),[5] and his improvement in skin-grafting (1874),[6] was a prominent contributor to surgical pathology.

Richard **von Volkmann** (1830–89), of Leipzig, son of the well-known Halle physiologist, and professor of surgery in the latter city (1867–89), also did much to introduce antisepsis during the Franco-Prussian War, was the first to excise the rectum for cancer (1878),[7] described the so-called ischemic contractures or paralyses (1881)[8] and cancer in paraffin-workers, and founded the well-known *Sammlung klinischer Vorträge* (1870), which contains some of the most valuable monographs of recent times. He was a man of aristocratic appearance, a poet ("Richard Leander"), and his "Dreams by French Firesides"[9] is a charming book.

Friedrich **von Esmarch** (1823–1908), of Tonning, Schleswig-Holstein, a pupil of Stromeyer and Langenbeck, who became professor at Kiel (1857–99), was a great military surgeon, having served through the campaigns of 1848–50, 1864–66, and 1870–71. He is most memorable for his introduction of the first-aid bandage on the battle-field (1869–70),[10] and for standardizing surgical hemostasis

---

[1] Czerny: Wien. med. Wochenschr., 1881, xxxi, 501; 525.
[2] Wölfler: Centralbl. f. Chir., Leipzig, 1881, viii, 705–708.
[3] Thiersch: Der Epithelialkrebs, Leipzig; 1865.
[4] Thiersch: De maxillarum necrosi phosphorica, Leipzig, 1867.
[5] Handb. d allg. u. spez. Chir. (Pitha-Billroth), 1867, i, 2. Abth., No. 3.
[6] Verhandl. d. deutsch. Gesellsch. f. Chir., Berlin, 1874, iii, 69–75.
[7] Volkmann: Samml. klin. Vortr., Leipzig, 1878, No. 131 (Chir. No. 42), 1113–1128.
[8] Centralbl. f. Chir., Leipzig, 1881, viii, 801–803.
[9] Träumereien an französischen Kaminen, Leipzig, 1871.
[10] Esmarch: Der erste Verband auf dem Schlachtfelde, Kiel, 1869.

by the "Esmarch bandage" (1873).[1] He did much to improve
the status of military surgery through his contributions on resection after gunshot wounds (1851), the proper locale for field
hospitals and bandaging stations (1861), surgical technics (1871),
first aid to the wounded (1875), and on first aid in accidents (1882).
He was the pioneer and founder of the so-called *Samariterwesen*,
for military nursing, in Germany, and, through his marriage with
a royal princess, became the uncle of the present emperor.

Ernst **von Bergmann** (1836–1907), of Riga, Russia, graduated at Dorpat in 1860, served in the Prussian army in the
wars of 1866 and 1870–
71, and on the Russian
side in the War of 1877–78,
after which he became a
prominent figure in Ger-
man medicine. He was
called to the chair at
Würzburg in 1878, and
succeeded Langenbeck at
Berlin (1882), where he remained for the rest of his
life. He greatly advanced
cranial surgery in his
memoirs on head injuries
(1873)[2] and surgical treatment of cerebral diseases
(1888),[3] and is also notable for his works on the
surgery of the joints
(1872–78), ligation of the
femoral vein (1882), dis-
eases of the lymphatic

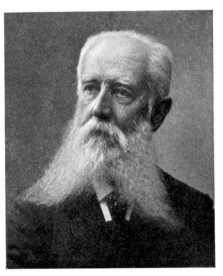

Friedrich von Esmarch (1823–1908).

glands (1881), and his various contributions to surgical pathology.
His letters of 1866–77 were edited by A. Buchholz (1911).

Ernst Julius **Gurlt** (1825–99), of Berlin, where he became professor in 1862, took part in all the German wars of the period,
wrote with ability on a great variety of themes, and holds a high
place in medical literature as the historian of surgery *par excellence.*
He was one of the most learned surgeons of his time, and his
Geschichte der Chirurgie (1898), dealing with the history of the

---

[1] Samml. klin. Vortr., Leipzig, 1873, No. 58 (Chir. No. 19), 373–384.

[2] Bergmann: Handb. d. allg. u. spez. Chir. (Pitha-Billroth), Erlangen,
1873, iii, 1. Abth., 1. Abschn.

[3] Die chirurgische Behandlung bei Hirnkrankheiten, Berlin, 1888.

subject down to the Renaissance period, is to surgery what Haeser is to medicine, unrivaled for scholarship, exhaustive treatment, and accurate bibliography. It is a work which stands quite apart as one of the greatest monuments of German thoroughness.

In **orthopedics**, especial distinction was attained by the Heine family, all of whom were expert mechanicians, in particular Jacob von Heine (1799–1879), of Cannstatt, who first described poliomyelitic deformities (1840) and wrote an important treatise on dislocations (1842), Gustav Simon (1868), Adolf Lorenz (1854–   ), of Weidenau, Silesia, who introduced the bloodless method of reducing congenital dislocations of the hip-joint by forcible manipulation, Julius Wolff (1836–1902), of West Prussia, author of a great monograph on the pathological transformations of bones (1892), and Albert Hoffa (1859–1907), who introduced a well-known operation for congenital hip dislocations (1890), and is founder and editor of the *Zeitschrift für orthopädische Chirurgie* (1891).

Of original operations by German surgeons of the nineteenth century, we may mention those of colostomy by Karl Maydl (1888), thoracotomy for empyema by Ernst Küster (1889), resection of the rectum by Paul Kraske (1891), excision of the Gasserian ganglion by Fedor Krause (1893), and excision of the stomach by Carl Schlatter (1897).

Of the French surgeons of the period, Aristide-Auguste **Verneuil** (1823–95), of Paris, who held many hospital appointments and trained many good pupils, made no original discoveries, but is remembered by such procedures as forcipressure in hemorrhage (1875), dry bandaging, treatment of abscesses with iodoform, and by the *Revue de chirurgie* (1881), of which he was one of the founders and editors. He wrote no large monographs, and his works are all contained in the six volumes of his *Mémoires de chirurgie* (1877–88).

Édouard **Nicaise** (1838–96), surgeon at the Laënnec Hospital (1880–96), was, like Malgaigne, especially learned in the history of his subject, issued superb modern editions of Guy de Chauliac (1890), Henri de Mondeville (1893), and Pierre Franco (1895), and wrote many fascinating essays.

Félix **Guyon** (1831–   ), a native of the Island of Réunion, professor of genito-urinary surgery at the Paris Faculty (1890), was one of the great teachers of this specialty in his time, and his clinics at Necker were followed by students from all over the world. His lectures on genito-urinary diseases (1881) and surgical diseases of the bladder and the prostate (1888) are his most important works. Bigelow's litholapaxy was perfected by Thomson and by Guyon, who was succeeded, and perhaps surpassed, by his brilliant pupil, Joaquin **Albarran** (1860–1912), another exotic, born at Sagua la Grande, Cuba, who was twice a gold medalist of the Paris Faculty (1888–89), and professeur agrégé in 1892, and, in his short life, became a star of the first magnitude as a teacher and through his many valuable innovations in the diagnosis of intrapelvic conditions by the urine. His works on exploration of the renal functions (1905) and surgery of the urinary passages (1909) are his masterpieces.

Other French surgeons of note were Charles Sédillot (1804–83), who performed the first gastrostomy (1849), Paul Berger (1845–   ), who wrote an exhaustive monograph on the interscapulo-thoracic amputation (1887), Mathieu Jaboulay, who first described the inter-ilio-abdominal amputation (1894), and wrote an authoritative monograph on the surgery of the sympathetic system and the thyroid gland (1900), Edmond Delorme (1847), who introduced the operation of decortication of the lungs for chronic empyema (1894–1901), Ulysse Trélat (1828–93), professor at the Hospital Necker, Louis-Felix Terrier (1837–1908), and Louis-X.-E.-L. Ollier (1825–1900). The Italian surgeons did some bold operating on the heart, the first in this field being Guido Farina, who sutured the right ventricle on June 8, 1896.[1] The first successful suture of the heart was done by L. Rehn at Frankfort on the Main in 1896.[2] Cardiolysis was proposed by Brauer in 1902. Of the Swiss surgeons, Jacques-Louis Reverdin (1842–   ) and Theodor Kocher are memorable for their operations on the thyroid gland, and August Socin (1837–1899) for his work in military surgery (1872), surgical diseases of the prostate (1875).

Sir James **Paget** (1814–99), of Great Yarmouth, England, graduated from St. Bartholomew's Hospital, with which he was all his life associated, and was serjeant surgeon to the Queen, receiving his baronetcy in 1871. A warm friend of Virchow, Paget was, like Brodie, a great surgical pathologist, his best works being his *Lectures on Tumours* (1851), *Surgical Pathology* (1863), *Clinical Lectures and Essays* (1875), the catalogue of the Pathological Museum of the Royal College of Surgeons (1882), of which he was president (1875), and his original descriptions of eczema of the nipple, with subsequent mammary cancer (1874),[3] and the trophic disorder, osteitis deformans (1877–82).[4] He also made an early note of erythromelalgia (Weir Mitchell's disease), and his lifework illustrates how the surgeon proper can be a good clinical observer.

Sir Jonathan **Hutchinson** (1828–1913), of Selby, Yorkshire, also a St. Bartholomew's man, surgeon to the London Hospital (1859–83), and professor of surgery at the Royal College of Surgeons (1879–83), was also an able surgical pathologist, and is especially memorable for his description of the notched, peg-shaped incisor teeth in congenital syphilis (1861),[5] of varicella gangrenosa (1882)[6] and other skin diseases, and for his views of the causation of leprosy, which he attributed to eating fish. His *Archives of*

---

[1] Farina: Bull. d. r. Accad. di med. di Roma, 1896–7, xxiii, 248.

[2] L. Rehn: Arch. f. klin. Chir., Berlin, 1907, lxxxiii, 723–778; Rehn's case was alive when he wrote this paper, ten and one-half years after the operation had been performed.

[3] Paget: St. Barth. Hosp. Rep., London, 1874, x, 87–89.

[4] Med.-Chir. Tr., London, 1876–7, lx, 37: 1881–2, lxv, 225.

[5] Hutchinson: Brit. Med. Jour., London, 1861, i, 515–519.

[6] Med.-Chir. Tr., London, 1881–2, lxv, pp. i–ii.

Surgery (1889–99) consist of ten volumes, issued in periodical form, the entire contents written by himself, forming a great storehouse of original observations on disease which will some day be studied like the works of John Hunter.

Sir William **MacEwen** (1848–   ), of Rothesay, Scotland, professor of surgery at the University of Glasgow (1892), is notable for his methods of osteotomy for genu valgum (1881), radical cure of oblique inguinal hernia (1887), treatment of aneurysm by acupuncture (1890), and his monograph on "Pyogenic Infective Diseases of the Brain" (1893), which sums up his brilliant work on the surgery of the brain and spinal cord.

Sir William **MacCormac** (1836–1901), of Belfast, Ireland, saw a great deal of military surgery in the Franco-Prussian and Turco-Servian wars, and early applied Listerian principles with success to the surgery of the joints and the abdomen, particularly in his pioneer operations for intraperitoneal rupture of the bladder (1886).[1]

Sir Victor **Horsley** (1857–   ), of Kensington, England, has been a pioneer in experimental and neurological surgery, particularly in his operations on the ductless glands (1884–86) and in his initial operation on the spinal cord (with Gowers, 1888),[2] after which, as Cushing says, "certain neurologists began to do their own surgery."

Sir Frederick **Treves** (1853–   ), of Dorchester, England, is widely known for his works on surgical anatomy (1883), intestinal obstruction (1884), appendicitis, and peritonitis, his System of Surgery (1895), and (with Lang) a very valuable dictionary of German medical terms (1890). He played an important part in the Transvaal war, has written some charming travel sketches, and performed the operation upon King Edward VII in 1902.

Two American surgeons whose life-work extended over into the Listerian period were Bigelow and Gross.

Henry Jacob **Bigelow** (1816–90), of Boston, Massachusetts, who became surgeon to the Massachusetts General Hospital (1846) and professor of surgery in the Harvard Medical School, was the leading surgeon of New England during his life-time. He was the first to excise the hip-joint in America (1852),[3] and, in his monograph on dislocation and fracture of the hip (1869),[4] he first described the mechanism of the iliofemoral or Y-ligament, emphasizing its importance in reducing dislocation by the flexion method.

---

[1] MacCormac: Lancet, London, 1886, ii, 1118–1122.

[2] Sir W. R. Gowers and Horsley: Med. Chir. Tr., London, 1887–8, lxxi, 377–430.

[3] Bigelow: Am. Jour. Med. Sc., Phila., 1852, xxiv, 90.

[4] The Mechanism of Dislocation and Fracture of the Hip, Philadelphia, 1869.

He also introduced the surgical procedure of litholapaxy or lithotrity for rapid evacuation of vesical calculus (1878).[1]

Samuel David **Gross** (1805–84), of Easton, Pennsylvania, professor of surgery at Louisville, Ky. (1840–56), and at the Jefferson
Medical College, Philadelphia (1856–82), was the greatest American surgeon of his time. He wrote the first exhaustive treatise on
pathological anatomy in English (1839),[2] which passed through three
editions and was highly thought of, even by Virchow. He also
wrote an authoritative treatise on diseases of the genito-urinary

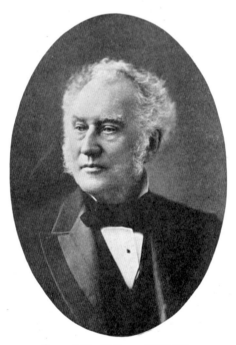

Samuel David Gross (1805–84).

organs (1851), containing the first account of the distribution of
urinary calculus; the first systematic treatise on foreign bodies in
the air-passages (1854); and an important two-volume system of
surgery (1859), all these works being extensively illustrated.
Gross invented many new instruments, made original experiments
upon the effects of manual strangulation (1836) and wounds of the
intestines (1843) in animals, dissected and described specimens of

---

[1] Bigelow: Am. Jour. Med. Sc., Phila., 1878, lxxv, 117–134.

[2] Gross: Elements of Pathological Anatomy, Boston, 1839.

molar pregnancy (1839), introduced deep stitches in wounds of
the abdominal wall, performed laparotomy for rupture of the
bladder, myotomy for wry-neck (1873), and first described prostat-
orrhea (1860). He knew the literature of his subject well, and his
histories of Kentucky surgery (1851) and of American surgery down
to the year 1876 are authoritative and accurate monographs. His
biographies of Drake, McDowell, John Hunter, Richter, Paré,
Mott, and others are all attractive reading. Gross was a strong
personality, a stalwart figure, with a beautiful, benignant countenance. His works were crowned, as the inscription on his funeral
urn reads, by "the milk-white flower of a stainless life." His
statue stands by the Army Medical Museum, Washington, D. C.
He was the greatest of the German-American physicians.

William Williams **Keen** (1837–   ), of Philadelphia, professor
of surgery at the Jefferson Medical College (1889–1907), is the
author of an important work on the surgical complications and
sequels of typhoid fever (1898), and has been a brilliant and skilful operator, particularly in diseases of the brain. He did much
for linear craniotomy (1891) and the inter-ilio-abdominal operation
(1904). He is well known by his American Text-book (1899–1903)
and his System of Surgery (1905), which are probably the best
American works of their kind. Among his historical essays, his
"Early History of Practical Anatomy" (1870) is most valuable
for its accuracy and thoroughness.

Nicholas **Senn** (1844–1909), of Buchs, Switzerland, settled in
the United States in 1852, graduated from the Chicago Medical
College (1868), and became professor of surgery at the Rush
Medical College of that city. Senn was a highly trained, scientific
surgeon, who made valuable experimental contributions to the study
of air embolism (1885), the surgery of the pancreas (1886), gunshot
wounds, and intestinal anastomosis, in which he introduced the use
of decalcified bone-plates. He was, in fact, a great master of intestinal surgery, especially in the treatment of appendicitis. He
devised a method of detecting intestinal perforation by means of
inflation with hydrogen gas (1888), and was the first to use the
Röntgen rays in the treatment of leukemia (1903). Senn played
an important part in the Spanish-American War, founded the
Association of Military Surgeons of the United States (1891), and,
at his death, left a fine collection of medical books to the Newberry
Library, and other handsome bequests to the city of his adoption.

Other prominent American surgeons of the Listerian period
are D. Hayes Agnew (1818–92), of Philadelphia, professor of surgery at the University of Pennsylvania, who was prominent in the
case of President Garfield, and one of the few surgeons who practised
medicine and surgery together; John Thompson Hodgen (1826–

82), of Kentucky, who devised many instruments and apparatus, in particular, his wire suspension splints for fracture of the femur and forearm, which are still in use; Henry Orlando Marcy (1837–), of Otis, Massachusetts, who introduced antiseptic ligatures in the radical cure of hernia (1878), and wrote important treatises on hernia (1889) and the surgery of the perineum (1889); Charles McBurney (1845–1913), of Roxbury, Massachusetts, who discovered "McBurney's point" as a sign for operative intervention in appendicitis (1889); Robert Abbe (1851–   ), of New York City, who introduced catgut rings in intestinal anastomosis and suturing (1892); Frank Hartley (1856–1913), of Washington, who originated intracranial neurectomy of the second and third divisions of the third nerve for facial neuralgia (1892); George Michael Edebohls (1853–1908), of New York, who introduced the operation of renal decapsulation in the treatment of chronic nephritis and puerperal eclampsia (1901); George Ryerson Fowler (1848–1906), who first performed thoracoplasty (1893); Roswell Park (1852–   ), of Pomfret, Connecticut, prominent in connection with President McKinley's case, and author of a textbook of surgery (1896) and an attractive history of medicine (1897); and the brothers, Charles Horace and William James **Mayo,** of Minnesota, whose genius for method and system at their hospital at Rochester, Minn., has made Listerian surgery almost as reliable a science as bookkeeping.

Prominent in orthopedic and plastic surgery were Frank Hastings Hamilton (1813–86), of Wilmington, Vermont, who was a pioneer in skin-grafting for ulcers (1854), and wrote an important treatise on fractures and dislocations (1860); and Louis Albert Sayre (1820–1900), of New Jersey, who performed the second excision of the hip-joint in America (1855) and introduced the method of suspension in a plaster-of-Paris jacket for Potts' disease (1877).

The **gynecology** of the post-Listerian period was, in the main, a brilliant development of the operative principles which had been established by McDowell, Sims, Emmett, and Battey in America, Koeberlé in France, Gustav Simon in Germany, and Sir Thomas **Spencer Wells** (1818–97) in England. The latter, one of the greatest of the ovariotomists, was a native of Saint Albans, Hertfordshire, a pupil of Stokes and Graves in Dublin, and of Travers in London. After serving for fifteen years as surgeon in the Royal Navy (1841–53), including an experience in the Crimean War, he settled in London, and, in 1858, performed his first successful ovariotomy, which was followed by a large number of favorable experiences with the same operation. Phenomenal luck attended all his improvements in technic, and, in a few years, he was known to his colleagues and sought by patients all over the world as an absolutely safe operator in ovarian conditions. His work was summed up in his treatise on *Diseases of the Ovaries* (1865–72). He was professor of surgery and pathological anatomy and president of the Royal College of Surgeons, and surgeon to the Queen's household, receiving his baronetcy in 1883.

A gynecologist of wider scope and even greater success was Robert **Lawson Tait** (1845–99), of Edinburgh, who settled in Birmingham in 1871, and made that city another Mecca for female patients seeking operative relief.   Tait's success in

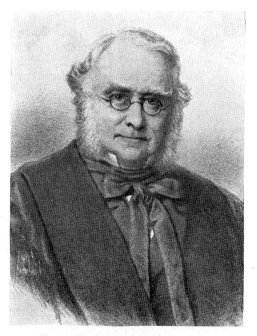

Sir Thomas Spencer Wells (1818–97).

operating, as judged by his statistics, was marvelous. He rolled up ovariotomies[1] and other abdominal sections by the thousands, with scarce a death, yet, strange to say, he was a violent and even truculent opponent of Lister, declining to see any causal relation between bacteria and disease, and pointing, with exaggerated

---

[1] Tait performed his first ovariotomy, July 29, 1868; removed an ovary for abscess, February 2, 1872; excised the uterine appendages to arrest the growth of a bleeding myoma, August 1, 1872; performed his first hysterectomy for myoma in 1873, removed a hematosalpinx, June 21, 1876; performed his first cholecystotomy, and removed his first pyosalpinx and hydrosalpinx, in 1879; and did a successful operation for ruptured tubal pregnancy, January 17, 1883.

scorn, to the fact that he never used any antiseptic precautions in his operations beyond simple cleanliness. The secret of his success was undoubtedly his wonderful skill, plus the use of warm or boiled water to flush out the abdomen, which was, of course, asepsis. Tait performed the first successful operation for ruptured tubal pregnancy (January 17, 1883), was the first to work out the pathology and treatment of pelvic hematocele, and, in his "Lectures" on these subjects (1888),[1] he points out that the first authoritative treatise on extra-uterine pregnancy was written by John S. Parry (1843–76), of Philadelphia (1876). In 1879 Tait excised the normal ovaries,[2] along the lines laid down by Battey (1872–73), but claimed that in none of his cases were the uterine appendages normal. This, with the similar operation of Alfred Hegar in 1877, developed, says Kelly, "the whole field of pelvic operations for diseases of the organs other than gross ovarian and fibroid tumors." "The peri-uterine phlegmons of Emmet and Thomas became recognized as tubal inflammations and abscesses." In 1879, Tait performed cholecystotomy, excision of hydrosalpinx and pyosalpinx, introduced his flap-splitting operation on the perineum, and his methods of dilating the cervix and of replacing the inverted uterus.

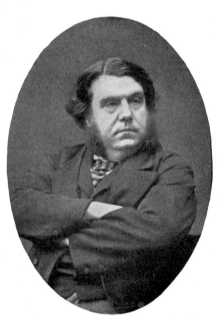

Lawson Tait (1845–99).

In 1880, he introduced hepatotomy, and, in 1881, he devised the special operation for excision of the uterine appendages by securing the pedicle with a silk ligature, tied by means of his invention, the "Staffordshire knot."[3] His method of "flap-splitting" in plastic repair of the perineum was a valuable inno-

[1] Tait: Lectures on Ectopic Pregnancy and Pelvic Hæmatocele, Birmingham, 1888.

[2] Brit. Med. Jour., London, 1881, i, 766.

[3] Ibid., 1881, i, 766.

vation (1879),[1] but it was not taken up in America for a long
time. Tait left interesting summaries of conclusions from his
operative statistics, treatises on diseases of the ovaries (1873) and
diseases of women (1879–1889), and highly original essays on rape
and other subjects connected with medical jurisprudence. In all
these productions, he is a forcible, effective, frequently coarse, but
always amusing, writer.

Of prominent innovations in operative gynecology, we may mention the
different methods of excising or enucleating uterine tumors introduced by
Eugène Koeberlé (1864), August Martin (1876), Karl Schröder (1878–84),
and Vincenz Czerny (1881); of excising the uterus, by Wilhelm Alexander
Freund (1878), Benjamin Franklin Baer (1892), Fernand Henrotin (1892),
and Jean-Louis Faure (1897); of treating uterine displacements, by James
Alexander Adams and William Alexander (1882), Robert Olshausen (1886),
Howard A. Kelly (1887), and George Michael Edebohls (1901).   The technic
of Cæsarean section was improved by Ferdinand Adolph Kehrer (1882),
particularly by Max Sänger (1882), by Edoardo Porro (1876), who first performed Cæsarean section with excision of the uterus and adnexa (1876), and
by Alfred Dührssen, who introduced the vaginal operation (1898).   Excision
of the vagina was introduced by Robert Olshausen (1895), the plastic reformation of the vagina by Alwin Karl Mackenrodt (1896), and a flap operation
for atresia of the vagina by George Henry Noble (1900).   Cæsarean section
in puerperal convulsions was introduced by Tjalling Halbertsma (1889).
Pubiotomy as a substitute for symphysiotomy is associated with the name of
Leonardo Gigli (1902).   Extra-uterine pregnancy was studied by John S.
Parry (1876); Lawson Tait, who performed the first successful tubal operation
(1883), by Richard Werth (1887), Joseph Eastman (1888), Joseph Price (1890),
John Clarence Webster (1892), and B. J. Kouwer, who first described ovarian
pregnancy (1897).   Much of the history of gynecology up to recent times has
been described by Playfair as a series of "crazes," a tendency to follow pre-
vailing fashions.   First of all came the uterine displacement craze, when
Graily Hewitt in England, Velpeau in France, Hodge in America, championed
the cause of the pessary for the treatment of backache or pelvic pain, and
every gynecologist felt himself called upon to invent one or to modify some one
else's; the unfortunate uterus all the while being, as Allbutt says, either "im-
paled on a stem or perched on a twig."   The pelvic cellulitis craze had its
origin in the fact that, in 1857, Gustave Bernutz found a case of peri-uterine
abscess due to inflammation of the pelvic cellular tissue, after which Bernutz
and Goupil published their famous memoir on pelvic cellulitis (1862).   This view
of pelvic pathology was widely taken up until Gaillard Thomas exploded it in
1880, by showing that much of alleged cellulitis is really peritonitis, and that
the former condition is rare in virgins.   In like manner oöphorectomy, clitori-
dectomy, inflammation of the os and cervix uteri, excision of the uterus and
its appendages, operations for extra-uterine pregnancy, and Cæsarean section
all had their day, according to the dictates of fashion.   Meanwhile very substantial work was done on the pathological side by C. A. Ruge and Johann Veit,
who described erosions of the cervix uteri (1877), by A. J. C. Skene on the para-
urethral glands (1880), by August Breisky on kraurosis vulvæ (1885), by Max
Sänger on decidual sarcoma of the uterus and other decidual tumors (1889–93),
by J. Whitridge Williams on papillary cystoma of the ovary (1891) and decidu-
oma malignum (1895), by Thomas S. Cullen on hydrosalpinx (1895), cancer of
the uterus (1900), and adenomyoma of the uterus (1908), and by Georg Winter
on gynecological diagnosis (1896).   The importance of latent gonorrhea in
women was first emphasized by Emil Noeggerath (1872), and the general sub-

[1] Obst. Jour. Gr. Brit., London, 1879–80, vii, 585–588. Brit. Gynæc. Jour.,
London, 1887–8, iii, 366: 1892, vii, 195.

ject developed by Ernst von Bumm (1885), Max Sänger (1889), and Ernst Wertheim (uterine and vesical gonorrhea, 1895–96). The treatment of uterine tumors by faradization was introduced by Georges Apostoli in 1884.[1]

Howard Atwood **Kelly** (1858–   ), of Camden, New Jersey, professor of gynecology in the University of Pennsylvania (1888) and the Johns Hopkins University (1889), who founded the Kensington Hospital in Philadelphia (1883), is a recognized leader of his science in America.

He was a pioneer in the use of cocaine anesthesia, in the treatment of retroflexion of the uterus by suspension (1887), in the introduction of the operations of nephro-ureterectomy, nephro-uretero-cystectomy, vertical bisection of the uterus in hysterectomy, bisection of fibroid or ovarian tumors, horizontal bisection of the cervix for tumors and inflammation, and ideal appendicectomy; the procedures of aëroscopic examination of the bladder and catheterization of the ureters, exploration of the rectum and sigmoid flexure, diagnosis of ureteral and renal calculi by wax-tipped bougies, diagnosis of hydronephrosis by injection and measurement of the capacity of the renal pelvis, operating on the kidney by the superior lumbar triangle, treatment of malignant tumors by radium, and various improvements in the treatment of vesico-vaginal fistulæ. He is the inventor of the Kelly pad, new rectal and vesical specula, and his Operative Gynecology (1898) and Medical Gynecology (1908), both illustrated with Max Brödel's drawings, are full of improvements in his science which have made these books among the best American treatises of the time.

He is also known by his valuable historical contributions on hypnotism, American gynecology, appendicitis, vesico-vaginal fistula, medical botanists, medical illustration, and American medical biography (1912). His "Stereo-Clinic" (1910–13) is a permanent photographic record of recent surgical procedures.

The tendency of recent gynecology to become merged into general abdominal surgery has been wittily signalized by Dr. Kelly as follows:

"The vital question which now affects gynecology is this, is she destined to live a spinster all her days? For we see her on one hand courted by her obstetrical ancestor, who seeks to draw her once more into an unholy, unfruitful alliance, destined to rob her of virility, to be rocked into innocuous desuetude for the rest of her days in the obstetric cradle, sucking the withered ancestral finger in the vain hope of nourishment (with apology for mixed metaphor). On the other hand, we see her wooed by a vigorous, manly suitor, General Surgery, seeking to allure her from her autonomy into his own house, under his own name, obliterating her identity."

Although antisepsis, and even asepsis, had been introduced into **obstetrics** before the time of Lister, the principle did not begin to take hold until surgeon and obstetrician alike began to cleanse their hands in carbolic or bichloride solutions. The first to employ the carbolic solution in obstetrics was Étienne **Tarnier**

---

[1] For bibliographical references to modern gynecology, see Index Catalogue, Surgeon General's Library, 1912, 2. series, xvii, 163–166.

35

546 HISTORY OF MEDICINE

of Paris (1881),[1] the inventor of the well-known axis-traction forceps (1877)[2] and the introducer of milk-diet in pregnancy.

Important features of the pre-antiseptic period were the artificial induction of premature labor by Carl Wenzel (1804), the use of ergot by John Stearns, of Massachusetts (1808), the establishment of the contagiousness of puerperal fever by Holmes (1843) and Semmelweis (1847–61), the first findings of albuminous urine in connection with puerperal convulsions by John C. W. Lever, of Guy's Hospital (1843),[3] Credé's *Handgriff* (1854), the introduction of combined cephalic version by Marmaduke Burr Wright, of Ohio (1854), and of combined podalic version by Braxton Hicks in 1864. In the early part of the century, the two French midwives, Mme. Boivin (1773–1841) and Mme. La Chapelle (1769–1821), published noteworthy treatises on obstetrics (1812 and 1821–25). Mme. La Chapelle's book, with its statistical deductions from 40,000 labor cases, had a good deal to do with the establishment of a proper norm or canon of obstetric procedure at the time. It was followed by such works as those of Velpeau (1829), Cazeaux (1840), and Dubois (1849) in France; Casper von Siebold (1841), Michaëlis (1842), Kiwisch (1851), Scanzoni (1852), and Carl Braun von Fernwald (1857) in Germany and Austria; Fleetwood Churchill (1834) and Francis Henry Ramsbotham (1841) in England; W. P. Dewees (1824), H. L. Hodge (1864), and W. T. Lusk (1882) in America. The best recent American treatise is that of John Whitridge Williams (1903).

Morphological study of the deformed pelvis and of spinal deformity in relation to difficult labor has been almost exclusively in the hands of the German obstetricians. The obliquely contracted pelvis (Naegele pelvis) was first described by Franz Carl Naegele in 1839, and the oblique ovoid pelvis by Carl C. T. Litzmann in 1853, the latter variety including the coxalgic, scoliotic, and kyphoscoliotic forms. The straight narrow pelvis, due to defective development of the sacrum, was described by Robert in 1842. The osteomalacic pelvis was first observed by William Hunter and described by the younger Stein. The rachitic or pseudo-osteomalacic type was described by Smellie, Sandifort, and the younger Stein, and named by Michaëlis (1851). The spondylolisthetic pelvis was described by Rokitansky in 1839, and carefully studied by Kilian as "pelvis obtecta" (1854). Rokitansky also introduced the term "kyphotic pelvis." Baudelocque was the first to observe and describe the funnel-shaped pelvis. The spinous pelvis (pelvis spinosa) was described and figured by Kilian in 1854, while Michaëlis and Litzmann first studied the flat pelvis (pelvis plana Deventeri) and its rachitic variety. Congenital cleft of the symphysis pubis was observed by Bonnet (1724) and Creve (1795), and described by Litzmann (1861). All these different varieties were carefully described by Gustav Adolf **Michaëlis** (1798–1848) in *Das enge Becken* (1851) and in *Die Formen des Beckens* (1861), by Carl Conrad Theodor Litzmann.

After Semmelweis, the most prominent obstetricians of modern times were Simpson, Credé, and Braxton Hicks.

Sir James Young **Simpson** (1811–70), of Bathgate, Scotland, became professor of obstetrics at Edinburgh in 1840, and soon acquired an enormous practice through his great ability and fascinating personality. As the first to employ chloroform in obstetrics and labor (1847), he made a great name for himself in the history of his science. He introduced iron wire sutures (1858), the long obstetric forceps, acupressure (1860–64), and many new "wrinkles" in gynecology and obstetrics, such as the uterine sound

[1] Tarnier: Tr. Internat. Med. Cong., London, 1881, iv, 390.
[2] Ann. de gynéc., Paris, 1877, vii, 241–261.
[3] Lever: Guy's Hosp. Rep., London, 1843, 2. s., i, 495–517.

(1843), the sponge tent, dilatation of the cervix uteri in diagnosis, "Simpson's pains" in uterine cancer (1863), version in deformed pelves. His memoirs on fetal pathology and hermaphroditism are noteworthy; and he also made valuable contributions to archeology and medical history, particularly on leprosy in Scotland (1841–42). He introduced village or pavilion hospitals, and, by his statistical investigations of the results of major operations (Hospitalism, 1869), did much to improve the status of hospitals. Although not without a certain touch of religious fanaticism, which may account for his somewhat bigoted opposition to Lister,

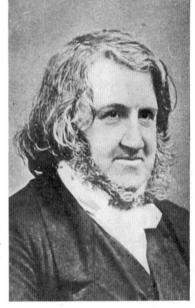

Sir James Young Simpson (1811–70).

he exerted a wonderful influence over his patients, and was, all in all, one of the most remarkable personalities of his time.

Carl Siegmund Franz **Credé** (1819–92), of Berlin, director of the obstetric and gynecological wards of the Charité (1852), and professor of obstetrics at Leipzig, introduced two things of capital importance in obstetric procedure, — the method of removing the placenta by external manual expression (1854–60),[1] and the prevention of infantile (gonorrheal) conjunctivitis by instillation of silver ni-

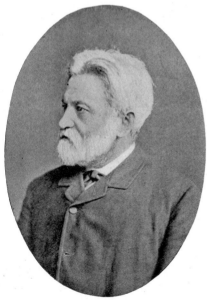

Carl Siegmund Franz Credé (1819–92).

[1] Credé: Klin. Vortr. über Geburtshülfe, Berlin, 1854, 599–603.

HISTORY OF MEDICINE

trate solution into the eyes of the new-born (1884).[1] He was editor of the *Monatsschrift für Geburtskunde* (1853–69), and of the *Archiv für Gynäkologie* (1870–92). He was an admirable teacher and a good organizer, having founded the obstetric and gynecologic polyclinic at Leipzig. The two innovations associated with his name entitle him to the permanent gratitude of mankind.

John Braxton **Hicks** (1825–97), of London, a famous teacher who held many honorable places, made an epoch in the history of obstetric precedure by the introduction of podalic version by combined external and internal manipulation (1863),[2] which forms a connecting link across the ages with Ambroïse Paré's famous paper. Hicks' priority has been disputed in favor of Marmaduke Burr Wright, who, however, employed or recommended external handling in *cephalic* version (1854). Hicks's observations on the condition of the uterus in obstructed labor (1867),[3] and on accidental concealed hemorrhage (1872),[4] are also highly esteemed by the practitioners of his art.

In the post-antiseptic period, Adolf Gusserow (1836–1906) described pernicious anemia in pregnancy (1871), Christian Wilhelm Braune (1831–92) studied pregnancy in frozen sections (1872), Gustav Adolf Walcher (1856–   ) introduced the hanging posture (*Hängelage*) in the conduct of normal labor (1889), L. M. Bossi originated the induction of premature labor by forced dilatation of the cervix (1892), Albert Döderlein studied the relation of the vaginal secretions to puerperal fever (1892), Fritz Momburg (1870–   ) and F. LaTorre introduced the use of the abdominal ligature to prevent uterine hemorrhage (1908).

Ophthalmology and the surgery of the eye were put upon a scientific basis mainly through the labors of three men, Helmholtz, Albrecht von Graefe, and Donders. When the ophthalmoscope was invented, von Graefe exclaimed: "Helmholtz has opened out a new world to us" (*Helmholtz hat uns eine neue Welt erschlossen*), and the usefulness of the instrument is sufficiently indicated by the fact that nearly every prominent eye specialist of recent times has tried to add some improvement to it. Not only did it elucidate the disorders of the uveal tract, but even such obscure diseases as those of the brain, the kidneys, and the pituitary body. Bouchut, in 1863, called the process "cerebroscopy."

Before the time of von Graefe, the infectious forms of granular conjunctivitis had been described by Baron Larrey (1802), John Vetch (1807), and Jacob Christian Bendz (1855); hyoscyamin and atropin had been used in examination by Franz Reisinger (1825); test-types had been introduced by

---

[1] Die Verhütung der Augenentzündung der Neugeborenen, etc., Berlin, 1884.

[2] Hicks: Tr. Obst. Soc. London (1863), 1864, v, 219–259 (Appendix), 265.

[3] *Ibid.* (1867), 1868, ix, 207–227 (Appendix), 229–239.

[4] Brit. Med. Jour., London, 1872, i, 207.

Heinrich Küchler (1843), Eduard Jaeger von Jaxtthal (1854), and Hermann Snellen (1862); Kussmaul had described the color phenomena in the fundus (1845); J. Mery (1704), Brücke (1845), and William Cumming (1845) had considered the significance of luminosity of the eye in vertebrates and man; Philipp Franz von Walther had described corneal opacity (1845); the mechanism of vision had been studied by Thomas Young (1801), Sir Charles Wheatstone (1838–52), Sir David Brewster (1842), William Mackenzie (1845), Johann Benedict Listing (1845), and Helmholtz; and good treatises on eye diseases had been written by Antonio Scarpa (1801), James Wardrop (1808), Georg Joseph Beer (1813–17), Benjamin Travers (1820), John Vetch (1820), George Frick (1824), William Mackenzie (1830), Sir William Lawrence (1833), C.-J.-F. Carron du Villards (1813), Friedrich August von Ammon (1838–41), Karl Himly (1843), Louis-Auguste Desmarres (1847), Carl Stellwag von Carion (1853–58), and Carl Ferdinand von Arlt (1854–6). The surgery of the eye had been advanced by George James Guthrie (1823), J. F. Dieffenbach (strabismus, 1842), Thomas Wharton Jones (1847), L.-A. Desmarres (1850), and particularly by Sir William Bowman (artificial pupil, 1852; lacrimal obstruction, 1857).

Albrecht von Graefe (1828–70), of Berlin, the creator of the modern surgery of the eye, and indeed the greatest of all eye surgeons, was the son of Carl Ferdinand von Graefe. After graduating in Berlin in 1847, he was urged to specialize in ophthalmology by Arlt in Prague, and, having followed the clinics of Sichel and Desmarres in Paris, the Jaegers in Vienna, Bowman and Critchett in London, he soon obtained phenomenal success in his native city, becoming professor at the University in 1857. In 1854, he founded the *Archiv für Ophthalmologie*, which contains most of his important discoveries and inventions and has remained the leading organ of his specialty to date. The first volume alone contains his papers on the disorders of the oblique eye muscles, the nature of glaucoma, keratoconus, mydriasis, diphtheritic conjunctivitis, and on double vision after strabismus operations. Von Graefe introduced the operation of iridectomy in the treatment of iritis, iridochoroiditis and glaucoma (1855–62),[1] made the operation for strabismus viable (1857),[2] and improved the treatment of cataract by the modified linear extraction (1865–68),[3] which reduced the loss of the eye from 10 to 2.3 per cent. He applied the ophthalmoscope to the study of the amblyopias in functional disorders with extraordinary success; made a brilliant diagnosis of embolism of the retinal artery as the cause of a case of sudden blindness (1859),[4] and proceeded to point out that most cases of blindness and impaired vision connected with cerebral disorders are traceable to optic neuritis rather than to paralysis of the optic

---

[1] Graefe: Arch. f. Ophth., Berlin, 1855–6, ii, 2. Abth., 202: 1857, iii, 2. Abth., 456: 1858, iv, 2. Abth., 127: 1862, viii, 2. Abth., 242.

[2] *Ibid.*, 1857, iii, 1. Abth., 177–386.

[3] *Ibid.*, 1865, xi, 3. Abth., 1: 1866, xii, 1. Abth., 150: 1868, xiv, 3. Abth., 106.

[4] *Ibid.*, 1859, v, 1. Abth., 136–157.

nerve (1860),[1] as had been maintained before his time. Graefe was also the founder of modern knowledge of sympathetic ophthalmia (1866)[2] and the semeiology of ocular paralyses (1866),[3] described conical cornea, or "keratoconus" (1854),[4] and first noted the stationary condition of the upper eyelid, when the eyeball is rolled up or down, in exophthalmic goiter (Graefe's sign, 1864).[5] Graefe's clinic became famous all over the world, and was followed, not so much by students as by practising physicians, who had come

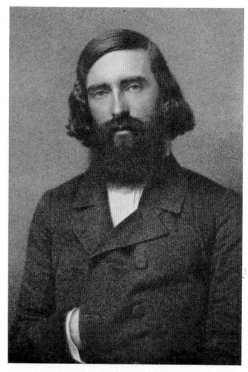

Albrecht von Graefe (1828–70).

to Berlin to learn ophthalmology from its greatest master. He was a man of refined, spirituel type, a *Johanniskopf*, as the Germans say, and his health did not long withstand the strain of such tremendous work as he accomplished in so short a life. Graefe was

[1] Arch. f. Ophth., Berlin, 1860, vii, 2. Abth., 58–71.
[2] *Ibid.*, 1866, xii, 2. Abth., 149–174.
[3] Symptomenlehre der Augenmuskellähmungen, Berlin, 1867.
[4] Arch. f. Ophth., Berlin, 1854–5, i, 1. Abth., 297–306.
[5] Deutsche Klinik, Berlin, 1864, xvi, 158.

fond of pranks and practical jokes, even after his youthful days were over, and many pungent witticisms attributed to him are still quoted and remembered.

Frans Cornelis **Donders** (1818–89), of Tilburg, Holland, was educated as an army surgeon, but became a professor in the Utrecht Faculty in 1848, and, after 1862, devoted himself exclusively to ophthalmology. To this field belong his studies of the muscæ volitantes (1847), the use of prismatic glasses in strabismus (1848), the relation between convergence of the visual axes and accommodation (1848), regeneration of the cornea (1848), anomalies of refraction as a cause of strabismus (1863), the invention of the ophthalmotonometer (1863), and, above all, his great work on *The Anomalies of Refraction and Accommodation*, which was published, not in Dutch, but in English, by the New Sydenham Society (1864). As a contribution to physiological optics, this book ranks with the labors of Helmholtz. It contains Donders' explanation of astigmatism, of the relations between strabismus and hypermetropic or myopic conditions, and his discovery of hypermetropia. It has been the main source of knowledge on the improvement of disorders of vision by spectacles up to the time of Gullstrand. It is said that, while impatiently waiting for one of Helmholtz's ophthalmoscopes, Donders contrived one for himself in which the silvered mirror with central perforation, now in use, was substituted for the superimposed glass plates of the Berlin master's instrument. In 1845, Donders became editor of the *Nederlandsch Lancet*, and in 1851 he established the Netherlandish Hospital for Diseases of the Eye (*Nederlandsch Gasthuis voor Oogleiden*); but his labors were not entirely confined to the eye. In 1863, he succeeded Schroeder van der Kolk as professor of physiology at Utrecht, and, in 1866, established the new Physiological Laboratory in the same city. His most important contribution to physiology was the first measurement of the reaction-

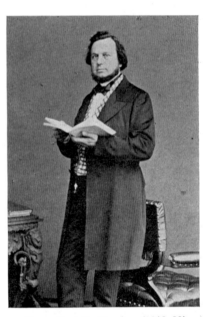

Frans Cornelis Donders (1818–89).

time of a psychical process (1868).[1] In 1845 he wrote on metabolism as the source of heat in animals and plants, and his contributions on the physiology of speech (1864–70)[2] are of great importance. Donders was highly accomplished, speaking English, French, and German like a native, yet modest to the point of diffidence. His earlier military avocations gave him a polished *tenue* which, with his natural personal charm, made him known all over Europe as one of the most attractive specialists of his time.

Prominent among von Graefe's pupils were his nephew **Alfred Karl Graefe** (1830–99), who made a clinical analysis of disordered movements of the eye (1858), invented a special "localization ophthalmoscope" for extracting deep-lying cysticerci, wrote a monograph on the treatment of infantile conjunctivitis by caustics and antiseptics (1881), and, with Saemisch, edited the well-known Graefe-Saemisch Handbuch der Ophthalmologie (1874–80); Julius **Jacobson** (1828–89), of Königsberg, who made a great improvement in the operative treatment of cataract by his peripheral incision under chloroform anesthesia (1863), reducing the loss of the eye from 10 to 2 per cent., and further improving the operation by extraction within the capsule (1888), originated the operative treatment of trachoma and trichiasis (   ), wrote a fine memoir on the work of his friend von Graefe (1885), and enjoyed the largest consulting practice in eastern Europe, patients streaming in even from Russia; the brothers Alexander (1828–79) and Hermann **Pagenstecher** (1844–   ), the former of whom made his mark in the history of cataract by the extraction of the lens in the closed capsule through a scleral incision (1866); Edwin Theodor **Saemisch** (1833–1909), of Luckau, who first described serpiginous ulcer of the cornea and its treatment (1870) and vernal conjunctivitis or *Frühjahrskatarrh* (1876), and edited the above-mentioned Handbuch with the younger Graefe; Julius **Hirschberg** (1843–   ), of Potsdam, whose name is associated with the introduction of the electromagnet into ophthalmology (1885), with a dictionary of ophthalmology (1887), and with the most complete and scholarly history of his science which has ever been written (1899–1911); Theodor **Leber** (1840–   ), who studied the diabetic disorders of the eye (1875) and the disorders of circulation and nutrition of the eye (1876); Ludwig **Laqueur** (1839–1909), who introduced the use of physostigmin in glaucoma (1876); Richard **Liebreich** (1830–   ), of Königsberg, who introduced lateral illumination in microscopic investigation of the living eye (1855), and published the first atlas of ophthalmoscopy (1863), in which he was followed by Jaeger von Jaxtthal (1869); and Hermann Jakob **Knapp** (1832–1911), of Dauborn, Hesse-Nassau, who became one of the leading ophthalmologists of New York city, founded the *Archives of Ophthalmology and Otology* (New York, 1869), and wrote valuable memoirs on curvature of the cornea (1859) and intra-ocular tumors (1869) and other subjects.

Of works relating to the normal eye we may mention Max Schultze's memoir on the anatomy and physiology of the retina (1866); the theories of vision of Helmholtz (1867), Edward Hering (1872–75) and Christine Ladd Franklin (1892); Willy Kühne's investigations of visual purple (1877), and Johannes von Kries' memoir on the function of the rods in the retina (1895). The examination of the eye was furthered by such inventions as the astigmometer (1867) of Emile **Javal** (1839–1907), of Paris; by the Javal-Schiötz ophthalmometer (1881); by the method of retinoscopy introduced by Ferdinand Cuignet (1873), and by the keratoscope invented by A. Placido (1882). Color-blindness was investigated by the Swedish physiologist Alarik Frithiof **Holmgren** (1831–97), who introduced the wool-skein test (1874) and gave special consideration to color-blindness under railway and maritime conditions (1878).

---

[1] Arch. f. Anat., Physiol. u. wissensch. Med., Berlin, 1868, 657–681.

[2] De physiologie der spraakklanken, Utrecht, 1870.

The relation of eye-strain and astigmatism to headaches and other neurotic symptoms was first investigated by S. Weir Mitchell (1874) and William Thomson (1879), and applied extensively to morbid psychology by George M. Gould (1888). The relation of eye diseases to general and organic diseases of the body was especially treated by Richard Förster (1877) and Hermann **Schmidt-Rimpler** (1898), who was also, with Hermann **Cohn** (1838–1906), a pioneer in the examination of the eyes of school-children. The bacteriology of the eye was especially advanced by Robert Koch, who discovered the bacilli of two different forms of Egyptian conjunctivitis (1883); by John E. Weeks, who found the same organism as the cause of "pink-eye" (1886); by Henri **Parinaud** (1844–1905), of Paris, who described an infectious conjunctivitis transmissible from animals to man (1889), and a lacrimal pneumococcic conjunctivitis in new-born infants (1894), both associated with his name; and by Victor Morax and Theodor Axenfeld, who simultaneously described the diplobacillary form of chronic conjunctivitis (1896–97). Apart from the Graefe-Saemisch Handbuch, perhaps the best modern treatise on ophthalmology is the monumental work of Louis de Wecker (1832–1906) and Edmond Landolt (1846–   ), published 1880–89. Another good work is that of the Greek, Photinos Panas (1894), whose name is especially associated with an operation for congenital and paralytic ptosis (1886). Besides the Americans already referred to, we may mention Henry Willard Williams (1821–   ), who introduced the treatment of iritis without mercury (1856) and a method of suturing the flap after cataract extraction (1866); Cornelius Rea Agnew (1830–88), who described a method of operating for divergent squint (1866), and Henry Drury Noyes (1832–1900), who first investigated retinitis in glycosuria (1867). Aside from the great work of Julius Hirschberg (1899–1911), good histories of ophthalmology have been written by August Hirsch (1877), P. Pansier (1903), and Carl Horstmann (1905), while Hugo Magnus (1842–   ) has dealt especially with the history of cataract (1876) and ancient ophthalmology (1901), Victor Deneffe with the Gallo-Roman oculists of the third century (1896), Pansier (1901) and Emil Bock (1903) with the history of spectacles, and Alvin A. Hubbell (1846–   ) with the developments of ophthalmology in America from 1800 to 1870 (1908).[1]

Laryngology and rhinology were specially advanced by the introduction of laryngoscopy by Benjamin Babington (1829), Robert Liston (1837), Manuel Garcia (1855), Ludwig Türck (1858–60), and Johann Czermak (1858); of rhinoscopy by Philipp Bozzini (1773–1809), in 1807, and (successfully) by Czermak (1859); of autoscopy of the larynx and trachea without the mirror by Alfred Kirstein (1863–   ), of Berlin, in 1895, and of direct bronchoscopy by Gustav Killian (1860–   ), of Mainz, in 1898. Suspension-laryngoscopy (*Schwebelaryngoskopie*) was introduced by Killian in 1912. The anatomy of the larynx and the physiology of the voice and speech were investigated by Johannes Müller (1839), Ernst von Brücke (1856), F. C. Donders (1870), Hubert von Luschka (1873), and Carl Ludwig Merkel (*Anthropophonik*, 1876). Max Schultze investigated the histology and nerve-endings of the Schneiderian membrane (1863), Emil Zuckerkandl the anatomy and pathology of the accessory sinuses (1882–92), and Hendrik Zwaardemaker the physiology of smell (1895). A perfected method of photographing the larynx was devised by Thomas Rushmore French in 1884. Important early treatises on laryngology were those of John Cheyne (1777–1836) on the Pathology of the Membrane of the Larynx and Bronchia (1809), William Henry Porter (1790–1861) on the surgical pathology of the larynx and trachea (1826), Armand Trousseau and Hippolyte Belloc on laryngeal phthisis, chronic laryngitis, and disorders of the voice (1837), Horace Green (1802–66) on diseases of the air-passages (1846), Samuel D. Gross on foreign bodies in the air-passages (1854), Sir Morell Mackenzie on laryngeal tumors (1871), and Francke Huntington Bosworth (1843–   ) on diseases of the nose and throat (1881). Intubation of the larynx in croup was introduced by Eugène Bouchut (1818–91) in 1858, first done in Paris in connection with

---

[1] For bibliographic references to this section see Surgeon-General's Catalogue, 1912, 2. s., xvii, pp. 168–171.

tracheotomy by Trousseau (1851–59), and perfected through the conscientious labors (1885–88) of the self-sacrificing Joseph P. **O'Dwyer** (1841–98), of Cleveland, Ohio, whose name stands with those of Semmelweis and Credé as one of the great benefactors of infant life. **Horace Green** (1802–66), of Crittenden, Vermont, was the pioneer of laryngology in the United States, the first to treat diseases of the throat by local applications (1838), and the author of important works on croup (1849) and the surgical treatment of polyps of the larynx (1852). The tonsillotome was invented by P. S. Physick (1828). Charles Henri Ehrmann (1792–1878) was the first to remove a laryngeal polyp (1844); Victor von Bruns (1812–83) first enucleated a laryngeal polyp by the bloodless method (1862), and was the pioneer of laryngoscopic surgery (1865); and Rudolph Voltolini (1819–89) first employed the galvanocautery in laryngeal surgery (1867) and performed the first laryngeal operation through the mouth with external illumination (1889). Paralysis of the vocal cords was first carefully studied by Carl Gerhardt (1833–1902) in 1863–72. The first important treatises on diseases of the nose were the Paris thesis of Jacques-Louis Deschamps *fils* (1804), and the "Ophrésiologie" (1821) of Hippolyte Cloquet (1787–1840), which were followed by such nose and throat treatises as those of Horace Green (1846), Carl Seiler (1879), E. F. Ingals (1881), Sir Morell Mackenzie (1880–84), C. E. Sajous (1885), O. Chiari (1887), R. Voltolini (1888), Lenox Browne (1890), and F. H. Bosworth (1890–92). Benjamin Löwenberg was the first to consider the nature and treatment of ozena (1885), and Ludwig Grünwald (1863–   ) the surgical treatment of nasal suppuration and disease of the ethmoid and sphenoid (1893). Ephraim Fletcher Ingals (1848–   ), of Lee Centre, Illinois, treated deflections of the nasal septum by partial excision in 1882, and this operation was finally perfected by Robert Krieg in 1889, Otto T. Freer in 1902, and Gustav Killian in 1904. Killian also originated the radical operation for chronic inflammation of the frontal sinus (1903). The best histories of laryngology and rhinology are those of Louis Elsberg (1879–80), Gordon Holmes (1887), Jonathan Wright (St. Louis, 1898), and the monumental work of C. Chauveau on the history of diseases of the pharynx (Paris, 1901–06).[1]

The foundations of **otology** were the catheterization of the Eustachian tubes through the mouth by Guyot (1724) and Cleland (1741), the mastoid operations of Petit (1774) and Jasser (1776), Cooper's perforation of the tympanic membrane for deafness (1800), and the monographs of Valsalva, Cotugno, Scarpa, and others. The first treatise on diseases of the ear was written by Jean-Marc-Gaspard **Itard** (1775–1838), of Oraison (Provence), in 1821, and this important work was followed by such treatises as those of Joseph Toynbee (1860), Anton Friedrich von Tröltsch (1866), Lawrence Turnbull (1872), Sir W. B. Dalby (1873), St. John Roosa (1873), Adam Politzer (1878–82), Victor Urbantschitsch (1880), and Friedrich Bezold (1906). Max Schultze described the nerve-endings in the labyrinth (1858), Helmholtz the mechanics of the ossicles and membrana tympani (1869), Goltz the physiological significance of the semicircular canals (1870), the elder [Magnus Christian] Retzius wrote an important monograph on the vertebrate ear (1884), Julius Richard Ewald studied audition in birds deprived of the labyrinths, and Stanislav Stein the functions of separate parts of the labyrinth (1894). Adam **Politzer** (1835–   ), of Alberti, Hungary, was the first to obtain pictures of the membrana tympani by illumination (1865), which he afterward illustrated in an atlas of 14 plates and 392 pictures (1896). The transmission of sounds through the cranial bones in diagnosis of aural diseases was first studied by Johann C. A. Lucae (1870), and great advances in exploration were made by Friedrich **Bezold** (1842–1908), of Rothenburg an der Tauber, who gave the first clear description of mastoiditis (1877), introduced new tests for audition in deafmutism (1896) and in unilateral deafness (1897). Among other advances were the Weber and Rinné tests, Hartmann's diapasons, and Sir Francis Galton's whistle for determining the superior limits of audition. The pioneers of aural

---

[1] For bibliographic references to this section see Surgeon-General's Catalogue, 1912, 2. s., xvii, pp. 171, 172.

surgery in the nineteenth century were Sir Astley Cooper (1801) and Sir William Wilde (1843–53), and after their time the most important English work on the subject was that of James Hinton (1827–75), of Guy's Hospital (1874). The modern surgery of the ear and mastoid has been mainly the work of the Germans. In 1873, Hermann **Schwartze** (1837–1910) and Adolph **Eysell** described the method of opening the mastoid by chiseling (*typische Aufmeisselung*). This operation was further improved by Emanuel **Zaufal** (1884) and Ernst **Küster** (1889), while Ludwig **Stacke** introduced excision of the ossicles (1890) and greatly improved the surgery of the middle ear (1892–97). Aural vertigo was first described by Prosper **Ménière** (1799–1862) in 1861, was again noted by Charcot as "vertigo ab aure læsa" (1874), while the relations between nystagmus and vestibular or cerebellar disease had been noted by Purkinje and Flourens, and have been developed, in the twentieth century, by Robert Bárány. An authoritative history of otology by Adam **Politzer** has just been completed (1907–13).[1]

Neither the English nor the French **clinical medicine** of this period had the purely scientific tendency which characterized the German. In England, pathology was little studied after the time of Bright, Hodgkin, and Addison, although the English talent for careful clinical observation was amply illustrated. The brightest phase of French medicine in the second half of the nineteenth century was its neurology. With the exception of Charcot, most of the French clinicians of the time were brilliant and elegant expositors of internal medicine, as Helmholtz has described them, rather than original workers in pathology.

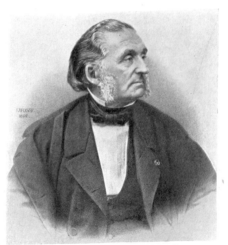

Armand Trousseau (1801–67).

Indeed, as we shall see, there are no professional pathologists in French medical schools, their places being supplied by physicians practising in hospitals.

Of the French clinicians, Armand **Trousseau** (1801–67), of Tours, a pupil of Bretonneau, professor in the Paris Faculty (1850) and physician at the Hôpital St. Antoine (1839) and the Hôtel Dieu (1850), occupied about the same position in French medicine as Bright and Addison, Stokes and Graves over the Channel. He received the prize of the Academy of Medicine for his classical trea-

---

[1] For bibliographic references to this section, see Surgeon General's Catalogue, 1912, 2. s.; xvii, 172, 173.

tise on laryngeal phthisis (1837), was the first to perform tracheotomy in Paris, and was a pioneer in the introduction of intubation (1851). He first described gastric vertigo and a diagnostic sign of infantile tetany, consisting of the voluntary reproduction of the paroxysms during the attack by compressing the affected parts. His *Clinique médicale de l'Hôtel Dieu* (1861), which passed through three editions, contains his best work, much of which has silently taken its place in the text-books. He was a man of big personality, a great master of clinical delineation, and a generous interpreter of the ideas of other men, particularly of the diseases described by Bretonneau, Addison, Hodgson, and Duchenne of Boulogne.

Georges **Dieulafoy** (1839–1911), of Toulouse, who wrote the most readable French treatise on internal medicine in his day (1880–84),[1] and is otherwise remembered by his employment of the trocar in the treatment of pleurisy, hydatids, etc., was a fiery clinical orator of the meridional type, who never bothered himself about scientific questions, but built up a large clientèle and otherwise enjoyed the expression or exploitation of his personality in the clinics. Handsome and gay (*le beau Dieulafoy*), he was gifted with great powers of elocution and mimicry, a natural born actor, with the gestures and intonations of an Italian tenor,—*des gestes qui implorent et qui caressent*,—and he always succeeded in posing his diagnosis in a way to excite the greatest admiration. Nevertheless, he was a physician of alert intelligence and fascinating personality, who at least endeavored to make his teaching anything but dull. He excelled in coining such expressions as "*le foie appendiculaire*," which illustrate his virtuosity in the use of the French language, but convey nothing very definite to the mind.

Sigismond **Jaccoud** (1830–1913), of Geneva, was another prominent Paris internist, whose treatise on practice (1871) and clinical lectures (1867–88) enjoyed about the same reputation as Dieulafoy's.

Jean-Alfred **Fournier** (1832–   ), of Paris, professor in the Paris Faculty, whose name is associated with the great venereal clinic at the Hôpital St. Louis, is reputed as a teacher of great power, possessed of a clear, harmonious voice, full of the finest delicacy and courtesy to patients or pupils, universally liked, and penetrating even the dullest minds by his luminous intelligence and clear, effective mode of expression. With Diday, of Lyons, Fournier did most to develop the subject of congenital syphilis, in which he brought "order out of chaos." Practically all his life has been devoted to the study of this disease, to every phase of which he added something of clinical importance, as also to its social aspects

---

[1] Dieulafoy: Manuel de pathologie interne, Paris, 1880–84.

(*Syphilis et mariage*, 1890). His statistics on the causal relation of lues to ataxia and paresis (1876–94)[1] are, with those of Erb, the most important contribution to the subject. Fournier is described as a keen-eyed, close-cropped military figure, looking like an old artillery officer.

Henri **Huchard** (1844–1910), of Auxon (Aube), was a clinician of the same effective type. He is especially remembered for his studies in therapeutics, his *Traité des névroses* (with Axenfeld, 1883), his great monograph on disorders of the circulation (1889), and particularly by his work on the clinical forms of arteriosclerosis (1909), which he did most to develop.

Among the original contributions of French clinicians are J.- A. Villemin's proof of the inoculability of tuberculosis (1868), the theses of L.-A. Thaon and J.-J. Grancher on the unity of phthisis (1873), Joseph Dumoutier's account of sleeping sickness (1868), Paul Lorain's delineation of sexual infantilism (1871), the descriptions of chronic interstitial hepatitis (1874) by Georges Hayem (1841–   ), of cirrhotic jaundice (1875) by Victor-Charles Hanot (1844–96), of primary endotheliomatous hypertrophy of the spleen by P.-C.-E. Gaucher (1882), of enteroptosis and gastroptosis by Frantz Glénard (1885), of primitive cancer of the pancreas by Louis Bard and Adrien Pic (1888), of cyanotic polycythemia by Henri Vaquez (1892); Ch. Bouchard (1887) and A. Combe (1907) on autointoxication; and the pediatric treatises of C.-M. Billard (1828–33); and of Rilliet and Barthez (1838–43), which contains an early account of poliomyelitis.

German clinical medicine in the second half of the nineteenth century includes such names as Frerichs, Traube, Kussmaul, Gerhardt, Ziemssen, Leyden, Senator, Naunyn, and Friedrich Müller.

Friedrich Theodor von **Frerichs** (1819–85), of Aurich, graduated at Göttingen in 1841, and soon achieved a reputation as an ophthalmologist, but afterward went over to scientific and internal medicine and became one of the founders of experimental pathology. He received his professorship at Göttingen in 1848, afterward holding chairs at Kiel (1850) and Breslau (1852), succeeding Schönlein at Berlin in 1859. Frerichs seems to have attained the summit of his profession in a surprisingly short while, and his course from Göttingen to Berlin has been likened by Naunyn to a triumphal progress. Students hung upon his lips, and his colleagues revered his wonderful precision in diagnosis. At forty, he had already done his best work, his great monograph on digestion in Wagner's Dictionary of Physiology, his discovery of leucin and tyrosin in the urine of acute yellow atrophy of the liver (1855),[2]

---

[1] Fournier: Les affections parasyphilitiques, Paris, 1894.
[2] Frerichs: Deutsche Klinik, Berlin, 1855, vii, 341–343.

his pathological studies of cirrhosis of the liver, pernicious malarial fever, and melanemia, and his books on Bright's disease (1851)[1] and diseases of the liver (1858).[2]   Yet, at Berlin, as his pupil, Naunyn, tells us, Frerichs seemed, at the height of his reputation, to undergo a sort of spiritual and intellectual blight.   Apart from his students, of whom he had always a large following, he became secluded, reserved, and querulous, and wrote little.   The second volume of his work on diseases of the liver (1868) is said to show a distinct

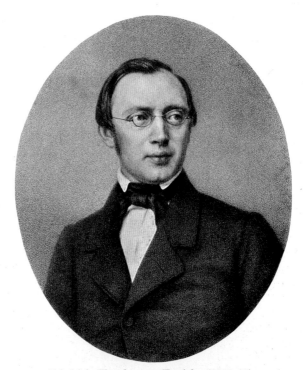

Friedrich Theodor von Frerichs (1819–85).

falling off of talent, although his lectures were always highly esteemed for their beautiful concision and accuracy, and he enjoyed an enormous consulting practice.   This change in Frerichs' personality was due, Naunyn thinks, to his extreme sensitiveness to criticism; to the opposition which he encountered in Berlin, especially from his mistakes about the origin of the bile-pigments and acids; to his falling out with Traube, his colleague at the

---

[1] Die Bright'sche Nierenkrankheit, Braunschweig, 1851.
[2] Klinik der Leberkrankheiten, Braunschweig, 1858.

Charité, and to the aggressive enmity which he encountered at the hands of Virchow. So strong was Virchow's personality that even Graefe and Langenbeck lined up with him in official opposition to Frerichs, whose productiveness was soon sterilized by this professional jealousy. It was only under the sympathetic influence of Leyden, who came on at the Charité in 1876 and eventually succeeded him, that he brightened up again and produced a monograph worthy of his fame, his work on diabetes (1884), based upon 400 cases and 55 autopsies. The clinical lectures of Frerichs, which he delivered offhand, are described by Naunyn as of classic perfection of phrase, clear and plastic in the delineation of disease, and as having a rare freshness from the number of facts drawn from his own experience. His diagnoses, which he made offhand, directly upon seeing the cases, were usually intuitive, always developed as a disturbance of physiological function, and never admitted to be wrong. Like Skoda, Frerichs was indifferent to patients, even to students, caring only for the scientific aspects of the disease itself, although he always condescended to outline a course of treatment, including a prescription. In person he was tall and ungainly, yet imposing through his style of delivery, which was frequently dramatic. The interest of Frerichs is that he developed scientific clinical teaching in Germany. His pupils include some of the brightest spirits of modern times, such men as Ehrlich, Naunyn, Leyden, and von Mering.

Ludwig **Traube** (1818–76), of Ratibor, Silesia, was a pupil of Purkinje, Johannes Müller, Skoda, Rokitansky and Schönlein, becoming the latter's assistant in 1849 and professor at Berlin in 1857. Traube early made his mark as one of the founders of experimental pathology by his investigation of the pulmonary disorders occasioned by section of the vagus nerve. This was followed by studies of suffocation (1846–47), the pathology of fever, the effect of digitalis, the relation of cardiac and renal disorders, and particularly by his *Beiträge zur experimentellen Pathologie* (1871–78), which gave him a wide reputation. Traube was one of the first of the Jewish physicians to receive official recognition after the events of 1848, and his clinics at the Charité soon became very popular on account of his exact methods and his honest, sincere attitude toward his patients. His long-standing difference with Frerichs was due to the usual disputes about clinical material, of which the latter, as physician-in-chief, had the lion's share.

Adolf **Kussmaul** (1822–1902), of Graben, near Karlsruhe, began as an army surgeon, becoming later professor at Heidelberg (1857), Erlangen (1859), Freiburg (1863), and Strassburg (1876). His earlier studies were upon the changes of color in the eye (1845), the effect of the circulation upon the movements of the iris (1856), the relation between anemia and epileptiform convulsions (1857). Of greater importance were his monographs on the psychology of the new-born infant (1859), on mercurial salivation and its relation to constitutional syphilis (1861), and on disorders of speech (1877). He was the first to describe "periarteriitis nodosa" (1866),[1] progressive bulbar paralysis (1873), and diabetic coma with acetonemia (1874),[2] and added much to the knowledge of tetany and osteomyelitis. Equally brilliant were his contributions to diagnosis and therapeutics. He introduced the concept of "pulsus paradoxus" (1873),[3] was the first to diagnose mesenteric embolism in the living subject (1864), the first to attempt esophagoscopy and gastroscopy (1869),[4] the first to wash out the stomach with the stomach-pump for gastric dilatation (1867–69), to treat gastric ulcer with large doses of bismuth, and to employ thoracentesis (1868).[5] His *Jugenderinnerungen* (1899) is one of the best of medical autobiographies, containing interesting sidelights on the palmy days of the New Vienna School. On Christmas day, 1893, he distributed among his friends a volume of poems, privately printed under the pseudonym "Dr. Oribasius."

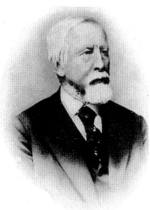

Adolf Kussmaul (1822–1902).

Carl **Gerhardt** (1833–1902), of Speyer, professor at Jena (1861), Würzburg (1872) and Berlin (1885), devoted himself mainly to pediatrics and laryngology. He made important contributions on laryngeal croup (1859), paralysis of the vocal cords (1863–72), laryngeal tumors (1896), syphilis of the larynx and trachea (1898), and was the author of treatises on auscultation and percussion (1890), diseases of children (1880) and the editor of a handbook of pediatrics (1887).

In connection with the name of Gerhardt, we may mention the pediatricians, Eduard Heinrich **Henoch** (1820–1910), of Berlin,

---

[1] With Rudolf Maier: Deutsches Arch. f. klin. Med., Leipzig, 1866, i, 484–518.

[2] *Ibid.*, 1874, xiv, 1–46.

[3] Samml. klin. Vortr., Leipzig, 1873, No. 54 (Innere Med., No. 62), 1637–1674.

[4] Deutsche Ztschr. f. Chir., Leipzig, 1900–1901, lviii, 500–507, 1 pl. (Communicated by G. Killian.)

[5] For references to these and other contributions of Kussmaul see Deutsches Arch. f. klin. Med., Leipzig, 1902, lxxiii, 1–89.

a pupil of Schönlein and Romberg, who wrote a masterly treatise on children's diseases (1861) and described Henoch's purpura (1874), and the Viennese, Alois **Bednar** (of Bednar's aphthæ), whose treatise on diseases of infants (1850–53) is equally well known.

Hugo **von Ziemssen** (1829–1902), one of Virchow's pupils, was professor of clinical medicine at Erlangen (1863), and (after serving in the Franco-Prussian War) at Munich (1874), where he directed the city hospital and founded the first clinical institute for instruction in the specialties (1877). Ziemssen was one of the great medical encyclopedists, whose fame rests largely today upon his Handbook of Special Pathology and Therapeutics in seventeen volumes (1875–85). He edited handbooks of therapeutics (1880–84), hygiene (1882–86), and skin diseases (1883–84), and made innumerable contributions to many different subjects.

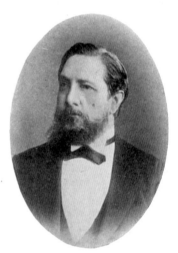

Ernst von Leyden (1832–1910).

Ernst von **Leyden** (1832–1910), of Danzig, a pupil of Schönlein and Traube, succeeded the latter at Berlin in 1876, and also succeeded to Frerichs' clinic upon his death (1885). In 1894, he was called to the Russian court to treat Czar Alexander, for which he received a patent of nobility in 1895. In 1879 he founded, with Frerichs, the *Zeitschrift für klinische Medizin*, and, in the later years of his life, was an active coeditor of several other journals. He acquired a great reputation in Berlin and specialized in neurology, his most famous work being his clinical studies of tabes dorsalis (1863–1901), respiration in fever (1870), diseases of the spinal cord (1874–76), poliomyelitis and neuritis (1880) and prognosis in heart disease (1889). He did most to promote the movement for hospitalization of phthisical patients in Germany.

Hermann **Nothnagel** (1841–1905), a pupil of Traube and Virchow, Leyden's assistant at Königsberg (1865–8), and professor at Freiburg (1872), Jena (1874) and Vienna (1882–1905), wrote an authoritative treatise on therapeutics (1870), made many excellent contributions to neurology, and is especially memorable for his encyclopedic Handbook of Special Pathology and Therapeutics in 24 volumes (1894–1905).

36

Hermann **Senator** (1834–1911), of Gnesen, Polish Prussia, a pupil of Johannes Müller, Schönlein, and Traube, became one of the directors of the Charité in 1881, and after Frerichs' death he was given a separate medical clinic and the University polyclinic (1888). He made his reputation by his investigations of the pathology of fever and its treatment (1873), diabetes (1879), albuminuria in health and disease (1882), which was translated for the New Sydenham Society (1890), and diseases of the kidneys (1896). He also described infectious peri-pharyngeal phlegmon (1888).

Bernard **Naunyn** (1839–   ), son of a burgomaster of Berlin, was Frerichs' clinical assistant for seven years, afterward professor of clinical medicine at Dorpat (1859), Bern (1872), and Königs-

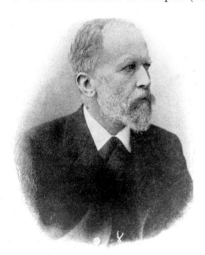

berg (   ), finally succeeding Kussmaul at Strassburg in 1888. With Klebs and Schmiedeberg, he founded the *Archiv für experimentelle Pathologie und Pharmakologie* in 1872, and, with Mikulicz, the *Mittheilungen aus den Grenzgebieten der Medizin und Chirurgie* (1896). Of all Frerichs' pupils, Naunyn and Ehrlich have best followed the master's bent in experimental pathology and pathological chemistry. Aside from his earlier investigations of hydatids and the chemistry of the transudates, Naunyn has devoted his whole life to the study of metabolism in diabetes and in diseases of the liver and the pancreas, his most important works being his clinical study of gall-stones (1892)[1] and his monograph on diabetes (1898).[2] In the former, he introduced the new concept of "cholangitis" as an inflammation of the lining membrane of the smallest bile-ducts causing obliteration of their lumina, explaining catarrhal jaundice and syphilitic hepatitis as primary and secondary forms of infectious cholangitis and regarding biliary calculi as the effect rather than the cause of the same disease. His treatment of the condition by drainage of the bile tract shows how the modern clinician may think surgically as the surgeon clinically. He opposed Flint's idea that cholesterin is a specific product of the liver

Bernard Naunyn (1839–   ).

---

[1] Naunyn: Klinik der Cholelithiasis, Leipzig, 1892.
[2] Der Diabetes mellitus, Vienna, 1898.

secretions or of metabolism. With his pupil, Stadelmann, he introduced the concept of diabetic coma as a fatal acidosis. When Naunyn went to Strassburg, his aggressive Prussian temperament excited a great deal of prejudice and opposition among the Alsatian population and it took him thirteen years to succeed, where even the suave Kussmaul had failed, in having the ancient city hospital (built 1718) converted into the splendid new building (1901). In spite of an attractive call to Vienna, he fought it out in Alsace, where his splendid clinical abilities, his stern fidelity to duty, his love of truth, his polished wit and sarcasm, did not fail of recognition in the end. On the social side, he was known as a man of widest culture, especially in music. His promised autobiography, if we may judge from the fascinating fragment published in 1908, should be the most interesting book in its class. His pupils number such distinguished pathological chemists as Ernst **Stadelmann** (1853–), of Insterburg, who investigated the relation of β-oxybutyric acid to diabetic coma (1883), the effect of alkalies on metabolism (1890) and peptonuria (1894), and, with M. Afanassyeff (1883), worked out the experimental pathology of toxemic and hemolytic jaundice (1891)[1]; Oscar **Minkowski** (1858–), of Alexoten, Russia, who described congenital acholuric jaundice with splenomegaly and urobilinuria (1900),[2] studied the presence of oxybutyric acid in diabetic urine (1884), the effect of excision of the liver on metabolism (1885), and, with Joseph von Mering, the production of diabetes by excision of the pancreas (1889–93); Max **Schrader** (1860–), who made valuable studies on the inhibitory center of the heart (1886) and the comparative physiology of the brain, and Adolf **Magnus Levy** (1865–) whose name is particularly associated with diabetic coma and its treatment (1899–1909). Naunyn and his pupils did the best recent work in chemical and experimental pathology.

Joseph **von Mering** (1849–), of Cologne, a pupil of Frerichs and Hoppe-Seyler, investigated phlorizin diabetes (1886) and collaborated with Minkowski in his experimental work on pancreatic diabetes (1889).

Carl **von Noorden** (1858–), of Bonn, professor at Frankfort (1893) and Nothnagel's successor at Vienna (1906), has made important studies of albuminuria in health (1885), disorders of metabolism (1892–95) and the treatment of the same (1909). His pupils, H. Eppinger, W. Falta and C. Rüdinger, have done much

---

[1] Stadelmann: Der Icterus (etc.), Stuttgart, 1891.

[2] Minkowski: Verhandl. d. Cong. f. inn. Med., Wiesbaden, 1900, xviii, 316. A non-congenital hemolytic icterus was described by F. Widal and P. Abrami (1907).

to develop the doctrine of the correlation of the internal secretions of the ductless glands (1908–9).

Friedrich **Müller** (1858–   ), of Augsburg, a pupil of Voit and Gerhardt, succeeded Biermer at Breslau (1890), and has held chairs at Marburg (1892), Basel (1899) and at Munich (1902), where his clinic is now one of the most largely frequented in Europe. An able internist and neurologist, he is perhaps the most scientific teacher of internal medicine today.

Karl Anton **Ewald** (1845–   ), of Berlin, an assistant of Frerichs and Senator's successor at the Augusta Hospital (1886), is known everywhere for his great work on disorders of digestion (1879–88), his use of intubation in exploring the contents of the stomach (1875) and his "test-breakfast," which he devised (1885) with his pupil, Ismar **Boas** (1858–   ), of Exin, Posen, whose treatises on diseases of the stomach (1890–93) and the intestines (1899) are also highly esteemed.

Ernst **Finger** (1856–   ), of Vienna; Hermann von **Zeissl**

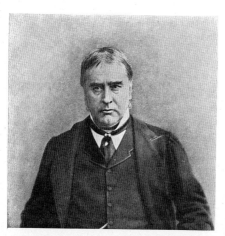

Sir William Withey Gull (1816–90).

(1817–84), of Zwittau, Moravia, and his son, Maximilian von Zeissl (1853–   ), of Vienna, have distinguished themselves in the field of genito-urinary and venereal diseases.

The most prominent clinicians and pathologists at Guy's Hospital during the later period were Gull, Wilks and Hilton Fagge. Sir William Withey **Gull** (1816–90), of Colchester, England, graduated in medicine from the University of London (1846) and soon became associated with Guy's, where he taught medicine for the rest of his life. He was one of the first to note the posterior spinal lesions in locomotor ataxia (1856–58),[1] described intermittent hemoglobinuria (1866),[2] myxedema (1873),[3] and, with Sutton, the "arteriocapillary fibrosis" in chronic nephritis (1872),[4] which

---

[1] Gull: Guy's Hosp. Rep., London, 1856, 3. s., ii, 143: 1858, iv, 169.
[2] Ibid., 1866, 3. s., xii, 381–392.
[3] Tr. Clin. Soc. London, 1873–74, xii, 180–185.
[4] Med.-Chir. Tr., London, 1871–72, lv, 273–326, 2 pl.

showed that the concept "Bright's disease" is something more than a local renal affection. He also wrote upon vascular obstructions, cerebral abscess, "anorexia nervosa," factitious urticaria, and described, with Addison, "vitiligoidea" or xanthelasma (1851–52).[1] He was one of the pioneers in the use of male fern in tenia (1855) and of static electricity in the treatment of nervous diseases (1852).[2] He was one of the greatest practitioners of his time, Napoleonic in appearance, witty, genial, attractive, and a beautiful lecturer. He is said to have fascinated his patients, to whose cases he gave unstinted time and pains, but, although adored by his pupils, he sometimes repelled his colleagues by his magisterial manner and his imperious temper. His clever epigrams "Savages explain, science investigates," and "You are a healthy man out of health," intended to soothe a troublesome hypochondriac, are often quoted. He defined a neurotic woman as "Mrs. A. multiplied by four," and to another he said, "Madame, you have a tired heart." He opposed surgical anesthesia with similar flippancies, and affected a sort of therapeutic nihilism, although he was, in reality, remarkably skilful with such drugs as he used. "The road to medical education," he said, "is through the Hunterian Museum and not through an apothecary's shop." He left a fortune of £344,000, almost unprecedented in the history of medicine.

Sir Samuel **Wilks** (1824–1911), of Camberwell, England, was associated with Guy's Hospital all his life and, in his charming "Biographical Reminiscences" (1911), he appears as its loyal historian, recounting the discoveries of his colleagues with scrupulous fidelity and settling many points of priority. The writings of Wilks really gave the diseases called after Bright, Addison and Hodgkin their place in English medicine. He himself introduced the term "enteric fever," was one of the first to study visceral syphilis (1857–63),[3] left clear accounts of such rare conditions as osteitis deformans (1868),[4] acromegaly (1869),[5] gave a classical account of alcoholic paraplegia (1868),[6] and, as dermatologist, described the "lineæ atrophicæ" on the skin (1861)[7] and dissecting-room warts (verrucæ necrogenicæ), or subcutaneous tuberculosis (1862).[8] Wilks was a personality of rare kindliness and charm, described by Osler as one of the handsomest men in London in his

[1] Guy's Hosp. Rep., London, 1850–51, 2. s., vii, 265, 2 pl.: 1852–3, viii, 149, 1 pl.

[2] *Ibid.*, 1852–53, 2. s., viii, 81.

[3] Tr. Path. Soc. London, 1857–58, ix, 55: 1860–61, xii, 216. Guy's Hosp. Rep., London, 1862–63, 3. s., ix, 1–63, 4 pl.

[4] Tr. Path. Soc. London, 1868–69, xx, 273–277.

[5] Wilks: Biog. Reminiscences, London, 1911, 188.

[6] Med. Times and Gaz., London, 1868, ii, 470.

[7] Guy's Hosp. Rep., London, 1861, 3. s., vii, 297–301.

[8] *Ibid.*, 1862, viii, 263–265.

time, with "a splendid head and merry blue eyes, a man whose
yea was yea and whose nay, nay." His lectures on pathological
anatomy (1859, re-edited by Walter Moxon, 1875), and on diseases
of the nervous system (1878) were standard sources of knowledge
among English students of his time.

Charles Hilton **Fagge** (1838–83), of Hythe, England, editor of
the Guy's Hospital Reports, was an able pathologist and clinician,
an authority on heart disease, an investigator of cretinism and
rickets, and an expert dermatologist. He translated Hebra for
the Sydenham Society (1866–68), grouped keloid, morphea and
spurious leprosy under the category "scleriasis" (1867), and gave
the classical description
of gastromesenteric ileus
(1869),[1] first noticed by
Rokitansky. His "Prin-
ciples and Practice
of Medicine" (1885–86),
which was completed by
Pye-Smith and Wilks after
his death, is one of the
solid books of the time.

Golding Bird (1814–
54), of Downham, Nor-
folk, described oxaluria
(1842), wrote an import-
ant book on "Urinary
Deposits" (1844), and was
a pioneer in electrotherapy
(1841–49).

Frederick William
Pavy (1829–1911), of
Wroughton, Wiltshire,
who graduated from the
University of London

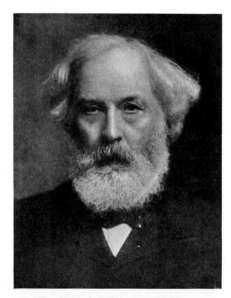

Sir Samuel Wilks (1824–1911).

(1850–53) and lectured at Guy's Hospital from 1856 to 1877, had
worked with Claude Bernard in 1853, and devoted his whole life
to the thesis that the liver is not a storehouse of available carbohydrates.

He started from his initial discovery that blood drawn from the inferior
vena cava of an animal, immediately after it has been killed by a sharp blow
on the head, contains no sugar; from which he inferred that the excess of sugar
which Bernard obtained from the liver was entirely due to postmortem changes
in that organ. Pavy maintained that sugar is decomposed and converted into

---

[1] Guy's Hosp. Rep., London, 1869, 3. s., xiv, 321–339. Tr. Path. Soc.
London, 1875–76, xxvii, 157–160.

fats and proteins in the intestines and reaches the liver only when it is in excess. By many ingenious arguments based largely upon original experimental work, he showed that the liver does not change glycogen into sugar during life, that oxygen does not destroy sugar in the blood and that glycogen itself exists in the blood; but, as his knowledge of the subject advanced, his views unconsciously adjusted themselves to those finally held by Bernard. Gowland Hopkins records the pathetic and ironic fact that the last experiment which Pavy performed indicated that more than 150 grams of dextrose per hour could be injected into the blood without appearing in the urine, which explodes the principal argument upon which he based his theory. Pavy was undoubtedly right, however, in holding that too much stress has been laid upon the liver as the sugar producer. He was the first to describe cyclic or postural albuminuria (1885) and the typhoidal arthritis known as "Pavy's joint" and is also remembered by his substitution of ammonia for caustic potash in Fehling's solution (Pavy's blue fluid), which, as Pavy's pellets, was one of the first preparations to be made in tabloid form. He had probably the largest practice in London in diabetic cases, in the treatment of which he was particularly successful, and his "Treatise on Food and Dietetics" (1874) is an index of his reputation as an investigator of metabolism.

Sir William **Jenner** (1815–98), of Chatham, England, professor at the University College, London, and physician to Queen Victoria, was Gull's great rival in practice, in which he was so successful that he left behind him a fortune of £375,000. He was a solid, able man, whose fame today rests upon the fact that, from a rigid clinical and pathological examination of thirty-six cases, he separated typhus from typhoid fever (1849),[1] although ten years later than Gerhard in America. Other prominent English practitioners of the time include John Hughes Bennett (1812–75), who described leukemia (1845); Charles J. B. Williams (1805–89), who was, in his day, an authority on consumption and diseases of the chest; Thomas Blizard Curling (1811–88), who first noted myxedema (1850); Sir Alfred Baring **Garrod** (1819–1907), who introduced the "thread test" in gout (1848–54),[2] and wrote an important treatise on the subject (1859); William Brinton (1823–67), who described plastic linitis, in his work on "Diseases of the Stomach" (1859); Sir Thomas **Barlow** (1845–), who first described infantile scurvy (Barlow's disease, 1876–82),[3] and George Frederick Still (1868–), who described arthritis deformans in children (Still's disease, 1896).[4]

Sir Thomas Clifford **Allbutt** (1836–), Regius Professor of Physic at the University of Cambridge, gave an early description of the joint symptoms in locomotor ataxia (1856–58),[5] is the author of the Goulstonian lectures on the visceral neuroses (1884), the

---

[1] Jenner: Month. Jour. Med. Sc., Edinb., 1849, ix, 663–680.

[2] Garrod: Med.-Chir. Tr., London, 1848, xxxi, 83: 1854, xxxvii, 49.

[3] Barlow: *Ibid.*, 1882–83, lxvi, 159–219. Early cases were described by J. O. L. Möller (1856–60), who did not consider the pathology of the condition.

[4] Still: *Ibid.*, 1896–97, lxxx, 47–59.

[5] Allbutt: Guy's Hosp. Rep., London, 1856, 3. s., ii, 143: 1858, 3. s., iv, 169.

Lane lectures on diseases of the heart (1896), and is especially known by his System of Medicine (1896–1907) and his valuable historical contributions on medieval medicine (1901) and surgery (1905) and on Greek medicine in Rome (1909).[1]

Sir William **Osler** (1849–   ), of Bond Head, Canada, Regius Professor of Medicine at the University of Oxford (1904), was professor at his alma mater, McGill University (1874–84), the University of Pennsylvania (1884–89) and at the Johns Hopkins University (1889–1904), where he did most to develop the scientific teaching of internal medicine in the hospital wards.   He was one of the earliest investigators of the blood-platelets (1873); described the visceral complications of erythema multiforme (1895), a form of multiple telangiectasis (1901), and chronic cyanosis with polycythemia and enlarged spleen (1903); devoted special monographs to the cerebral palsies of children (1889), chorea (1894), abdominal tumors (1895), angina pectoris (1897), cancer of the stomach (1900), and has done much *Filigranarbeit*, such as the description of the erythematous swellings (Osler's spots) in malignant endocarditis (1908).   His "Principles and Practice of Medicine" (1892) is the best English text-book on the subject in our time.   His essays on Linacre (1908), An Alabama Student (1908), Servetus (1910), and other subjects are among the most attractive of modern contributions to the history of medicine.   In this field, he is especially memorable for his studies of the work of the earlier American clinicians, whose modern status he has done most to establish.   He is also the editor of "Modern Medicine" (1910).

In Osler's clinic at the Johns Hopkins, much important work was done, such as the studies of malarial fever by W. S. Thayer and others (1886–1902), the investigation of amebic dysentery by William T. Councilman and Henri A. Lafleur (1890–91), the finding of the microörganisms in gonorrheal endocarditis and septicemia by W. S. Thayer and George Blumer (1896), the studies of eosinophilia in trichinosis by Thayer and Thomas R. Brown (1897–98), the demonstration of sexual conjugation in the malarial parasites by William G. MacCallum and Eugene L. Opie (1897–98), and the exhaustive study of pneumothorax by Charles P. Emerson (1903).

Lewellys Franklin **Barker** (1867–   ), of Norwich, Ontario, who succeeded Osler as physician-in-chief at the Johns Hopkins Hospital, has done much to advance the study of anatomy in America by his works on the nervous system (1899) and anatomical nomenclature (1907), his translation of Spalteholtz's Hand Atlas

---

[1] Brit. Med. Jour., London, 1909, ii, 1449; 1515; 1598.

(1900), and his Laboratory Manual (1904), and has added much to the literature of neurology and clinical pathology. In 1896, he described a unique case of "circumscribed unilateral and elective sensory paralysis," analogous in its bearings to the auto-observation of Henry Head, and with Frederick M. Hanes (1909), the eye signs in chronic nephritis. With F. J. Sladen, he has also made interesting clinical and pharmacological studies of the autonomic visceral nerves in relation to the mechanism of internal secretion and hormonic equilibrium—the vagotonic and sympathicotonic phenomena postulated by Eppinger and Hess (1910–13).

William Sidney **Thayer** (1864–   ), of Milton, Massachusetts, professor of clinical medicine at the Johns Hopkins University, has made extensive investigations of malarial fever (1895–97) and typhoid fever (1904), the observations on gonorrheal endocarditis and trichinosis above referred to, and made the first clinical notation of the third sound of the heart (1908).

Of other American practitioners, Austin **Flint**, Sr. (1812–86), of Petersham, Massachusetts, was, in his life-time, an authority on clinical medicine and auscultation, particularly in his treatises on practice (1866), percussion and auscultation (1876), and medical ethics (1883). His son, Austin Flint, Jr., was an eminent physiologist.

Alfred L. **Loomis** (1831–1895), of Bennington, Vermont, who settled in New York city, wrote the best American text-book on "Physical Diagnosis" (1873), which, even today, is sometimes consulted.

William **Pepper** (1843–98), of Philadelphia, Pennsylvania, described the changes in the bone-marrow in pernicious anemia (1875), wrote many good papers, and edited the first large American "System of Medicine" (1886), but, apart from his great practice, his activities were mainly devoted to the University of Pennsylvania, of which he became provost (1881–94), and where he greatly improved the facilities for medical education.

Jacob M. **Da Costa** (1833–1900), of Philadelphia, wrote a standard treatise on diagnosis (1864), and much upon functional diseases of the heart. He described irritable heart in soldiers (1862–71), which was also noted by Alfred **Stillé** (1813–1900), who played an important part in establishing the individuality of typhus and typhoid fevers (1838) and was a prominent teacher of pathology.

Nathan Smith **Davis** (1817–1904), of Chicago, perhaps the leading practitioner of that city in his day, was the father of the American Medical Association, and the author of a good History of Medical Education and Institutions in the United States (1851).

James **Tyson** (1841–   ), of Philadelphia, professor of pathol-

ogy (1876–89) and practice (1899–1910) in the University of Pennsylvania, is widely known for his admirable works on the cell doctrine (1870), examination of the urine (1875), physical diagnosis
(1891), practice (1896), and, in particular, his monograph on
Bright's disease and diabetes (1881).

Abraham Jacobi (1830–   ), of Hartum, Westphalia, a graduate of Bonn (1851), was held in detention for his participation in
the German revolution of 1848, and settled in New York in 1853,
where he is now honored and revered as one of the leading practitioners in this country and the Nestor of American pediatrics, a
subject which he taught in different medical schools of New York
for forty-two years.   He was a founder and editor of the American
Journal of Obstetrics (1868–71), and is the author of works on disorders of dentition (1862), infant diet (1872, 1875), diphtheria
(1876, 1880), diseases of the thymus gland (1889), and pediatrics
(1896–1903).   He has played a prominent part in the advancement
of American medicine, and has written many discourses, distinguished by quaint wit, varied learning, and true wisdom (Collec-
tanea Jacobi, 1909).   He has also written the authoritative
monograph on the history of American pediatrics (Baginsky-
Festschrift, 1913).

    Much good work has been done in America by such teachers and practi-
tioners as the Jacksons, the Shattucks, the Bowditches, the Minots, James J.
Putnam, R. C. Cabot (Boston); Charles L. Dana, L. E. Holt, T. Mitchell
Prudden, Frank P. Foster, Joseph Collins, M. Allen Starr (New York); the
Mitchells, James M. Anders, Wharton Sinkler, John H. Musser, Alfred Sten-
gel (Philadelphia); Eugen F. Cordell, Frank Donaldson, Thomas B. Futcher,
H. B. Jacobs, Henry M. Thomas (Baltimore); Samuel C. Busey, W. W. Johnston, D. S. Lamb (Washington, D. C.); James B. Herrick, Frank Billings (Chicago); Charles F. Hoover (Cleveland); George Dock, W. J. Calvert (St. Louis),
Joseph Jones, Edmond Souchon (New Orleans); Charles D. Spivak (Denver),
and, in Canada, by such men as Robert Palmer Howard, James Bovell, George
Ross, A. D. Blackader and J. George Adami, to mention only a few names.
    Of the many important advances in diagnostic procedure we may mention
the graphic method of investigating the pulse introduced by Karl Vierordt
(1855), A. Stich's suggestion of the use of reflexes in diagnosis (1856), the
sphygmograph of Étienne-Jules Marey (1860), the sphygmomanometers of
Ritter von Basch (1887) and Scipione Riva-Rocci (1896), the tonometer of
Gustav Gaertner (1899), the introduction of esophagoscopy by Kussmaul
(1868), cystoscopy, urethroscopy, and rectoscopy by Max Nitze (1877), gastroscopy by Mikulicz (1881), gastrodiaphany by Max Einhorn (1889), autoscopy
of the air-passages by Alfred Kirstein (1895), direct bronchoscopy and suspension laryngoscopy by Gustav Killian (1898–1912); above all the X-rays by
Wilhelm Conrad Röntgen (1893); Kernig's sign in cerebrospinal meningitis
(1884), Henry Koplik's sign in measles (1898), Pietro Grocco's triangle in
pleurisy (1902), the differentiation of pericardial pseudocirrhosis of the liver
(Pick's disease) by Bamberger (1872) and F. J. Pick (1896), and such phases
of urinary analysis as Fehling's test for sugar (1848), Bence Jones's proteid
(1848), indicanuria (Max Jaffe, 1877), Ehrlich's diazo-reaction (1882), Rudolf
von Jaksch on acetonuria and diaceturia (1885), Matthew Hay's test for bile
(1886), F. Gowland Hopkins' mode of estimating uric acid (1893), cryoscopy,
introduced by Sandor Koranyi (1894), Ernst Salkowski on pentosuria (1895),
the test of Percy John Cammidge in pancreatic disease (1904), Albarran's

experimental polyuria (1905), L. Ambard's urea constant (1910), and the phenolphthalein test in renal disease described by L. G. Rowntree and Geraghty (1910). Max Einhorn (1862–   ), of Grodno, Russia, a Berlin graduate and professor in New York, has made many ingenious additions to gastro-enterology, e. g., gastrodiaphany (1887), stomach-buckets (1890), an esophagoscope (1901), radiodiaphany (1904), the bead test (1907), duodenal buckets (1908), and dilators for the cardia (1909) and pylorus (1910).

Modern **neurology** is mainly of French extraction and derives from Duchenne, of Boulogne, through Charcot and his pupils.

In the eighteenth century, Johann Peter Frank had filed a special brief for the study of diseases of the spinal cord (1792); Fothergill had described facial neuralgia (1773); Whytt, tubercular meningitis (1768); Cotugno, sciatica (1770); Pott, pressure paralysis from spinal deformity (1779); Lettsom, the drug habit and alcoholism (1786); Nikolaus Friedreich, facial hemiplegia (1797), and John Haslam, general paralysis (1798). In the early nineteenth century, cerebral dropsy was described by George Cheyne (1808), delirium tremens by Thomas Sutton (1813) and John Ware (1831), tetany by J. Clarke (1815), S. L. Steinheim (1830), and J. B. H. Dance (1832); paralysis agitans by Parkinson (1817), alcoholic neuritis by James Jackson (1822), neuroma by W. Wood (1829), and electric chorea by Angelo Dubini (1846). Epilepsy and spinal hemiplegia have been known since the Greeks and chorea since the time of Sydenham. Tabes dorsalis had been vaguely considered by Schelhammer (1691) and Brendel (1749), and was the subject of the dissertations of Ernst Horn's pupils, Loewenhard (1817), von Weidenbach (1817), Schesmer (1819), Gossow (1825), but these last, Max Neuburger thinks, really deal with cases of prostatic neurasthenia. Horn's own view of the disease, faulty as to pathology and semeiology, is given in the dissertation of his son, Wilhelm von Horn (1827). In 1844 Steinthal gave a remarkably exact and complete description of the characteristic gait, the paresthesia, the electric pains, the gastric and vesical crises and the amaurosis, but this was soon forgotten.[1]

The first real advance in the diagnosis of ataxia was made by Moritz Heinrich **Romberg** (1795–1873), of Meiningen, who graduated at Berlin in 1817 (his thesis being a classical description of achondroplasia), and became professor there in 1838. His Lehrbuch der Nervenkrankheiten (1840–46) was the first formal treatise on nervous diseases, and made an epoch by its careful collation of hitherto scattered data, its clear, precise clinical pictures and its attempt to systematize treatment. It contains (p. 795) the well-known "pathognomonic sign" that ataxics cannot stand with their eyes shut (Romberg's sign), and a description of "ciliary neuralgia."

Romberg's "propædeutic clinic" at Berlin, instituted in 1834, was much frequented for the advantages derived from diagnoses made by physical examination.

Guillaume-Benjamin-Amand **Duchenne** (1806–75), who, as Collins says, found neurology "a sprawling infant of unknown parentage which he succored to a lusty youth," was descended from a long line of seafaring people at Boulogne, and it was an in-born

---

[1] Martin Steinthal: Jour. f. prakt. Heilk., Berlin, 1844, xcviii, 1. St., 1–56; 2. St., 1–84, cited by Neuburger.

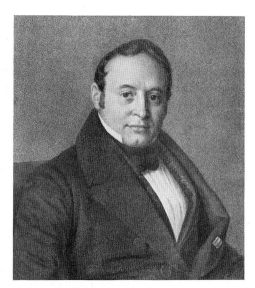

Moritz Heinrich Romberg (1795–1873).

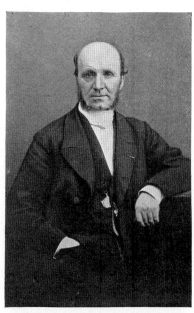

Guillaume-Benjamin-Amand Duchenne, of Boulogne (1806–75). (From
a carte de visite photograph in the Surgeon-General's Library.)

love of science which prevented
him from complying with his
father's wish that he should
become a sailor. Coming up
to Paris, he studied under
Laënnec, Dupuytren, Magendie and Cruveilhier, graduated
in 1831, and after practising
for some years in Boulogne,
settled in the capital and devoted the rest of his life to
neurology and electrophysiology. His method of prosecuting his studies was peculiar.
A strange, sauntering, mariner-
like figure, he haunted all the
larger Parisian hospitals from
day to day, delving into case-
histories, holding offhand arguments with the internes and
physicians-in-chief, who frequently laughed at him for his
pains, and following interesting cases from hospital to hos-

pital, even at his own expense. All this was done in an unconventional and eccentric way, which at first laid him open to suspicion and exposed him to snubs, but the sincerity of the man, his transparent honesty, and his unselfish devotion to science for itself, soon broke down opposition, and, in the end, when his reputation was made, he was greeted everywhere with the warmest welcome. Being timid and inarticulate in relation to public speaking, he was aided by his friend, the fair-minded and generous Trousseau, who, out of fondness for Duchenne, often voiced his ideas with effect in medical societies.

Duchenne was led to study nervous diseases through his interest in electricity, and he first set out to classify the electrophysiology of the entire muscular system, studying the functions of isolated muscles in relation to bodily movements, and summarizing his results in De l'électrisation localisée (1855). He started with the observation that a current from two electrodes applied to the wet skin can stimulate the muscles without affecting the skin, and it was his brilliant application of this principle to pathological conditions that brought out so many fine points in the diagnosis of nervous disorders and made him the founder of electrotherapy, in which he was followed by Remak, Ziemssen and Erb. His electrophysiological analysis of the mechanism of facial expression under emotion, illustrated by many striking photographs (1862),[1] is approached only by Darwin's work on the observational side. He was the first to distinguish between the different forms of lead palsy and of facial paralysis from lesions of the brain or nerves, including the rheumatic and lacrimal forms. But his great field was the spinal cord. In 1840, Jacob von Heine (1800–79), of Canstatt, had described infantile paralysis as a spinal lesion,[2] but in the face of his description, it was usually regarded as an atrophic myasthenia from inactivity. Duchenne pointed out that such a profound disorder of the locomotor system could only come from a definite lesion, which he located in the anterior horns of the spinal cord (1855), his view being afterward confirmed by Gull, Charcot, Cornil, and Vulpian. He also described anterior poliomyelitis in the adult as due to atrophic lesions of the ganglion cells of the anterior horns, and his name is permanently connected with spinal progressive muscular atrophy of the "Aran-Duchenne type" (1847–61). In 1850, F.-A. Aran, of the Hôpital St. Antoine, published some cases of spinal progressive muscular atrophy which had been worked out by Duchenne.[3] The latter, in his exhaustive study of the whole matter, at first regarded the disease as a primitive alteration of the muscles, then assumed a lesion in the anterior horn of the spinal cord, finally, under pressure of current opinion, returned to his original view of a primitive muscular atrophy.[4] He described the initial pseudohypertrophies in detail, but did not interpret them, as Erb did. The most definite thing which Duchenne described was the bulbar or glosso-labio-lingual paralysis (1860),[5] which is known by his name, as also the pseudohypertrophic form of muscular paralysis (1868).[6] Although the latter is simply one of the many forms of muscular dystrophy now recognized, it was Duchenne's careful work in the hospital

---

[1] Duchenne: Mécanisme de la physionomie humaine (etc.), Paris, 1862.

[2] Heine: Beobachtungen über Lähmungszustände der unteren Extremitäten (etc.), Stuttgart, 1840.

[3] Aran: Arch. gén. de méd., Paris, 1850, 4. s., xxiv, 4; 172.

[4] Duchenne's final account of the disease is given in his De l'électrisation localisée, 2. éd., Paris, 1861, 437–547.

[5] Arch. gén. de méd., Paris, 1860, 5. s., xvi, 283; 431.

[6] Ibid., 1868, 6. s., xi, 5; 179; 305; 421; 552.

wards which first opened up the whole subject. In his work on locomotor ataxia, Duchenne labored under one great disadvantage. He cared little for book knowledge, and knew nothing of the work of Steinthal and Romberg, let alone the fact that Edward Stanley had described disease of the posterior columns of the spinal cord in 1839 and Sir William Gull in 1856–58. In 1858–59,[1] Duchenne described the disease at full length, differentiating it from the paralyses, demonstrating the lesion in the cord and pointing out that it is due to lues. When he heard of the work of the German clinicians, he contended that the ataxies observed by them were not the same as those he had seen, and so obscured his subject in controversy.

In appearance, Duchenne was a deep-chested, broad-shouldered, sailor-like man, whose ruddy, contented, humorous countenance has been well preserved in the many photographs in his work on physiognomy. He was at once jolly, expansive, and absent-minded, brusque yet cordial, disputatious yet tactful, and he attributed his success in bearding the lions of the hospitals to his combination of poise and insensitiveness. The last four years of his life were clouded by arteriosclerosis of the brain, and he died forgotten and unhonored, except by a corporal's guard of old friends at his grave; but he is, with Charcot and Marie, one of the greatest neurologists of France. The best account of him in English is the sympathetic study of Joseph Collins (1908).[2]

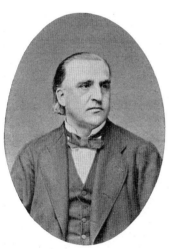

Jean-Martin Charcot (1825–93).

Contemporary with Duchenne and far greater in the scope and scientific accuracy of his work was Jean-Martin **Charcot** (1825–93), of Paris, who graduated in 1853 with a thesis on arthritis nodosa, and in 1862 became physician to the great hospital of the Salpêtrière, with which his name will always be associated. Here, from small beginnings, he created the greatest neurological clinic of modern times, which was followed by enthusiastic students from all parts of the world.

Charcot was not only a great neurologist, but early made his mark in his lessons on senile and chronic diseases (1867), diseases of the liver, the biliary passages, and the kidneys (1877). He left memorable descriptions of chronic pneumonia, gout and rheumatism, endocarditis, and of tuberculosis, in the dual nature of which he did not believe. He made important physio-

[1] Arch. gén. de méd., Paris, 1858, 5. s., xii, 641: 1859, xiii, 36; 158; 417.

[2] Collins: Med. Record, New York, 1908, lxxii, 50–54.

logical studies of the localization of functions in cerebral disease (1876), and (with Albert Pitres) on the cortical motor centers in man (1895). The five volumes of his lessons on nervous diseases delivered at the Salpêtrière (1872–93) are a good summary of his work, much of which was, as with Ludwig, conveyed through the medium of his pupils. Thus, in 1866, he described, with Henri Bouchard, miliary aneurysms, emphasizing their importance in cerebral hemorrhage; with Georges Delamarre, the gastric crises in locomotor ataxia (1866); with Bouchard, the ataxic *douleurs fulgurantes* (1866); with Alexis Joffry, the lesions in muscular atrophy (1869); with Pierre Marie, the peroneal form of muscular atrophy (1886); and his ideas on hysteria and hystero-epilepsy were set forth in the clinical studies of Richer (1879–85) and Gilles de la Tourette (1891). He defined hysteria as a psychosis superinduced by ideation, the touchstone being the subject's capacity for responding to suggestion. He considered "the phases of the major attack, the innumerable psychic and somatic manifestations, the phenomena of transference on the application of metals, the sensory changes in hemianesthesia and hemianalgesia, the motor phenomena of contracture and spasm, the visual features, the relation of hysteria to traumatism, its frequency in the male—these and a score of related problems" (Osler). In muscular atrophy, he differentiated between the ordinary wasting or Aran-Duchenne type and the rarer amyotrophic lateral sclerosis (1874); and described, with Marie, the progressive neural or peroneal type (1886), which was also described, in a Cambridge graduating dissertation, by Howard Henry Tooth (1886). He differentiated the essential lesions of locomotor ataxia and described both the gastric crises and the joint affections (Charcot's disease). He separated multiple sclerosis from paralysis agitans, although the "intentional tremor" which he signalized as a differential sign had been noted by Bernhard Cohn in 1860. "No writer," says Osler, "has more graphically described the trophic troubles following spinal and cerebral disorders, particularly the acute bedsore." Like Babinski after him, Charcot regarded hypnotism as a neurotic condition, akin to, if not identical with, hysteria, and there was a long-drawn battle between the school of the Salpêtrière and that of Nancy (under Liébeault and Bernheim) as to the part played by suggestion, which, in the hands of the latter, some say, became mere brow-beating. Charcot was not deceived by the feigning of some of his patients, and, in the end, regarded hypnotism as a doubtful therapeutic measure. The soundness of his view is borne out in the modern tendency to merge the procedure into psychotherapy. Charcot was a purely objective investigator, cared little for the special psychology of neurotic patients, and so was saved from some of the subjective exaggerations of the Freudian school. "For purely psychological investigation," says Havelock Ellis, "he had no liking, and probably no aptitude. Any one who was privileged to observe his methods of work at the Salpêtrière will easily recall the great master's towering figure; the disdainful expression, sometimes, even, it seemed, a little sour; the lofty bearing, which enthusiastic admirers called Napoleonic. The questions addressed to the patient were cold, distant, sometimes impatient. Charcot clearly had little faith in the value of any results so attained."

Apart from his clinical work, Charcot was an artist of talent, and the creator of the study of medical history in the graphic and plastic arts. With Paul Richer, he published two fascinating monographs on demonomania in art (1887), and on the deformed and diseased in art (1889), while many valuable studies by his pupils, Henri Meige, Richer, and others, appeared in his *Iconographie photographique de la Salpêtrière*, begun in 1876 and continued to the present time. Through his wife, who was a lady of wealth, Charcot lived in easy circumstances, but his clinical genius, his keen, clear mind, his poise and dignity, would have made him a commanding figure in any station in life.

Pierre **Marie** (1853–   ), of Paris, Charcot's ablest pupil, graduated in 1883, and became professor in the Paris Faculty in 1889. In 1886, he described, with Charcot, the peroneal type of muscular atrophy,[1] and has made at least four original delineations of new forms of nervous disease. These are his descriptions of acromegaly, pointing out the pituitary lesion (1886),[2] hypertrophic pulmonary osteoarthropathy (1890),[3] hereditary cerebellar ataxia (1893),[4] and the so-called rhizomelic spondylosis or Strümpell-Marie type of spinal arthritis deformans (1898).[5] He has also made an assault of destructive criticism upon Broca's conception of aphasia, maintaining that the third left frontal convolution has no special rôle in spoken language (1906), and upon the identity of the Aran-Duchenne type of muscular atrophy, which he challenges (1897).

The ablest German neurologist, after Romberg, is Wilhelm Heinrich **Erb** (1840–   ), of Winnweiler, Bavaria, a pupil of Nikolaus Friedreich, who became professor at Heidelberg (1880). He followed Duchenne in the extensive development of electrotherapy (1882), wrote important hand-books on diseases of the cerebro-spinal nerves (1874) and of the spinal cord and medulla (1876), and did much to establish the modern theory of the muscular dystrophies, which he described and classified (1891). He also described brachial palsy (1874),[6] syphilitic spinal paralysis (1875),[7] the juvenile type of muscular atrophy (1884),[8] and the so-called asthenic bulbar paralysis or myasthenia gravis (1878),[9] also described by Willis (1685) and by Goldflam in 1893 (Erb-Goldflam symptom-complex). Simultaneously with Westphal (1875), Erb discovered the significance of the knee-jerk in locomotor ataxia[10] and, with Fournier, he did most to establish a statistical causal relation between tabes and syphilis.

Other German neurologists of the period were Nikolaus **Friedreich** (1825–82), of Würzburg, who described hereditary ataxia (1863–76)[11] and paramyoclonus multiplex (1881),[12] diseases which

---

[1] Marie: Rev. de méd., Paris, 1886, vi, 97–138.   [2] *Ibid.*, 1886, vi, 297–333.
[3] *Ibid.*, 1890, x, 1–36.   [4] Semaine méd., 1893, xiii, 444–447.
[5] Rev. de méd., Paris, 1898, xviii, 285–315.
[6] Erb: Verhandl. d. naturh.-med. Ver. zu Heidelberg, 1874–77, n. F., i, 130–137.
[7] Berlin. klin. Wochenschr., 1875, xii, 357–359.
[8] Deutsches Arch. f. klin. Med., Leipz., 1883–84, xxxiv, 467–519.
[9] Arch. f. Psychiat., Berlin, 1878–79, ix, 172.
[10] Arch. f. Psychiat., Berlin, 1875, v, 792; 803.
[11] Friedreich: Arch. f. path. Anat. (etc.), Berlin, 1863, xxvi, 391; xxvii, 1: 1876, lxviii, 145; lxx, 140.
[12] *Ibid.*, 1881, lxxxvi, 421–430.

are sometimes eponymically confused; Carl Friedrich Otto **Westphal** (1833–90), of Berlin, who described agoraphobia (1871), signalized the knee-jerk in diagnosis (1875)[1] and did important work in psychiatry (1892); Heinrich **Quincke** (1842–   ), who described angioneurotic edema (1882),[2] which had also been noted by John Laws Milton as giant urticaria (1876); and Adolf **Strümpell** (1853–   ), of Neu-Autz, Courland, who is well known for his treatise on internal medicine (1883) and who described spondylitis deformans (1897) and pseudosclerosis of the brain (Westphal-Strümpell disease).

The leading English neurologists of the period were John **Hughlings Jackson** (1834–1911), of Yorkshire, who did much to establish the use of the ophthalmoscope in diagnosing brain diseases (1863), made valuable studies of aphasia (1864), described unilateral convulsions or Jacksonian epilepsy (1875),[3] and originated the doctrine of "levels" in the nervous system (1898); Sir William Richard **Gowers** (1845–   ), of London, who is well known for his treatises on diseases of the spinal cord (1880), epilepsy (1881), diseases of the brain (1885) and the nervous system, did much good work on the finer anatomy of the nervous system, and described ataxic paraplegia; and Sir Victor **Horsley** (1857–   ), of Kensington, England, who did admirable work on the physiology of the nervous system, the functions of the ductless glands, and, with Gowers, was the first to remove a tumor of the spinal cord (1888).

In America, George Miller Beard introduced the concept of neurasthenia or nervous exhaustion (1869), outlined by Eugene Bouchut as *nervosisme* (1860); George Huntington described hereditary (Huntington's) chorea (1872); William Alexander Hammond (1828–1900), once Surgeon-General in the United States Army, made his mark with his "Physiological Memoirs" (1863), described athetosis (1873), and wrote a good book on nervous diseases (1871); Thomas G. Morton described metatarsalgia (1876); Bernhard Sachs (1858–   ) described amaurotic family idiocy (1887–96), the ocular manifestations of which had been noted in 1880 by Waren Tay (Tay-Sachs disease); William F. Milroy, of Omaha, Nebraska, described persistent hereditary edema of the legs, or "Milroy's disease" (1892); Charles Karsner Mills (1845–   ) described unilateral progressive ascending paralysis (1900) and unilateral descending paralysis (1906); and James

---

[1] Westphal: Arch. f. Psychiat., Berlin, 1875, v, 803–834.

[2] Quincke: Monatsh. f. prakt. Dermat., Hamburg and Leipzig, 1882, i, 129–131.

[3] Jackson: Brit. Med. Jour., London, 1875, i, 773.

37

J. Putnam, of Boston, with Charles L. Dana and others, differentiated primary combined sclerosis.

Silas **Weir Mitchell** (1830–   ), of Philadelphia, the leading American neurologist of his time, is a graduate of the Jefferson Medical College, Philadelphia (1850). In 1859, with Hammond, he investigated the arrow poisons, corroval and vao, and he was the first, after the Abbe Fontana and Bonaparte, to investigate serpent venoms (1870–86). With Edward T. Reichert, he isolated the diffusible globulins of the venoms, his studies having an important bearing upon the more recent work of Fraser (1896), Calmette (1896), Kyes (1902–03), Flexner and Noguchi (1909). In 1869, he pointed out the coördinating functions of the cerebellum, and, with Morris J. Lewis, demonstrated that the knee-jerk can be reënforced by sensory stimulation (1886). During the Civil War, he was in charge of Turner's Lane Hospital, Philadelphia, where he established a special ward for nervous patients, and here, with George R. Morehouse and William W. Keen, he made those studies of gunshot and other injuries of nerves (1864) which were afterward expanded in his important work, on "Injuries of Nerves and Their Consequences" (1872). This book contains the earliest distinct accounts of ascending neuritis, the treatment of neuritis by cold and splint-rests, the psychology of the amputated and other data which have been absorbed in the text-books. Mitchell was the first to describe erythromelalgia, or red neuralgia (1872–78),[1] and postparalytic chorea (1874),[2] and he was (with William Thomson) the first to emphasize the importance of eye-strain as a cause of headache (1874).[3] In 1875, Mitchell introduced a treatment of nervous disease by prolonged rest in bed, with such adjuvants as optimum feeding, massage, and electricity, the so-called "rest cure," or Weir Mitchell treatment, which is now used everywhere. His ideas on the subject were summed up in his classical monograph, "Fat and Blood" (1877), which has been translated into French, German, Spanish, Italian, and Russian. Mitchell was also the first to study the effect of meteorological changes upon traumatic neuralgias, particularly in old amputation stumps (1877). He has made a large number of minor investigations of highly original character, and is well known in the world of letters by his charming contributions to poetry and fiction.

Other innovations in neurology besides those already mentioned were the original descriptions of unilateral paralysis with crossed anesthesia by Brown-Séquard (1851), acute ascending paralysis by Octave Landry (1859),

---

[1] Amer. Jour. Med. Sc., Phila., 1878, n. s., lxxvi, 17–36.
[2] *Ibid.*, 1874, lxviii, 342–352.
[3] Med. and Surg. Reporter, Phila., 1874, xxxi, 67–71.

congenital cerebral spastic paraplegia by William John Little (1861), symmetrical gangrene by Maurice Raynaud (1862), disease of the crura cerebri (Weber's syndrome) by Hermann Weber (1862), alcoholic paraplegia by Sir Samuel Wilks (1868), plexiform neurofibroma (*Rankenneuroma*) by Paul Bruns (1870), myotonia, described in his own person, by Julius Thomsen (1876), syringomyelia with trophic disturbances by Augustin-Marie Morvan (1883), impulsive tic or saltatory spasm (jumping, latah, myriachit) by Georges Gilles de la Tourette (1884), subacute combined degeneration of the spinal cord by Otto Leichtenstern (1884) and Ludwig Lichtheim (1884), astasia-abasia by Paul Blocq (1888), progressive interstitial hypertrophic neuritis of infants by Jules Déjérine and Jules Sottas (1893), infantile progressive muscular atrophy by Guido Werdnig (1890–94) and Johann Hoffmann (1894), meralgia paræsthetica by Max Bernhardt and Vladimir Karlovich Roth (1895), and amyotonia congenita by Hermann Oppenheim (1900). Herpes zoster was first ascribed to a lesion of the spinal ganglia by Friedrich von Bärensprung (1861–63), and was further localized as an acute hemorrhagic inflammation of the posterior spinal and cranial ganglia by Henry Head and A. W. Campbell in 1900. Megrims and all mental disturbances coming under the description of brain-storms or nerve-storms were described by Edward Liveing in 1873. The visceral neuroses were investigated by Sir Clifford Allbutt (1884), and the pathology of the cerebral circulation by Leonard Hill (1896). Aphasia, first described and localized by Bouillaud (1825),[1] defined as "aphemia" by Broca (1861), has been further studied by Hughlings Jackson (1866), Carl Wernicke (1874), Adolf Kussmaul (1877), Ludwig Lichtheim (1885), and Pierre Marie (1906), who has contested the part played in aphasia by Broca's convolution, insisting that the true lesion is a lenticular zone in the left temporoparietal lobe (Wernicke's zone), which is also in dispute. Aphemia, anarthria, verbal amnesia, and other phases of the subject were elucidated by Henry Charlton Bastian (1897–98), word-blindness (dyslexia) was described by Rudolf Berlin (1887), and apraxia (motor asymbolia) by Hugo Karl Liepmann (1900).

After the time of Pinel and Reil, the **treatment of the insane** without mechanical restraints (open-door method) was advanced by John **Conolly** (1856) and by the Tukes, of whom Daniel Hack **Tuke** (1827–95) collaborated with John Charles Bucknill in a "Manual of Psychological Medicine" (1858), which played a great part in its day. Another advocate of the no-restraint system was Wilhelm **Griesinger** (1817–68), of Stuttgart, a pupil of Schönlein, a clinical assistant of Wunderlich, and ultimately Romberg's successor at Berlin (1865–67), who, apart from his work in psychiatry, distinguished himself by his early description of hook-worm infection as "tropical chlorosis" (1866), and did much, in Germany at least, to clear up the status of typhus, typhoid, relapsing and malarial fevers, in his monographs on infectious diseases (1857–64). Griesinger's "Pathology and Therapy of Psychic Disorders" (1845) did away with much of the mysticism of the past, gave clear and unmistakable clinical pictures based upon rational psychologi-

---

[1] Erich Ebstein points out that cases of aphasia had been described by Van Swieten (1753), Goethe: *Wilhelm Meister*, vii, ch. 6, and *Wanderjahre*, iii, ch. 13 (1796). These had, however, been preceded by the case of Linnæus (1742). Thomas Hood (Phrenol. Tr., 1822, iii) is said to have given a case with autopsy before Bouillaud, but the latter, who had made 700 by 1848, will always be credited with the classical account of the disease. According to Trousseau, the term "aphasia" was devised by the celebrated Hellenist, Crisaphis. See Ebstein, Zeitschr. f. d. ges. Neurol., Berlin, 1913, xvii, 58–64.

cal analysis, aimed to connect the subject with pathological anatomy and advocated the open-door and the psychiatric clinic. Since Griesinger's time, the scientific study of insanity has been mainly in the hands of the Germans.

Theodor **Meynert** (1833-92), of Dresden, professor of neurology and psychiatry at Vienna (1873-92), editor of the *Jahrbücher für Psychiatrie* (1889-92), made many investigations of the anatomy and physiology of the brain (1865-72), described amentia, and wrote on insanity as "Diseases of the Fore-Brain" (1884).

Karl **Wernicke** (1848-1905), of Tarnowitz, Upper Silesia, professor at Berlin (1885) and Breslau (1890), described sensory aphasia, including alexia and agraphia (1874), diseases of the internal capsule (1875), acute hemorrhagic polioencephalitis (1881), and presbyophrenia (1900); wrote treatises on brain diseases (1881-83) and insanity (1894-1900), and issued a splendid atlas of the brain (1897-1904).

Emil **Kraepelin** (1856-   ), of Neustrelitz (Mecklenburg), professor of psychiatry at Dorpat (1886) and Heidelberg (1890), was the pioneer of psychoanalysis in psychiatry (1896)[1] and his "Kompendium" (1883) and thirty lectures on psychiatry (1901) introduced a new and simple classification of insanity, emphasizing the affective, precocious, involutional, katatonic and maniacal forms, introducing the concepts "dementia præcox" and "manic-depressive insanity," and bringing about many simplifications by clever grouping of related varieties.

Paul Eugen **Bleuler** (1857-   ), of Switzerland, has expanded Kraepelin's original concept of "dementia præcox" to include a group of "schizophrenias" (1910) which imply many things not regarded by Kraepelin, in particular "autism," or the mental life of the individual which is kept apart from the outside world.

Adolf **Meyer** (1866-   ), of Switzerland, professor of psychiatry at the Johns Hopkins University (1910), has also maintained the psychogenic origin of dementia præcox—that it is functional rather than organic.

Richard **von Krafft-Ebing** (1840-1902), of Mannheim, a pupil of Friedreich and Griesinger, professor at Strassburg (1872), Graz (1873), and Vienna (1889), wrote the best German work on forensic psychiatry (1875), also a treatise on psychiatry based upon clinical experience (1879), and is especially known for his *Psychopathia sexualis* (1886), which classifies and describes the various forms of sexual inversion and perversion, especially in their medicolegal relations. Albert Moll is another writer on this theme.

New methods of psychopathological investigation were introduced by Robert Sommer (1899). Psycho-analysis was introduced by Kraepelin (1896),

[1] Kraepelin: Psychol. Arb., Leipzig, 1896, i, 1-91.

Sigmund Freud, and C. G. Jung (1905). General paralysis of the insane was described by John Haslam (1798) and Calmeil (1826), moral insanity by James Cowles Prichard (1835), circular insanity by Jean-Pierre Falret (1854), hebephrenia by K. Kahlbaum (1863) and Hecker (1871), katatonia by Karl Kahlbaum (1874), psychasthenia by Pierre Janet (1903), presenile dementia, with placques in the brain, by Alois Alzheimer (1911). Alcoholic paraplegia, already noted by James Jackson (1822) and Sir Samuel Wilks (1868), was described as a polyneuritic psychosis by Sergiei Korsakoff (1887). Heinrich Laehr (1820–1905), editor of the *Allgemeine Zeitschrift für Psychiatrie* (1858–   ), made valuable directories of the insane asylums of the Germanic countries (1852–82), an unrivaled bibliography of the literature of psychiatry, neurology, and psychology from 1459 to 1799 (1900), and a calendar of psychiatry (1885) containing, day by day, all the important events connected with the history of the subject. Otto Mönkemöller has written well on the history of psychiatry (1903–10).

The later nineteenth century marks the scientific or parasitic period of **dermatology,** in which many cutaneous diseases were directly traced to microscopic organisms, especially under the leadership of Sabouraud and Unna.

Hebra's work was completed and extended by his son, **Hans von Hebra** (1847–   ), of Vienna, who wrote a text-book on skin diseases in relation to diseases of the entire organism (1884), described rhinoscleroma (1870) and rhinophyma (1881), and by his pupil, the Hungarian Moriz **Kaposi** (1837–1902), who completed the elder Hebra's text-book, besides writing one of his own (1879), and described pigmented sarcoma of the skin (1872), diabetic dermatitis (1876), xeroderma pigmentosum (1882), lymphoderma perniciosa (1885), the various forms of lichen ruber (1886–95), and ultimately put Hebra's impetigo herpetiformis upon a definite footing (1887). Dermatology was popularized by Sir William James **Erasmus Wilson** (1809–84), who made an early reputation with his "Dissector's Manual" (1838), "Anatomist's Vademecum" (1840), and anatomical plates, his "Diseases of the Skin" (1842), dermatological "Atlas" (1847), and his Royal College of Surgeons lectures on dermatology (1871–78), particularly by his gift of £5000 for founding a chair of dermatology in the latter institution and the extensive collection of dermatological preparations which he made for the same. Wilson classified cutaneous disorders as diseases of the true derma, of the sudoriparous and sebaceous glands, the hair and follicles, and he was the first to describe dermatitis exfoliativa (1870). The parasitic etiology of skin diseases had been introduced by the Arabians, by Cosimo Bonomo, who described the parasite of scabies (1687); by John Hunter, who gave a clinical description of the disease; by Wichmann, of Hamburg, who established its parasitic nature (1786); by Schönlein, who described the achorion fungus of favus (1839); by David Grüby (1809–98), who described a contagious tinea sycosis or mentagra (porrigo decalvans or phytoalopecia), due to a fungus (1841–43), and by Carl Eichstedt, who established the relation between scabies and Microsporon furfur (1846). Grüby's work received little attention until the **bacteriologic and parasitologic period,** when it was taken up by Raymond **Sabouraud** (1864), of Paris, who made extensive studies of the different varieties of trichophyton (1894), the etiology of eczema (1899–1900), of pityriasis, and the "pellicular alopecias" (1904). Sabouraud did the best work on the mycotic diseases of the skin. In 1881, Thin had shown that trichophyton is distinct from ordinary fungi. Eczema marginatum of the groin and axilla (dhobie itch) has been traced to the Epidermophyton inguinale, pityriasis versicolor to Microsporon furfur, and tropical imbricata to another ring-worm fungus. Meanwhile extremely valuable work was done on the pathological, bacteriological, and therapeutic side by Paul Gerson **Unna** (1850–   ), of Hamburg, who was severely wounded as a volunteer in the Franco-Prussian War, and afterward founded a private clinic (1881) and a hospital for skin diseases (1884) in his native city. He published valuable works on the anatomy (1882) and histopathology of the

skin (1894) and the treatment of skin diseases (1898), founded the *Monats-
hefte für praktische Dermatologie* (1882) and *Dermatologische Studien* (1886),
and edited an international atlas (1889) and a histopathological atlas (1894)
of skin diseases. Unna, a most prolific writer, described seborrheic eczema
(1887–93), the morococci of eczema (1892–97), the different cocci of favus
(1892–99), phlyctænosis streptogenes (1895), pustulosis staphylogenes (1896),
described the pathology of leprosy (1910), and introduced ichthyol and resorcin
(1886), and specially coated pills for local absorption in the duodenum (1884).

Among the original descriptions of skin diseases in the modern period
are those of porrigo (1864), dysidrosis (1873), and hydroa (1880) by Tilbury
Fox (1836–79), colloid milium by Ernst Wagner (1866), dermatitis exfoliativa
by Erasmus Wilson (1870), giant urticaria (angioneurotic edema) by John
Laws Milton (1876), angiokeratoma by Wyndham Cottle (1877), infantile ex-
foliative dermatitis by Ritter von Rittershain (1878), neurofibroma by F. D.
von Recklinghausen (1882), epidermolysis bullosa by Alfred Goldscheider
(1882), varicella gangrenosa by Sir Jonathan Hutchinson (1882), xeroderma
pigmentosum (1882), lymphoderma perniciosa (1885), lichen ruber monile-
formis (1886) by Moriz Kaposi (1837–1902), who also established the definite
status of impetigo herpetiformis (1887), lichen ruber planus (1895), and pem-
phigus vegetans (1896); erythema elevatum by Judson S. Bury (1888), fol-
licular psorospermosis by Jean Darier (1889), acanthosis nigricans by Sigmund Pollitzer and V. Janowsky (1890), angiokeratoma and porokeratosis
(1893) by Vitterio Mibelli (1891), hyperkeratosis by Emilio Respighi (1893),
benignant sarcoid by Carl Boeck (1899), chronic atrophic acrodermatitis by
J. Herxheimer and Kuno Hartmann (1902), granulosis rubra nasi by Josef
Jadassohn (1901), parapsoriasis by Louis Brocq (1902) and lichen nitidus by
Felix Pinkus (1907). Of Americans, Robert William Taylor described idiopathic progressive atrophy of the skin (1876); Louis A. Duhring, dermatitis
herpetiformis (1884); Andrew Rose Robinson, hydrocystoma (1884); Thomas
Caspar Gilchrist, blastomycetic dermatitis (1896); Benjamin R. Schenck,
sporotrichosis (1898); and Jay F. Schamberg, the progressive pigmentary
dermatitis which goes by his name (1900–01).[1]

The work of Magendie in experimental **pharmacology** was ably
continued by Alexander Crum Brown and Thomas Richard Fraser,
who first investigated the relation between the chemical constitution of substances and their physiological action ("anchoring the
molecules") (1867),[2] in which they were followed by Sir Thomas
Lauder Brunton (1892), and by J. T. Cash and W. R. Dunstan
(1893). Friedrich Walter investigated the actions of acids upon
the animal organism (1877), Ernst Stadelmann the action of
alkalies upon metabolism (1890). Admirable text-books on materia medica and therapeutics were written by such men as Sydney
Ringer in England (1869) and H. C. Wood in America (1874), both
of whom aimed to establish the status of drugs on the clinical side,
while Buchheim, Schmiedeberg, and Binz in Germany, Brunton
and Cushny in England, have done brilliant experimental work
on animals. The latter names have been particularly associated
with the destructive and critical pharmacodynamics of the
present time, the aim of which is to apply a rigorous sifting

[1] For bibliographical references to these diseases see Index Catalogue
(S. G. O.), 1912, 2 s., xvii, 150–152.

[2] Tr. Roy. Soc. Edinb., 1867–9, xxv, 151–203.

process to the vast numbers of alleged remedies listed in the various formularies and pharmacopeias, on the principle of "Prove all things, hold fast to that which is good." The effect of this destructive criticism has not only been admirable in reducing the gigantic vegetable materia medica of the past to reasonable proportions, but, in the face of the huge output of coal-tar products by the German chemists, initiated by Perkin's discovery of aniline dyes (1856), it became absolutely necessary. "The period of constructive pharmacology," Cushny declares, "has scarcely dawned" and he points out that remedies may now "be numerated in units where they were once counted in scores." The French clinicians Henri Huchard and Charles Fiessinger, for instance, have limited actual drug therapy to some 20 remedies or groups of remedies, viz.: opium, mercury, quinine, nux vomica, digitalis, arsenic, phosphorus, ergot, belladonna, chloral, bismuth, the bromides, the hypnotics, the purgatives, the antiseptics, the anesthetics, the antipyretics, the nitrites, the sera and vaccines, the animal extracts, each of which has a specific therapeutic intention. The whole tendency of recent pharmacology is in the direction of simplification and specificity, but it is rightly contended by the therapeutists of the older school that human beings are not necessarily rabbits and guinea-pigs of a larger growth, since individual drugs have different effects, not only upon different animals, but upon different human beings. The only final test of the reliability of a drug is at the bedside.

The leading pharmacologists of the German school are Rudolf **Buchheim** (1820–79), of Bautzen, professor at Leipzig (1846), Dorpat (1849), and Giessen (1867), who published a text-book of materia medica in 1856 and investigated the action of potassium salts, of purgatives, cod-liver oil, ergot, the mydriatic alkaloids of the Solanaceæ, etc.; his pupil, Oswald **Schmiedeberg** (1838–), of Courland, professor at Dorpat (1870) and Strassburg (1872), who first investigated the action of poisons on the frog's heart (in Ludwig's laboratory, 1871), and did a great amount of critical and experimental work on muscarin and other drugs, the tendency of which is crystallized in his well-known elements of pharmacology (1883); and Karl **Binz** (1832–1912), of Bernkastel, a pupil of Virchow and Frerichs and professor at Bonn (1868), where he founded the Pharmacological Institute of the University (1869). Binz published a text-book on materia medica (1866) and |lectures on pharmacology (1884), made experimental investigations of the action of quinine, alcohol, arsenic, the ethereal oils, the halogen compounds, and the anesthetics, and wrote an admirable history of anesthesia (1896). Hans **Meyer** (1853–), of Insterburg, a pupil of Ludwig and Schmiedeberg, professor at Dorpat (1882), Marburg (1884), and Vienna (   ), and E. Overton, have devoted especial attention to the part played by lipoid solvents in narcosis.

In England, Sir Thomas Lauder **Brunton** (1844–   ), of St. Bartholomew's Hospital, is the author of a well-recognized text-book of pharmacology and therapeutics (1885), the Croonian Lectures upon the relation between chemical structure and physiological action (1892), monographs on disorders of assimilation (1901), and the therapeutics of the circulation (1908).

Arthur Robertson **Cushny** (1866–   ), of Scotland, who has been professor of pharmacology at Ann Arbor (1893–1905) and in the University of London (1905), was a pupil of Schmiedeberg, and his text-book of pharmacology and therapeutics (1899) is imbued with the spirit of his master. He has done admirable work on the effects of digitalis on heart-muscle (1912).

Horatio C. **Wood** (1841–   ), of Philadelphia, professor of botany (1866–76) and therapeutics (1876–1907), also professor of nervous diseases (1875–1901) in the University of Pennsylvania, made an important investigation of the pathology of sunstroke (1872), wrote a memoir on the Algæ of North America (1872), and is the author of a treatise on therapeutics (1874), in which the effects of the various drugs upon man in small doses were first discussed, then of experimentation upon animals, which, with the evidence of toxicology, was made the rationale of their use in disease. This book also contains a standard classification of drugs. Wood investigated amyl nitrite, discovered the physiological and therapeutic properties of hyoscine, and first systematized the treatment of accidents in anesthesia. He was editor of the *Philadelphia Medical Times* (1873–80), the *Therapeutic Gazette* (1884–90), the United States Dispensatory (1883–1907), and is the author of a book on nervous diseases (1887).

Good original work has been done by Torald **Sollmann** (1874–   ), of Cleveland, Ohio, who has written a noteworthy text-book of pharmacology (1901).

John Jacob **Abel** (1857–   ), of Cleveland, Ohio, professor of pharmacology at the Johns Hopkins University (1893), is editor of the *Journal of Pharmacology and Therapeutics* (1909), and has made valuable investigations of new substances. Among his pupils, Reid Hunt is known by his studies on experimental alcoholism (1907) and the thyroid (1909), L. G. Rowntree and J. T. Geraghty by their discovery of the phenolsulphonephthalein test in kidney disease (1910). At the Johns Hopkins, also, Samuel J. Crowe discovered that hexamethylenamin (urotropin) is excreted in the cerebrospinal fluid (1909), which led to its extensive use in membranous diseases caused by microörganisms.

The special action of magnesium salts upon tetanus was investigated in America by Samuel James Meltzer and John Auer (1905–6).

Among the many drugs introduced in recent times are chloral by Oscar Liebreich (1869), antipyrin (Knorr) by Wilhelm Filehne (1884), cocaine (as anesthetic) by Carl Koller (1884), salipyrin by Riedel (1884), ichthyol and resorcin by Paul Gerson Unna (1886), salol by Marcel von Nencki (1886), acetanilide by Cahn and Hepp (1886), sulphonal (Baumann, 1884) by Alfred Kast (1888), trional and tetronal by Baumann and Kast (1888), strophanthus hispidus by Thomas R. Fraser (1891), suprarenal extract by G. Oliver and E. A. Schäfer (1894–5), eucaine by Merling (1896), heroine by Dreser (1898), veronal (1904) and proponal (1905) by Emil Fischer and Joseph von Mering, novocaine by Alfred Einhorn (1905), scarlet red (Biebrichs, 1882) by B. Fischer (1906), bismuth paste by Emil J. Beck (1908), pantopon by Hermann Sahli (1909), and salvarsan ("606") by Ehrlich (1909).

Of other therapeutic measures, **electrotherapy** was modernized by Duchenne of Boulogne (1847–55), Robert Remak (1855–58), Hugo von Ziemssen (1857), Moriz Benedikt (1868–75), and Wilhelm Heinrich Erb (1882); static electricity was first employed at Guy's Hospital by Thomas Addison, Golding Bird, and Sir William Gull (1837–52); the double faradic current was used against uterine diseases and tumors by Georges Apostoli at Paris (1884), and the high-frequency current was introduced by Jacques-Arsène d'Arsonval (1892). The X-rays, discovered by Wilhelm Conrad Röntgen in 1893, soon became a most reliable aid in diagnosis, and, in the hands of experts, a useful therapeutic measure, as also radium.

The **hypodermic syringe** was introduced in Europe by Francis Rynd (1845), Charles-Gabriel Pravaz (1851), and Alexander Wood (1855), and, in America, by Fordyce Barker (1856).

In 1895, G. Forlanini introduced the treatment of phthisis by artificial pneumothorax; and the principle of employing deep alcohol injections in neuralgia was suggested by Pitres and Vaillard in 1887, and first employed by Karl Schloesser in 1903.

Hydrotherapy was popularized by Max Joseph Oertel and the Silesian farmer, Vincenz Priessnitz (1799–1851), whose cold packs and outdoor methods were followed up by the Bavarian pastor Kneipp; by C. Munde at Gräfenberg (1839); in England, by James Manby Gully at Malvern (1842); and, in the United States, by Russell Thacher Trall (1844), Joel Shew, and others. Scientific hydrotherapy is especially associated with the names of Ernst Brand (1827–1897), a practitioner at Stettin, who put Currie's forgotten cold bath treatment of typhoid fever upon a reliable working basis (1861–63), and Wilhelm Winternitz (1835–1905) of Josefstadt, Bohemia, professor at Vienna (1881), director of the hydropathic establishment at Kaltenleutgeben, and founder of the *Blätter für klinische Hydrotherapie* (1890), who wrote the best modern treatise on the subject (1877–80), based upon experimental as well as clinical investigation. Oskar Lassar in Berlin and Simon Baruch in New York have been the leading propagandists for public baths within the means of the people in large cities.

Dietetics and regimen were advanced by William Banting (1797–1878), of England, who introduced the cure of obesity by the general reduction of food, including the exclusion of fats and carbohydrates (1863), by Liebig, Wöhler, Beaumont, Moleschott, Pavy, Pavloff, Rubner, Chittenden, and the other investigators of nutrition and metabolism, by Boas and Ewald, who introduced test-meals in digestive disorders, by Debove, who originated forced feeding in phthisis, and latterly by Carl von Noorden, who has made a special study of dietetics in disorders of metabolism and introduced the oatmeal diet in diabetes. Special treatments of heart disease were introduced by the laryngologist Max Joseph Oertel (1835–1897), of Dillingen, Bavaria, whose method consists in proteid diet with reduction of liquids, free perspiration and graduated uphill exercises (1884) and by Theodor Schott (1852–   ) who, at Nauheim, discovered the beneficent effect upon weak hearts of carbonated baths (1883) combined with slow gymnastics, executed by the patient and resisted by the operator. Intubation of the stomach was introduced by Adolf Kussmaul (1869).

The scientific applications of **hypnotism** were principally studied by Charcot and his pupils at the Salpêtrière and by the two leaders of the Nancy school, Ambroise-Auguste Liebeault in his *Le sommeil provoqué* (1889) and *Thérapeutique suggestive* (1891) and Hippolyte Bernheim in *De la suggestion dans l'état hypnotique et dans l'état de vieille* (1884) and *Hypnotisme, suggestion, psychothérapie* (1891). These titles show the general tendency, away from hypnotic suggestion and toward mental and moral suasion or psychotherapy, which was implicit in Charcot's teaching. Psychotherapy was put upon a definite basis in such works as Paul Dubois' book on the moral treatment of psychoneuroses (1904), and *Isolement et psychotherapie* (1904) by Jean Camus and Philippe Pagniez. The treatment of neurotic persons by moral education became the word of ambition. It was applied with ability by Rev. Elmwood Worcester and his associates at the Emanuel Church at Boston.

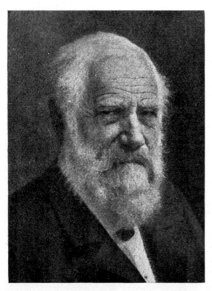

Max von Pettenkofer (1818–1901).

Gymnastics for therapeutic purposes were introduced as "Swedish movements" by Per Henrik Ling (1776–1839) about 1813, and have latterly been elaborated into such methods as mechanotherapy and kinesitherapy, particularly at the Zander Institute. The gospel of life and exercise in the open air, the feeling that external nature has a kindly healing side toward bodily and mental ills, was implicit in the teachings of Greek medicine, has been the theme of such modern writers as Thoreau, Walt Whitman, and John Burroughs, and has been applied with success in the treatment of phthisis everywhere and in neurasthenic states, by J. Madison Taylor and other specialists.

The founder of **experimental hygiene** was Max von **Pettenkofer** (1818–1901), of Lichtersheim, Bavaria, a pupil of Liebig and Bischoff, who became professor of "dietetic chemistry" at Munich in 1847, and professor of hygiene at the same university (1853), where, under his direction, the first Hygienic Institute was opened, in 1875. Pettenkofer's earlier work, as we have seen, was in the field of physiological chemistry and metabolism.

In 1844 he introduced the well-known test for bile acids and in 1863–4, with Voit, he made his classical investigations of metabolism in respiration.

He also investigated such substances as the sulphocyanates in sputum, hippuric acid, kreatin and kreatinin. From 1855 on, he devoted much attention to the etiology of cholera and typhoid fever, the spread of which he attributed to the condition of the soil and soil-water, latterly opposing the bacterial theory of infection to the extent of swallowing a culture of virulent cholera bacilli at seventy-four, in order to prove his thesis. In spite of his erroneous and arbitrary views, he all but rid the city of Munich of typhoid through the introduction of a proper system of drainage, a subject which frequently involved him in controversy with Virchow. Pettenkofer's most important contributions to experimental hygiene were his method of estimating carbon dioxide in air and water (1858), his investigations of the ventilation of dwelling houses (1858), and the relation of the atmosphere to clothing, habitations and the soil. He studied the relative advantages of stove and hot air heating, showed that air can pass through the thickest masonry, and investigated the contamination of the atmosphere from gases deep in the earth. He was ennobled in 1883 and became president of the Bavarian Academy of Sciences in 1889. In 1882, Pettenkofer published, with Ziemssen, the *Handbuch der Hygiene*, and he was one of the coeditors of the *Zeitschrift für Biologie* (1865–82) and the *Archiv für Hygiene* (1883–94). Experimental hygiene, as based upon the bacterial theory of infection, took a new start with the work of Koch and his associates in the Hygienic Institute at Berlin.

Perhaps the most important of the earlier treatises on **public hygiene** after the time of Johann Peter Frank were John Roberton's "Medical Police" (Edinburgh, 1808–9) and the treatises of François-Emmanuel Fodéré (1822–4) and Alexandre-J. B. Parent-Duchâtelet (1836), who also wrote an epoch-making work on prostitution in the city of Paris (1836). In the first half of the century, the subject was extensively cultivated in France. Various treatises were written by Molard (1841), Royer-Collard (1843), Bourdon (1844), Michel Levy (1844–5), Briand (1845), Foy (1845), Boudin (1846), while Parkes's Manual of 1864 set the pace for later works by L. Hirt (1876), E. Fazio (1880–86), G. H. Rohé (1885), Max Rubner (1888), E. Flügge (1889), J. Uffelmann (1889–90), W.｣Prausnitz (1892), L. Mangin (1892), Ferdinand Hueppe (1899), A. W. Blyth (1900), Charles Harrington (1901), W. T. Sedgwick (1902) and M. J. Rosenau (1913). Pettenkofer's great handbook (1862–94) was followed by similar cooperative works, edited by Thomas Stephenson and Shirley F. Murphy (1892–4), Theodor Weyl (1893–1901) and Max Rubner (1911). **Industrial hygiene** was advanced by Sir Humphry Davy (1779–1829), who invented the well-known safety lamp for coal miners (1818); by Charles Turner Thackrah (1795–1833) of Leeds, one of Sir Astley Cooper's pupils, who, in his treatise of 1832, first investigated brass-founders' ague, dust diseases, etc.; by Tanquerel des Planches (1809–62), who wrote an important work on diseases in lead workers (1839); by François Melier, who dealt with the hygiene of tobacco manufacturers (1849); by A.-L.-D.-Delpech, who investigated the rubber industry (1863), and, with J. B. Hillairet, the diseases of chromium manufacturers (1869–76). In Germany, Ludwig Hirt (1844–   ) of Breslau, wrote a monumental four volume treatise on occupational diseases (1871–78), which was followed by the *Handbücher* of H. Eulenburg (1876), H. Albrecht (1894–6) and Th. Weyl (1908). In England, Sir Thomas Oliver has paid especial attention to dust diseases, miners' and live-wire accidents (*Dangerous Trades*, London, 1902), and Leonard Hill investigated caisson disease (1912) and the general evils of stuffy atmosphere. Rudolf Virchow played an important part in the sanitation and sewage disposal of Berlin (1868–73) and was the originator of the modern movement for the hygiene and inspection of school-children (1869), which was ably carried forward by the labors of Edwin Chadwick (1871), Hermann Ludwig Cohn (1887) and a host of workers in recent times. The **sanitation of hospitals** was greatly forwarded by Florence Nightingale (1859), Lord Lister (1870), Sir Douglas Galton (1893), and by the object lessons gained in the construction of such fine modern structures as the Johns Hopkins Hospital in Baltimore (1889), the Hamburg Eppendorf pavilion (1889), or the Rudolf Virchow in Berlin (1906). The hygiene of habitations and the planning of towns is a subject of recent interest among architects and sanitary engineers. In 1874, Lord Kelvin said that there can be no proper hygiene of indoor life until "architecture becomes a branch of scientific engineering."[1]

Public hygiene in England was specially advanced by Sir Edwin **Chadwick** (1800–1890), and by **Sir John Simon** (1816–1904), whose famous "Public Health Report" (1887) and "English Sanitary Institutions" (1890) exerted great influence upon modern developments and legislation. The most important English treatise on hygiene is the manual of Edmund Alexander **Parkes** (1819–76), published in 1864, in the preparation of which he was aided by **Lord Sidney Herbert** (1810–61), of Lea, who was Secretary for War at the outbreak of the Crimean War (1854) and chairman of the Royal Commission on the sanitary conditions of the army and of military hospitals and barracks. Lord Herbert was in frequent consultation with Parkes as to the formation of the Army Medical School at Fort Pitt, Chatham, in 1860, which was transferred to the Royal Victoria Hospital, Netley, in 1863. It was the friendship of Lord and Lady Herbert for Florence Nightingale which led to the latter's passage to Scutari with forty nurses to look after the soldiers in the Crimean contest. It is said that all the recommendations made by the South African Royal Commission in 1901 had been made by Lord Herbert fifty-five years before. His colleague, Parkes, held the first chair of hygiene in England (at Fort Pitt, 1860), and the Parkes Museum of Hygiene was instituted in his memory, July 18, 1876, and opened on June 28, 1879.

Baron Mundy, of Vienna, called Parkes "the founder and best teacher of military hygiene in our day, the friend and benefactor of every soldier."

Perhaps the earliest modern work on **statistics** was the famous *Essay on the Principle of Population* (1803) of Thomas Robert Malthus (1766–1834), of Guildford, England, which maintains that food-supply and birth-rate increase in arithmetic and geometric ratios respectively, and has exerted a profound influence upon the postponement of marriage and the decrease in size of families down to the present time. Medical statistics were introduced by Louis (1835). The modern methods of arriving at the mortality of large cities and other data were blocked out by the Hungarian statistician Josef von Körösi (1873); the fallacies and other mathematical relations of vital statistics were studied by the English writers, Henry Wyldbore Rumsey (1875) and William Farr (1885). In America, John Shaw Billings (1838–1913) made valuable contributions, particularly in his Cartwright Lectures (1889) and his special reports on the United States Census. The statistical investigations of Jacques Bertillon (1851–   ) on the depopulation of France (1880–1911)[2] have had their effect upon other countries in which a falling off of the birthrate is noticeable. Karl Pearson's work belongs to the twentieth century.

In the department of **medical jurisprudence**, the treatise of François-Emmanuel Fodéré (1798, 1812) was the standard source of authority in France

---

[1] Lord Kelvin: Popular Lectures, London, 1884, ii, 211.
[2] J. Bertillon: La dépopulation de la France, Paris, 1911.

in the early part of the century. In Germany, Johann Ludwig Caspar (1796–1864), of Berlin, achieved a wide reputation through his works on medical statistics and state medicine (1825–35), judicial postmortems (1851–3), and his Practical Handbook of Legal Medicine (1856), which remained, for a long time, unsurpassed for its wealth of facts and sound judgments. The first treatises in English were written by the Americans, Theodoric Romeyn Beck (1823) and Isaac Ray (1839). William Augustus Guy (1810–85) was the first English writer on the subject (1844). Other American treatises of note were those by Francis Wharton and Moreton Stillé (1855), and John Ordronaux (1869), both of which deal with forensic medicine from the lawyer's point of view. The four volume treatise of Witthaus and Becker (1894–96) is a comprehensive modern encyclopedia, written by many hands. Heinroth (1825), Isaac Ray (1839), Krafft Ebing (1875) and Charles Arthur Mercier (1890) have dealt with the jurisprudence of insanity, Carl Ferdinand von Arlt with the medicolegal aspect of injuries of the eye (1875), M.-J.-B. Orfila (1813–15), Sir Robert Christison (1829), Auguste-Ambroise Tardieu (1867) and Georg Dragendorff (1868–72) with toxicology, Frank Hastings Hamilton with the jurisprudence of deformities after fractures (1855), and Krafft-Ebing with sexual perversion and inversion (1886–7). Theodore George Wormley wrote a sterling work on the microchemistry of poisons (1867) and Virchow's little handbook of postmortem technic (1876) was the standard in its day. In recent times, Paul Brouardel (1837–1906), of Paris, is memorable for a number of exhaustive monographs of value, in particular, those on death and sudden death (1895), hanging, strangulation, suffocation and drowning (1897) and infanticide (1897). The precipitin test (Bordet-Uhlenhuth) for blood-stains was introduced in 1901,[1] and the cobra-venom reaction in insanity (Much-Holtzmann) in 1909.[2]

From the time of Haller, the study of **medical history** has been mainly in the hands of German and French writers.

British scholars, such as Francis Adams (1796–1861), of Banchory, Scotland, William Alexander Greenhill (1814–94), of London, and others have made valuable translations of the greater Greek and Roman classics; and delightful books and essays, with the genuine flavor of letters, have been written by William MacMichael (The Gold Headed Cane, 1827), John Brown (Horæ Subsecivæ, 1858), J. Cordy Jeaffreson (A Book about Doctors, 1860), Wilks and Bettany (History of Guy's Hospital, 1892), Sir Benjamin Ward Richardson (Disciples of Æsculapius, 1900), particularly by the two Regius professors, Osler and Allbutt; yet no work on a large scale has been attempted in Great Britain or America which will measure up with the performances of Haeser or Daremberg, unless it be Charles Creighton's History of Epidemics in Britain (1894). Thomas Young's Introduction to Medical Literature (1813), an unfinished history of medicine by Edward Meryon (1861), a very readable one by Edward T. Withington (1894), the studies of John Flint South (1886), Sydney Young (1890), and D'Arcy Power (1899) on English surgery, Sir Clifford Allbutt's studies of medieval medicine and surgery (1901–05), J. F. Payne on Anglo-Saxon medicine (1904), Norman Moore on medical education in Great Britain (1908), and the illuminating essays of Sir William Osler and Raymond Crawfurd are among the best things that have been done in England. Up to the present time, American contributions have been meager in extent. The best are the essays of Joseph Meredith Toner, the historical survey entitled "A Century of American Medicine" (1876), the "Medical Essays" of Oliver Wendell Holmes (1883), Weir-Mitchell's history of instrumental precision in medicine (1892), James J. Walsh's studies of medieval medicine and

---

[1] Uhlenhuth: Deutsche med. Wochenschr., Leipzig and Berlin, 1901, xxvii, 86; 260.

[2] Much: Centralbl. f. Bakteriol. (etc.), Beil. zu 1. Abt., Jena, 1909, xlii, 48–50.

the history of nursing by Mary Adelaide Nutting and Lavinia L. Dock (1907–12). An excellent short history of medicine was written by Roswell Park (1897); the history of medicine in the United States has been treated by Francis Randolph Packard (1901) and James Gregory Mumford (1903); Jewish medicine by Charles D. Spivak and F. T. Haneman (1904); medical folk-lore by Robert Fletcher; medical botanists and medical illustrators by Howard A. Kelly.

The earliest German work of consequence in the nineteenth century was the *Geschichte der Heilkunde* of J. F. K. **Hecker** (1795–1850) which was followed by his collective monograph on the great epidemics of the Middle Ages (1865). The most scholarly and thoroughgoing medical history of modern times was written by Heinrich **Haeser** (1811–84), who became professor of medicine at Jena (1839), Greifswald (1849) and Breslau (1862). Haeser was the son of a music director at Weimar, was brought up in an atmosphere of culture and was one of the most learned physicians of his time. His earlier works on the history of epidemic diseases (1839–41) and his *Bibliotheca epidemiographica* (1843), with the valuable *Additamenta* by Johann Gottlieb Thierfelder (1843) demonstrate his talents for close investigation. These came to apt fruition in his *Lehrbuch der Geschichte der Medicin und der Volkskrankheiten* (1845), which, in its third edition (1875–82), had become an unrivaled storehouse of knowledge, wonderfully accurate as to dates and citations, although naturally there were a few errors here and there. The third volume, on the history of epidemics, contains original citations of many first-hand descriptions of disease from the old municipal and monkish chronicles, a field in which Haeser has been equalled only by Sudhoff. Haeser's masterpiece was followed in Germany by the histories of Wunderlich (1859), Johann Hermann Baas (1876), Julius Pagel (1898, 1901–6), and the Viennese professor, Max Neuburger (1906), all of them works of solid and sterling character. Meanwhile, Arabian medicine was treated by Heinrich Ferdinand Wüstenfeld (1840) and Karl Opitz (1906), the history of syphilis by Conrad Heinrich Fuchs (1843), Julius Rosenbaum (1845), and Iwan Bloch (1901–11), the history of medieval leprosy by Virchow (1860–61), German medicine by Heinrich Rohlfs (1875–82) and August Hirsch (1893), Viennese medicine (1884) and the history of medical education (1889) by Theodor **Puschmann** (1844–99), Thibetan medicine by Heinrich Laufer (1900), cuneiform medicine by Felix von Oefele (1902), the history of plague by Georg Sticker (1908–10), Persian medicine by the Norwegian, Adolf Mauritz Fonahn (1910), and Jewish medicine by Julius Preuss (1911). Julius **Pagel** (1851–1912), a busy practitioner of Berlin, who edited Mondeville (1889–92) and Mesue (1893), wrote a history of medicine in 1897 and issued a capital biographical lexicon (1900), an encyclopedic history of medicine (1901–6), and a useful medical chronology (1908). The work of Karl Sudhoff has a high place in the twentieth century. The ablest medical historian of France was Charles-Victor **Daremberg** (1817–72), of Dijon, who edited and translated Oribasius (1851–76), the Four Masters (1854), select works of Hippocrates (1843), Galen (1854–6) and Celsus (1859), made original investigations of Homeric medicine (1865), Hindu medicine (1867), medicine between Homer and Hippocrates (1869), and wrote an admirable history of medicine (1870), which is still consulted. Daremberg was a warm friend of Emile **Littré** (1801–81) of Paris, one of the greatest of medical philologists, who was the author of the splendid five-volume dictionary of the French language (1863–72), published the finest modern edition of Hippocrates, with French translation (1839–61), also of Pliny's natural history (1848–50), reëdited Nysten's medical dictionary and wrote many interesting historical essays. Other French contributions of value are the medical histories of Eugene Bouchut (1873) and Léon Meunier (1911), Maurice Raynaud's study of medicine in the time of Molière (1862), the splendid memorials of the Paris Medical Faculty by Auguste Corlieu (1896) and Noé Legrand (1911), and Ernest Wickersheimer's study of Renaissance medicine in France (1905). The study of medicine in relation to art was inaugurated by Virchow (1861), placed upon its feet by the extensive work of Charcot and his pupils and continued in such German works as Hermann Peters' "Der Arzt" (1900), Eugen Holländer on medicine in classical painting (1903), medical caricature and satire (1905) and medicine in the plastic arts (1912), and Robert Müllerheim on the lying-in chamber in art (1904). Medicine in ancient India was treated by Sir Bhagvat Sin Jee (1896) and August F. R. Hoernle (1907), medicine in Mexico by Francisco A. Flores (1886–88), medicine in Upper Canada by William Canniff (1894). Useful biographical dictionaries of medicine are those of Bayle and Thillaye (1855), August Hirsch and E. Gurlt (1884–88) and Pagel (1900). The notices in the "Dictionary of National Biography" (1885–1912) for English physicians; and for American physicians, James Thacher (1828), S. D. Gross (1861), W. B. Atkinson (1878), R. F. Stone (1894), Irving D. Watson (1896) and Howard A. Kelly (1912) are indispensable. In Italy, a good history of medicine was written by Francesco Puccinotti (1850–66), the Copenhagen manuscripts of the School of Salerno were edited by Salvatore De Renzi (Collectio Salernitana, Naples, 1853–59) and Piero Giacosa (1901) and an excellent history of dentistry was written by Vincenzo Guerini (1909).

Among the modern periodicals devoted to medical history are Hecker's *Litterarische Annalen der gesammten Heilkunde* (Berlin, 1825–35). *Janus*, edited by A. W. E. Th. Henschel (Breslau, 1846–8) and continued at Breslau (1851–53), Sir Benjamin Ward Richardson's *Asclepiad* (London, 1885–95), *Chronique médical* (Paris, 1894–1913), *Janus* (Amsterdam, 1896–1913), the *Medical Library and Historical Journal* (Brooklyn and New York, 1903–7), which had a short-lived successor, the *Æsculapian* (Brooklyn, 1908–9), and the *Archiv für Geschichte der Medizin* (Leipzig, 1907–13), founded and edited by Karl Sudhoff. The latter is by far the most important periodical on the subject which has yet appeared, the contents being devoted exclusively to original research. Several medical history societies are now publishing transactions, in particular, the Deutsche Gesellschaft für Geschichte der Medizin und der Naturwissenschaften at Leipzig (*Mittheilungen*, 1902–13), the Charaka Club, New York (*Proceedings,* 1902–10), the Société française d'histoire de médecine, Paris (*Bulletin,* 1903–13), the Società italiana della storia critica delle scienze mediche e naturali, Rome (Rivista, 1910–13), the Society of Medical History of Chicago (*Bulletin,* 1911–13) and the Historical Section of the Royal Medical Society of London (*Proceedings,* 1913). The *Bulletin* of the Johns Hopkins Hospital (1890–1913) is the literary organ of the Hospital Historical Club. The careful reviews in the Leipzig *Mittheilungen,* under the direction of Sudhoff and Siegmund Günther, afford a convenient clearing-house of all recent medico-historical literature.

As the modern period has been the great age of medical periodicals, so too it has been the age of **medical bibliography.**

In the past, Conrad Gesner did something of the kind as early as 1545. Haller was the leading medical bibliographer of the eighteenth century, and, in the nineteenth, Young (1813), Haeser (1862), Ploucquet, Forbes, Atkinson, Watts and others did good work; but the first attempt to give an indexed author catalogue of an entire period, including the contents of periodicals, was the *Medicinisches Schriftsteller-Lexicon* (33 volumes, 1830–45) of the Danish surgeon, Carl Peter **Callisen** (1787–1866). As a complete conspectus of the medical literature of the last half of the eighteenth century and the first third of the nineteenth, this production ranks with Haller's as one of the most wonderful things ever achieved by a single man. It is invaluable for scope and accuracy. Other works of equal value are the *Handbuch der Bücherkunde* (1828) of Ludwig Choulant (1791–1861), which, in its second edition (1841), is, with the indispensable *Additamenta* of Julius Rosenbaum (1842), the best check list we have of the different editions of the older medical writers. The *Repertorium bibliographicum* (1826–28) of Ludwig **Hain,** with the supplements of Walter Arthur Copinger (1895–1902) and Dietrich Reichling (1905–11), has been the standard catalogue of the incunabula.

The opportunity for a unique bibliography of the entire medical literature of the world was afforded by the building up of the Library of the Surgeon-General's Office at Washington, which, at the outbreak of the Civil War, consisted of some 1000 odd volumes and became, in time, the largest medical library in the world through the energy, perseverance and ability of its principal founder, John Shaw **Billings** (1838–1913), a native of Indiana, who had been a distinguished army surgeon in the Civil War. In 1876, Billings published a "Specimen Fasciculus" of a combined index catalogue of authors and subjects, arranged in a single alphabet in dictionary order, and, in 1880, he issued the first volume of the *Index Catalogue* of the library, in which he was assisted by Robert **Fletcher** (1823–

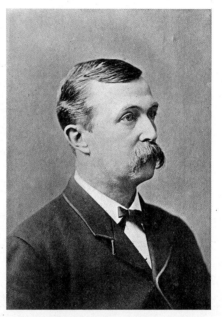

John Shaw Billings (1838–1913). (Courtesy of the National Academy of Sciences.)

1912), of Bristol, England. This work, the most exhaustive piece of medical bibliography ever undertaken, has now reached its thirty- fourth volume (second series, XVIII), and embraces the contents of a medical library of over 500,000 volumes. The selection of the material and the scientific classification in the first series (1880–95) were made by Billings; the careful proofreading was done by Fletcher; both classification and proofreading of the second series (1896) were done by Fletcher up to the time of his death (1912). This work, and the *Index Medicus*, a monthly bibliography of the world's medical literature, edited in the first series

(1879–99) by Billings and Fletcher, and revived, with Fletcher as editor-in-chief, by the Carnegie Institution of Washington, in 1903, are known to all physicians who use medical literature. Apart from his talents as a medical bibliographer, Billings was a man of all-round ability, an able operative surgeon in war-time, an authority on military medicine, public hygiene, sanitary engineering, statistics and hospital construction, the author of the most critical account of American medical literature (1876) and the best history of surgery that has been published in English (1895) and widely known as the designer of the Johns Hopkins and other modern hospitals. Altogether, Billings did a giant's work for the advancement of American medicine. Fletcher made many admirable contributions to anthropology and medical history.

Apart from the Index Catalogue, there were many valuable bibliographies of smaller scope, such as Hernandes Morejon's bibliographic history of Spanish medicine (1842–52), the Royal Society's Catalogue of Scientific Papers (1867–96), E. J. Waring's Bibliotheca Therapeutica (1878), R. Schmid's bibliography of public hygiene, 1898–1906, Heinrich Laehr's bibliography of psychiatry, neurology, and psychology from 1459 to 1799 (1900), the Index Catalogue of Medical Zoölogy by Charles Wardell Stiles and Albert Hassall (1902–12) and the International Catalogue of Scientific Literature published for the different countries by the Royal Society (1907–10).

THE TWENTIETH CENTURY: THE BEGINNINGS OF ORGANIZED PREVENTIVE MEDICINE

PRIMITIVE medicine, with its Egyptian and Oriental congeners, is essentially a phase of anthropology. Greek medicine was science in the making, with Roman medicine as an offshoot, Byzantium as a cold-storage plant and Islam as traveling agent. The best side of medieval medicine was the organization of hospitals, sick nursing, medical legislation and education: its reactionary tendencies are mainly of antiquarian interest. The Renaissance period marks the birth of anatomy as a science, with a corresponding growth of surgery as a handicraft. The best of seventeenth-century medicine was purely scientific. Eighteenth-century medicine was again retrograde in respect of system-making, but has to its credit the beginnings of pathology, instrumental diagnosis, experimental and physiological surgery, and acquires an added social interest in relation to the founding of preventive medicine and the extension of public hygiene. In the nineteenth century, the advancement of science was organized and scientific surgery was created. The interest of twentieth-century medicine is again social.

The most noticeable thing about recent medicine is the growth of coöperation and international solidarity, and the fact that nearly every important advance that has been made is prophylactic, that is, comes within the scope of preventing the occurrence, the recurrence or the spread of disease. Listerism; the gifts to mankind of Jenner, Pasteur, Semmelweis, Credé, and O'Dwyer; the chemical and bacteriological examination of air, water, food, soils, and drugs; the purification of sewage; cremation; the hygiene of occupations and habitations; the medical inspection and care of school-children and factory children; the Binet-Simon tests; vacation colonies; social surveys and settlement work; the war on the white-slave traffic; the police surveillance of perverts and criminal characters in great cities like Berlin; the Gothenberg method of regulating the liquor traffic; the revival of the old Greek ideal of athletics and personal hygiene; the displacement of the medieval ascetic view of the sexual instinct by the clear-eyed scientific view; the formation of societies for moral prophylaxis and eugenics; the proposed legal regulation of marriage and sterilization of degenerate stock; the intensive

594

study of alcoholism, the drug habit, syphilis, tuberculosis and cancer; the use of medical bibliography and statistics to get extensive
information as to pathological conditions in space and time; the
coöperation of universities, armies, public health services and private endowments in preventing tropical or parasitic diseases; international congresses; the Geneva Convention; even such things as
Banting, Bertillonage, Esmarch bandages, or sanitary towels and
drinking cups, are all features of preventive medicine or medicine
on a grand scale. It is evident that the misapplication of some
of these prophylactic measures might lead to social slavery worse
than that of feudalism, because, as Emerson said, "The race is
great, the ideal fair, the men whiffling and unsure." In the hands
of corrupt politicians, Johann Peter Frank's great concept of a
scientific medical police might easily become a stalking horse for
private vindictiveness, in the regulation of marriage, for instance.
As Allbutt has wittily said: "The Greek philosopher, like the modern socialist, would sacrifice man to the State; the priest would
sacrifice man to the Church; the scientific evolutionist would
sacrifice man to the race."

The tendency in all branches of recent science, even in zoölogy,
sociology, therapeutics, internal medicine and surgery, has been
to pass out of the descriptive into the experimental stage. The
aim of science to predict and control phenomena is shown in the
application of the equation in Mendel's law to the study of heredity,
in Loeb's proof that the fertilization and development of the embryo is a chemical process, in the consideration of the accessory
chromosome as the determinant of sex, in the conquest of such
diseases as typhoid and yellow fever or hookworm infection, in
the extravital cultivation and rejuvenation of tissues, in the more
exact knowledge of diseases of the heart, disorders of the internal
secretions, and diseases due to filterable viruses, and in the recent
developments of Hunterian or physiological surgery.

In 1865,[1] the Augustinian monk, Gregor Johann **Mendel**
(1822-84), abbot of Brünn, announced the results of certain experiments on hybridization in peas in the form of a law which sheds
much light upon inheritance and the origin of species. If we agree
to represent the generation of hybrids by the mathematical process of squaring, and if a represents the dominant or unchangeable
characters, and b the recessive or latent characters in the parents,
then Mendel's law becomes identical with Newton's binomial
theorem: $(a+b)^2 = a^2 + 2ab + b^2$; in other words, one-half of the
progeny will breed true to the parental characters $(2ab)$, while the

---

[1] Mendel: Versuche über Pflanzen-Hybriden, Verhandl. d. naturf. Ver.
in Brünn (1865), 1866, iv, 3-270.

other half will be divided equally between offspring possessing only the dominant (*a*) and the recessive (*b*) characters. In subsequent generations, the hybrid offspring will breed according to Mendel's law, while the dominants and recessives will breed true to their kinds. For at least thirty-five years, this unique approximation, printed in an obscure periodical, remained unnoticed, but in 1900, Hugo de Vries (1848–   ), C. Correns, and E. Tschermak simultaneously confirmed Mendel's results in every respect, while, in 1897, Francis Galton had arrived at a statistical "law of heredity," based upon his observations on the pedigrees of Basset hounds. From his experi-

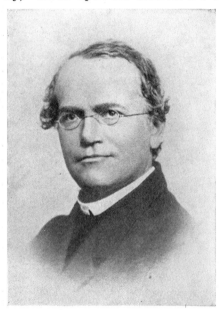

Gregor Johann Mendel (1822–1884).
(Courtesy of Professor William Bateson, London.)

ments with the plant Œnothera Lamarckiana, de Vries, advanced his "mutation" hypothesis of the abrupt or spontaneous origin of species from those permanent, transmissible variations or mutations which are to be differentiated from the Darwinian variations of the fluctuating, impermanent kind. The artificial production of new species *in extenso* has been carried out by Luther Burbank at his open-air laboratory in California. The effect of the theories of Mendel and de Vries upon recent biology has been to deprive Darwin's idea of natural selection of the supernatural and ethical attributes

which have been read into it by overzealous admirers, but no experiments to date have demonstrated that species originate by mutation alone. The trend of recent opinion is to the effect that the importance of mutation, which commonly obtains in plants only, has been somewhat exaggerated. Darwin perhaps overemphasized the significance of the *external* factor of environmental stress in the struggle for existence as originating species by long-continued (eventually) "natural" selection. Mendel and de Vries have indicated the *internal* biochemical forces at work in bringing about the mathematical permutations and combinations of the determinants in the supposed discontinuous origin of species *de novo* or *per saltum*. But whether evolution proceeds by slow gradations or by leaps and bounds or, what seems most likely, is capable of both continuous and discontinuous processes, it is probable that the apparently spontaneous results of saltatory or Mendelian variation had, in each case, "a long foreground," in the sense of being the end product of a complex series of physico-chemical changes. In other words, Mendelian mutations are probably latent factors or coefficients of a given species which crop out occasionally and breed true to their kind, and, in any case, represent the term and end of some physico-chemical process. Old Sir Thomas Browne,[1] the first to use the term, said that "mutations, however they began, depend upon durable foundations, and such as may continue forever," which seems the conclusion of the whole matter. Natural selection and mutation may "explain" the origin of structural adaptations, so that their transmutations can be verified, if need be, in the laboratory, but of the origin of organic and functional adaptations, such as the regeneration of tissues, automatic regulation of form, development of embryos from fractions of the ovum or by chemical activation (parthenogenesis), these theories tell us nothing, because the "power of adaptation" which is assigned as a reason is the very thing we are called upon to account for and explain. At most, we can only explain adaptation by harking back to the old Hallerian doctrine of the specialized "irritability" of individual protoplasmic tissues, which Ehrlich has declared to be one of the most obscure provinces of physiology.

In striking contrast with Mendelism stands the new statistical science of **biometrics,** which is the special creation of Francis Galton and his brilliant pupil, **Karl Pearson** (1857–   ). The theory of probabilities was first applied to sociological phenomena by the Belgian astronomer and statistician, Adolphe Quetelet (1796–1874),[2] but Galton's "Natural Inheritance" (1889) introduced the statistical study of biological variation and inheritance. Pearson, an English barrister, now director of the Laboratory for National Eugenics, founded by Galton, has applied the higher mathematics in the most ingenious way to the solution of these problems and has created a rational school of iatromathematics. His fascinating volumes on "The Chances of Death" (1897) opened out many new views as to the meaning of statistics as interpreted by algebraic curves, the significance of correlations, and the use of the same in obtaining accurate data as to the hidden causes of

---

[1] Pseudodoxia Epidemica, Book, vi, ch. x, "Of the Blackness of Negroes" (Bohn's ed., v. ii, p. 188) cited by Punnett.

[2] Quetelet: Sur l'homme, Brussels, 1836; Lettre   .   .   .   sur la théorie des probabilités appliquée aux sciences morales et sociales, Brussels, 1846; Loi de périodicité, Brussels, 1870, etc.

biological and social phenomena which cannot themselves be measured quantitatively. Galton used the term "regression" to indicate the extent to which an average biological unit is more like the
mean or mediocre level of the general stock than like its parent. By
correlation, Pearson means the logical opposite, viz., the extent to
which the offspring is more like its parents than to the average
unit of the species. If parent and offspring are exactly alike, in
respect of the quality under investigation, the correlation curve
will be a line making an angle of 45° with the abscissæ or the ordi-
nates. If the filial quality exists to a lesser degree than the parental, the curve will have a more insignificant slope, the degree of
slope ("correlation-coefficient") being the tangent of the angle
made with the horizontal. If there is no correlation, the curve will
be a horizontal line. By this means, Pearson has brought out
many new facts and bionomic theorems, particularly in the journal
Biometrika.[1] For example, he has shown that, in the case of tuberculosis, it is not the disease but the diathesis which is inherited,
not the seed but the soil; that there is no neurotic inheritance
from alcoholic parentage unless the stock itself be neurotic; that
the death-rate from disease is selective in a large per cent. of cases,
and that a higher infantile death-rate implies the survival of a
stronger and more enduring stock. Pearson believes that the
improvements of medical science and the tendency of nature to
insure the survival of the fittest are diametrically opposing forces,
and he contends, *e. g.*, from the surprising fertility of successive
generations of achondroplasic dwarfs, that the humane tendency
of modern medicine to preserve the diseased and deformed is not
only detrimental to the human species, but can only be set off or
obviated by preventing these defectives from breeding their kind.
He has indicated how Galton's law of ancestral inheritance can
be improved upon by selective breeding, so that regression, the
tendency to revert to a mediocre average, will in a few generations
be hardly sensible. He claims that tall women procreate faster
than small women, that dark-eyed people are more fertile
than the light-eyed, and has established the law of "assortative
mating," in virtue of which human beings, in most cases, mate, not
as usually believed, with their opposites in stature, complexion,
etc., but with their own kind. In this respect, he finds that hus-
band and wife are more nearly alike than uncle and niece or first
cousins, in accordance with the French proverb, *Les époux se res-
semblent.* The inference is that, according to Galton's law, the
strong tend to perpetuate and strengthen their kind by mating,
biologically speaking, in their own class. Similarly, it is held that a
greater amount of high-grade ability could be produced by select-

---

[1] Founded, in 1901, by W. F. R. Weldon, Francis Galton and himself.

ive breeding, since "the average genius we meet is more likely to be an exceptional variation of a mediocre stock than a common variation of an exceptional stock. This accounts for the fact that the sons of geniuses are often so disappointing." These theories of Galton and Pearson have met with no little opposition, not because they are incorrect, but because, as already stated, Darwinism has often a brutalizing effect upon shallow minds, who take theories too literally. According to Weismann's theory, acquired characters are not inherited, and the finest moral or mental traits in the parents will not benefit the offspring unless they have the right start in life. Oliver Twist may go to the bad in a den of thieves, and Bill Sykes may have it in him to steal and murder, even with the most careful upbringing. That morality is always an inhibition, showing, at least, the importance of "early training" (euthenics),[1] was sensed by the broad-minded Goethe, who declared himself capable of committing any crime. The studies of the Jukes family, the Hill Folk, and the Nams show one side of the shield, Galton's investigations of talented families the other, the record of the Kallikak family both. The work of Bateson, Punnett, of Charles B. Davenport and the experts at the Cold Spring Harbor Station, bears out the Mendelian axiom that, as the individuality of a living organism is established by the presence or absence of certain biological determinants, so qualities may be inherited, but not their absence. As brown eyes are due to the presence, blue eyes to the absence, of a certain pigment in the iris, as dancing mice differ from normal mice in lacking part of the internal ear, so brachydactyly (short fingers), presenile cataract, keratosis, xanthoma, hypotrichosis congenita, diabetes insipidus, night-blindness, and Huntington's chorea indicate the presence of certain factors in the germ plasm which may interdict the union of two such abnormals; but albinism, deaf-mutism, retinitis pigmentosa, congenital imbecility, and the tendency to respiratory and neurotic disorders are due to an inherent lack of something which may be supplemented by judicious cross-breeding with sound stock,[2] although Pearson contends that it is a waste of good material to employ sound stock for this purpose. Hence consanguineous marriages are not necessarily bad, if both units be sound. Nature's tendency to revert to the mediocre level of the common stock, to Walt Whitman's "divine average," will make the average a very low level indeed if it proceeds downward from poor or faulty material to start with. Thus eugenics, while attain-

---

[1] "The environment of to-day is the heredity of to-morrow" (Tredgold).

[2] C. B. Davenport: Eugenics, New York, 1910; Heredity (etc.), New York, 1911, *passim*.

able in animals, seems, in man, a desperate attempt to get a purchase on Nature and make her improve upon herself. Actual selection is often influenced by the bizarre caprices of "the unstable heart of man," and while individual propagandism could be made extremely effective, social control would be difficult of accomplishment without tyrannous espionage and surveillance. In the lower strata of society, marriage laws may not prevent illegitimacy or incest, vasectomy is dubious,[1] and selective pure-line breeding, without some striking quality to start with, might only result in a race of negative prigs.

Much time and energy have been expended in the long-standing controversy between **materialists and vitalists.** The trend of all recent biological, and especially physiological, thinking has been away from vitalism, because, like other forms of intellectual complacency, it only drives the subject into a blind alley and sidetracks the chances of further investigation. The materialist, who regards the living cell as a physicochemical unit, furnished with a center of oxidation (nucleus) and bounded by a semipermeable membrane, its physiological processes being looked upon as resultants of mechanical, physical and chemical laws, at least offers something which can be tried out experimentally to its last consequences. The vitalist has nothing to offer except sterile phrases like the "entelechies" of Driesch,[2] which only beg the question. In the laboratory, vitalism would seem to be on its last legs. Even the regeneration of substance and regulation of form in Murphy's autogenous bone-grafts probably depend, in the last analysis, upon some subtle chemical likeness. Carrel's experiment of making the excised viscera functionate extravitally for a definite time goes to show that, even in the higher animals, the separate organs have a mechanical autonomy of their own. There appear to be configurated phases of protoplasm which lie between plants, with a limited number of mechanical degrees of freedom, and animals, with an unlimited number, and also phases which, as King puts it, "are neither alive nor dead but between the two." The only true criterion of death is the thermodynamic, in which the substance is reduced, as Willard Gibbs said, to a "phase of dissipated energy,"

---

[1] The undesirable tendencies of mutilated or eunuchoid individuals, let loose upon society, are well known in the Orient and are frequently emphasized in the foot-notes of Sir Richard Burton's Arabian Nights.

[2] Driesch defines an entelechy as a non-spatial, non-perceptual agent which can suspend or modify physiological processes at will, so that two absolutely identical systems, may, if alive, behave differently under absolutely identical conditions (biological indeterminism). But he admits that he can produce no examples to prove his case and that his doctrine does not apply to actual experiment. As Jennings says, "he maintains in general what he denies in particular," which, of course, pulverizes his theory.

e. g., has become an inert mass, incapable of spontaneous change, because its free energy or chemical potentiality is practically *nil*. According to physico-chemical theory, an unfertilized ovum, a senile paramecium, an encysted ameba or an inactivated pathogenic bacillus are all in a temporarily insulated or "adiabatic" state, in which energy can neither go in nor out of them; and such "storehouses of energy" begin to functionate only when subjected to the catalytic influence of external physico-chemical agencies, which stimulate their surface energies. Examples of these phenomena are found in the experiments of Maupas and Calkins on the chemical rejuvenation of protozoa and of Loeb on the chemical activation of the ovum.

Jacques **Loeb** (1859–   ), a medical graduate of Strassburg (1884), who has been professor of biology and physiology at Bryn Mawr (1892–1900), University of Chicago (1900–1902), University of California (1902–1910), and is now head of the department of experimental biology in the Rockefeller Institute, has been a brilliant investigator in many branches of physiology, but his most characteristic work is that upon the dynamic or chemodynamic theory of living processes. In his work on the physiology of the brain, he made original researches on the chain reflexes, and overthrew Munk's position that the Rolandic area is made up of cellular "sensory spheres," by showing that the particular paralysis occasioned by each cortical excision will be abolished as soon as the wound is healed. He was one of the first to settle the question: of what order of magnitude is the smallest particle that can show all the phenomena of life? (1893)[1] and the experiments made by himself and pupils upon temperature coefficients have established other important criteria of physiological processes. He has made extensive investigations of the effects of electrolytic, thermal and radiant energy upon living matter, and he founded the theory of "tropisms" (1890)[2] as the basis of the psychology of the lower forms of life, purely mechanical and chemical data displacing the old theory of purposeful instinctive reactions. Even for the higher forms, his main position is that all actions of fundamental importance are instinctive, and have nothing to do with states of consciousness, and even these may have a chemical basis. In 1899, he caused the unfertilized eggs of the sea-urchin to develop into the swimming larvæ by treating them with hypertonic sea water (*i. e.*, in which the concentration has been raised by the addition of salt or sugar). Similar results had been published by Tichomiroff (1886), who claimed to have developed unfertilized silkworm eggs

---

[1] Loeb: Arch. f. d. ges. Physiol., Bonn, 1894–95, lix, 379–394.

[2] Der Heliotropismus der Thiere, Würzburg, 1890, and later publications.

by rubbing them gently with a brush or by temporary immersion in concentrated sulphuric acid. Bataillon got similar effects by needle-punctures (1911). Loeb carried his imitation of normal fertilization further by a preliminary treatment with butyric acid, producing an artificial fertilization membrane with complete development, following immersion of the eggs in a hypertonic solution before returning them to normal sea water. The formation of the membrane is supposed to accelerate oxidation, which Loeb regards as the criterion of a living process. Thus the ovum can be activated just as a protozoön can be rejuvenated or an asphyxiated body resuscitated, by purely physico-chemical means, although the result is an organism whose somatic cells lack one-half the normal number of chromosomes.

In 1902, Clarence Erwin McClung stated that the accessory chromosome, which Henking and Montgomery had located in certain spermatozoa, is the determinant of sex.[1] In McClung's view, each animal produces two kinds of spermatozoa in equal proportions, one set of which possesses the accessory chromosome. This has been found to be true of many animals by Edmund B. Wilson, who holds that all unfertilized eggs contain a sex chromosome, and that, after fertilization, those which acquire two by the process produce females, those which remain with one only, males. This has been confirmed by T. H. Morgan, who has shown that in organisms like plant-lice, in which fertilized eggs produce females only, the egg is always fertilized by spermatozoa containing an accessory chromosome, because the other kind cannot live to maturity. Also, twins always have the same sex, as being developed from cells with the same number of accessory chromosomes. Hence, as Loeb says, "it is impossible to influence the sex of a developing embryo by external influences." Morgan's experiments on sex-limited inheritance in Drosophila indicate that the accessory chromosomes are also the transmitters of the hereditary qualities which predominate in each sex. All these experiments tend to do away with the untenable theories of sex determination which have been advanced in the past.

Two features of recent **physiology** may be especially signalized, the doctrine of the hormones and the application of advanced instrumental methods in the study of diseases of the heart. In 1902, William M. Bayliss and Ernest H. Starling announced to the Royal Society that the secretion of pancreatic juice which is caused by introduction of acid into the duodenum is not a local reflex,[2] but is produced by a substance (secretin) thrown out from

---

[1] Biol. Bull., Boston, 1902, iii, 43–84.

[2] This phenomenon had been ascribed by Pavloff and his pupils to an "acid reflex," proceeding by a reflex arc of which the vagus was regarded as the efferent nerve.

the intestinal mucous membrane under the influence of the acid
and carried thence by the blood-stream to the glands, as shown by
experiment. Pavloff's subsequent discovery of enterokinase confirmed the views of Bayliss and Starling and the latter have developed the theory of the chemical control of the body by means of
"hormones" or chemical messengers, which pass from the organs
and glands by the blood channels to other parts of the body. This
theory had already been advanced, *quâ* theory, by Bordeu in the
eighteenth century; the idea was inherent in Darwin's "pangenesis,"
and it has been admirably adapted to explain the many clinical
phenomena produced by disturbances of the ductless glands, and
the general theory of treatment by animal extracts. In 1903,
Charles E. de M. Sajous, a mathematician by training, had already
erected a system of medicine upon the doctrine of the internal
secretions, a *tour de force* based upon pure deduction from a large
number of related facts. The old notion of "diathetic diseases"
is now giving place to the more definite concept of disorders of
metabolism, many (perhaps all) of which are bound up with some
bouleversement of hormonic equilibrium or some disturbance of
function in the ductless glands. Operative surgery has played the
most important part in working out the physiology and pathology
of these glands, a branch of internal medicine which has, indeed,
been almost entirely developed by scientific experimentation.

The starting-point of the doctrine of internal secretions was Claude
Bernard's work on the glycogenic function (1848–57) and Addison's account
of disease of the suprarenal capsules (1849–55). The former was thrown
into striking relief through von Mering and Minkowski's experimental production of diabetes by excision of the pancreas (1889) and the later studies of E. L.
Opie (1901), Ssoboleff (1902), and W. G. MacCallum (1909), showing that the
presumable source of this pancreatic glycosuria is in the islands of Langerhans. Addison's description of the suprarenal syndrome led Brown-Séquard
to excise the adrenals in 1856, reproducing fatal symptoms resembling Addison's disease, and his result was repeatedly confirmed by Tizzoni (1886–89),
Abelous and Langlois (1891–93), Schäfer, and others. In 1894–95, Oliver and
Schäfer found that injection of the watery extract of the suprarenal gland into
the blood produced marked slowing of the heart and rise of blood-pressure. The
active principle was obtained in crystalline form by Jokihi Takamine in 1901.
The description of hyperthyroidism or exophthalmic goiter by Parry
(1786), Graves (1835), and Basedow (1840), and of hypothyroidism or
myxedema by Curling (1850), Gull (1875) and Ord (1877), emphasized the
mysterious importance of the thyroid gland, which was excised with fatal
results (in the dog) by the Geneva physiologist, Moritz Schiff, in 1856.
In 1882, Reverdin of Geneva produced experimental myxedema by total or
partial thyroidectomy and, in 1883, Theodor Kocher of Bern reported that
30 out of 100 thyroidectomies were followed by a "cachexia strumipriva." In
1884, Schiff produced 60 cases of fatal excision in dogs, and pointed out that
the animals could be saved by a previous graft of part of the glands, which led
Murray and Howitz to the treatment of myxedema with thyroid extract,
with wonderfully successful results. Horsley's observations on monkeys and
the collective investigations of Sir Felix Semon showed that cretinism, myxedema and cachexia thyreo-strumipriva are one and the same. The part played
by the internal secretion was first pointed out by Schiff, and the isolation of

iodothyrin by Baumann, in 1896, indicated its relation to iodine metabolism. In
1906, Erwin Payr transplanted a bit of thyroid from a woman to the spleen of
her myxedematous daughter, with successful result. The parathyroid glands
were described by Ivar Sandstrom in 1880 and, in 1891, Eugene Gley showed that
negative thyroidectomies in certain animals would be rendered speedily fatal if
the four parathyroids were also removed. This was confirmed by Vassale and
Generali (1896). Transplantation of the parathyroids was then essayed by
von Eiselsberg (1892), Leischner (1907), and W. S. Halsted (1909), and it
was shown that tetany will be produced if a transplanted gland is removed and
per contra that the tetanic spasms will disappear after injecting the saline extract of the gland or after parathyroid feeding or transplantation. In 1908,
W. G. MacCallum and C. Voegtlin showed that exhibition of calcium salts will
remove tetany, even in man, which seems to connect the parathyroids with
calcium metabolism. The function of the thymus gland was first investigated
by Friedleben (1858), but the effects of its excision or of the injection of its extracts are still obscure. Felix Platter (1614) and Kopp (1830) described early
cases of thymus death in infants. The status lymphaticus was first sketched
out by Richard Bright (1838) and more fully described by Paltauf (1889).
Henderson got retarded atrophy of the gland on castration (1904) and Paton
found that thymectomy increases the growth of the testes. The first experiment
in physiological surgery upon human beings was made by the gynecologist,
Robert Battey, who excised the normal healthy ovaries for the relief of neurotic
and non-menstruating women in 1872. The rationale of this operation, in
relation to a supposed internal secretion from a specialized set of ovarian cells,
has since been justified in many remarkable ways, particularly in osteomalacia
and by the experiments of Starling and Lane-Claypole, which show that section
of the mammary nerves or of the spinal cord in rabbits does not produce the
inhibitory effect of Battey's operation upon pregnancy or lactation. The
relation of the Sertoli cells in the testis to internal secretion is *sub judice*, the
most significant experiments so far being those of Brown-Séquard (1889–91)
and Poehl (1896–97) upon the injection of testicular extracts. In the last
twenty years, much attention has been paid the pituitary body. Fatal excisions
of the gland in animals had been made by Marinesco (1892), Vassale and
Secchi (1894), and others, but Nicholas Paulesco of Bucharest was the first
to point out that removal of the anterior lobe is fatal and removal of the posterior lobe negative (1908). Meanwhile Mohr had described obesity with
pituitary tumor (1840), Pierre Marie had shown the relation of the pituitary to
acromegaly and gigantism (1886), Fröhlich described pituitary tumor with
obesity and sexual infantilism (1901), and Harvey Cushing and his associates at
the Johns Hopkins Hospital actually produced an experimental pathological re-
version to the Fröhlich syndrome by partial excision of the anterior lobe in adult
dogs (1908). Cushing has shown that the anterior lobe secretion influences
normal growth and sexual development, while the posterior lobe has to do with
metabolism of carbohydrates and fats, the high tolerance of sugars in posterior
lobe insufficiency yielding to treatment with pituitary extract. Cushing and his
pupils have also shown the relation of the hypophysis to diabetes (1912) and
hibernation (1913). These experiments upon the ductless glands indicate the
important part they play in regulating the chemical equilibrium of the body.

The doctrine of the correlation of the different internal secretions has been especially emphasized by the Viennese clinicians,
Hans Eppinger, W. Falta, and C. Rüdinger (1908–9). Eppinger
and Leo Hess[1] have also applied the ideas of Gaskell, Langley and
Sherrington as to the opposing functions of the two "autonomics"
of the sympathetic system in the elucidation of the complex
mechanism of physiological equilibrium, and of visceral neurology

---

[1] Eppinger and Hess: Die Vagotonie, Berlin, 1910.

(1910). They postulate two opposing diathetic conditions, vagotonus and sympathicotonus, the semeiology of which can be thrown into relief by certain pharmacodynamic tests. These have been likened to "tuning keys by means of which we can operate upon the complicated stringed instrument of the body, and voluntarily make one string tighter to increase its vibrations, or another looser to dampen its function."[1] Eppinger and Hess also assume that the pancreas secretes a hormone, "autonomin," which antagonizes adrenaline, the hormone governing the sympathetic autonomic. While much of this is in dispute, it seems probable that the chemical hormones act *viâ* the blood upon the central nervous system, while the two opposing autonomics of the sympathetic system control the ductless glands and the visceral organs made up of smooth (involuntary) muscle.

The trend of recent thinking in regard to the heart's action is overwhelmingly in favor of the myogenic theory of Gaskell and Engelmann, which received its strongest support from embryology.

In 1893, Wilhelm His, Jr. (1863–   ), and, a little earlier, Stanley Kent (1892), discovered a narrow band of muscle, an embryonic rest between the auricles and ventricles, now called the auriculo-ventricular bundle of His, which acts as a bridge for contractile impulses, in accordance with Gaskell's theory that this cardiac phenomenon is due to the inherent contractility of its muscles alone. Later, Arthur Keith and Flack (1907) discovered a tissue-rest of fine, pale, faintly striated fibers in the heart wall, supplied with arterioles and connected with the Purkinje fibers and nerve terminals, the so-called Keith-Flack or sino-auricular node, now dubbed "the pacemaker of the heart." S. Tawara traced out the muscular ramifications from the His bundle and discovered another muscular (atrioventricular) node in close relation to it (1908). If the His bundle is destroyed in the dog, the contractile impulse will no longer pass from the auricle to the ventricles, and the latter will immediately assume their own autonomy, beating at a much slower rate, while the auricles, controlled by the vagus, will go on as before. This is the condition known in pathology as complete heart block or Stokes-Adams disease, which His produced experimentally in 1895. At the Johns Hopkins Hospital, Erlanger, by means of a clamp compressing the His bundle, in the dog, thus blocking the auricular impulse, has been able to produce two-time, three-time and four-time rhythms, finally passing into complete heart block. Further light upon the intimate pathology of cardiac disturbance was thrown by the string galvanometer invented by Willem Einthoven of Leyden in 1903.[2] In 1889,[3] Augustus D. Waller conceived the idea of measuring and figuring the variation of the action currents in the living heart by leading them off through electrodes placed upon the moist skin, connected with a galvanometer, the curves being obtained by photographing the movements produced by the mercury of a Lippmann electrometer. Owing to the lag or inertia of the mercury meniscus, the curves in Waller's method were not true curves and had to be corrected by mathematical computations. The process was rendered accurate by the sensitive instrument of Einthoven, which consists essentially of an extremely delicate thread of platinum or of quartz coated with silver, which is strung, like a violin-string, midway between the poles

---

[1] Januschke: Cited by L. F. Barker.

[2] Einthoven: K. Akad. v. Wetensch. te Amst. Proc. Sect. Sc., 1903–04, vi, 107–115, 2 pl.

[3] A. D. Waller: Phil. Tr., 1889, London, 1890, clxxx, B, 169–194.

HISTORY OF MEDICINE

of a stationary electromagnet. This reverses the ordinary conditions in galvanometers, in which the magnet is movable and the measurable current passes through stationary coils. When the feeble heart currents pass through the delicate string, they cause deflections which are smaller and shorter, or greater and longer, in proportion to its state of tension. The pictures of cardiac excitation which are thrown off in this way Einthoven calls "electrocardiograms," or telegrams from the heart, in that they give an accurate bulletin of its electromotive condition. Although his instrument is expensive, it has been of material assistance in analyzing and even diagnosing such conditions as valvular disease, heart block, auricular fibrillation, paroxysmal tachycardia, pulsus alternans, pulsus bigeminus, three- and four-time gallops and other rhythmic changes. The pioneer in the graphic study of cardiac disease was the Scotch practitioner, James Mackenzie, who first made simultaneous records of the arterial and venous pulses to elucidate the clinical condition of the heart; and by raising the question, "How much work can the heart do?" concentrated future investigation upon the energetics of heart-muscle (1893–4). Mackenzie first investigated the multiform arrhythmias, and differentiated the "nodal rhythm," which James Lewis afterward defined as "auricular fibrillation" and identified with the "pulsus irregularis perpetuus" of Hering, producing the condition experimentally by sewing electrodes into the auricle of an animal. Mackenzie also demonstrated the wonderful efficiency of digitalis in auricular fibrillation (1910), and the use of this drug is now interdicted in the sinus arrhythmias, heart-block, paroxysmal tachycardia and pulsus alternans. Cushny showed the value of the electrocardiogram in checking up the effects of digitalis, which apparently depresses the conductivity of the bundle of His. Thus the view of Schmiedeberg, that digitalis not only slows the heart by vagal stimulation, but stimulates the cardiac muscle (1874), has given place to the older, classical view of Bouillaud, that, clinically, digitalis is a true "opium of the heart" (1835). Many other investigations have been made, and the new English periodical, *Heart* (London, 19), has been founded for such studies. In 1906, Einthoven laid wires between the Leyden Hospital and his laboratory and was able to take cardiac tracings from ward patients at a distance of more than a mile. Further, it has been found possible to obtain graphic figurations of the rhythm of the heart sound (phonocardiograms) by means of a stethoscope and a Marey tambour, the receiver being a microphone or such devices as manometric flames, or the Weiss phonoscope, the receiver of which is a soap-bubble. These records can be placed in juxtaposition with curves of the carotid pulse for comparison. The electrical telephone-stethoscope of S. G. Brown intensifies the heart sounds 60 times and by connecting this with the long-distance service, heart sounds in London have been heard distinctly by physicians in the Isle of Wight, a distance of about 100 miles.[1]

The problem of the **synthesis of proteins** from their amino-acid constituents will always be associated with the great name of **Emil Fischer** (1852–   ), of Euskirchen, Rhenish Prussia, who, as professor of chemistry at Munich (1879), Erlangen (1882), Würzburg (1885), and Berlin (1892), has devoted his whole career to this work. Fischer has discovered, isolated and formulated a host of new substances, such as phenylhydrazin (1875), the aliphatic hydrazins (1875–77), mannose, isomaltose, and the drugs veronal (1902), proponal (1905), saiodin (1905), elarson (1913). He has made vast researches in the synthesis of the purin compounds, including caffein, xanthin, theobromine (1879–95); and has developed a

---

[1] For a full account of these instruments, with illustrations, see the admirable résumé by Professor L. F. Barker, Johns Hopkins Hosp. Bull., Baltimore, 1910, xxi, 358–389.

"family tree" of gout, demonstrating the purin nucleus as a sort of germ-plasm common to all the metabolic products of the disease. He has synthetized most of the sugar groups (1883–94), including the six hexoses derived from mannitol and fourteen out of the sixteen possible isomeric aldohexoses predicted by van't Hoff and Le-Bel; and, in his studies of the polypeptides (1899–1906),[1] he has linked together great chains of amino-acid substances to form these compounds, which are essential parts of the different protein molecules. Liebig believed that there is only one aboriginal protein. Paul Schützenberger and other recent chemists have shown that individual proteins differ from each other in respect of the various amino-acids produced by hydrolysis. Fischer has devised quantitative methods for isolating these, and he has shown that there is an amido group or nucleus common to all the proteins. His investigations of the enzymes (1894) show that they are specific in action, affecting only certain chemical substances, to which, as he puts it, they are related as a key to a lock or a glove to a hand, an analogy which Ehrlich has cleverly applied in his side-chain theory. A brilliant stroke of genius was

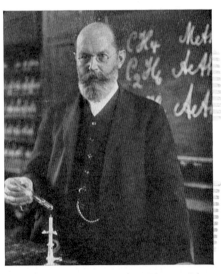

Emil Fischer (1852–   ). (From a photograph in the Surgeon General's Library.)

Fischer's deliberate attempt to produce a reliable hypnotic, ending in the synthesis of veronal (1904).[2] No chemist of modern times has better deserved the honor of the Nobel prize, which he received in 1902.

Emil **Abderhalden** (1877–   ), of St. Gall, Switzerland, a pupil of Emil Fischer, professor of physiology at Halle, is the author of a bibliography of alcoholism (1897) and a text-book of physiological chemistry (1908), and is the editor of a hand-book of biochemical technic (1909–10), to which he has added many

[1] Fischer: Untersuchungen über Aminosäuren, Polypeptide und Proteine, Berlin, 1906.

[2] Therap. d. Gegenwart, Berlin, 1904, xlv, 145.

new procedures. He has made a vast number of investigations of metabolism and food-stuffs, adopting Carl Ludwig's method of publishing his researches in collaboration with his many pupils. His special field is the integration and disintegration of albuminoids and nucleic acids in the animal body, the metabolism of the cell (1911), the synthesis of its *Bausteine* (1912), and the synthesis of artificial food-stuffs, as tried out experimentally upon animals. He holds that the individual cells of animal and vegetable foods are made up of a number of chemical or phasic units which, in digestion and metabolism, are split up and transformed into other substances, to be assimilated by the body cells, according to their needs. In his attempt to synthetize an artificial food, he has shown that dogs can be successfully fed upon the amino-acid constituents of albumen, that tryptophan is essential to nutrition, but glycocoll is not, that grape-sugar can be substituted for complex carbohydrates, that glycerin and fatty acids can take the place of fats, and that nucleic acids can be replaced by their split products (nucleosides, etc.). Abderhalden has recently taken up the study of the protective ferments of the animal body and has already evolved a biochemical test for pregnancy and other conditions by a ferment reaction (1912).[1]

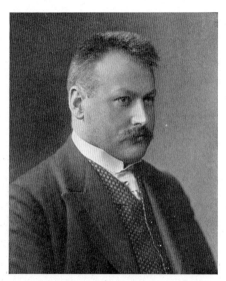

Emil Abderhalden (1877–   ).

In America Thomas B. Osborne and Lafayette B. Mendel have also done important experimental work on artificial or synthetic foods (1911).

Of late years, there has been an amazing increase in the literature of **psychology,** normal, morbid and comparative, including such related subjects as pedagogics, psychoanalysis, psychotherapy, epistemology, the scientific aspects of evidence and the relation of everyday thinking to border-line insanity. Comparative psychology turns mainly upon Loeb's theory of tropisms in the

---

[1] Ztschr. f. physiol. Chem., Strassburg, 1912, lxxvii, 249; lxxxi, 90.

lower forms (or the views of those who, like H. S. Jennings, oppose it), and the study of "behavior" in the higher animals. The mental development of the newborn infant has been specially studied by Kussmaul and Preyer. Pedagogics and juvenile psychology have been treated by Binet, Claparède, Stanley Hall, Seguin Maria Montessori, and others. Among the leaders in morbid psychology is Pierre **Janet** (1859–   ), professor at the Collège de France, who developed the theory of psychologic automatism (1889), the relations between neuroses and fixed ideas (1898)[1] described psychasthenia (1903), and made extensive investigations of the mental status of hysteric patients (1903–08). In 1905–8, Alfred **Binet** (1857–1911) and Th. Simon introduced a remarkable eries of graded tests for mental retardation by which it is pos- sible to localize the developmental status of a patient's mind in re- lation to his age and the growth of his body, thus enabling school- teachers or school inspectors to segregate defective or "unusual" children. Another characteristic development is the exhaustive or intensive study of sexual psychology, with which modern writers, from scientific students like Krafft-Ebing and Havelock Ellis, down to insane men of letters like Nietzsche and Weininger, have been vastly preoccupied. The atmosphere of the present time, its art, poetry, fiction, and drama, is saturated with sexualism. Poets like Goethe, Swinburne, and Walt Whitman did much to dispel the ancient theological nightmare of the sinfulness of normal sexuality in men and women, and were forerunners of the scientific view that the instinct, guided by proper ethical restrictions, is an all-im- portant part in normal human development which has to be either recognized or reckoned with. Schopenhauer wrote on the subject with bitter and unsparing realism, and latterly women of such high repute as Rahel Varnhagen, Ellen Key, and Helen Putnam have considered the matter from a higher viewpoint, on account of its importance in connection with such problems as the proper hygiene and well-being of growing children, the growth of prostitution and commercialized vice, the social enslavement of women in crowded communities, and other degradations of a purely indus- trial age. In Germany, several periodicals are devoted to the sexual instinct alone, and the problem of biological teaching of school-children in these matters is under consideration. On the pathological side, there is the question of sexual perversion and the crimes resulting from it, for which, in young, healthy frontier communities like the United States, no special provisions had been necessary in criminal procedure until the crowded conditions of

---

[1] Année psychol., Paris, 1905–08, *passim*.

modern cities brought the unsavory subject to the surface.[1] The part played by suppressed or repressed sexuality in the development of neurotic conditions has been especially studied by Sigmund **Freud** (1856–   ), of Freiberg in Moravia, a pupil of Charcot, and professor of neurology at Vienna. Charcot, as we have seen, threw the sexual theory of hysteria into disrepute, but Janet, from 1889 on, emphasized the view that the disease is primarily of emotional causation, and, advancing from this viewpoint, Breuer and Freud have explained the mechanism of its development as the result of a psychic traumatism or nervous shock, usually of sexual nature, in the first instance, leading to morbid brooding and a kind of mental involution. The basic idea of Freud's theory is that a large number of even ordinary mental processes come from hidden sources, unknown or unsuspected by the individual. In this way he has interpreted the significance of dreams (*Traumdeutung*), witticisms, infantile amnesia and auto-erotism, unconscious memories, absent-minded actions, anxiety-neuroses, and other aspects of the "psychopathology of everyday life." He believes that there is a rigid determinism of psychical effects and that many complex mental processes never attain to consciousness and can only be elicited by a long process of "psychoanalysis," the technic of which was largely developed by his pupil, C. G. Jung. Freud's first successful case, that of the patient "Dora," was of this kind, and the correctness of his reasoning seems borne out by the successful treatment of hysteria through the disburdening of the mind or other appropriate psychotherapy. Some phases of Freud's teaching, such as the "Œdipus myth," are based upon formal literary analogies, and the long-winded exaggerations or distortions of his doctrine by some of his disciples are surely not scientific. But he has given neurologists a new instrument for exploring subconscious states which, in competent and temperate hands, may be effective. In America, his ideas have been followed by J. J. Putnam, A. A. Brill, W. A. White, and others, and such variants as Bleuler's theory of normal "autistic thinking" go to show the very thin partitions which sometimes divide sanity from insanity.

Parasitology and Chemotherapy.—In the last decade of the nineteenth century, as a result of the many improvements in microscopic and bacteriological technic, physicians began to study

---

[1] J. L. Caspar, in his Practical Handbook of Legal Medicine (1856), regarded these crimes as among the "strange bubbles which sometimes rise from the low life of towns." Their modern study is due to Krafft-Ebing (1886) and to Leopold von Meerscheidt-Hüllesem, chief of police at Berlin, who showed the necessity of the segregation and surveillance, under humane restrictions, of perverted individuals in large cities, if only on account of blackmail and the homicidal tendencies which these characters are known to develop.

the animal and vegetable, and particularly the protozoan, parasites as causes of disease, but the greatest triumphs in this field belong to the twentieth century.

Before this time, Bassi had found the pathogenic organism of silkworm disease, or muscardine (1837), Schönlein, the achorion of favus (1839), Donné, the Trichomonas vaginalis (1837), Johannes Müller, the psorosperms (1841), David Grüby, the Trypanosoma sanguinis in frogs (1843), Davaine, the Cercomonas hominis (1857), Malmsten, the Balantidium coli (1857), Lambl, the Lamblia intestinalis (1859). The first group of parasitic diseases to be investigated was that of the protozoan dysenteries, the amœbæ of which had been seen by Lambl in 1860, by Lewis in 1870, and by Loesch (1875), who made drawings of both the innocuous and pathogenic forms, with the latter of which he was able to infect dogs. Koch and Kartulis, in Egypt, differentiated between endemic dysentery due to amœbæ, and epidemic, due to bacteria. The term amebic dysentery was introduced by W. T. Councilman and H. A. Lafleur at the Johns Hopkins Hospital in 1891, two types of parasites being recognized, the harmless Amœba coli, and the pathogenic Amœba dysenteriæ. These views were confirmed by Casagrandi and Barbagallo (1897), and particularly by Fritz Schaudinn, who styled the harmless form Entamœba coli and the pathogenic form Entamœba histolytica (1903). These species were first confirmed by Craig, who afterward found Viereck's pathogenic Entamœba tetragena in the Philippines and discovered a new species of diarrheal parasite, Craigia (Paramœba) hominis (1906), which Calkins regards as a new genus. Other pathogenic species of amebæ have been described by various observers, and diarrheal and dysenteric infections have also been found to be associated with Laverania, Leishmania, Balantidium coli, and the above-mentioned flagellate forms, Cercomonas, Trichomonas, and Lamblia. Meanwhile the question of bacillary dysentery had been settled by the discovery of bacilli by Shiga in Japan (1898), Kruse in Germany (1900), and Flexner at Manila (1900). The pathogenic strain usually found in America is known as the Flexner-Harris type.

The symptoms of hook-worm infection were vaguely outlined in the Egyptian papyri, and for centuries the disease was variously known as Egyptian or tropical chlorosis, miner's or bricklayer's anemia and St. Gothard tunnel disease. The parasite was described as Anchylostoma duodenale by Angelo Dubini (1843), and its causal relation to the disease was pointed out by Wilhelm Griesinger (1866). In 1900, Captain Bailey K. Ashford, U. S. Army, discovered the great prevalence of the disease in Porto Rico, and it was soon found to be very common among the rural population of the Southern States (U. S.) by Charles Wardell Stiles (1867–   ), of Spring Valley, New York, who discovered that the parasite of the American infections is a new species, which he called Uncinaria americana (1902) and later Necator americanus. Stiles, who had already made his reputation in parasitology by his work on revision of species and nomenclature and his contributions to descriptive zoology, has since devoted himself, as professor of zoölogy in the U. S. Public Health and Marine-Hospital Service, to the task of exterminating the disease in the South, in connection with the Rockefeller Commission established for this purpose in October, 1909. Under the able and tactful guidance of its administrative secretary, Mr. Wickliffe Rose, this Commission, in the face of much opposition at the start, has succeeded in awakening the South, through its newspapers, boards of health, schools and medical men, to looking after its own interest in the matter, so that open-air clinics at stated intervals are now widely attended. In three years (1910–12), no less than 393,566 persons have been treated for hook-worm in the Southern States. In 1898, Arthur Looss made the important discovery that the hook-worm larva can penetrate the skin, reaching the intestines by a devious route, and this fact has enabled Stiles and Ashford to devise effective means of prophylaxis among rural populations. In Ashford's campaign against the disease in Porto Rico (1903–04), some 300,000 out of a population of a million have been treated, with a reduction of 90 per cent. in the mortality from anemia. Pellagra, another disease which has latterly been identified in America, has been closely studied by

Marie, Sambon and others in Europe, and by Ames W. Babcock, Claude H. Lavinder and other southern physicians in the United States. Its cause is still unknown, some regarding it as due to a parasite transmitted by the Simulium fly, others as a food-intoxication, like ergotism or beri-beri, others as due to the action of photodynamic substances. Pellagra has recently appeared in England.

In 1911, Laveran's malarial parasite was obtained in pure cultures *in vitro* by Charles C. Bass, of New Orleans.

The trypanosomes discovered by David Grüby (1809–98) in the frog (1843) and by Lewis in the rat (1878) were non-pathogenic, but a new interest in these organisms was awakened when Griffith Evans, in 1880, discovered in India that surra, a disease of horses, mules, camels and cattle, is caused by a variety which was afterward named by Steel and Crookshank, Trypanosoma evansi (1885–86). In 1894, Sir David Bruce (1855–   ) found that the tsetse fly disease or nagana of Zululand is due to the Trypanosoma brucei (Plimmer and Bradford, 1899), which he proved experimentally to be conveyed from the blood of big game animals to cattle and horses by this fly (*Glossina morsitans*). In the same year (1894), Rouget discovered T. equiperdum (Doflein, 1901) as the cause of dourine or mal du coït in horses; in 1901 Elmassian found T. equinum (Vosges, 1902) as the cause of mal de caderas in South American dogs and horses; Theiler, in 1902, found T. theilieri (Bruce, 1902) in the bovine gall-sickness or galziekte of South Africa and T. dimorphon (Laveran and Mesnil, 1904) was found to be the cause of another animal disease in equatorial Africa by Dutton and Todd in 1904. The most important find, however, was that of T. gambiense in the blood of man by J. Everett Dutton in 1901, which was afterward seen by Aldo Castellani in the cerebrospinal fluid and blood of five cases of African sleeping sickness (1903). It was then shown by Bruce and Nabarro, of the Royal Society Commission, that the tsetse fly is the vector of the disease, and that Gambia fever, the disease first seen by Dutton and Todd in 1902, and sleeping sickness are two stages of the same infection. A Brazilian variety of human trypanosomiasis, due to T. cruzi and transmitted by a bug (*Conorhinus sanguisuga*), was described by Carlo Chagas in 1909. Another remarkable organism was found in 1900 by Sir William Boog Leishman (1865–   ) in a postmortem film from a case of fever at Dum Dum, near Calcutta, and afterward described by him, in May, 1903, as possibly a trypanosome. In July, 1903, Major C. Donovan found the same bodies in blood taken in life from splenic punctures. In July, 1904, Leonard Rogers announced the development of these parasites into flagellates and, in 1906–07, Walter Scott Patton described their development into flagellates in the bedbug. All these discoveries have associated the Leishman-Donovan bodies with the tropical splenomegaly, dumdum fever or kala-azar. In 1903, James Homer Wright found similar parasites (Leishmania tropica) in Oriental endemic ulcers and in 1908 Charles Nicolle found Leishmania infantum in infantile kala-azar. In 1888, Victor Babes (1854–   ), a Roumanian physician, discovered a small protozoön in the blood of sheep suffering from an epizoötic disease called "carceag," and the genus was called in his honor Babesia by Starcovici (1893), the term Piroplasma having been proposed by Patton in 1895. A similar parasite was claimed by Babes as the cause of hemoglobinuric fever of European cattle and in the same year Theobald Smith (1859–   ) found the organism "Pyrosoma bigeminum" in Texas fever, which, with F. L. Kilborne, he demonstrated to be transmitted by the tick. This was the first demonstration, after Manson's, of the transmission of infection by a blood-sucking insect, and after this time knowledge of the different piroplasmoses or babesioses grew apace, the best known being the canine form (Piroplasma or Babesia canis, Piana and Galli Valerio, 1895), the life cycle of which has been carefully traced by G. H. F. Nuttall and Graham Smith. The so-called Piroplasma hominis, assumed to be the cause of spotted fever of the Rocky Mountains, was shown by Craig to be an artefact in the erythrocytes (1904). In like manner, the bodies found in the central nervous system in hydrophobia by Adelchi Negri (1876–1912) are still *sub judice*. Cytoryctes variolæ, a protozoön found in the skin lesions of smallpox, was described by Giuseppe Guarnieri (1894) and its life history was traced by Gary N. Calkins (1904), while similar bodies were found in variola by W. T. Councilman and others in 1903 and by Mallory in scarlatina in 1904. Histoplasma capsulatum found in a tropical splenomegaly on the Isthmus of Panama by S. T. Darling in, 1906 is said to be a yeast. The spirochæte or spirillum of relapsing fever, discovered by one of Virchow's assistants, Otto Obermeier (1843–73) in 1873, was to open out the most important phase of parasitic diseases yet known, viz., the conquest of syphilis by Schaudinn, Wassermann and Ehrlich. In 1904, the spirochete of African relapsing fever (tick fever) was discovered independently by Nabarro, Ross and Milne in Uganda and by Dutton and Todd in the Congo and was called Spirochæte duttoni, in honor of Dutton, who died from the disease, after he had proved its transmission by a tick (Ornithorodoros moubata). The spirochete of the American variety of relapsing fever was discovered by Frederick G. Novy in 1907.

The most telling advances in **protozoölogy** and the most striking applications of this science to medicine were made by Fritz Schaudinn (1871–1906), the son of an East Prussian inn-keeper, who took his doctor's degree in zoology in Berlin in 1894, and, after some studies of the Foraminifera, devoted the rest of his life to the Protozoa. As a descriptive zoölogist, he isolated many new species, such as Amœba binucleata (1895), Paramœba eilhardi (1896), Eimeria schubergia (1900), and Cyclospora caryolitica, the cause of pernicious enteritis in the hedgehog (1902), but his most important work was in the development of the life cycles of different protozoa as distinctive or differential criteria of species, and the bearings of the same upon disease.

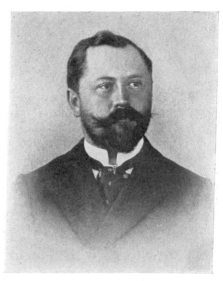

Fritz Schaudinn (1871–1906).

In his classical researches on the Coccidia (1897) and Eimeria (1900), he showed a sexual fusion of differentiated gametes, not unlike the union of spermatozoön and ovum, and his work gradually overthrew the notion that the protozoa are "immortal" through any simple process of asexual cell-division. In establishing the difference between the harmless Entamœba coli of Lösch and the pathogenic Entamœba histolytica (1903), he showed that, in the former, over and above asexual multiplication, the nucleus sometimes divides into two daughter nuclei, which undergo chromatin reductions and eventually fuse and fertilize each other; in the latter, he thought that reproduction is accomplished by fission, gemmation or formation of spores with nuclei derived from the parental chromidia, but this has recently been shown to be erroneous, in that E. histolytica is now known to reproduce itself by the formation of cysts containing four daughter nuclei. In his work on two new species of bacteria, B. bütschlii and B. sporonema, Schaudinn demonstrated that there is a similar autogamy of spores in the former and spore formation in the latter, when the possibilities of transverse fission have become exhausted. Thus it became clear that, even in plant organisms like the bacteria, a species may wear itself out and become extinct unless rejuvenated and reinvigorated by sexual conjugation, a view which has been strikingly confirmed for protozoa for such observers as Gary N. Calkins (1869–   ), who has carried Paramecium through several hundred generations by this means (1902). In investigating the alternation of generations and of hosts in Halteridium noctuæ and Trypanosoma noctuæ, Schaudinn showed that the former, which is parasitic in the red blood-corpuscles, and the latter, a parasite of the plasma, are really phases of a single life-cycle, the sexual period of which occurs in the mosquito. This has led many observers to believe that the Hæmosporidia and the Trypanosomata are members of a single order of flagellates. In addition to his work on amebic dysentery, which he carried out experimentally upon animals, Schaudinn confirmed the work of Ross and Grassi upon the malarial parasite, identifying Plasmodium vivax (Grassi and Feletti) as the cause of tertian fever (1902) and also confirmed Looss's demonstration of hook-worm infection through the skin (1904).

In May, 1905, working with Erich Hoffmann, Schaudinn crowned his life-work by the discovery of the Spirochæta pallida of syphilis,[1] and in a valuable paper of his own (October, 1905),[2] he described the morphology of the spirochetes, that of syphilis justifying the establishment of a new genus, Spironema or Treponema. Schaudinn's discovery of this almost invisible parasite was due to his incomparable skill in technic and staining methods and the causal relation was rapidly established by thousands of confirmatory observations made by enthusiastic microscopists all over the world. Schaudinn was Privatdocent at Berlin (1898) and director of protozoölogy in the Kaiserliches Gesundheitsamt (1904) and the Institut für Schiffs- und Tropenhygiene at Hamburg (1906). In 1903 he founded the Archiv für Protistenkunde, the literary organ of protozoölogy, which he had found in the descriptive stage and left an experimental science.

The first steps in the conquest of syphilis had thus been made by professional zoölogists, Metchnikoff and Schaudinn. The next advances were made by an investigator who, although educated as a physician, has practically worked out his results as a chemist and pharmacologist.

Paul **Ehrlich** (1854–   ), of Strehlen, Silesia, was a clinical assistant of Frerichs (1878–85) and Gerhardt (1885–89), Privatdocent (1889) and professor (1890) at Berlin, where he became an assistant in Koch's Institute. In 1896 he was entrusted with the directorship of the newly founded Institut für Serumforschung at

---

[1] Arb. a. d. k. Gesundheitsamte, Berlin, 1905, xxii, 527–534.

[2] Deutsche med. Wochenschr, Leipzig u. Berlin, 1905, xxxi, 1665–1667.

Steglitz, which was transferred, under his direction, to the *Institut für experimentelle Therapie* at Frankfort on the Main (1899).

At Breslau, Ehrlich was but an indifferent student, occupying his time mainly with experiments on dye-stuffs and tissue staining, but the results of his labors soon appeared in his improved methods of drying and fixing blood smears by heat, his triacid stain, his detection of the granulations in mast cells by basic aniline staining (1877), his division of the white blood-corpuscles into neutrophilic, basophilic and oxyphilic, his fuchsin stain for tubercle bacilli, based upon the discovery that they are acid-fast (1882), his diazo-reaction of the urine, used in the diagnosis of typhoid fever (1882),[1] his method of intravital staining (1886),[2] in all of which he has been a great pioneer in merging descriptive cellular pathology into experimental cellular chemistry. This is particularly the case in his study of the oxygen requirements of the organism (1885), in which he applies the idea of a selective affinity between chemical substances and body tissues to protoplasmic chemistry and first outlines his "side-chain theory." This theory was suggested by August Kekulé's hypothesis of the closed benzene ring (1865), in which the six carbon atoms of this compound (C_6H_6) are assumed to form a stable hexagonal nucleus among themselves, while their fourth affinities are linked with unstable "side-chains" of easily replaceable hydrogen. Hoppe-Seyler had assumed that the emission and absorption of light in chlorophyll are accomplished not by the entire molecule itself but by certain specialized groups of peripheral atoms. In like manner, Ehrlich assumed that the living protoplasmic molecule consists of a stable nucleus and unstable peripheral side-chains or chemo-receptors, which enable it to combine chemically with food substances and neutralize toxins or other poisons by throwing out detached side-chains into the blood. In spite of the enormous amount of criticism which has

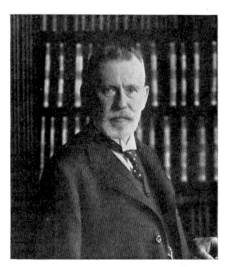

Paul Ehrlich (1854–). (Courtesy of Captain Henry J. Nichols, United States Army.)

been heaped upon this theory and its author, it may safely be affirmed that, as based upon a fundamental postulate in organic chemistry, it has proved to be a valuable "heuristic principle" in developing the science of immunity and serum reactions. Thus, August **von Wassermann** (1866–) did not hesitate to affirm that without it he could never have hit upon the special and extremely reliable hemolytic diagnosis of syphilis with which his name is associated and which was discovered one year after Schaudinn had found the parasite of the disease (1906).[3] Although the original Wassermann reaction has been much simplified by such ingenious modifications as those of Hideyo Noguchi (1909),[4]

---

[1] Ztschr. f. klin. Med., Berlin, 1882, v, 285–288.

[2] Deutsche med. Wchnschr., Leipzig u. Berlin, 1886, xii, 49–52.

[3] Deutsche med. Wchnschr., Leipzig u. Berlin, 1906, xxxii, 745.

[4] Noguchi: Jour. Exper. Med., New York, 1909, xi, 392–401.

particularly his "luetin" reaction, based upon pure cultures of the Treponema (1911),[1] yet it is plain that no such advances could have been made upon a purely physical or mechanical hypothesis. From the discoveries of Schaudinn and Wassermann, it became known that such immunes as come under Colles' and Profeta's law have the syphilitic spirochetes in their blood, whence Ehrlich reasoned that protozoan diseases cannot be treated by special antitoxins, but must be handled by drugs which can at once sterilize the patient's body of the parasites without injuring the body tissues. In attempting to treat trypanosomiasis in mice with certain specific dyes, he found that if the doses were too small to completely sterilize the animal of the parasite, a race of trypanosomes could be bred which proved permanently "fast" or resistant to the effects of the drug. This power of parasites to immunize themselves and their descendants against the action of drugs was the *Leitmotif* of the long series of "trial and error" experiments to find a *therapia sterilisans* against syphilis, and it proved to be the weak point in their final result, "606," or salvarsan. This drug, which was first tried out by Ehrlich's Japanese assistant, S. Hata (1910), and has since been tested in thousands of cases, is, in itself, as reliable a specific as quinine in malarial infection, and is moreover a valuable prophylactic, in that it rapidly cleans up the ugly luetic sores and eruptions and sterilizes the blood, thus minimizing the possibility of infecting others. But the fact that it does not appear to reach some of the spirochetes, which, like the gonococcus, burrow into the deep tissues, is responsible for disconcerting relapses, while "606" itself sometimes causes severe collateral effects upon the eye or the nervous system. The merits of "neo-salvarsan" ("914" in Ehrlich's experimental series) are now on trial, but it is hardly likely that any drug will prove a complete sterilizer under the above conditions. Salvarsan is said, however, to be an ideal *therapia sterilisans* in the case of Treponema pertenue, the parasite of yaws. Of the other features of Ehrlich's scientific work, his introduction of such remedies as methylene-blue for quartan fever, trypan red for bovine piroplasmosis, arsenophenylglycin for the trypanosomiases; his proof that animals can be quantitatively immunized against vegetable poisons like abrin and ricin; his improvement of Behring's diphtheria antitoxin and his establishment of an international standard of purity for the same; his demonstration that cancer can be changed into sarcoma in animals by successive inoculations, and that the growth of cancer depends upon the presence of certain food substances in the body; his vast researches in the whole field of serology and immunity, can only be mentioned.

In his skill in improvising hypotheses to meet the opponents of his theories, Ehrlich resembles Galen. In his predilection for quaint and archaic Latin phrases, he is like Paracelsus. But he has done the most effective work since Pasteur and Koch in the science of infectious diseases, and he has added new territory to the domain of experimental pharmacology and therapeutics by his genius for research and his wonderful industry.

Jules **Bordet,** Director of the Institut Pasteur de Brabant (Brussels), has been a great pioneer in the theory of serology and immunity reactions, for the phenomena of which he gives a simple and purely physical explanation. He discovered bacterial hemolysis (1898),[2] and, with Octave Gengou, fixation of the complement (1900–1901),[3] and, with the latter, he also discovered

[1] Jour. Exper. Med., N. Y., 1911, xiv, 557–568, 3 pl.

[2] Ann. de l'Inst. Pasteur, Paris, 1898, xii, 688: 1899, xiii, 273.

[3] *Ibid.*, 1900, xiv, 257: 1901, xv, 289: 1902, xvi, 734. Deviation of the complement was discovered by A. Neisser and Weichsberg (München. med. Wochenschr., 1901).

the specific bacillus of whooping-cough (1906),[1] the causal relation of which has recently been demonstrated, according to Koch's postulates, by F. B. Mallory and others (1913).[2] As compared with Ehrlich's complex terminology, Bordet's theory of serum reactions is simplicity itself. He assumes that the toxin is neutralized by an antitoxin through absorption, comparable with that shown by a fabric in taking up dyes. Complete neutralization would be like complete saturation of the fabric with the dye-stuff, but if the toxin be added in divided doses, the last portion of the toxin could not be absorbed, because its first portions have become supersaturated with the antitoxins and can take up no more of them. Similarly, he assumes a *substance sensibilisatrice* in antitoxic sera which sensitizes the red blood-corpuscles for bacteria to the action of the alexins, as a mordant does for a dye-stuff. The disputes between Bordet and Ehrlich turn upon the simple fact that the former explains what he has seen in terms of physics, the latter in terms of structural chemistry.

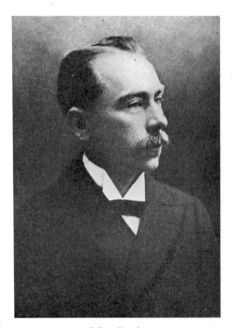

Jules Bordet.

Apart from the work of Metchnikoff, Bordet and Ehrlich, there have been many advances in **serology** of great practical value, notably the discovery of agglutination and its application to the diagnosis of typhoid fever (1896) by Ferdinand Widal (1862–) and A. Sicard; the diagnostic use of tuberculin by the conjunctival reactions of Albert Calmette (1907) and Alfred Wolff-Eisner (1907), and the cutaneous reactions of Clemens von Pirquet (1907) and Ernst Moro (1908); Sir Almroth E. Wright's preventive inoculation against typhoid fever by dead cultures of the bacillus, with the opsonic index as a guide (1900); the cobra venom reaction in insanity (Much-Holtzmann, 1909); the discovery that water can be sterilized by ultraviolet rays by Victor Henri, André Heilbronner and Max Recklinghausen (1910); Emil Abderhalden's enzyme reaction in the diagnosis of pregnancy (1912); and the theory of filterable viruses. Many new modes of treatment with bacteria

---

[1] Ann. de l'Inst. Pasteur, Paris, 1906, xx, 731, 1 pl.: 1907, xxi, 720.

[2] Mallory, Horner and Henderson: Jour. Med. Research, Boston, 1913, xxvii, 391–397, 2 pl.

or bacterial products abound, such as Besredka's sensitized vaccines, Carl Spengler's employment of the bovine type of tubercle bacillus, and the use of bacilli attenuated in the cold-blooded animals against tuberculosis (Klebs, Friedmann), all of which are now on trial.

The theory of filterable viruses as a cause of disease was first put upon a definite basis through the discovery of Friedrich Löffler and Paul Frosch that the inoculable virus from foot and mouth disease will pass through the finest filters (1898). Shortly afterward, Beijerink discovered the same phenomenon in the mosaic disease of the tobacco plant, and down to the present time, a large number of filterable viruses have been found, notably in the pleuropneumonia of cattle by Edmond Nocard (1899), in African horse sickness by Allan MacFadyan (1900), in yellow fever by Reed, Carroll and Agramonte (1901), in cattle plague by Nicolle and Adel Bey (1902), in fowl diphtheria or epithelioma contagiosum by Marx and Stocker (1902), in hog cholera by Dorest, Bolton and McBryde (1905), in molluscum contagiosum by Julius Berg (1905), in dengue by Ashburn and Craig (1907), in trachoma by Bertrelli and Cecchetto (1908), in three day or Pappataci fever by Doerr and Russ (1908), in typhus fever by Nicolle (1910), in tabardillo by Howard Taylor Ricketts (1911), in measles by Goldberger and Anderson (1911), and in chicken sarcoma by Peyton Rous (1911–12).[1] Some of these viruses, such as those of rabies, molluscum contagiosum, verruca vulgaris, chicken sarcoma and probably trachoma, require an abrasion of the surface for infection, others simply contact with the mucous membrane; and some, such as variola, measles, scarlatina, rabies, trachoma, etc., exhibit specific cell inclusions (Prowazek's chlamydozoa). As in the case of such minute organisms as Bordet's whooping-cough bacillus, or the organism recently claimed by Flexner in infantile poliomyelitis, it is probable that all filterable viruses will eventually turn out to contain filtered microscopic organisms not yet visible by present modes of investigation.

Great practical advances in the science of infectious diseases have been made in recent times through the coöperation of army surgeons. The work of Alphonse Laveran on malarial fever, of Ferdinand Widal on typhoid fever, of Friedrich Löffler and Emil Behring on diphtheria, of Major Sir Ronald Ross on malarial fever, of Surgeon General Sir David Bruce on Malta fever and sleeping sickness, of Lieut. Colonel Sir William B. Leishman, Major Donovan and Major Leonard Rogers on kala azar, will compare favorably with what John Hunter or Helmholtz accomplished during their period of military service. In the United States Army the labors of such men as Beaumont, Woodward, Otis, Billings, Woodhull, Smart and Huntington have set an example which has been followed by a number of able workers in recent times. The first American army surgeon to take up the study of bacteriology was Surgeon General George M. Sternberg (1838–   ), who isolated the diplococcus of pneumonia simultaneously with Pasteur (1880)[2] and published valuable treatises on bacteriology (1896) and disinfection (1900). During his administration, Major Walter Reed (1851–1902), of Virginia, who had studied under Welch at Johns Hopkins and had

---

[1] For a full account of present knowledge of the filterable viruses, see S. B. Wolbach in Jour. Med. Research, Boston, 1912–13, xxvii, 1–25, 1 tab.

[2] Sternberg: Rep. Nat. Bd. Health, 1881, Washington, 1882, iii, 87–92.

done good work on the pathology of typhoid fever in his laboratory (1895), was detailed as the head of a Board consisting of James Carroll, Artistide Agramonte and Jesse W. Lazear, to study yellow fever in Cuba, then occupied by the American army (1900). Josiah Clark Nott and Carlos Finlay (1833–) had already advanced the theory that the disease is transmitted by the mosquito, but when Reed went to Cuba, the Bacillus icteroïdes of Sanarelli held the field. Reed and his associates soon disproved Sanarelli's theory of causation, and proceeded at once to attack the problem of transmission by mosquitos. During the course of their experiments,[1] twenty-two cases of yellow fever were produced experimentally, fourteen by infected mosquito-bites, six by the injection of blood, and two by the injection of filtered blood-serum, thus proving the existence of a filterable virus (1901),[2] confirmed by Rosenau at Vera Cruz in 1903, while seven enlisted men disproved the fomites theory of transmission by sleeping in infected bedding. Carroll was the first to submit to mosquito inoculation and came through an attack of yellow fever successfully. Lazear died from the effects of an accidental mosquito bite. Thus it was proved, according to the most rigorous conventions of formal logic, that the cause of yellow fever is either an ultra-microscopic organism or a filterable virus which is transmitted to man by a particular species of mosquito, the *Stegomyia fasciata* or *calopus*. With reference to the conditions under which the experiment was performed, particularly the period of development in the body of the mosquito, the demonstration of Reed and Carroll is one of the most brilliant and conclusive in the history of science. Its economic importance is indicated by the immense saving of life and money through the eradication of yellow fever in the United States and the West Indies, if not throughout the entire world. In February, 1901, shortly after Reed had proved his case, Major William C. Gorgas, United States Army, as chief sanitary officer of Havana, Cuba, began to screen yellow fever patients and destroy mosquitos, and, in three months, Havana was freed from the disease for the first time in 150 years. In connection with the work on the Panama Canal, Colonel Gorgas has freed that part of the Isthmus, not only from yellow fever, but from all dangerous infections, and through this great triumph in sanitation, Panama, formerly a notorious plague spot of disease, the "White Man's Grave," as it was called, is now one of the healthiest communities in existence. The investigations of typhoid fever incidence in camp during the Spanish-American War (1898) by Major Walter Reed, Victor C.

[1] Reed (*et al.*), Philadelphia Med. Jour., 1900, vi, 790–796.
[2] Tr. Ass. Am. Phys., Philadelphia, 1901, xvi, 45–72.

Vaughan and Edward O. Shakespeare demonstrated the transmission of the disease by flies. During the American occupation of Porto Rico, the island population was vaccinated and freed from small-pox under Colonel John Van R. Hoff, and shortly afterward Captain Bailey K. Ashford discovered the presence of hook-worm infection in the Island (1900)[1] and has since devoted himself to the task of stamping it out. Captain Charles F. Craig (1872–) demonstrated that intra-corpuscular conjugation in the malarial plasmodia is the cause of latency and relapse and that there are malaria carriers (1902–05);[2] showed that the so-called Piroplasma hominis of Rocky Mountain spotted fever is really an artefact in the erythrocytes (1904); and, in the Philippines, demonstrated with Percy M. Ashburn that the cause of dengue is a filterable virus transmitted by the mosquito Culex fatigans (1907).[3] Craig also discovered two new parasites, Paramœba hominis (1906)[4] and (with Ashburn) Microfilaria philippinensis (1906),[5] and is the author of extensive monographs on the malarial fevers (1901, 1909) and the parasitic amebæ in man (1911). Captain Henry J. Nichols collaborated with Ehrlich in his initial work on salvarsan (1910) and has since investigated the experimental production of yaws (1910–11). Under the administration of Surgeon-General George H. Torney, Major Frederick F. Russell, in 1909, began the huge experiment of vaccinating the United States army against typhoid fever, after the methods advocated by Chantemesse and Widal in France (1888), Pfeiffer and Kolle in Germany (1896) and Sir Almroth Wright in England (1896). From a morbidity of 173 (16 fatal) cases of typhoid in 1909, Russell was able to bring his statistics down to 9 cases of the disease with one fatality in 1912, while at present the army is absolutely free from typhoid. The mobilization of United States troops on the Mexican border in 1912[6] gave Major Russell an opportunity, such as never came even to Jenner or Pasteur, viz., that of testing his vaccine at a huge outdoor clinic consisting of some 20,000 men. The absolute success of his experiment is now a matter of history.

Intimately connected with the history of infectious diseases is the illustrious bead-roll of its medical martyrs. With Servetus and Semmelweis, who died for their opinions, should be classed such names as Daniel A. Carrion (verrugas), Jesse W. Lazear (yellow

[1] Ashford: New York Med. Jour., 1900, lxxi, 552–556.

[2] Craig: Am. Med., Philadelphia, 1905, 982; 1029.

[3] Craig and Ashburn: Philippine Jour. Sc., Manila, 1907, B. ii, 93–146.

[4] Am. Jour. Med. Sc., Philadelphia, 1906, cxxxii, 214–220.

[5] Ibid.: 435–443.

[6] Russell: Harvey Lecture, 1913.

fever), A. Yersin and Hermann Franz Müller (bubonic plague), Tito
Carbone (Malta fever), Allan MacFadyen (typhoid and Malta
fever), J. Everett Dutton (African relapsing fever), Howard Taylor
Ricketts (tabardillo), and Thomas B. McClintick (Rocky Mountain fever), all of whom lost their lives in investigating the diseases
with which their names are associated.

The **surgery** of the twentieth century has been devoted mainly
to refinements, inventions and improvements in procedure, such as
Arbuthnot Lane's treatment of fractures by plates and screws
(1892–1905) and his method of treating intestinal stasis from
"Lane's kink" (1903–9), the operations for the excision of the
prostate by P. Johnston Freyer, of the Indian Medical Service
(1901), and Hugh Hampton Young (1903), of Baltimore, the use
of bismuth paste in the treatment of chronic tubercular sinuses
and cavities by E. Beck (1906), the injection affording at the
same time a complete radiogram of the ramifications of the cavity;
the treatment of cancer by a bombardment with high-frequency
sparks of wide dimensions (fulguration), introduced by de Keat-
ing-Hart, of Paris (1910), the many instruments invented by
Eugène Doyen, of Paris, the use of the "Cargile membrane" in
preventing postoperative intestinal adhesions (1912), etc.

August **Bier** (1861–   ), von Bergmann's successor at Berlin
(1907), introduced intraspinal anesthesia with cocaine (1899), a
new method of treating amputation stumps (1900), and active
and passive hyperemia as an adjuvant in surgical therapy (1903).[1]
In cocaine anesthesia by the spinal route, Bier was preceded by
James Leonard Corning (1855–   ), of New York city, in 1885.[2]

Ernst Ferdinand **Sauerbruch** (1875–   ), of Barmen, Rhenish Prussia, professor at Marburg (1907), while working in Mikulicz's clinic at Breslau, greatly advanced the possibilities of intra-
thoracic surgery by his invention of the pneumatic chamber at
reduced atmospheric (negative) pressure for the prevention of
pneumothorax (1903–04). The idea of using differential pressure
was first conceived by Quénu and Tuffier in 1896. Sauerbruch
also devised the positive pressure cabinet in which a patient
breathes compressed air, while the pleural cavity is opened at
ordinary atmospheric pressure. The earlier cabinets were clumsy
and had many inconveniences, but, with the modern improvements,
Sauerbruch, Willy Meyer and others have made great advances in
the surgery of the esophagus and the chest. Positive pressure by
means of intubation (the Fell-O'Dwyer method) was recommended

---

[1] Bier: Hyperämie als Heilmittel, Leipzig, 1903.
[2] Corning: New York Med. Jour., 1885, xlii, 317–319.

by Rudolph Matas in 1899. In 1909,[1] Samuel James Meltzer and John Auer, of the Rockefeller Institute, greatly simplified matters by the method of intratracheal insufflation of air through a tube passed into the trachea, producing "continuous respiration without respiratory movements." Maintenance of respiration in a strapped animal by means of a bellows had been demonstrated by Vesalius and Robert Hooke, but the ingenious Meltzer-Auer experiment made the procedure viable and was a true advance in physiological surgery.

Much effective work in visceral surgery has been done by Eugène Doyen (Paris), César Roux (Lausanne), Emil Werner Körte (Berlin), A. W. Mayo Robson (London), Sir Berkeley G. A. Moynihan (Leeds), John B. Murphy (Chicago), Charles H. Mayo and William J. Mayo (Rochester, Minnesota), and John M. T. Finney (Baltimore); in the surgery of the head by von Bergmann, MacEwen, W. W. Keen, H. Schloffer, Harvey Cushing; in the surgery of the vascular system by Erwin Payr (Innsbruck), W. T. Halsted, J. B. Murphy, Alexis Carrel; in osteoplastic and orthopedic surgery by Albert Hoffa, Erich Lexer, E. Lorenz, J. B. Murphy, John B. Roberts, Edward H. Bradford, and by Joel Ernest Goldthwait, of Marblehead, Massachusetts, who has done much to simplify the complicated subject of "rheumatic disorders" by his classification of arthritis into the villous, infectious, atrophic and hypertrophic varieties (1904).

As in eighteenth century Paris, modern cities abound with able operators whose innovations have been principally along the lines of technical procedure. This is particularly the case with the Parisians—Tuffier, Terrillon, Chassaignac, Faure, Hartmann, Pozzi, Delbet, Albarran—many of whom have included gynecological work as part of their specialty.

The last few years are remarkable for a revival of Hunterian or physiological surgery. Even as Marion Sims and Billroth in their specialties greatly advanced the clinical pathology of diseases of the abdominal and pelvic viscera, so we find Kocher, Horsley, von Eiselsberg, Halsted, Crile, Cushing, Carrel, Murphy, not only thinking physiologically in their work, but making many new departures by means of experimentation on animals. Hunter, Merrem and Sir Astley Cooper did this, as also Jameson and Gross in America, but since their day the method has been almost nonexistent.

At the head of the surgical profession today stands, by common consent, the honored name of Theodor **Kocher** (1841–   ), of Bern, Switzerland, who was a pupil of von Langenbeck and Billroth, and has held the chair of surgery in his native town since 1872. Kocher is known for his method of reducing dislocations of the shoulder-joint (1870),[2] for his contributions on hernia, osteomyelitis, his operations for artificial anus, etc., his hydrody-

---

[1] Meltzer and Auer: Jour. Exper. Med., New York, 1909, xi, 622–625.
[2] Berlin. klin. Wochenschr., 1870, vii, 101–105.

namic theory of the effect of gunshot wounds, and especially for his work on the thyroid gland. He was the first to excise the thyroid for goiter (1878),[1] and he has performed this difficult operation over 2000 times with only four and a half per cent. mortality. In 1883,[2] he published his description of the "cachexia strumipriva," which he had found as a sequel in 30 out of his first 100 thyroidectomies, and which, in connection with the pioneer experiments of Moritz Schiff on dogs (1859) and the work of the Reverdins and Horsley, inaugurated the physiology and physiological surgery of the ductless glands. Kocher has also applied experimental surgery to the physiology of the brain and spinal cord. He is described as a slow, careful, precise and absolutely skilful operator, a typical scientific surgeon, who obtains the completest clinical history of his patients before beginning, and with whom success is an almost foregone conclusion. He maintains an absolutely aseptic field of operation and is a master of minute dissecting. His text-book of operative surgery (1894) is an index of his great learning. In appendicitis à chaux and à froid, he is said to be excelled by his pupil, César Roux, of the Canton de Vaud, whose post-haste, sleight-of-hand methods, sometimes to the exclusion of anesthesia and

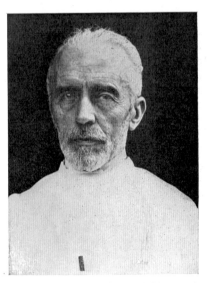

Theodor Kocher (1841–   ). (Courtesy of Professor Harvey Cushing, Harvard University.)

antisepsis, can scarcely be recommended for imitation. The same thing is true of the sensational, cinematographic methods of Doyen in Paris, and, in general, the less showy the operating, the better the patient's chances.[3]

---

[1] Cor.-Bl. f. Schweiz. Aerzte, Basel, 1878, viii, 702–705.

[2] Arch. f. klin. Chir., Berlin, 1883, xxix, 254–337.

[3] As Professor Harvey Cushing says, in his recent address before the International Medical Congress (London, 1913): "The accurate and detailed methods, in the use of which Kocher and Halsted were for so long the notable examples, have spread into all clinics—at least into those clinics where you or I would wish to entrust ourselves for operation. Observers no longer expect to be thrilled in an operating room; the spectacular public performances of the past, no longer condoned, are replaced by the quiet, rather tedious

Anton **von Eiselsberg** (1860–   ), of Steinhaus, Austria, professor of surgery at Utrecht (1893), Königsberg (1896) and Vienna (1901), is a pupil of Billroth. He was one of the first to notice the appearance of tetany after goiter operations (1890), and, in 1892, he produced tetany experimentally by excising a cat's thyroid which he had successfully transplanted into the abdominal parietes.[1] He has also studied the metastases of thyroid cancer and has recently been a prominent worker in the surgery of the pituitary body.

William Stewart **Halsted** (1852–   ), of New York, is professor of surgery in the Johns Hopkins University (1889). He was the first to ligate the subclavian artery in the first portion with success (1892);[2] he devised the well-known supraclavicular operation for cancer of the breast (1889),[3] and, simultaneously with Bassini, the modern operation for hernia (1889).[4] He has done much work in experimental surgery, particularly on circular (1887) and bulkhead (1912) suturing of the intestines, occlusion of the aorta and larger arteries by means of a metal band as a substitute for ligation (1909),[5] and in auto- and iso-transplantations of the parathyroid glands (1909),[6] which, in connection with H. Leischner's classical paper of 1907, have had much to do with establishing the functional status of these organs. In aid of a strictly aseptic technic he introduced fine black silk sutures and rubber gloves, silver foil, gutta-percha tissue in drainage and has devised a number of new sutures and stitches. Quietly and unobtrusively, Halsted has taught the delicate art of the perfect healing of wounds, which has been nowhere more beautifully demonstrated than at his clinic.

George W. **Crile** (1864–   ), of Chile, Ohio, professor of clinical surgery in the Western Reserve University since 1890, is the author of highly original experimental researches on surgical shock (1899), blood-pressure in surgery (1903), hemorrhage and transfusion (1909), which procedure he has carried almost to perfection by his skill and technic. He has introduced various new operations for cancer of the lip, uterine prolapse, etc., and he was the first to perform a major operation with intraneural injections of cocaine as an anesthetic (1887). He has worked with particular

---

procedures which few beyond the operator, his assistants, and the immediate bystander can profitably see. The patient on the table, like the passenger in a car, runs greater risks if he have a loquacious driver, or one who takes close corners, exceeds the speed limit, or rides to admiration." Brit. Med. Jour., London, 1913, ii, 294.

[1] von Eiselsberg: Wien. klin. Wochenschr., 1892, v, 81–85.

[2] Halsted: Johns Hopkins Hosp. Bull., Baltimore, 1892, iii, 93.

[3] Tr. Am. Surg. Ass., Phila., 1898, xvi, 144–181, 5 pl.

[4] Johns Hopkins Hosp. Bull., Baltimore, 1893, iv, 17–24, 3 pl.

[5] J. Exper. Med., N. Y., 1909, xi, 373–391, 3 pl.

[6] Ibid., 175–199, 2 pl.: 1912, xv, 205–215, 2 pl.

ability in minute "block dissections" of the lymphatics in cancer. His operations on the head and neck for this condition (1908) are comparable with the Halsted breast excision or the Wertheim-Clark operation for uterine cancer. His theory of "anoci-associa-tion," the blocking of shock in operations by the combination of general and loca anesthesia (morphia and scopolamine followed by nitrous oxide and novocaine), has been referred to.

Harvey **Cushing** (1869-   ), of Cleveland, Ohio, professor of surgery at the Johns Hopkins (1902–11) and Harvard Universities (1912), has devoted himself latterly to neurological surgery, and par-ticularly to the surgery of the head and the pituitary body. He has done much original work in experimental physiology, pathology and surgery, such as experimental production of gall-stones (1899), experimental production of valvular heart lesions in the dog, with successful operative treatment of the same (1908), successful treat-ment of facial paralysis in man by anastomosis of the spinal acces-sory and facial nerves (1903); he has introduced various new proce-dures—anesthetic nerve-blocking (1898), a special suture, lumbar drainage in hydrocephalus, cross-bow incision in opening the base of the brain, and has developed decompressive operations, particularly in intracranial hemorrhages in the new-born (1905) and inaccessible tumors (1905). In his work on the pituitary body, he has thrown much light on its physiological functions by the experimental pro-duction of sexual infantilism in animals, by the study of pituitary metabolism in disease, pregnancy, hibernation and other conditions, and by the general consideration of its disorders as "dyspituitar-ism." His monograph on this subject (1912)[1] contains his mode of operating and is an exhaustive study of the condition as approached from the physiological, pathological, clinical, and surgical sides.

Great advances in **vascular surgery** have been made by the experimental method.

Indeed, the first case of a successful venous suture was the celebrated "Eck fistula" (1877), which has since been applied by Pavloff and others in experiments requiring the physiological exclusion of the liver. In 1881, Vin-cenz Czerny tried to suture an eroded jugular vein, with fatal results, but Schede succeeded in suturing the femoral vein, and, by 1892, had 30 success-ful cases. In 1889, Jassinovski made 26 experimental arterial sutures upon animals, all lateral, and was followed by Dörfler (1890), who, like Murphy and Silberberg before him, employed a suture passing through all three arterial coats. By proceeding aseptically, he avoided thrombosis, and, in 1891, Dur-ant applied the method with success in two cases of arterial suture in man. These were all lateral sutures. The first end-to-end suture of veins was at-tempted with success upon a dog by Hirsch in 1881, and, in 1898, Jaboulay and Briau successfully applied their U-suture to the severed carotid artery of a donkey, to be followed with equal success upon animals by Salomoni and Tom-aselli. The first successful circular suturing of blood-vessels in man was done by

---

[1] The Pituitary Body and its Disorders, Philadelphia, 1912.
40

John Benjamin **Murphy** (1857–   ), of Appleton, Wisconsin, professor of surgery in the Northwestern University, Chicago (1895), who, after many experimental end-to-end resections of wounded arteries and veins, successfully united a femoral artery, severed by a gunshot wound, in 1896.[1] Murphy had already done epoch-making work in the production of "cholecysto-intestinal, gastro-intestinal, entero-intestinal anastomosis and approximation without sutures" by means of a special button (1892),[2] which was preceded by the decalcified bone-plates of Nicholas Senn, potato and turnip plates, etc. Meanwhile, Robert Abbe (1851–   ), of New York, had introduced catgut rings for intestinal suturing (1892),[3] and had attempted prothetic union of blood-vessels by means of a fine glass tube (1894), which was improved upon by Erwin Payr's device of absorbable magnesium cylinders (1900). In 1897,[4] Murphy introduced end-to-end suture of blood-vessels by means of invagination, the intima being brought into apposition with the adventitia, but, although there was no hemorrhage, the circulation was restored in only four cases out of thirteen, on account of the narrowing of the lumen of the vessels, with consequent thrombosis. This was finally obviated by the triangular suture of Carrel (1900). Before this innovation, Höpfner and others had transplanted pieces of artery or vein by means of Payr's magnesium rings, and Ullmann had tried to transplant a kidney in the dog in 1902. All these experiments fell through, however, on account of septic complications, and even Carrel succeeded only by dint of the most refined asepsis. Murphy has developed anastomosis of the intestines by invagination and has had remarkable results with bone-grafts, which, curiously, do not succeed, as a rule, unless the sliver of tissue used is autogenous—from the patient himself. The graft will, in time, reproduce the exact contour of the defective bone, in accordance with Driesch's morphological law of the "totipotency of protoplasm."

Rudolph **Matas** (1860–   ), of New Orleans, has greatly improved the operation for the radical cure of aneurysm by his procedure of aneurysmorrhaphy (1902),[5] *i. e.,* closing the mouths of the blood-vessels entering into the aneurysm.

Alexis **Carrel** (1873–   ), of Sainte-Foy-les-Lyon, France, a graduate of the University of Lyons (1900), who came to America in 1905 and is now an associate member of the Rockefeller Insti-

---

[1] Murphy: Med. Record, New York, 1897, ii, 73–88.

[2] Murphy: *Ibid.*, 1892, xlii, 665–676.

[3] Abbe: *Ibid.*, 1892, xli, 365–370.   [4] Murphy: *Ibid.*, 1897, li, 73–88.

[5] Matas: Tr. Am. Surg. Assoc., Phila., 1902, xx, 396–434, 16 pl.

tute, has revolutionized the surgery of the vascular system and made great advances in physiology and physiological surgery, for which he was made a Nobel prizeman in 1912. In 1902, he published his first paper on vascular anastomoses and visceral transplantation,[1] in which he showed that perfect end-to-end anastomosis of blood-vessels can be secured by inserting in the opposing ends a triple-threaded suture, which, when drawn tightly, converts the round lumen of the vessel into an equilateral triangle, thus securing closest apposition, without leakage, preserving the continuity of the lumen, and so avoiding thrombosis. Before Carrel's time, a wounded artery was treated only by ligation in continuity. From end-to-end anastomosis of arteries he advanced, by means of specially invented needles and rigid asepsis, to the substitution of a lost piece of an artery by pieces of artery or vein, and thence to the transplantation of organs from animal to animal. Thus, he has transplanted a kidney, with its vascular supply, from cat to cat, secretion of urine beginning before the end of the operation, and this feat has not only been proved successful in man, but extended to other viscera also. Transplantations in mass of blood-vessels, organs, viscera, and limbs have been also successful.[2] Carrel's investigations of the latent life of arteries (1910)[3] led to the preservation of portions of blood-vessels in cold storage for days or weeks before using them in transplantation. Latterly, he has applied the principle of R. G. Harrison's experiment on extravital cultivation of nerve-cells (1910) to the extravital cultivation and rejuvenation of tissues (1911),[4] culminating in his remarkable experiment of keeping the excised viscera of an animal alive and functionating physiologically *in vitro* (1912).[5] He has also succeeded in activating and accelerating the growth of connective tissue by dressings of thyroidal, splenic, embryonic and other animal extracts (1913).

The Nobel prize in medicine for 1911 was awarded to Allvar **Gullstrand** (1862–   ), of Landskrona, Sweden, professor of **ophthalmology** in the University of Upsala (1894), for his mathematical investigations of dioptrics or the science of the refraction of light through the transparent media of the living eye. As Willard Gibbs founded the chemical theory of heterogeneous substances, so Gullstrand has founded the dioptrics of heterogeneous media.

[1] Carrel: Lyon méd., 1902, xcviii, 859–864.

[2] Jour. Am. Med. Assoc., Chicago, 1908, li, 1662–1667.

[3] Jour. Exper. Med., New York, 1910, xii, 460–486.

[4] Jour. Am. Med. Assoc., Chicago, 1911, lvii, 1611.

[5] Jour. Exper. Med., New York, 1913, xviii, 155–161.

Formerly, the image in the eye was regarded as a schematic, "collinear," or point-for-point affair, like that studied on the lenses of optical instruments. Gullstrand took up the study of the ocular image from the viewpoint of reality, clearly differentiating its actual formation from its optical projection. By applying the methods of mathematical physics, especially those of Sir William Rowan Hamilton, he treated the problem as one concerning a set of widely diffused bundles of rays, refracted through a system of continually curving planes, and showed that, during accommodation, the index of refraction of the lens is augmented by an actual change in its structure. His principal works on this theme are his General Theory of Monochromatic Aberrations (1900),[1] and his essays on dioptrics of the crystalline lens (1908) and the real optic image (1906). In 1889, he introduced a practical method of estimating corneal astigmatism by a single observation, an advantage possessed by a single instrument, the Sutcliffe ophthalmometer. In 1892, he introduced a photographic method of locating a paralyzed ocular muscle. He also introduced a micrometric method of estimating the photographed corneal reflex, as giving the most exact knowledge of the form of the normal and diseased cornea. His work in this field is not unlike Burdon-Sanderson's photographic determinations of reaction time in muscle. In 1907, he showed that the yellow color of the macula in the retina is a cadaveric phenomenon, not existing in life; and, as above stated, he discovered the intracapsular mechanism of accommodation.[2] He also devised the reflexless stationary ophthalmoscope (1912), which excludes all light not belonging to the ophthalmoscopic image, and is thus free from all reflections from the mirror or the eye itself, giving a better image, better stereoscopic effect, and a wider field of vision. He has invented corrective glasses with aspherical lenses for those operated on for cataract, which give cleaner cut and more luminous images, with wider range of vision, than spherical lenses with the same focal distance.

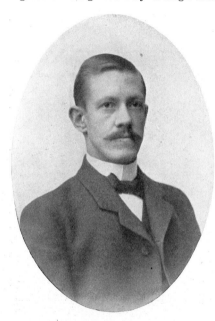

Allvar Gullstrand (1862–   ).

Two prominent innovations in **eye surgery** of recent times have been made by officers of the Indian Medical Service. The operation of extraction of cataract within the capsule was introduced by Lieut. Colonel **Henry Smith** in 1900,[3] and his success

---

[1] Gullstrand: Allgemeine Theorie der monochromatischen Aberrationen, Upsala, 1900.

[2] Arch. f. Ophth., Berlin, 1912, lxxii, 169–190.

[3] H. Smith: Indian Med. Gaz., Calcutta, 1900, xxxv, 240: 1901, xxxvi, 220; 1905, xl, 327.

with it has been remarkable. As a benefactor of humankind, he is known all over northern India, where the reflection of the pitiless sunlight from the dusty plains tells with terrific force upon the eyes of the natives. His clinic at Jullundur, in the Punjab, is frequented not only by streams of blind people, coming by every mode of travel, but by ophthalmic surgeons, even from the western United States, who travel across the world to learn his methods. He averages about 3000 extractions a year, and, by 1910, he had 24,000 to his credit, of which 20,000 were done by the intracapsular method. Another new operation, that of sclerocorneal trephining for glaucoma, was introduced by Major Robert Henry **Elliot,** I. M. S., in August, 1909.[1] The oper-
ation of von Graefe had held the field for half a century, Lagrange and Herbert had emphasized the value of sclerectomy, and even corneal trephining had been essayed by Argyll Robertson, Blanco, Fröhlich, and Freeland Fergus, but Elliot has made the operation his own by many improvements and has made it viable.

Great advances in the diagnosis and treatment of disease of the **internal ear** have been made by Robert **Bárány** (1876–   ), of Vienna, Privatdocent at the University, who has

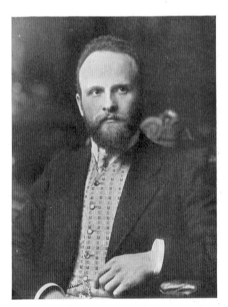

Robert Bárány (1876–   ). (From a photograph in the Surgeon General's Library.)

done much to clear up the hazy subject of aural vertigo, or Ménière's disease, especially in differentiating it from allied or adjacent lesions in the cerebellum, from epilepsy, or from ordinary nystagmus (1906).[2] Labyrinthine vertigo or "vestibular nystagmus" is interpreted by Bárány as a disturbance of function of the vestibular nerve or the organs to which it is distributed, and he has traced its origin to a

---

[1] Elliot: Ophthalmoscope, London, 1909, vii, 804–808.

[2] Bárány: Arch. f. Ohrenh., Leipzig, 1906, lxviii, 1–30, and later publications.

large number of different causes with which it might be confused. He has introduced a number of ingenious differential tests, such as production of nystagmus by irrigation of the external meatus with cold or warm water (caloric test), or by having a patient try to point at an object with his eyes shut after having previously touched it (static test), and he has been able to prove his case by successful operations on the cerebellum or the internal ear. He has also devised a "noise machine" for testing paracusis Willisii, and other diagnostic novelties.

The last ten or twenty years have witnessed an unusual growth of interest in the **history of medicine.** Many admirable mono-

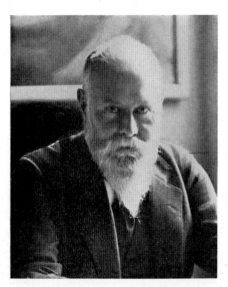

Karl Sudhoff (1853–   ). (From a portrait in the Surgeon General's Library.)

graphs and essays have appeared, societies have been formed in Germany, France, England, Italy, and the larger American cities, expositions of rare objects, books, and pictures have been held, and many modern physicians have made valuable private collections of the same. The most important advance of recent years was the foundation of the *Institut für Geschichte der Medizin* at Leipzig, in 1905, under the direction of Professor Sudhoff, for whom a special chair of the subject was created in the University (1905). This Institute and its publications are supported by a special endowment of 500,000 marks left for this purpose by the widow of the late Professor Theodor Puschmann, and in accepting the directorship Professor Sudhoff stipulated that a separate home for the new specialty should be erected. Karl **Sudhoff** (1853–   ), of Frankfort on the Main, who had practised medicine for many years before this event, and is entirely self-taught in medical history, began his studies with his important investigations of Paracelsus (including a thorough study of the Paracelsus manuscripts), begun in 1876, and published 1887–99, which are sto-authoritative. He has written exhaustive and scholarly monill graphs on the iatromathematicians of the fifteenth and sixteenth centuries (1902), manuscript and other fifteenth century medical illustrations (1907), the early history of anatomical illustration (1908), German medical incunabula (1908), the Greek papyri of the Alexandrian period (1909), ancient balneology (1910), and the early history of syphilis (1912). These are all original researches of the highest order, and, in addition, Sudhoff has published a host of minor investigations of value, particularly in the *Archiv für Geschichte der Medizin*, which he founded in 1908. He has made many of the rarer medical texts accessible to German readers through his *Klassiker der Medizin*, a series of inexpensive reprints which, in style and *format*, are like Ostwald's well-known editions of scientific classics. His method of investigation is a new departure. With the financial resources at his command, he travels far and wide in search of rare or unprinted medical manuscripts and illustrations in the European libraries, private and public, and, by photographing these and collating them, he has been able to apply the inductive method with signal ability in bringing out many new facts, settling disputed points, and exploding much of the traditional *Papierwissenschaft* which has been slavishly accepted to date. Thus he has shown, by collation of unprinted manuscripts, that up to the time of Vesalius, anatomical and other illustrations were for centuries based upon servile tradition and almost devoid of any signs of original observation. No one has written more effectively upon anatomical illustration since Choulant. Sudhoff has also developed the whole science of the *Lasstafelkunst*, against which Paracelsus brayed with such obscene vigor in his Liber Paragranum (1589), and, during this research, he discovered the first medical publication to be set in type, Guttenberg's purgation calendar of 1462, in the Bibliothèque nationale in Paris. His philological researches on the Alexandrian papyri (1909) throw much light on the status of Egyptian medicine in this period, and his recent investigation of the early history of syphilis (1912), which we have already described, furnishes a formidable argument against the theory of the American origin of the disease. He has also added much to our knowledge of the advancement of state medicine during the Middle Ages. His original investigations and reproductions of the medieval laws and ordinances, to prevent leprosy, plague and syphilis, go far beyond the labors of Haeser in this field. To look through his wonderful catalogue of the Dresden Historical Exhibit (1911) is to realize how little one knows about medical history. Sudhoff believes that classical philologists who have exhausted the possibilities of the secular literature of Greece and Rome, should try their teeth on the older medical writings and help to elucidate them. His exhaustive study of the German medical incunabula (1908) supplements and completes the work of

Choulant, and is a forerunner of the movement, now in progress in Prussia, to get up an international catalogue of all the medical incunabula in public and private libraries, in order to decide the many unsettled points as to time, place of publication and authorship.

With the work of this distinguished scholar, this sketch of recent medicine may fitly close.

CULTURAL AND SOCIAL ASPECTS OF MODERN MEDICINE

READERS of Lecky's "History of European Morals" will recall the impressive pages in which this eminent philosophical writer discusses the effects of the modern spirit of industrialism upon ethical relations, even upon sexual morality. Two types of character, he says, are apt to be produced—the thrifty and cautious, which has "all that cast of virtues which is designated by the term 'respectability'"; and the speculative, enterprising type, which is "restless, fiery, and uncertain, very liable to fall into great and conspicuous vices, impatient of routine, but by no means unfavorable to strong feelings, to great generosity or resolution." The first type is prevalent in poor, isolated communities, the second among the busy marts of commerce. These phases of the great industrial movement of modern life have not been without their effect upon medical practice. During the nineteenth century, we see the physician becoming more and more impersonal, more of a business man and not so much influenced by the social and ethical obligations which were certainly a characteristic of the eighteenth century physician. The "family doctor" of the past has well-nigh disappeared, except in small communities, and, in the modern period, we find the city physicians, under stress of competition, creating everywhere local codes of medical ethics. The reasons for this are not far to seek. They have been set forth at sufficient length in Mr. Bernard Shaw's clever but superficial tirades on the commercialization of the medical profession. Otto Jüttner, in his interesting life of Daniel Drake, tells of a certain gruff physician in the Western Reserve in the early thirties who, when summoned to see any patient of whose financial status he was ignorant, always demanded, on entering the room: "Who pays this bill?" This is a crude instance, yet compare it with what Abraham Flexner says about the careers of the two Hunters, Matthew Baillie, Bright, Addison, and Hodgkin:

"These men all ran substantially the same course. As unknown youths they became assistants in the dead-house or the out-patient department of the hospital. This was their opportunity; obscurity was their protection. They spent years in working out, on both pathological and clinical sides, the important problems with which their names are severally associated. When, at the close of a decade, they had achieved scientific eminence, they were whirled off into busy practices. The rest of their active lives they spent as prosperous consultants, visiting the hospital and teaching in its medical school, of course, but without the leisure, environment, or stimulus requisite to further scientific pursuit. The hospital as an institution was indifferent; other inducement there was none. Fifteen or twenty unproductive years followed. Thus men blossomed early, but they left no seed; they had no scientific heirs; they established no line." [1]

Flexner is apparently not familiar with John Hunter's pupils, with the actual facts about Addison and Hodgkin as "prosperous consultants," nor with the successors of Bright and Addison at Guy's Hospital; yet it is not unlikely that a good consulting practice, a comfortable berth in Harley Street, has been a prominent ambition of the London practitioner in the modern period. Even in Germany, Flexner is disposed to admit "a growing suspicion that the idealism of the clinical professors is yielding to the temptation, perhaps the need, of increased income. . . . The scale of living has been altered by industrial prosperity; new ideals, material in character, are creeping in." From the days of John Hunter's unwilling quest after "that damned guinea" to the disputes of our own time about "fee-splitting," contract practice, lodge doctors, *Krankenkassen*, patent medicines, unqualified practitioners and general surplus of doctors, the necessity of struggling for a competence, instead of having it assured by family practice, as in the eighteenth century, has wrought a change in the modern physician. The ideal is scientific and impersonal, to be as efficient as an engineer and to look and act like one.

In spite of themselves, men are influenced by the social conditions which impinge upon them. It is a noticeable fact that the pictures of Americans of the Civil War generation have a more sincere and ideal look than those of the present time. The modern type everywhere is one of clean-cut business efficiency. In the advancement of science this has been an immeasurable gain. Modern science has done away with the idea of personal infallibility, has centered itself upon results and has a fine probity of its own. "The scientific gentleman," said Billings, "is the blue-ribbon of our day." It is to the credit of modern medicine that, in spite of intense competition, thousands of physicians have continued to practise their profession along the old honorable lines, giving largely and nobly of their time to the poor, although, in the crowded streets of finance, a man whose heart is better than his head is a fool by definition. The most enlightened physicians of today are advancing preventive medicine, which tends to do away with a great deal of medical practice. "Certainly men who regularly render a large part of their services gratuitously and are constantly striving to eradicate their own means

---

[1] A. Flexner: Medical Education in Europe, New York, 1912, 13.

of livelihood cannot be convicted of being altogether mercenary."[1]

As Harvey Cushing quaintly puts it: "Dr. Pound of Cure Lane is being superseded by his young disciple, Dr. Ounce of Prevention Street."[2]

The increased cost of living, the automobile, expensive office appointments and instruments, foreign study and travel, make heavy inroads on the modern physician's income, and, hence, have almost tripled the rate of **medical fees.** In other words, the purchasing power of money is steadily declining. According to the laws of economics, the greater the supply of gold, the more it becomes a commodity and the fewer the things it will buy. It is easier to get money nowadays than unadulterated food and raiment or unscamped labor.

At the end of the eighteenth century (1798) the professional charges of "practitioners of physic and surgery in the State of New York"[3] were $1 for an ordinary visit or $1.25, with a single dose of medicine, 12 cents each for pills and powders, $5 for a consultation ("verbal advice") or a night visit, $1 to $2 for bloodletting, $4 for cupping, $100 each for amputating a joint, excising an eye, operating for aneurysm, while operating for hernia, stone, or cataract cost $125; an ordinary labor case was $15 to $25; a difficult one, $25 to $40. S. C. Busey, commencing practice in Washington, D. C., in 1849, got $1 a visit, and "many times the bill was settled with a fraction, and often a small fraction, of that amount."[4] At present, the average bill for a city visit is $3 ($2 in some localities), and consultations and obstetrical and surgical cases are paid in proportion. In England, the average consultant's fee is one or two guineas; in the country districts, or among the poor, visits may be variously ten shillings, five shillings, eighteen pence, or sixpence. In France, during the Napoleonic wars, a cabinet consultation or a city visit was 10 sous (1805–39); by 1850 it was 1 franc. Bloodletting was 1 livre; an accouchement, 12 livres. In Prussia (1906), physicians and patients make whatever bargain they choose: 2 to 20 marks for an office visit, 1 to 10 marks for a subsequent visit or a consultation, 4 to 10 marks for a confinement, with half as much again for twins, 3 to 15 marks for removing a tonsil, 10 to 30 marks for setting a fracture. In 1892, over half the physicians of Berlin were making less than 3000 marks annually; about one-tenth were making over 10,000. At Berlin, in 1908, the salary of a professor ordinarius was 4800 marks, with increases of 400 marks every four years, up to a limit of 7200 marks at the end of twenty-four years' service. Outside Berlin, it begins with 4200 and ends with 6600 marks. A salaried extraordinarius gets 2600 marks to start with, with 4800 marks as the limit. In Austria, the extraordinarius starts with 3200 kroner and reaches 4000 kroner in a decade. Flexner says that a prominent German professor disclosed the sources of his income as "$300 as hospital physician, paid by the city; $2000 as professor, paid by the state; $5000 in student fees. He also does some consultant practice in the afternoon."[5]

Modern art, like that of the seventeenth century, has represented medical subjects in varied and manifold ways. One prominent

---

[1] J. B. Nichols: "Medical Sectarianism," Wash. Med. Ann., 1913, xii, 12.

[2] Cushing: Brit. Med. Journal, London, 1913, ii, 291.

[3] J. J. Walsh: "Physicians' fees down the ages," Internat. Clin., Phila., 20 s., iv, 259–275.

[4] Samuel C. Busey: Personal Reminiscences, Washington, 1895, 63.

[5] Flexner: Op. cit., pp. 148, 293–299.

characteristic of modernity, "the strange disease of modern life," is to seek what is odd and new, and, in art, to find inspiration in ugliness. Goya's canvases in the Prado, for instance, and particularly his etchings, are triumphs of the *macabre*. His figurations of teratology, idiocy, insanity, death by violence and general bloodshed, show the curious interest in the horrible, the solemn delight in death which the Goncourts thought essentially Spanish: "*Le génie de l'horreur, c'est le génie de l'Espagne.*" The Musée Wiertz in Brussels affords another example of this tendency. Infanticide, suicide, premature burial, and eroticism are the special themes of this artist. A more recent development is the *scabreux*, which has been exhaustively treated by modern cartoonists and caricaturists, like Gavarni, and in the canvases of the German Secessionists, some of whom have represented childbirth, for instance, with appalling frankness. Every recent *Salon des réfusés* at Paris has had something of this kind. Along more conventional lines there have been plenty of canvases representing doctors at the bedside or surgeons operating in clinic; and of pictures of the old-fashioned literary type, which tell a story, such as E. Hamman's Vesalius; Germain Colot cutting for stone in the presence of Louis XI (1414), by Rivoulon; Paré operating on the outskirts of a besieged town by L. Matout; the "Pestiferes de Jaffa" of Antoine-Jean Gros; Feyen-Perrin's "Leçon de Velpeau"; or Péan demonstrating hemostasis by forcipressure (L. Gervex). Others, such as Andrea Cefaly's dentist (1875), Edelfelt's "Pasteur in his laboratory," or the picture of Charcot demonstrating a hysterical case at the Salpêtrière, show the tendency toward realistic or photographic representation, as of something "caught in the act." Carolus Duran, Sargent, Cecilia Beaux, and others have made many excellent oil portraits of recent physicians. Many modern medical men have illustrated their own works, in particular the Bells, Henle, His, Leidy, and Lister. Paul Richer made a beautiful drawing of Charcot, and Charcot himself was a talented draughtsman and decorator of porcelain. His pencil followed the lead of the comic and the fantastic, and his caricatures of the Paris Faculty, as friends in council (*L'Aréopage*) and in Indian file (*en queue*), are delicious. Sir Seymour Haden, the surgeon, was one of the most accomplished of modern etchers. In sculpture, we have Alfred Boucher's bas relief of Tobias restoring his father to sight (Musée de Troyes), Falguière's full-length statue of Charcot (Salpêtrière, 1898), and the more conventional figures of English and American physicians in various localities. Rodin has made a large number of curious shorthand notations of human anatomy, as preparatory to his peculiar mode of treating marble. Of the many recent monuments to

Servetus, we may mention the figure on the funeral pyre in the Place de Montrouge (Paris) by Jean Baffier, the contemplative Servetus, in doctor's cap and gown, in the vestibule of the Museo Velasquez at Madrid, the statue of the martyr in prison by Roch (Annemese), the Rodinesque nude by Joseph Bernard at Vienne (Isère) and the expiatory plinth of rough-hewn granite at Geneva. Servetus has also been commemorated in a play by the Spanish dramatist and physician, José Echegaray (*La muerte en los labios*).[1]

As modern physicians have been abundantly caricatured in the graphic arts, so the business-like tendencies of the profession in our own time have afforded liberal opportunities for literary satire. Baas has hit off the early nineteenth century doctors of this type as characterized "by the fashionable cut of their clothing, their universal greetings and rapid gait, their imperturbable amiability, and the thermometer, stethoscope, percussion hammer, etc., peeping out of their coat pockets."[2] All this implies a somewhat sweeping survey of a whole period, but we find similar traits of smartness in such characters as Dickens' Dr. Slammer in Pickwick or Dr. Jobling in Martin Chuzzlewit, and Charles Reade's Dr. Aberford in Christie Johnstone. Thackeray's Dr. Firmin and Wilkie Collins's Dr. Downward represent types of a craftier and more dubious kind. The best imaginative portrait of the high-bred physician of intellectual type is that of Lydgate, in George Eliot's "Middlemarch," a novel which, on the whole, affords the most effective side-light on English medicine in the late Georgian and early Victorian periods. The keenest edge of the author's satire is reached in the medical gossip of the gentlewomen in the tenth chapter. Mrs. Cadwallader likens Casaubon, the fossil bridegroom of the beautiful Dorothea, to a dose of medicine, "nasty to take and sure to disagree"; and Lady Chettam, in discussing Lydgate's superior family connections, observes: ·

"One does not expect it in a practitioner of that kind. For my own part, I like a medical man more on a footing with my servants; they are often all the cleverer. I assure you I found poor Hicks's judgment unfailing; I never knew him wrong. He was coarse and butcherlike, but he knew my constitution."

The same note is sounded in Major Pendennis's horror lest a lady marry her uncle's doctor, which would seem a far cry from the present esteem in which physicians are held. Henry James's "Washington Square" (1880) opens with an amusing assurance of their superior status in the United States. Balzac immortalized

---

[1] Osler mentions another: "The Reformer of Geneva" (privately printed, 1897), by Professor Shields (Princeton).

[2] Baas: *Op. cit.*, p. 770.

the French country doctor,[1] but his Horace Bianchon is a fancy portrait. Gustave Flaubert, Samuel Warren, Charles Lever, Oliver Wendell Holmes, Weir Mitchell have all approached the subject from different angles. Mitchell has made a clever study of a quack.[2] The medical students of Dickens, Albert Smith, and others are sufficiently well known. Turgenieff's Bazaroff,[3] the agnostic, anarchistic student of Eastern European type, is a genuine creation.

The conditions of **medical education** in modern times may be briefly stated as follows: The teaching of medicine as a science, as something of larger scope than its practice, began with the foundation of laboratories and with the gradual assemblage of specialties as units in university instruction. From Boerhaave's time on, great teachers have always had a limited number of brilliant pupils, who had it in themselves to be what they were, but the average medical student did not begin to come into contact with the actual working facts and experiences necessary for his "education," until he was given an opportunity to test and try things for himself, and this was only possible, even in anatomy, when practical work was substituted for routine didactic lecturing, often based upon fantastic theories emanating from the teacher's brain. German university teaching was for a long time didactic, but with the foundation of such laboratories as Purkinje's at Breslau (1824), Liebig's at Giessen (1825), or Virchow's at Berlin (1856), there was a new departure; and, although it took a long time for the new movement to get under way, yet, since the advent of Virchow and his contemporaries, the modern world has been going to school to Germany in the sciences upon which medicine is based, while England and France have mainly excelled in the organization of hospital and clinical teaching. As late as 1842, Helmholtz, graduating as an army surgeon, discussed, among other theses, a surgical operation which, like Haller in the past, he had never seen or tried. While German medicine was in the throes of "Nature Philosophy," Laënnec and Louis, Bright and Addison, Graves and Stokes, Dupuytren and Astley Cooper, were turning out crowds of competent clinicians and surgeons. At the present time, German medical education is based upon the sound assumption that all the specialties, even dentistry or obstetrics, are so many phases of physics and chemistry, and there is hardly one of her eminent teachers who has not done original work in some fundamental branch of medicine at the beginning of his career.

---

[1] Balzac: Le médecin de campagne (1833).

[2] Weir Mitchell: The Autobiography of a Quack, New York, 1900.

[3] Turgenieff: Fathers and Sons (1862).

In the United States, conditions were entirely different. In colonial times, the medical student, however poorly educated, had, at least, the advantage of being under a preceptor, and thus coming into actual contact with the details of medical practice. But in the stress and competition of a growing democracy, this custom was soon discontinued, and while one or two medical schools maintained a certain level of excellence, a vast number of inferior schools were permitted to spring up which had no reason for existence. In the first half of the century, ambitious and enterprising American students, who had the means, were going to Paris to study under Louis, or to Astley Cooper in London; in the later period, they were swarming to Virchow in Berlin, to Charcot in Paris, or to Billroth in Vienna. It was only toward the end of the nineteenth century, under the direction of Eliot at Harvard, Billings, Welch, and Osler, at the Johns Hopkins, and Pepper in Philadelphia, that medical teaching began to be true university teaching, in the sense of training a student to make use of his own mind as a substitute for blind acceptance of dogma. In the early period, scores of able American physicians, it is true, came out of inferior schools and learned their medicine by practising it, but what they accomplished was due to themselves and not to the conditions from which they sprang.

On the continent, clinical medicine was ably taught by Corvisart, Laënnec, Louis and Trousseau in Paris, Schönlein and Frerichs in Berlin, Skoda and Oppolzer in Vienna. At this time, "snap diagnoses," like sleight-of-hand surgery, were the fashion. Corvisart once remarked that the subject of an oil painting must have been a victim of heart disease and it proved to be so. Frerichs was so infatuated with this cult that he never admitted a diagnosis to be wrong. Yet the most exact methods known were employed in the clinics. Corvisart was the reviver of percussion. The stethoscope, in Laënnec's hands, was the means of developing the science of diseases of the chest. Louis and the Irish clinicians introduced pulse timing by the watch. Piorry invented the pleximeter. Wunderlich put clinical thermometry upon a scientific basis. The stethoscope was first mentioned in the Harvard Catalogue in 1868–9, the microscope in 1869–70. Wilks tells us that the clinical thermometer was regarded as a novelty at Guy's Hospital as late as 1870. Neither Keen nor Tyson saw a clinical thermometer or a hypodermic syringe during 1862–5. Billings, however, in taking care of the wounded from the seven days before Richmond (1862), had provided himself with both.[1]

---

[1] J. S. Billings: Tr. Coll. Phys., Phila., 1905, 115–116. Clinical thermometry was popularized in the United States by Édouard Séguin's books of 1873 and 1876.

In 1840, Schönlein introduced the novelty of lecturing in German at the Charité, while Geheimrat Wolff, his Berlin rival, conducted in opposition a "*lateinische Klinik*," where there was neither percussion nor auscultation, and this pedantry was not suspended until shortly before Schönlein's retirement in 1857. Schönlein's clinics, as described by Naunyn,[1] were of the highest scientific order. Upon entering the ward, the short, fat Schönlein would sink into a comfortable arm-chair beside the patient's bed, while his assistant read the case-history with the necessary details of auscultation and percussion and all the chemical and microscopical findings. He would then rise and examine the patient, and, dropping into his chair again, proceed to develop his diagnosis upon pathological grounds, and then discuss the case from the point of view of etiology and therapy. If a patient died, there was an autopsy with an "epicrisis" in which possible errors in diagnosis were discussed. After Schönlein came Frerichs (1859), who kept up the same traditions. He would examine new cases directly upon entering, and, if he found that his assistants had thoroughly studied them, the histories would be read, with all the accessory data of examination of urine, excreta, sputum, larynx, even the fundus of the eye; while microscopic slides would be demonstrated and pictures (often from his private collection) handed about among the students. He never nagged or bullied his assistants, treating them, Naunyn says, as if they were essential organs of his own body. His recapitulation of the case, with diagnosis, sometimes theatrical, was esteemed a masterpiece. It rested upon a rigorous scientific basis, yet, in closing with his subject, Frerichs favored the minute bedside casuistry of the English; and the patient, if not removed in time, sometimes heard a bad prognosis. Therapy was carefully considered by Frerichs and prescriptions forthcoming, as part of the subject, although, Naunyn thinks, the results did not greatly concern him. Upon the recovery or death of the patient, Frerichs gave a vivid and instructive epicrisis and, at the end of each semester came the "general epicrisis" in which all the cases gone over were carefully reviewed.[2] Upon such teaching as this was based the German development of internal medicine as a science, even down to the great clinics of Naunyn or Friedrich Müller. Traube, who became clinical director of the other wing of the Charité in 1853, was also esteemed for his exact diagnoses.[3] He

---

[1] B. Naunyn: Die Berliner Schule vor 50 Jahren (Samml. klin. Vortr., No. 478), Leipzig, 1908, 210, 211.

[2] Naunyn: *Op. cit.*, 212, 215–218.

[3] For example, that of aortic aneurysm by laryngoscopic detection of paralysis of the left vocal cord. Osler relates that on one occasion, when a postmortem did not confirm his views, Traube simply said "*Wir haben nicht richtig gedacht!*"

was more conscientious and sincere in bedside examination, more interested in his patients than Frerichs, and was consequently better liked in private practice; but, according to Naunyn, he knew little chemistry, was an almost servile follower of Virchow in pathology, and, in his efforts to make clinical medicine subservient to physiology, sometimes went into wire-drawn subtleties and superfine distinctions. Virchow favored Traube and hated Frerichs, so that their relations were never cordial. Naunyn relates[1] that it was a common circumstance for the two great clinicians to stalk by at the head of their classes in the Charité without taking the slightest notice of each other, and their pupils were tacitly forbidden to associate in public. Meanwhile Virchow was the bright particular star of the Berlin school, a political revolutionary in his youth, an intellectual tyrant in old age. His public lectures, at which he was often late for political reasons, were diffuse, tedious, and difficult to follow, on account of his lengthy, often involved, sentences, but he was a brilliant master at the postmortem table and merciless in examining students.[2] To the north of the old Charité stands the new Charité, an ugly, gloomy building with grated windows containing the insane, the syphilitic, and a "combined station," the patients of which were sick convicts taken from the prisons. Of this "combined station" Virchow was physician-in-chief, and here, most assiduous in his duties, he actually posed as a "clinician."[3] At Vienna, Skoda was all for auscultation, Rokitansky all for postmortems, and Oppolzer was the best all-round teacher. In England, Addison was easily the greatest clinical lecturer of his time, handsome, brilliant, and eloquent, but feared by his students on account of his cold, arbitrary manners and his martial outside. The genial, even-tempered Bright ran him an easy second, and although not so imposing in the lecture room, did more scientific work in the end and had a much larger practice. With these men, and with Hodgkin, pathology and clinical medicine went hand in hand. After them came Gull, Wilks, and Fagge, all attractive teachers. In France, Trousseau was the most vivid and picturesque lecturer of the period, setting the pace for Dieulafoy, Marie, and other teachers of the courteous, quick-minded French type. Charcot's public clinics were unique of their kind, and designed to meet the needs of the great throngs who followed them. In order to throw his

---

[1] Naunyn: *Op. cit.*, 219.

[2] His occasional bitterness Naunyn attributes to the hardships of his early youth.

[3] "Die Assistenzärzte jener Abteilung erzählten oft, wie regelmässig und ausführlich er dort die Visite mache, und wie gern er den Arzt spiele," Naunyn, *op. cit.*, 215, 222.

41

teaching into stronger relief, he demonstrated his cases in a miniature theater, the stage of which was furnished with footlights and all
the scenic accessories of illumination from different angles. The
patients stood before the footlights or in the limelight, if necessary,
while Charcot, from the side of the stage, elucidated their cases in
a slow, distinct manner, for the benefit of foreigners. When the
patient was dismissed, the pathological lesion would immediately
be thrown upon a screen at the back of the stage, and this theatrical
effect never failed of impressing his large audience. Charcot's
wonderful lectures were always carefully written out in his own
hand and handed to his assistant, as he passed out, to be published
in due course. His screen effects have now given place to the
epidiascope and the cinematograph, which has been utilized by
some modern surgeons as the only way of making a large concourse
of students see the details of an operation.[1] In the earlier American schools, clinical teaching was largely didactic, most of the
schools lacking true clinical facilities, and hospital work being usually accessible only to those who obtained positions as internes or
externes. These deficiencies were set off, in the later period, by the
postgraduate school, in which the teaching was entirely practical,
and which Flexner has satirically described as "an undergraduate
repair shop."[2] Private preceptors and quiz-masters were employed by those who could afford it during their medical courses.
A good example is to be had in Busey's account of the private
teaching of George B. Wood, of Philadelphia, about the middle
of the nineteenth century. Wood, a grave, dignified Quaker
who had a private botanic garden, spent $20,000 on diagrams
and models, and gave over $60,000 in endowments to the University
of Pennsylvania and the College of Physicians of Philadelphia,
would meet his students nightly at his private house, around a
table lighted by a silver candelabra, and here he would examine
them, line by line, precept by precept, through the two volumes
of his book on practice of medicine.[3] This method was fairly
typical of American teaching in the period. Its defects were that
it was a mere pedagogic rubbing in of what had already been
heard in routine lectures, with hardly any practical clinical experiences whatever. W. W. Keen says that the Philadelphia clinics,
"until Da Costa, in the session of 1866–67, took hold of them,
were about as inane and useless as one could imagine."[4] What

---

[1] Naunyn, for instance, has likened Langenbeck's clinic in Berlin to an arena
in which one saw Langenbeck himself, a number of backs, and great streams
of blood, a common enough experience in the larger surgical amphitheaters.

[2] Flexner: Medical Education in the United States, New York, 1910, 174.

[3] Busey: Op. cit., 31–37, 45–46.

[4] W. W. Keen: Jeffersonian, Philadelphia, 1912, xiv, 3.

clinical teaching should be is seen in Flexner's spirited account of Friedrich Müller's clinic at Munich:

"A path is opened in order to wheel the patient in. The professor reads the history, displays on the blackboard the temperature chart, then, in quick, clear fashion, explores the patient, pointing out what he finds, discoursing on its significance, suggesting alternative explanations, until he settles down on the most probable diagnosis. This furnishes the topic for development and further illustration. The etiology, the pathology, the therapeutics, of the condition are set forth with wonderful vigor and lucidity . . . A master mind at work is exhibited daily to two hundred students or more."[1]

Teaching of this type depends upon the man, and, other things being equal, has existed in the past here and there. The means of its more general extension in the present were afforded by the liberality of monarchical governments in Europe and of million-aires in America. So far as original research is concerned, brilliant investigators have seldom failed of obtaining laboratories or institutes in the end, as witness the cases of Purkinje at Breslau (1824), Liebig at Giessen (1825), Buchheim at Dorpat (1849), Virchow at Berlin (1856), Bowditch at Harvard (1871), Petten-kofer at Munich (1872), Schmiedeberg at Strassburg (1872), Liebreich at Berlin (1883), Welch at Baltimore (1884), Pasteur at Paris (1888), Koch at Berlin (1891), and Ehrlich at Frankfort (1896), or such American institutions as the laboratories established in Philadelphia by William Pepper (1895), the Rockefeller Institute in New York (1901), the Memorial Institute for Infectious Diseases in Chicago (1902), the Henry Phipps Institute for Tuberculosis in Philadelphia (1903), The Carnegie Institution of Washington (1903), the Rudolf Spreckels Laboratory (1910) or the Henry Phipps Psychiatric Clinic of Baltimore (1913). In 1859, the Chicago Medical College introduced the novelty of a three years' graded course of study, but the requirements were not rigidly adhered to. The first real reform in American medical education was made, in 1871, by President Charles W. Eliot, of Harvard, who raised the entrance requirements of the Harvard Medical School, lengthened its curriculum to three years, and graded it, providing at the same time better facilities for clinical and laboratory instructions. In 1880, the three years' course, of nine months each, was extended to four years; in 1892–93 it was made obligatory; and an academic degree was required for admission in 1901. The three years' graded course was introduced in the medical departments of the Universities of Pennsylvania and Syracuse in 1877, to be followed by Ann Arbor (1880) and others. In 1893, the Johns Hopkins Medical School, organized by President Daniel C. Gilman, John S. Billings, Henry Newell

---

[1] Flexner: Medical Education in Europe, p. 170.

Martin, and William H. Welch, was opened, and with it came the opportunity for teaching scientific medicine by modern methods. Billings's original recommendations for the Johns Hopkins Hospital, made in 1875,[1] included not only the care of the sick poor, but the graded accommodation of pay and private patients in rooms or suites of rooms, proper education of physicians and nurses, and, above all, the promotion of "discoveries in the science and art of medicine, and to make these known for the general good." He insisted that the out-patient department should be connected with the building set apart for the instruction of students, and separated from the administration buildings; that clinical instruction should be mostly given in the wards and out-patient department, and not in an amphitheater, except in the surgical unit; that medical cases should not be brought from beds to an amphitheater; that there should be two pharmacies and a training-school for nurses; and that a perfect system of records, financial, historical, and clinical, should be kept. With Osler as physician-in-chief, Welch, Halsted, and Kelly in the chairs of pathology, surgery, and gynecology, a brilliant and efficient medical faculty was soon developed, with actual work in wards, clinics, dispensaries, laboratories, and dead-house as the basis of teaching. A bachelor's degree is required for admission, the students serve as clinical clerks and surgical dressers, after the Scotch and English fashion; the laboratories and clinics coöperate as hospital units, as in Germany. Billings lectured on medical history before the hospital was opened, the subject being furthered by Osler's evenings with his students at his home and by the meetings of the Hospital Historical Club. Osler required his students to read and report on the foreign medical journals, and otherwise develop the art of self-direction. The example of Johns Hopkins soon set the pace for Boston, Philadelphia, New Haven, Ann Arbor, Chicago, and elsewhere. At the University of Pennsylvania, a fourth year course of entirely practical work was introduced in 1892–93, laboratories of hygiene (1892) and clinical medicine (1895) were added through William Pepper's efforts, and, in 1903, the Phipps Institute for Tuberculosis was added as a clinical plant. On September 25, 1906, the Harvard Medical School acquired a magnificent set of new buildings. Such American schools as the Jefferson (Philadelphia), the University of Michigan (Ann Arbor), the Rush and Northwestern (Chicago), the University of Minnesota (St. Paul), have now very good laboratory and clinical facilities, and there is much prospect of improvement in the South. The Medical Department at Washington University

---

[1] Hospital Plans, five essays, New York, 1875, 3–11, *passim.*

(St. Louis) has recently acquired a handsome endowment, and St. Paul, Minnesota, is equally well off in this respect. The two leading Canadian schools, McGill (Montreal) and the University of Toronto, are organized on the English plan and are of a high grade of excellence.

In 1909–11, Abraham Flexner, at the instance of the Carnegie Foundation for the Advancement of Teaching, made two close and comprehensive studies of the status of medical education at home and abroad,[1] and his strictures on American conditions excited a storm of comment and criticism. In a work of this small compass, it is not proposed to go into details. Flexner's descriptions of what he saw are truthful and sincere, and therefore authoritative. Many inferior medical schools, brought face to face with the fact that "An unpleasant truth is better than a pleasant falsehood," doubtless resented an invitation to go out of business if they could not improve themselves. That there have been too many American medical schools—39 in Illinois, 14 in Chicago, 42 in Missouri, with 12 survivors, 43 in New York, with 11 survivors, 27 in Indiana, with 2 survivors, 20 in Pennsylvania, with 8 survivors, 18 in Tennessee, with 9 survivors, 20 in Cincinnati, 11 in Louisville—was an inevitable resultant of conditions of growth in a democracy, as also the amazing overplus in the number of physicians—one doctor on the average for every 640 persons in the entire United States, 1 : 460 in New York, 1 : 580 in Chicago, 1:245 in Washington, D. C., as against 1:2000 in the whole German Empire and 1 : 1000 for its larger cities. The surface explanation is simple. There are more people in the world, consequently more physicians, American conditions indicating a definite lack of restrictive requirements. Billings, in his survey of American medicine in 1876, accepted these conditions philosophically for two important reasons, viz., that a young man who has spent so many years "in the study of medicine as it ought to be studied, that is to say, in preparing himself to study and investigate for the rest of his life, will not settle in certain districts," and that to set a definite standard for medical matriculation, graduation and registration would be hazardous in a country of such wide extent, since, to be uniform, it must necessarily, be made a low one.[2] Moreover, the financial and other resources for improving medical education on a grand scale were not at that time forthcoming in this country. The present ideal is summed up in Weir Mitchell's aphorism that "the rate of advance in medicine is to be tested by what

---

[1] Flexner: Medical Education in the United States and Canada, New York, 1910. Medical Education in Europe, New York, 1912.

[2] J. S. Billings, Am. Jour. Med. Sc., Phila., 1876, n. s., lxxi, i, p. 480.

the country doctor is," in other words, the people of the United States should see to it that they have the same highly trained physicians that every peasant can have in Germany. Of his early student days in the Western Reserve (1857–60), Billings wrote: "They taught us medicine as you teach boys to swim, by throwing them into the water"; and, in 1878, he believed that it would be long before the annual number of medical graduates at the Johns Hopkins exceeded 25. Yet, in the third year, there were 32, and today many are settling in the smaller localities of the South and elsewhere, showing that advantages for income and investigation have materially improved since the Centennial year. The future of American medical education is, like all other higher developments, simply in the hands of the only aristocracy we strive for— the aristocracy of an enlightened public opinion. One ideal of our country, what Emerson called its "mysterious destiny," is the old ideal of the democratic New England community—the "conversion of raw material into efficiency," and its results and failures can only be properly judged by this standard. The difficulties encountered in providing adequate medical assistance for vast tracts of territory are well illustrated in the case of Russia, where all accredited physicians have to be university medical graduates. The deficiency is supplied by the institution of "civil Feldscherism," which came into being with the emancipation of the serfs (February 19, 1861), and has been a subject of heated dispute. The military Feldschers were originally those pupils of Peter the Great's medical school at Moscow, who had suffered a *capitis diminutio* for insubordination or inefficiency and were abased to the level of playing regimental barber or nurse to the barrack hospital. The civil Feldscher has been defined as the "leib-medik of the moujik," in other words, he is a half-fledged, half-educated medical assistant, who is deputized by the government to take care of the vast numbers of peasants, of whom the *mirs* or village communities of Russia are largely made up.[1] The village doctor receives the peasant at stated intervals, the Feldscher looks after him the rest of the time, while "flying corps" of oculists and other specialists are occasionally sent across the Caucasus into Siberia or wherever needed. The Feldscher is thus a sort of *pis aller*, and the reason for his existence is a tacit agreement that it is better to have a half-doctor than no doctor at all.

The tendencies of German, French, and English medical teaching have been determined by the racial and national characteristics of these peoples, which are as definite as the physical configuration or the chemical composition of their bodies. For cen-

---

[1] Lancet, London, 1897, ii, 359–361.

turies, German university teaching has followed the ideal of academic freedom. Education being, as Flexner says, a game in which the student must make the first move, he is left to think and act for himself, and if he becomes a poll-parrot, it is his own fault. German professors and students alike migrate from town to town, as in the Middle Ages, and university appointments are not local, but based solely upon fitness and ability. The medical Faculty of Berlin is made up of outsiders. When the student has passed his university and state examinations, he may practise or, if he has distinguished himself by original research, become a Privat Docent, with the *venia legendi* or right to teach on his own account, from which status he may, if he builds up his reputation, rise through the various grades of professorship. Conditions like these make for original research and it seems natural that the very idea of public scientific laboratories or institutes for hygiene or psychiatry should have originated in Germany. Add to this the sharply drawn distinctions between *Wehrstand, Lehrstand,* and *Nährstand,* and the singular fitness of the race for classifying and coördinating knowledge. The faults of the German system are mainly along practical lines and are summed up in the phrase "survival of the fittest." The nurses, as in France, are of poor quality, but there is no dearth of clinical material, only the difficulty of making it available for large bodies of students, who are usually taught, not in the wards, but in the amphitheater. "The dullest rustic," says Flexner, "has long since grasped the idea that the professor is chosen for his skill and learning." The hospitals are full of patients, but to get in close touch with them, one must be either a *Hospitant* (Famulus) or a *Praktikant,* and the former has the advantage. The *Hospitant* can follow his chiefs through the wards and examine patients, but otherwise, as a professor's fag, engaged in recording cases, examining urine, preparing slides, and other things which Sir Clifford Allbutt designates as "merely clerks' work," his opportunities are not overwhelmingly sought for by German students. The *Praktikant* is "a non-resident interne of vague status,"[1] abruptly chosen from his class and pitchforked into the clinical arena, where, as a raw student, his ignorance is thrown into the limelight, and his chief has little time to correct his fumbling. He must sink or swim on his own merits. The German professor, a high priest of his science and its teaching, his brain stored with classified knowledge, sometimes acquires, it is said, a heaviness of mind which may degenerate into topheaviness, and his autocratic position may sometimes be manifested as a "stiff *Vornehmheit,*" an unpleasantly impersonal manner

---

[1] Flexner: *Op. cit.,* 163.

toward pupils or patients,[1] which is in odd contrast with the easy informality of the best modern English, French and American traditions. The advantages of modern French and English clinical teaching are precisely in the latter direction. The relations between teacher and pupil, professor and patient, are less official and formal, and the ideal is, in Huxley's phrase, to make the greatest possible number fit to survive. Parisian patients are even said to contribute much to the success of clinical instruction by their quick, intelligent replies.[2] In Paris, the hospitals, being public charities, are thrown open to students everywhere, and the whole aim of French teaching is bedside instruction. Ward teaching is cleverly exploited by means of *stagiaires* or student assistants, of whom each professor has to instruct a large number, and to whom two or three beds each are allotted for instruction. Stagiaires, externes and internes, are quizzed, in succession, by a running fire of questions from the chief, as he considers each case, and, so informal is procedure that it is no discourtesy for even an outsider to ask pertinent questions.[3] Clinical study is optional in the first year and obligatory from the second on. Upon graduation, the student must write and publish a thesis and it is open to him to compete for the position of *agrégé* or assistant professor by means of the *concours* or public examination. The French graduating theses differ from the German or Russian in that, as a rule, they are exceedingly clever and well-written *résumés* of what is known rather than records of original work. They are invaluable for reference. As with the French, the strong point of English medical teaching is clinical instruction. Emerson said of the English that "theirs is a logic that brings salt to soup, hammer to nail, oar to boat," and, necessarily, the physician to the bedside. The English hospitals are not, as with the Germans and French, governmental institutions or public charities, but are supported by voluntary contributions, and, with the exception of Oxford, where medical teaching is academic, and Cambridge, where it is confined to the fundamental sciences, the English type of instruction is that of the hospital medical school. Here, the student is given the same clinical advantages that obtain in Paris, the nursing system is the finest in the world, but the institutions not being connected with universities, little opportunity for post-graduate or other instruction for outsiders has been afforded until recently. Of the English clinical teacher, Flexner says, "No matter who or how many attend his lectures, his pupils are specifically those with whom he talks at the bedside." These make

---

[1] This may be regarded as of little moment, since the general testimony is in accordance with Flexner's view that, all things considered, patients and pupils are very fairly treated in Germany.

[2] Flexner: *Op. cit.*, 229–230.   [3] Flexner: *Op. cit.*, 229–230.

their rounds daily with the house physician, rendering complete case histories with microscopic findings. All are put through their paces twice weekly, in a rigorous but urbane, informal spirit, by the senior physician. The same thing obtains at the final examinations, which are a severely practical grilling, although the bearing of the examiners is said to be "informal, sympathetic, and easy, even to the point of joining in tea with the onlookers who happen to be present when that national function becomes due."[1]

In modern teaching of the fundamental sciences, the principal drawback has been the descriptive or expository lecture. In anatomy, this vogue was started by the eighteenth century men, the so-called "surgeon-anatomists," and particularly by the Monros at Edinburgh, of whom the "evergreen *tertius*," up to 1846, "unconcernedly at noon ate cranberry tarts in the midst of grinning students at a small pastry cook's, and with digestion unimpaired the next hour read his grandfather's essays on hydrophobia as part of an anatomical course."[2] Honest John Bell tilted vainly against these ineptitudes of "the windy and wordy school," pointing out that "in Dr. Monro's class, unless there be a fortunate succession of bloody murders, not three subjects are dissected in the year," while "nerves and arteries which the surgeon has to dissect at the peril of his patient's life" were demonstrated on a subject fished up from the bottom of a tub of spirits and exhibited at a distance of a hundred feet.[3] But even after Bichat, Bell and Knox, and the Warburton act of 1832, anatomy was still treated as the handmaid of surgery (or of the fine arts) until the modern Germans—Henle, Gegenbaur, Waldeyer—correlated it with histology, morphology and embryology. The dingy, ill-lighted, malodorous dissecting room, where, as Flexner says, "eight or ten inexpert boys hack away at a cadaver until it is reduced to shreds," still survives in some localities in the United States. The anatomical laboratory or institute, such as the Clover-Leaf Hall at Munich, with 500 students dissecting at once under the eye of the professor, or Mall's series of separate rooms at the Johns Hopkins, or Harvard, with its extensive cold-storage plants, is an innovation of recent date. Dearth of material and too many students are the great handicaps, and, even in Germany, Flexner argues, the most scientific lecturing will never compensate for insufficient experience in dissecting. In England, where the utilitarian view has prevailed, it is significant that there have been no great anatomists since the time of Sir Charles Bell. Horner, Holmes, Harrison Allen, Leidy and Dwight were able teachers in America, but the modern scientific methods were introduced by Minot at Harvard and by Mall at the Johns Hopkins. Mall has isolated his students in separate rooms and done away entirely with didactic, descriptive lectures.[4] France has had no physiologists of the first rank since Claude Bernard, unless we regard Pasteur as an example. In England, Foster at Cambridge and Burdon-Sanderson at Oxford, both pupils of Sharpey, set the pace in physiological teaching. In America, advanced instruction began when Bowditch opened the first physiological laboratory at Harvard in 1871 and Huxley brought Newell Martin to the Johns Hopkins (1890), the traditions being ably kept up by Porter in Boston, Howell in Baltimore and others. Two of the most original

[1] Flexner: *Op. cit.*, 188–205, 282.

[2] Lonsdale: Cited by Stirling (Some Apostles of Physiology, London, 1902, 119).

[3] John Bell: Letters on Professional Character and Manners, Edinburgh, 1810, cited by Flexner.

[4] For a full account of the status of anatomy and its teaching in America, see C. R. Bardeen, Bull. Univ. Wisconsin, Madison, 1905 (No. 115), scient. ser. iii, No. 4, 85–208.

of American physiologists, Beaumont and Weir Mitchell, had no affiliations with European teaching whatever. German physiological teaching, the highest development of the century, grew out of the great laboratories of Johannes Müller at Berlin, Ludwig at Leipzig and Voit at Munich, but, even in Germany, it is urged that there is too much elaborated lecturing and too little laboratory work (Flexner). In pathology, all Europe sat at the feet of Virchow and his pupils, of whom Cohnheim was the teacher of Welch, who, with Prudden, brought experimental pathology and bacteriology to America. He established a research laboratory at the Johns Hopkins in 1884. The French indifference to pathology is shown by the fact that two neurologists, Charcot and Marie, held the chair for years, the former succeeding Vulpian in 1872. Marie was appointed to Victor Cornil's chair, "very much," as Osler puts it, "as if Allan Starr or Dana were selected as successor to Prudden." Bacteriology has been best taught in France at the Pasteur Institute and its branches; in Germany, at the institutes of Koch, Ehrlich, von Behring and others; in Belgium, by Bordet; in America, by Welch, Simon Flexner, Vaughan, Novy, Abbott, Ernst and others. "Bacteriology," says Flexner, "transformed hygiene from an empirical art into an experimental science," and the teaching of the two has gone hand in hand since the foundation of Koch's Institute. Experimental pharmacology was first taught by Magendie in France and by Buchheim, Traube, and Schmiedeberg in Germany. Brunton, Ringer, Langley and Cushny in London, Fraser in Edinburgh, represent the height of English teaching. Wood founded clinical pharmacology in America. Cushny at Ann Arbor, and Abel at the Johns Hopkins introduced the modern German methods. Legal medicine is best taught at Vienna, where all judicial autopsies, coroner's cases, and anything medical connected with court-room procedure, is under the control of the university professor; in Paris and Lyons, in connection with the admirable service of the Prefectures of Police; and at Edinburgh, where the professor is also police surgeon. It is ably argued by Abraham Flexner that the most scientific lecturing in all the subjects mentioned will be imperfectly assimilated if the student has not received proper preliminary instruction in physics, chemistry, and general biology. In clinical medicine, not even the splendid lectures of a Charcot or a Friedrich Müller can take the place of bedside teaching, which it is one of the chief merits of English medicine to have consistently followed.

America, beginning with Elizabeth Blackwell's graduation in 1849, was the pioneer in **medical education for women.** In the United States and Canada, women can now study medicine anywhere on the same terms as men. The Woman's Medical College of Pennsylvania (Philadelphia) was organized in 1850, and the Woman's Medical College of Baltimore in 1882. The English Medical Register of 1858 contains the name of a single lady graduate of Geneva, and a second was examined and qualified in 1865. In 1874, the London School of Medicine for Women was opened with fourteen students; and, in 1896, they acquired the privilege of resident posts at the Royal Free Hospital. In the same year, the Royal College of Physicians in Ireland and the London University admitted them to the privilege of examination. No other London hospital schools are open to women, but the universities of Durham, Manchester, Liverpool, Birmingham, Leeds, and Bristol are co-educational. At Glasgow, Aberdeen, Dundee, and St. Andrew's they are given every facility, but there has been much opposition in Edinburgh. On the continent, the Swiss universities took the lead in 1876, the German states followed, one by one, Prussia being the last to throw open the right of university instruction and graduation to women in 1908. Paris, Vienna, Rome, Brussels, Upsala, and Copenhagen are all co-educational. The faculties of Paris and Bern are the most frequented. Crowds of enthusiastic young Russian Jewesses flock to the latter, and turn out huge annual batches of inaugural dissertations. The number of women graduates who get into practice is said to be relatively small, probably by reason of marriage.

Of the many admirable **hospitals** constructed in the modern period, the pavillion system attained a high plane of development in the Johns Hopkins Hospital, planned by J. S. Billings and opened in 1889, and the Hamburg-Eppendorf pavillion, opened in the same year. In hygienic advantages and economy of administration, these structures marked a great advance upon the huge, many-storied buildings of the past. The Peter Bent Brigham Hospital at Boston (1913), also originally planned by Billings, follows the same idea. With the opening of the Rudolf Virchow Hospital at Berlin (1906) a new idea was introduced, that of a community of separate pavillions as detached hospital units, and upon this plan are based such hospitals as the new Allgemeines Krankenhaus at Vienna and the Cincinnati General Hospital, both in process of construction.

The first sanitarium for phthisical patients was established at Görbersdorf, in the Waldenburg Mountains, by Hermann Brehmer in 1859. It still exists, and its success has led to the foundation of many similar institutions in mountain and winter resorts, notably those of Karl Spengler at Davos and Edward L. Trudeau at Saranac Lake in the Adirondacks. In 1876, Peter Dettweiler founded the sanitarium at Falkenstein in the Taunus, introducing the reclining chair for rest-cure in the open-air, portable receptacles for sputa, and other novelties. The sanitarium movement in Germany was especially fostered by Ernst von Leyden and there are now thousands of these institutions all over the world. Besides the mountain and winter resorts, like Asheville or Sankt Moritz, the climatic treatment includes the arid and semi-tropical, like Arizona or Yalta in the Crimea, and the maritime, like the Riviera and Algiers. The seashore sanitaria also include those for scrofula, with which the coast-lines of countries like Italy and Norway are dotted. The first international congress for tuberculosis was held July 25–31, 1888, at Paris, and, after the sixth (1901), an International Association was formed, which holds annual "conferences" in different cities and prepares for the now triennial international congresses, of which three have already been held at Paris (1905), Washington (1908), and Rome (1911). A French society of similar title exists in Paris, and publishes a

Revue. Since the gift of the Phipps Institute in 1903, the subject has awakened keen interest in America, especially through the labors of Trudeau, Vincent Y. Bowditch, L. F. Flick, Arnold Klebs, S. A. Knopf, Henry Barton Jacobs, Frank Billings, and others. The **nursing** of the sick at the hands of trained, well-bred women is an institution of modern times. The period from the latter part of the seventeenth century up to the middle of the nineteenth has been called the "dark age" of sick nursing, in which the status and competence of female attendants had sunk as low as the hospitals in which they served. Outside the Roman Catholic orders, in which discipline and decency still prevailed, this was almost universally the case. The pudgy, slatternly, dowdy looking female, of drunken and dubious habits, was the type from the old colored prints to the time of Sairey Gamp. In 1857, the servant nurses in the larger London hospitals were referred to in the *Times* as follows:

"Lectured by Committees, preached at by chaplains, scowled on by treasurers and stewards, scolded by matrons, sworn at by surgeons, bullied by dressers, grumbled at and abused by patients, insulted if old and ill-favored, talked flippantly to if middle-aged and good-humoured, tempted and seduced if young and well-looking—they are what any woman might be under the same circumstances."[1]

The idea of training nurses to attend the sick in a special school for the purpose originated with Theodor **Fliedner** (1800–64), pastor at Kaiserswerth on the Rhine, and his wife Friederike, who, in 1833, turned the garden-house of their pastorate into an asylum for discharged female prisoners, and in October, 1836, founded the first school for deaconesses (*Diaconissenanstalt*), which became the model for similar institutions in Germany and elsewhere. To the Fliedners came, in 1840, Elizabeth Fry, famous for her extension of John Howard's work in reforming prisons, and later **Florence Nightingale** (1823–1910), an English lady, born at Florence, Italy, who devoted her whole life to sick nursing and, indeed, made it the model institution which it is in English-speaking countries today. When the Crimean war broke out in March, 1854, Miss Nightingale, at the instance of Lord Sidney Herbert, then Secretary of War, went out with a body of nurses to take charge of the barrack hospital at Scutari, where her ministrations and reforms soon became a matter of history. In the face of the indifference of public officials and the opposition of narrow bureaucrats, she received the loyal support of Lord Raglan and the hardworking army surgeons, and, within ten days, was feeding nearly 1000 men from her diet kitchen, and, in three months, was pro-

---

[1] London Times, April 15, 1857. Cited by Nutting and Dock, History of Nursing, New York, 1907, i, 505.

viding 10,000 men with clothes and other necessities from her own supplies. The effect of her unexampled success was such that after her return to England a sum of £50,000—the Nightingale fund—was raised to establish a school for nurses at St. Thomas's Hospital, which was opened on June 15, 1860, with fifteen probationers, who were scientifically trained as "new style nurses." These soon filled up vacancies in the larger hospitals, which brought about a wholesale regeneration of English nursing. Nightingale nurses were sought for everywhere. The adoption of the Geneva Convention, in 1864, created the necessity for better nursing on the continent; and, in America, the movement was especially furthered by Marie Zakrzewska and Elizabeth Blackwell, the first training-school for nurses in the United States having been founded by the former in 1873. Elizabeth Blackwell (1821–1910), of Bristol, England, the first lady medical graduate (1849), Clara Barton (1830–   ), of Oxford, Massachusetts, and Louise Lee Schuyler were instrumental in organizing sick nursing and medical aid during the Civil War. In 1873, three training-schools were established at the Bellevue, New Haven, and Massachusetts General Hospitals, and the Johns Hopkins Training-School for Nurses was superintended by Miss M. Adelaide Nutting, who, with Miss Lavinia L. Dock, wrote a "History of Nursing" (1907). Miss Nightingale's "Notes on Hospitals" (1859) and "Notes on Nursing" (1860) are true medical classics, distinguished by the rarest common sense and simplicity of statement. She defined nursing as "helping the patient to live," introduced the modern standards of training and *esprit de corps*, and early grasped the idea that diseases are not "separate entities, which must exist, like cats and dogs," but altered conditions, qualitative disturbances of normal physiological processes, through which the patient is passing. While she did not know the bacterial theory of infectious diseases, she realized that absolute cleanliness, fresh air, pure water, light and efficient drainage are the surest means of preventing them.

Since the time of Pinel and Reil, Tuke and Conolly, the proper study and care of the insane has been an object of ambition, often dimly realized. When Esquirol succeeded Pinel at the Salpêtrière, in 1810, he made great reforms in housing and regimen, traveled all over France to carry out Pinel's ideas, founded ten new asylums and was the first to lecture on psychiatry (1817). Gardner Hill introduced the idea of "no restraint" at Lincoln Asylum, England, in 1836, and in 1839, in the face of bitter opposition, John Conolly discarded all mechanical restraints at the Hanwell Asylum. The abuses attending the commitment and care of the insane in private asylums were vigorously attacked by Charles Reade in "Hard

Cash" (1863). Early American institutions were the Blooming-dale Asylum, New York (1809), now the Bloomingdale Hospital at White Plains, the Friends Asylum, at Frankford, outside Phila-delphia (1817), the McLean Hospital, Boston (1818), the Hartford Retreat (1824), the South Carolina Hospital at Columbia (1828), and the New Jersey State Asylum at Trenton (1848). The latter was established through the propagandism of Miss Dorothea Lynde Dix, of Maine, whose work in ameliorating the condition of the insane in America is similar to John Howard's prison and hospital reforms. She is said to have been instrumental in found-ing no less than thirty-two asylums. With the opening of the Utica State Hospital in 1843, began what Hurd calls "the era of awakening,"[1] and by 1850 the movement for State provision for the insane was well on its way. The State asylums at Willard (1869) and Binghamton, New York (1881), were founded to set off the barbarities in the treatment of the chronic insane in county asylums. Pliny Earle, in 1867, emphasized the importance of suitable employment for the insane. In 1885, Daniel Hack Tuke made a sweeping attack on American and Canadian asylums, and in 1894,[2] Weir Mitchell pointed out the deficiencies in the proper care and treatment of the insane, discussed the general "woodenness" of boards, the evils of political control, and indicated the absolute lack of any scientific study of insanity in American hospitals. The latter idea originated with the Germans. The very first article which Griesinger penned for his *Archiv* (1868)[3] proposed a reorganization of the German hospitals and outlined the idea of a psychiatric clinic, where the patients should be studied and treated, as in hospital, before commitment or discharge. In Berlin, Ideler had demonstrated cases at the Charité in 1832, to be followed by Griesinger (1866), Westphal (1869), and Jolly (1890). Psychiatric clinics were opened at Strassburg (1872), Basel (1876), Breslau (1877), Bonn (1882), Freiburg (1887), Halle (1891), and elsewhere, the movement culminating in the fine insti-tution opened by Kraepelin at Munich November 7, 1904. On April 16, 1913, the Psychiatric Clinic, donated to the Johns Hopkins Uni-versity by Henry Phipps, and modeled along the German lines, was opened at Baltimore under the direction of Professor Adolf Meyer.

In the development of national and international regulation of **public hygiene,** necessity has been the mother of invention. There was nothing spontaneous about the movement. It was

---

[1] H. M. Hurd: Am. Jour. Insanity, 1913.

[2] S. Weir Mitchell: Proc. Am. Med.-Psychol. Ass., 1894, Utica, N. Y., 1895, i, 101–121.

[3] W. Griesinger: Arch. f. Psychiat., Berlin, 1868–69, i, 8–43.

simply forced upon the attention of legislators by the modern outbreaks of epidemic disease and by the evils resulting from crowded cities and slums, factories, ateliers, and the like, and its developments have been slow. The first big scare came from the invasion of Asiatic cholera (1826–37), which had been endemic in India for centuries, was pandemic in Asia during 1816–30, had spread over Russia by 1830, skirted Northeastern Germany in 1831, reaching England in June of the same year, and Calais, March, 1832, and invaded America *viâ* Quebec and New York. Heinrich Heine has left a graphic and memorable account of its outbreak in Paris. On the twenty-ninth of March, the night of *mi-carême*, a masked ball was in progress, the *chahut* in full swing. Suddenly, the gayest of the harlequins collapsed, cold in the limbs, and, underneath his mask, "violet-blue" in the face. Laughter died out, dancing ceased, and in a short while carriage-loads of people were hurried from the *redoute* to the Hôtel Dieu to die, and, to prevent a panic among the patients, were thrust into rude graves in their dominoes. Soon the public halls were filled with dead bodies, sewed in sacks for want of coffins. Long lines of hearses stood *en queue* outside Père Lachaise. Everybody wore flannel bandages. The rich gathered up their belongings and fled the town. Over 120,000 passports were issued at the Hôtel de Ville. A *guillotine ambulante* was stalking abroad, and its effect upon the excitable Parisians reduplicated the scenes of the Revolution or the plague at Milan. With signal intelligence, Heine puts his finger upon the chief obstacle which public health movements have ever encountered, viz., the dread of disturbing private business. In this case, an *émeute*, with barricades, was stirred up among the rag-pickers, who resented the removal from the streets of the piles of offal from which they derived their livelihood. The suspicion of secret poisoning was raised, as a counter-theory to that of infection, the cry *"à la Lanterne"* was heard, and six persons were murdered and naked corpses dragged through the streets, under this belief. Finally the public press quieted the panic, and the *Commission sanitaire* was able to accomplish something.[1] Similar panics, such as the shot-gun quarantines at the South during yellow fever, with the lugubrious "Bring out your dead!" have led to the necessity of enlightened organized control of public health.

Cholera was again pandemic in 1840–50, 1852–60, 1863–73, and at later intervals in Europe. It is still wide-spread in the Far East. Cerebro-spinal fever appeared periodically at the intervals 1805–30, 1837–50, 1854–74 and 1875 to the present time; influenza, in 1830–33, 1836–37, 1847–48, and

---

[1] Heine: Französische Zustände, letter of April 9, 1832 (Sämmtliche Werke, Cotta ed., xi, 88–102).

1889–90; yellow fever in the Southern States in 1853, 1867, 1873, 1878, and 1897–99. Typhus fever was rife during the Napoleonic wars and smote Ireland severely in 1817, 1819, and 1846. Typhoid, scarlatina, measles, and other infections appeared at intervals. Bubonic plague was spread from Hong Kong all over the world from 1894 on, and without modern sanitation, the pandemic would probably have attained to mediæval proportions. Politics came near wrecking the situation in San Francisco in 1907–8, and it was only through the Marine Hospital Service experts, who diagnosed the disease and destroyed the rodent carriers, that the city, perhaps the country, was saved. The epidemic character of poliomyelitis was first noted by Medin in Sweden (1887), and its incidence in the Scandinavian countries, Austria, and the United States (1907–10) has been severe. Its pathology was ably investigated by Simon Flexner, who isolated a germ in 1913. In 1762, a sanitary council was established in every Prussian province, but it was not until the second pandemic of cholera (1840–50) that France and England began to wake up to the task of organizing public health. In 1840, a national organization of *Conseils d'hygiène* for the cities with special committees for the provinces was formed in France, the essence of which still survives. Early English legislation, such as the Peel Act of 1802, to preserve the "health and morals" of cotton-spinners and factory hands, was directed mainly toward the hygiene of occupations, particularly child labor (1836). In 1848, Parliament passed the Public Health Act based upon the startling returns of the Health of Towns Commission (1844) and constituting a General Board of Health, with sanitary inspectors to report upon the health of cities. This was followed by a long line of progressive legislation, including the Common Lodging Houses Acts (1851, 1853), the Nuisances Removal Act (1855), the act of 1858 transferring the powers of the General Board of Health to the Privy Council, the organization of the Local Government Board (1871), the Public Health Act of 1875, the Infectious Diseases (Notification) Acts of 1889 and 1899, the Infectious Diseases (Prevention) Act (1890), the Contagious Diseases (Animals) Act (1891), the Public Health (London) Act (1891), the Isolation Hospitals Act (1893), the Local Government Act of 1894, the Public Health (Ports) Act (1896), the Vaccination Acts of 1898 and 1907, the Rivers Pollution Prevention Act (1898), and the Notification of Births Act (1907). The investigations and reforms instituted by Lord Ashley (1833) in regard to child labor led to a succession of acts (1844–1912) which have raised the age limit of employment to twelve years. Children were forbidden to work in white lead in 1878, the factory acts of 1864, 1867, 1870 and 1878 were extended to workshops in 1891, a Coal Mines Regulation Act was passed in 1896, Workmen's Compensation Acts in 1897 and 1906, and, in 1901, medical officers of health were required to keep registers of workshops and report upon them annually. The *loi Roussel* of December 23, 1874 (France) for the protection of friendless children was a great advance in humanitarian legislation. In the reforms of prisons, insane asylums and dangerous trades, the effect of the writings of Charles Dickens and Charles Reade should not be forgotten. England has now a very efficient corps of medical officers of health, a body which is almost extinct in France. Every German university has now a hygienic institute, and the German *physikus* is at once a public health official and an expert in legal medicine. In the United States, there were no advances in public hygiene beyond a few stray smallpox regulations, until after the second cholera pandemic, when a sanitary survey of Massachusetts was made in 1849. A State Board of Health for Louisiana was established at New Orleans in 1855, to be followed by Massachusetts (1869), California (1870), and the other states of the union. In 1901, only ten states had a satisfactory system of vital statistics (Kober). The American Public Health Association was organized in 1872. The cholera epidemic of 1872–73 led to the appointment of a Cholera Commission and the yellow fever epidemic of 1878 to the creation by Congress of a National Board of Health (March, 1878), which died out from lack of appropriations. Its place has been taken, since 1883, by the United States Marine Hospital Service, now the Public Health Service (1912). The latter has a good Hygienic Laboratory and its experts have done much admirable work. In such matters as the supervision of milk supply, child hygiene, and the close and accurate registration of disease—the sanitary surveys for diagnosing the condition of a sick-community which Paul M. Kellogg has likened to "blue-prints"—the best recent work has been done by the State Boards of Massachusetts and Penn-sylvania and by the Department of Health of New York City. The latter is now of especial importance in relation to the great overplus of foreign popula-tion in the Borough of Manhattan. Hygienic improvements in nearly all countries and cities have produced a very striking diminution in the death rate and a corresponding increase in the mean duration of life. The celebrated Paris sewers were installed in 1854–6, those of Hamburg about the same time, to be followed by Frankfort (1867), Danzig (1869), Berlin (1873), and Munich (1880). In England, where sewage is commonly discharged into the sea, filtra-tion beds were first employed at Wimbledon in 1876. The improvements in sewage disposal, such as those of Pettenkofer in Munich and Virchow in Berlin, or the bacterial system of purification, introduced in England by William J. Dibdin (1896), have had great effect upon the mortality of typhoid fever and other water-borne diseases, as also the purification of the water-supply by sand filtration, notably in the cases of Lawrence, Mass. (1894), the Belmont filtra-tion plant of Philadelphia (1893), and Washington, D. C. (1905). In Ger-many, the great filtration plants of Berlin and Hamburg, as, also, the ingenious "Imhof System" of sewage purification, employed in the Emscher Thal, are worthy of special note. Prussia has probably the best system of preventing the adulteration of food and drugs, punishing such offenses, not by fines, but by actual imprisonment. There was no pure food legislation in the United States until 1881, when laws were passed simultaneously by New York, New Jersey, and Michigan, and no adequate national legislation until the passage of the Food and Drugs Act of June 30, 1906, and the Meat Inspection Act of the same year, which still seems upon a somewhat unsatisfactory basis. For a long time, progressive legislation in public hygiene in the United States has been blocked by individuals or corporations who do not want their business interfered with, if they can help it, and who regard American citizenship as conferring a mysteri-ous "right" to do as they please, irrespective of their neighbors. The impudent claims of white-slave traders along these lines were quashed by the ruling of the Supreme Court of February 24, 1913, which explicitly denies the existence of any private right in itself, particularly the right of crooks to do wrong. The broad distinction, made by Tacitus, Milton and Goethe, between "license" and "liberty," as upheld by a tribunal of this eminence, has an important bearing upon our future developments in state medicine.[1]

Sectarianism and quackery flourish apace in modern life, often under strange guises. According to Flexner, "the homeopath is the only sectarian found at all in Great Britain or on the Continent," because a qualified physician, no matter what he may call himself, must pass the necessary examinations in order to practise. The proportion of homeopaths was 211:30,558 in Germany in 1909, and 193:31,154 in Great Britain in 1907. In America, under existing legislation, every species of medical sect—oste-opathy, chiropraxis, Christian Science, eclecticism, botanic medi-cine, etc.—has been permitted to flourish. In 1909, there were 15 homeopathic, 8 eclectic, 1 physiomedical, and 8 osteopathic schools in the United States. There are no sectarian institutions in Canada. In respect of fiduciary allegiance to Hahnemann's original doctrines, the modern homeopath is often like a skeptical

---

[1] For a discussion of the legal aspects of this matter, see the paper by Dr. William C. Woodward, Health Officer, D. C., in the Georgetown Law Journal, Washington, 1913, i, No. 3.

or backsliding clergyman. Scientific medicine is neither homeopathic nor allopathic. Upon the subject of treatment, which is
often very much in the air, hinges the whole matter of tolerance
of sectarianism and quackery. In the past, as we have seen,
many important features of medical treatment were actually introduced by laymen. Therapeutics, in fact, began with herb-
doctoring. It is the purely experimental status of actual therapeutics which opens a loophole for the modern quack. "The
very candor of scientific medicine gives him his chance, for, just
where the scientific physician admits his inadequacy, the charlatan
is most positive" (Flexner). In the early part of the nineteenth
century, John St. John Long, a handsome impostor, who traded upon
his influence over women without meeting their advances, had
enormous success in England, and even Napoleon consulted the
pythoness Lenormand. In 1869, Germany made the serious
mistake of passing a statute abolishing the obligations of physicians to attend urgent calls and to treat the poor *gratis*, which
incidentally let down the bars to all unlicensed practitioners
who might profess merely to treat disease. The result of this
"*Kurierfreiheit*" was a tremendous outpouring of nature-healers,
faith healers, Baunscheidtists, exorcists, masseurs and masseuses,
and devotees of vegetarianism, Kneippism, *Nacktkultur*, blue and
green electricity, and occultism of all kinds. Police returns show
that there were 1013 registered quacks in Berlin, as against 28 in
1879, and 1349 quacks out of 3584 physicians in 1909. There were
6137 registered quacks in Prussia in 1905 and 2112 in Saxony.
In Great Britain, qualified physicians have been listed in the
Medical Register since the Medical Act of 1858, but there is no
police registration of quacks. As in Germany and the United
States, they may use the mails and advertise *ad libitum*. "The
newspapers, the billboards, and the 'bus give the charlatan easy and
continuous access" (Flexner). There were 31,592 licenses for the sale
and manufacture of proprietary remedies in 1894–95 at five shillings each, and 40,734 in 1904–05. The blue book report issued
by the Privy Council Office in 1910 shows that herbalists, bone-
setters, nature-healers, abortionists, venereal and consumption
specialists, hernia and cancer quacks abound. As in Germany,
they are punished when caught in heinous malpractice or murder,
but they are usually too shrewd to be caught.[1] The British Medi-

---

[1] The case against the "healers" of the novelist Harold Frederic, whose
death at the hands of these "Christian Scientists," in 1898, was, as Bernard
Shaw puts it, "a sort of sealing with his blood of the contemptuous disbelief
in and dislike of doctors he had bitterly expressed in his books," was reluctantly
dismissed by Justice Hawkins at the Central Police Court, London, on the
ground of insufficient evidence as to Frederic's own part in the transaction. The
supposed private "right" of a person to do imbecile things, even to his own

cal Journal devoted a whole number to the exposure of quackery in 1911. In France, there are better laws, but they are not rigidly enforced. America has been a paradise for quacks, from the time of Perkins down. Nowhere have patent medicine vendors made so much money. "What need of Aladdin's lamp when we can build a palace with a patent pill" was one of Lowell's witticisms, and it illustrates the easy-going, humorous, American tolerance of humbuggery and fraud. But so long as therapeutics is what it is, the subject is almost beyond the reach of legislation, and, as in France, rigid legislation might turn out to be a farce. The newspapers, reaping the harvests they do from advertising quackery, are indifferent, although the location, citation, and exposure of quacks and quack medicines have latterly afforded rare sport for keen-sighted journalists who are something more than pressmen. The only serious attempts to take up the cudgels on behalf of the public are those made by the British Medical Association and the American Medical Association.

The **British Medical Association** was organized on July 19, 1832, in the board room of the Worcester Infirmary, at the instance of the late Sir Charles Hastings, who was then physician to the Infirmary. Since its foundation, meetings have been held in different cities of Great Britain each year, and the Association now has many home and colonial branches. Its published transactions, 1832–53, and the Provincial Medical and Surgical Journal (1840–53), succeeded by the Association Medical Journal (1853–57), were also its organs until the British Medical Journal was founded in 1857. As representing the united profession of Great Britain, the Association has played an important part in the development of English medicine in the modern period, particularly in medical reform, looking after parliamentary bills relating to public health legislation and poor laws, and in the exposure and censure of quackery, patent nostrums, and other frauds. In 1909, it published "Secret Remedies," a convenient directory of current nostrums.

In 1847, the **American Medical Association** was organized, owing its inception to a national convention of delegates from medical societies and colleges called by the Medical Society of New York State, largely through the efforts of Nathan Smith Davis, to improve the then disgraceful status of medical education in the United States. During the first fifty years of its existence, its activities were confined to discussion rather than accomplishment, and its membership was limited to specially elected delegates. Since its reorganization at St. Paul, in 1901, membership in the Association has been based upon membership in the state medical societies, which are again based upon membership in the county societies. Both state and national organizations have a specially elected House of Delegates to transact business, which welds the whole profession of the country into an efficient organized body, capable of accomplishing things. Under the earlier dispensation, the aims of the Association were restricted mainly to the narrower problems of medical ethics; its present purpose is largely the direction of public opinion in regard to public hygiene and medical education. In spite of much opposition, the Association, in the last twelve years of its existence, has accomplished many important things, first and foremost, in checking, through its Council on Pharmacy and Chemistry, the exploitation of the medical profession by patent medicine makers and the

---

detriment or destruction, is a delicate point in legal and political casuistry, but it was decided adversely, as we have seen, by the U. S. Supreme Court, in the case of those who are in a way to become a public nuisance.

swindling of the people by quacks and quackery, special records of "New and Non-Official Remedies," proprietary medicines, diploma-mills and other frauds being kept and published for public use. It has vastly improved the status of the state medical societies as to increase in membership and efficiency, so that where formerly the state societies published meagre volumes of "transactions" at rare intervals, there were, by 1910, some twenty-two state society journals, a great improvement in the centralization of periodical literature. The Council on Medical Education (1905), has, through its propaganda in the last eight years, done much to decrease the number of low grade medical schools and consequently of incompetent or unscrupulous physicians. It has also done much to secure four year courses and "full time" professors for the more scientific disciplines. According to data recently supplied by the Association,[1] there have been some 308 medical colleges, with 118 other institutions of dubious character, in the United States during the period 1765–1913, of which there were 6 in existence in 1810, 162 in 1906, and 106 in 1912–13. Since 1904, 79 medical schools have ceased to exist, 47 by merger, 32 by extinction. During 1912–13, some 14 medical colleges were closed. In the same collegiate year, there were 17,015 medical students, as against 28,142 in 1904 and 18,412 in 1911: also 3,679 medical graduates for the year 1912–13, as against 5,747 in 1904 and 4,483 in 1912. These decreases indicate, of course, the prospect of a corresponding average improvement in quality. There are "fewer but better colleges," 55 of which have met the improved requirements for admission of the Association of American Medical Colleges (January 1, 1912). The present proportion of physicians to the total population of the United States is 142,190 : 91,972,266, or one physician to every 640 persons. In proportion to the actual population, North Carolina has the smallest supply of physicians (1 : 1,193) and the District of Columbia the largest (1 : 245). Thirteen State licensing boards have recently insisted on higher preliminary requirements. Finally, through its Council on Health and Public Instruction, the Association has now public speakers in practically every state of the Union, who instruct the people directly in regard to infectious diseases. The *Journal of the American Medical Association*, founded in 1883, and now under the able editorial management of George H. Simmons, has steadily advanced to a position corresponding with that of the *British Medical Journal* in England or the *Deutsche medicinische Wochenschrift* in Germany.

There is no modern science or group of sciences which has so many current **periodicals** as medicine. In striking contrast with the eighteenth century, which had hardly a medical journal to speak of, our own time, particularly our own country, has literally swarmed with medical journals, many of which are, as the Germans say, *Eintagsfliegen*—of ephemeral duration. Each of the latter has, or has had, its use in some particular locality or as subserving the interests of some theory or sect, some "ism" or "pathy." There are too many medical periodicals in the modern world. Mr. Charles Perry Fisher estimates some 1654 current up to January, 1913.[2] Of these, 630 are American, 461 German, 268 French, 152 British, 75 Italian, 29 Spanish. Mr. H. O. Hall, of the Surgeon General's Library, estimates some 1391, kept in the reading room during 1912–13. In the first series (1880–95) of the Index Catalogue, 4920 medical periodicals were indexed; at the end of the fiscal year, July 1, 1913, the total number indexed (1880–1913) was 7970.

---

[1] Jour. Amer. Med. Assoc., Chicago, 1913, lxi, 569–603, *passim*.
[2] Bull. Med. Library Assoc., Baltimore, 1913, n. s., ii, 22.

The great number of medical periodicals, as of medical societies, in the United States is due, not to social or scientific conditions, but, as in Russia, to the extent of national territory and to the expansion of cities.[1] All countries have periodicals which are obviously "home-grown" and intended for home consumption. As a rule, the journals of the larger cities—Boston, New York, Philadelphia, Chicago, New Orleans, and others—are of better quality and of more metropolitan character than those of the several States, but the latter are being graded up to a much higher standard by the centralization of State medical societies, through which the State medical journal is also the organ of the State medical society. This is now true of 22 States, and a similar improvement is noticeable in Canada, where the *Canadian Medical Association Journal* (1911–13), to which Osler often contributes a charming literary *causerie*, takes the place of the Montreal Medical Journal, now out of running (1888–1910).

Following the Medical Repository (1797–1824) came, in order of time, the Philadelphia Medical Museum (1804–11), the Philadelphia Medical and Physical Journal (1804–09), the Medical and Agricultural Register (Boston, 1806–07), the Baltimore Medical and Physical Recorder (1808–09), the American Medical and Philosophical Register (1810–14), the New England Journal of Medicine and Surgery (Boston, 1812–28), the American Medical Recorder (Philadelphia, 1818–29), and the Philadelphia Journal of the Medical and Physical Sciences, founded in 1820 by Nathaniel Chapman. In 1825, Chapman started a new series of the last journal under the title "American Journal of the Medical Sciences," which, under the subsequent editorship of Isaac Hays, I. Minis Hays and others, has been, for a long period, the best of the American monthly medical periodicals. Among the best of the medical weeklies have been the Boston Medical and Surgical Journal (1828–1913), which has been edited by such men as John Collins Warren, Francis Minot, George B. Shattuck, and others; The Medical News (Philadelphia, 1843–1905), founded by I. Minis Hays; The New York Medical Journal (1865–1913), which, of late years, has been edited with great ability by the late Frank P. Foster (1841–1911) and by Charles E. de M. Sajous; The Medical Record (1866–1913), edited by George F. Shrady, and, latterly, by Thomas L. Stedman. The Philadelphia Medical Journal (1898–1903) and American Medicine (Philadelphia, 1901–1913) were originally edited by George M. Gould. Among the best periodicals devoted to special subjects are The American Journal of Obstetrics (New York, 1868–1913), founded by Emil Noeggerath and Abraham Jacobi; The Annals of Surgery (1885–1913); The American Journal of Physiology (Boston, 1898–1913), The Archives of Ophthalmology and Otology (New York, 1869–1913), founded by Herman Knapp; The Journal of Experimental Medicine (New York, 1896–1913), founded by William H. Welch; The Journal of Infectious Diseases (Chicago, 1904–1913), founded by Ludvig Hektoen; The Journal of Biological Chemistry (New York, 1905–13), founded by Christian A. Herter; The Journal of Medical Research (Boston, 1896–1913); The Journal of Morphology

---

[1] In 1881, Dr. James R. Chadwick, late librarian of the Boston Medical Library, said: "In England, it is possible for those who are specially interested in gynecology and obstetrics to attend the meetings of the Obstetrical Society of London, as actually happens, whereas in America the distances to be traversed are so great as to render this impossible." (Boston Med. and Surg. Journal, 1881, cv, 245.) At the present time there are national American societies of all the specialties, which meet annually.

(Boston, 1887–1901), founded by the late Charles O. Whitman, and the Journal of Experimental Zoölogy (Baltimore, 1904–1913), edited by Ross Granville Harrison.

The better sort of medical periodicals may be roughly divided into three classes: those devoted exclusively to purely scientific and experimental researches; those devoted to the specialties; and those which include, along with clinical and surgical cases, papers, original or sophomorical, upon set subjects, reports of progress, abstracts, reviews, translations, historical tidbits, facetiæ, and medical gossip. In periodicals of the first class, Germany takes the lead in number. In respect of quality, the transactions of such learned bodies as the Royal Society of London, the scientific academies of France, Prussia, Saxony, Bavaria, Austria, Italy, or the *Société de biologie* of Paris, stand first, as regards occasional contributions to physiological science. Then come the publications of university laboratories and clinics, of medical societies, institutes, and other foundations, in relation to which, the titles *Annalen, Arbeiten, Archiv, Beiträge, Berichte, Centralblatt, Jahrbuch, Mitteilungen, Monatsschrift, Sammlung, Verhandlungen, Veröffentlichungen Vierteljahresschrift,* or *Zeitschrift* usually connote something of positive value, just as *Blätter, Correspondenzblatt, Calender, Organ, Repertorium, Wochenschrift,* or *Zeitung* have a more dubious implication. Of annual publications, *Ergebnisse* contain valuable résumés of current scientific work; *Jahresberichte,* the equivalents of our year-books, are useful for bibliographical reference or statistical compilation. As a rule, the periodicals devoted to anatomy, physiology, bacteriology, psychology, anthropology, surgery, or the different medical specialties are good of their kind in any country. Except in France, the veterinary journals are of better quality than the dental. Homeopathic journals are almost uniformly poor, and journals devoted to osteopathy, antivivisection, and other fads have no scientific value whatever. Of the general medical periodicals of the third class, the *Wochenschriften* of the larger Germanic cities,—Berlin, Munich, Vienna,—the *British Medical Journal, The Lancet,* and the journals of the larger cities of Great Britain— Edinburgh, Glasgow, Dublin, Bristol—are all of the best quality. The corresponding publications in the Latin, Scandinavian, and Slavic countries are of unequal value. Aside from decadent literature, almost anything printed in France is well written, and the witty *feuilletons* in the Parisian medical journals are no exception to the rule. Some, like the *Chronique médical,* are *capables de tout* in this respect. Many of the French and Italian weeklies are printed on large, inconvenient sheets like newspapers, which suggests the advantages of Ostwald's idea of a definite *Weltformat,* a uniform size and shape for all scientific books and periodicals. An undesirable feature of the smaller-sized Latin periodicals is the actual advertisement of nostrums within the text, or the binding of such advertisements between the leaves of the journal. Italy is practically the only country which glorifies the names of its great medical men eponymically by bestowing them upon medical periodicals,[1] as in the case of *Cesalpino, Fracastoro, Malpighi, Morgagni, Ramazzini, Tommasi*. Most of the Spanish medical journals are inferior even to those of South America in quality. The beautiful language of Spain is a social rather than a scientific medium, and much of her medical literature is taken up with rhetoric and *problemas para solucionar*. Printed with aniline inks upon inferior paper, most of our valued medical productions will have crumbled or their contents faded away in a century or more, and criticism of medical periodicals seems idle or ungracious. The slightest of them may subserve a useful purpose in setting some anxious inquirer upon the path of study or of original investigation. Walsh, in his studies of medieval medicine, has emphasized the fact that the human mind soon tires of difficult or insoluble problems, and may drop a subject for centuries. To insure continuity of interest there must be constant rejuvenation and restimulation, and in no phase of modern activity is it so imperative that the scientific spirit should burn and shine like a sacred fire, as in the field of medicine. The highest function of the medical journalist today is to introduce new currents of scientific ideas and to keep them in circulation. The public would be much better protected from quacks if our newspapers drew their information from reliable representatives of the medical press, instead of from reporters, untrained in science and with a mania for advertising the sensational.

One of the most striking features of modern medicine is the tendency toward **internationalism,** even on the field of battle. In 1862, Henri Dunant (1828–1910), a Swiss philanthropist, published his "Souvenir de Solferino," and this account of the barbarities of warfare led to the International Conference of the Red Cross Societies at Geneva in 1863, and to the signing, on August 22, 1864, of the Geneva Convention, in which fourteen different States pledged themselves to regard the sick and wounded, as also the army medical and nursing staffs, as neutrals on the battlefield. This movement was warmly supported by Queen Augusta of Prussia and the Grand Duchess Maria Pavlovna of Russia, and today its intention is carried out all over the civilized world.

---

[1] The Dutch journal, "Pieter Camper," is another case in point.

In 1867, the first international medical congress was opened at Paris, at the instance of Henri Guitrac, to be followed by those at Florence (1869), Vienna (1873), Brussels (1875), Geneva (1877), Amsterdam (1879), London (1881), Copenhagen (1884), Washington (1887), Berlin (1890), Rome (1890), Moscow (1897), Paris (1900), Madrid (1903), Lisbon (1906), Budapest (1909), and London (1913). It had already been preceded by international congresses on statistics (Brussels, 1851), hygiene and demography (Brussels, 1852), ophthalmology (Brussels, 1857), veterinary medicine (Hamburg, 1863), anthropology (Spezia, 1865), and pharmacy (Brunswick, 1865), and was followed by a series on otology (New York, 1876), laryngology (Milan, 1880), criminal anthropology (Rome, 1885), tuberculosis (Paris, 1888), dermatology (Paris, 1889), physiology (Basel, 1889), psychology (Paris, 1889), gynecology and obstetrics (Brussels, 1892), tuberculosis (Paris, 1895), leprosy (Berlin, 1897), dentistry (1900), care of the insane (Antwerp, 1902), milk (Brussels, 1903), school hygiene (Nuremberg, 1904), cancer (Heidelberg, 1906), pellagra (Turin, 1906), and epilepsy (Budapest, 1909). These are only a few of such international gatherings, which include almost every specialty.

Another sign of the international spirit is the award of the Nobel prizes for medicine to von Behring (1901), Ronald Ross (1902), Finsen (1903), Pavloff (1904), Koch (1905), Golgi and Ramon y Cajal (1906), Laveran (1907), Metchnikoff and Ehrlich (1908), Kocher (1909), Kossel (1910), Gullstrand (1911), Carrel (1912), as also to Röntgen for physics (1901), Emil Fischer for chemistry (1902), and Henri Dunant for promotion of peace (1901). In America, men of great financial resources, like Carnegie, Rockefeller, and Phipps, have outpaced foreign governments in liberal endowments for scientific and medical research.

"A new era has come in medicine," says Osler, "the age of cosmopolitanism. As in finance and trade, the world has become a single country." As Emerson observed long ago, "There is no fence in metaphysics discriminating Greek, or English, or Spanish science . . . To wave our own flag at the dinner table or in the university is to carry the boisterous dulness of a fire club into a polite circle." The concerted advancement of science implies the brotherhood of man, and the cosmopolitan spirit tends to put a quietus upon narrow racial or national exclusiveness. In the interest of universal peace, the busy modern world has little use for autolatry in the Englishman, *Deutschtümelei* in the German, *chauvinisme* in the Frenchman, spread-eagleism in the American, or the *Banzai* of Japan. In science, at least, the narrow racial or religious fanatic is apt to be looked upon as a public nuisance or a private bore. The aristocracy of science differs from that of the past in freedom from the prejudice of creed or race. Hence Renan said ironically, *La science est roturière.* Virchow, with finer intelligence, intimated that it is in bad taste to mix up private religious convictions with the ideals of scientific investigation: *Die Wissenschaft und der Glaube schliessen sich aus.* The aim of the dogmatic theologian in the past has been to enslave the human mind: the free thinker has cared too little about the development of reliable character—the eternal opposition indicated in Pope's lines:

"Is he a churchman? Then he's fond of power;
A smart free thinker?—all things in an hour."

That the dogmas of theology, as assuming absolute knowledge of the unknowable, have little to do with the sacred ministry of Christ's teaching is shown by the bloody wars and massacres they have caused, and by the judicial assassination of the martyrs of truth and honor. War is still *ultima ratio*, because nations, like individuals, as the English poet said, "begin to fight when they cease to think." The surest agent of universal peace is the steady advancement of science. "Aims, methods and persistency," says Jacobi, "are common to the medical profession of all countries. On its flag is inscribed what should be the life rule of all nations: Fraternity and solidarity."

Even in its warfare upon theology, science has been concerned with only one point—that we should judge people not by what they say (their professions or creeds), but by the things they do, and, as Sherrington points out, thought is itself an action. The specious verbiage with which the quack deceives his patients or the sharp practitioner his clients, in law, politics or finance, is based upon an initial insincerity of thought, upon intentional artistic lying. "Science," as Ostwald says, "may therefore be considered as the surest and most lasting part of the spiritual treasure which man possesses. Such predictions as are indorsed by science are accepted as the most reliable ones by the intelligent majority of men." Of the importance of scientific research in medicine, another great physicist, Rowland, has spoken with a force that is apocalyptic, especially in regard to "the discontinuity of the ordinary, indeed the so-called cultivated legal mind"[1]:

"The ordinary crude mind has only two compartments, one for truth and one for error; indeed, the contents of the two compartments are sadly mixed in most cases; the ideal scientific mind, however, has an infinite number. Each theory or law is in its proper compartment indicating the probability of its truth. As a new fact arrives, the scientist changes it from one compartment to another so as, if possible, to always keep it in its proper relation to truth and error. . . . Natural laws there probably are, rigid and unchanging ones at that. Understand them and they are beneficent: we can use them for our purposes and make them the slaves of our desires. Misunderstand them and they are monsters who may grind us to powder or crush us in the dust. Nothing is asked of us as to our belief; they act unswervingly and we must understand them or suffer the consequences. Our only course, then, is to act according to the chances of our knowing the right laws. If we act correctly, right; if we act incorrectly, we suffer. If we are ignorant, we die. What greater fool, then, than he who states that belief is of no consequence provided it is sincere. An only child, a beloved wife, lies on a bed of illness. The

---

[1] H. A. Rowland: Am. Jour. Sc., New Haven, 1899, 4. s., viii, 409–411.

physician says that the disease is mortal; a minute plant called a microbe has obtained entrance into the body and is growing at the expense of the tissues, forming deadly poisons in the blood or destroying some vital organ. The physician looks on without being able to do anything. Daily he comes and notes the failing strength of his patient and daily the patient goes downward until he rests in his grave. But why has the physician allowed this? Can we doubt that there is a remedy which shall kill the microbe or neutralize its poison? Why, then, has he not used it? He is employed to cure but has failed. His bill we cheerfully pay because he has done his best and given a chance of cure. The answer is *ignorance*. The remedy is yet unknown. The physician is waiting for others to discover it, or perhaps is experimenting in a crude and unscientific manner to find it. Is not the inference correct, then, that the world has been paying the wrong class of men? Would not this ignorance have been dispelled had the proper money been used in the past to dispel it? Such deaths some people consider an act of God. What blasphemy to attribute to God that which is due to our own and our ancestors' selfishness in not founding institutions for medical research in sufficient number and with sufficient means to discover the truth. Such deaths are murder. Thus the present generation suffers for the sins of the past and we die because our ancestors dissipated their wealth in armies and navies, in the foolish pomp and circumstance of society, and neglected to provide us with a knowledge of natural laws. In this sense they were the murderers and robbers of future generations of unborn millions and have made the world a charnel house and palace of mourning where peace and happiness might have been. Only their ignorance of what they were doing can be their excuse, but this excuse puts them in the class of boors and savages who act according to selfish desires and not to reason and to the calls of duty. Let the present generation take warning that this reproach be not cast on it, for it cannot plead ignorance in this respect. . . . All the sciences are linked together and must advance in concert. The human body is a chemical and physical problem, and these sciences must advance before we can conquer disease."

This pronouncement, of fifteen years ago, is now "ancient history" and may seem to many emotional and outmoded. But it should not be forgotten that the man who made it believed with intense conviction that scientific research implies "that love of truth, that care in its pursuit, and that humility of mind which makes the possibility of error always present." Let any one who regards the scientific spirit as overweening consider Goethe's satirical lines on Haller's materialism, Ronald Ross's poem on making his great discovery or the utterances of Rowland, and let him contrast these with the logic which affirms that God is good, yet denies, implicitly at least, that Darwin's work, Mendel's work, Loeb's work, Ehrlich's work was not placed in man's hands for the ultimate good of man. In the attempt to bridge over the vast gap between the microcosm which is accessible to our senses and the unknown universe which lies beyond our ken, the human mind reveals itself at every turn as a very feeble instrument of precision. Top-heaviness is not for science. For centuries, as Huxley said, "she has played the part of Cinderella." If she is to retain her charm and fascination, she must not become too vain, nor make unduly extravagant claims. As Baas has quaintly observed: "When the summit of anything is reached, all paths lead inevitably to the bottom."

The highest function of the physician is still the relief of human suffering, not merely to drug his patients, but to care for them; and, as the surgeon must know how to think clinically, the clinician to think surgically, at need, so it is possible that, some day, the word "cure" will, as part of the same Hippocratic ideal, be restored to its ancient meaning (*curare*). Meanwhile, it is recognized that the whole medical science includes its parts, is greater than its practice, applies to the ills of society as well as human ailments.

The aim of modern medicine, coördinate with the advancement of all the sciences, is the prediction and control of phenomena,

APPENDICES

I. MEDICAL CHRONOLOGY

B. C.

4500.	Dawn of Babylonian Civilization.
4000–3000.	Beginnings of Egyptian Civilization.
2830–2530.	Age of the Pyramid builders.
2500.	Surgical operations depicted upon tomb of Pharaohs at Saqquarah.
2250.	Code Hammurabi.
1500.	Ebers Papyrus.
1300.	Berlin Papyrus.
950.	Homer.
800.	Period of Brahminic medicine.
755.	Founding of Rome.
600.	Massage and acupuncture practised by the Japanese.
639–544.	Thales of Miletus.
580–489.	Pythagoras.
522.	Democedes founds a medical school at Athens.
504–443.	Empedocles.
500–428.	Anaxagoras.
490.	Battle of Marathon.
480.	Thermopylæ and Salamis.
461–430.	Age of Pericles.
460.	Hippocrates born.
431–404.	Peloponnesian War.
430–425.	Plague of Athens.
429–347.	Plato.
400.	Thucydides describes Athenian epidemic in his history.
384.	Aristotle.
370–286.	Theophrastus of Eresos.

338–323.	Alexander the Great.
300.	Alexandrian School. Euclid.
280.	Herophilus.
212.	Archimedes killed at capture of Syracuse.
146.	Siege of Corinth.
124.	Asclepiades of Prusa (Bithynia) born.
80.	Mithridates, King of Pontus, experiments with poisons.
50.	Themison.
31 B. C.–14 A.D.	Augustus Cæsar. Celsus.

A. D.

45.	Scribonius Largus.
54–68.	Nero. Dioscorides. Aretæus.
55–63.	Lucretius describes epidemic in "De rerum natura."
78.	Plague following eruption of Vesuvius.
98–117.	Trajan. Rufus of Ephesus.
117–138.	Hadrian. Soranus of Ephesus.
125.	Plague of Orosius.
131–201.	Galen.
164–180.	Plague of Antoninus.
251–266.	Plague of Cyprian.
302.	Eusebius, Bishop of Cæsarea, describes Syrian epidemic of smallpox.
303.	Martyrdom of Saints Cosmas and Damian.
326–403.	Oribasius.
335.	Constantine closes the Asclepeia and other pagan temples.

369. Hospital of St. Basil erected at Cæsarea by Justinian.

375. Plague Hospital at Edessa.

395–1453. Byzantine Empire.

400. Fabiola founds first nosocomium in Western Europe.

476. Fall of Western Roman Empire.

525–605. Alexander of Tralles.

527–565. Ætius of Amida (reign of Justinian I.).

529. Monte Cassino founded by Benedict of Nursia.

542. Nosocomia founded at Lyons by Childebert I and at Arles by Cæsarius.

570. Marius, Bishop of Avenche, employs the term "variola."

571. Mohammed born.

580. Hospital at Merida founded by Bishop Masona.

581. Gregory of Tours describes smallpox epidemic at Tours.

590. Epidemic of St. Anthony's fire (ergotism) in France.

600. Aaron, a Christian priest, describes smallpox in his "Pandectæ."

602. Mohammed's Hegira.

610. Hospital of St. John the Almsgiver at Ephesus.

625–690. Paul of Ægina.

651. Hôtel Dieu founded by Saint Landry, Bishop of Paris.

675. Monastic records of smallpox in Ireland.

732. Battle of Tours.

738. School of Montpellier founded.

750–1258. Eastern Caliphate.

786–802. Reign of Harun al-Rashid.

794. St. Albans Hospital (England).

799. Coronation of Charlemagne.

809–873. Johannitius.

825. Xenodochium at Mont St. Cenis.

829. Hôtel Dieu (Paris) first mentioned.

830–920. Isaac Judæus.

848–856. School of Salerno first heard of.

860–932. Rhazes.

962. Hospice St. Bernard.

980–1036. Avicenna.

1021. Dancing Mania.

1025. University of Parma founded.

1050. Albucasis.

1066. Battle of Hastings.

1073–1080. Gregory VII.

1096–1272. Crusades.

1099. Order of St. John of Jerusalem founded.

1101. Regimen Sanitatis written.

1110–1113. Universities of Paris and Bologna founded.

1126–1198. Averroes. Avenzoar.

1131. Council of Rheims forbids clerics to practise medicine.

1132. Holy Cross Hospital founded at Winchester.

1135–1204. Moses Maimonides.

1137. St. Bartholomew's Hospital (London) founded by Rahere.

1138–1254. Hohenstaufen Emperors.

1139. Lateran Council interdicts surgery among the higher clergy.

1140. Nicolaus Salernitanus ("Antidotarium").

 King Roger II of Sicily restricts medical practice to licentiates.

1145. Hospital of the Holy Ghost founded at Montpellier by William VIII. of Montpellier.

1161. Jewish physicians burned at Prague on charge of "poisoning wells."

1163. Council of Tours ("Ecclesia abhorret a sanguine").

1167–68. Migration of students from Paris to Oxford to form a "studium generale."

1180. Roger of Parma completes his "Practica chirurgiæ."

1181. Montpellier declared a free school of medicine.

1187. Mohammedans conquer Jerusalem.

1191. Teutonic Order approved by Clement III.

1193–1280. Albertus Magnus.

1197. St. Mary's Spital in London.

1198. Hospital movement inaugurated by Innocent III.

1201–1277. Saliceto.

1204. Innocent III opens Santo Spirito Hospital in Sassia.

1204. University of Vicenza founded (by migration of students).

1209. Migration of students from Oxford to Cambridge.

1210. Collège de St. Côme founded at Paris by Jean Pitard.

1211. Innocent III recognizes University of Paris.

1213. Salerno made a university by Frederick II.

1214. University of Palencia founded by Alphonso VIII.

1214–94. Roger Bacon.

1214. Ugo Borgognoni made city physician of Bologna at a fixed salary.

1215. Magna Charta.
St. Thomas's Hospital founded by Peter, Bishop of Winchester.

1222. University of Padua founded (migration of students from Bologna).

1223–1226. Louis VIII 2000 lazar houses in France.

1224. Frederick II issues law regulating the study of medicine and founds University of Messina.

1225. Frederick II founds University of Naples.

1227–1274. Thomas Aquinas.

1228. University of Vercelli founded (abolished, 1372).

1231. Salerno constituted a medical school by Frederick II.
Gregory IX issues bull *Parens scientiarum* authorizing faculties to govern universities.
Frederick II issues law authorizing a quinquennial dissection at Salerno.

1233. Apothecary shop at Wetzlar.
Gregory IX charters University of Toulouse as a "studium generale."

1234–1312. Arnold of Villanova.

1235–1315. Raymond Lully.

1241. Law of Frederick II favoring dissection and regulating surgery and pharmacy.
University of Siena founded.

1242. Roger Bacon refers to gunpowder.

1243.   University of Salamanca founded by Ferdinand III of Castile.

1247.   Hospital of St. Mary of Bethlehem founded as a priory by Simon Fitzmary.
Council of LeMans prohibits surgery to monks.

1248.   University of Piacenza founded by Papal charter (reconstituted, 1398).

1249.   University College (Oxford) founded by William of Durham.

1250-1320. Peter of Abano.

1250.   Roland of Parma, surnamed Capellati, edits the surgery of Roger of Palermo.
Joinville describes scurvy in troops of Louis IX at siege of Cairo.

1252.   Bruno of Longoburg.

1254.   Alphonso the Wise founds University of Seville.

1256.   Enfranchisement of serfs at Bologna.

1257.   Sorbonne founded at Paris.

1263.   Balliol College (Oxford) founded.

1264.   Merton College (Oxford) founded.

1265.   English House of Commons organized.

1265-1308. Duns Scotus.

1265-1321. Dante.

1266.   End of Western Caliphate.
University of Perugia founded.

1266   Teodorico Borgognoni teaches aseptic treatment of wounds.

1267.   Council of Venice forbids Jews to practise medicine among Christians.

1275.   Saliceto completes his treatise on surgery.

1284.   Peterhouse College (Cambridge) founded.

1282.   Sicilian Vespers.

1285.   Salvino degli Armati invents spectacles.

1287.   Plica Polonica in Poland after Mongol invasion.

1289.   University of Montpellier (1181) chartered by Nicholas IV as a "studium generale."

1295-96.   Lanfranc completes his treatise on surgery.

1300.   University of Lerida founded by James II of Spain.
Boniface VIII issues bull *De sepulturis*.

1302.   Creation of the States General in France.
First post-mortem for medico-legal purposes.

1303.   Boniface VIII charters universities of Rome and Avignon.

1304.   Henri de Mondeville teaches anatomy at Montpellier.

1305.   Clement V charters Universities of Orleans and Angers.
City Hospital of Siena established.

1308.   Clement V charters University of Perugia.

1309.   University of Coimbra chartered by King Diniz of Portugal (reconstituted, 1772).
Papal See removed to Avignon.

1312.   University of Palermo founded.
Henri de Mondeville's surgery completed.

1315.   Mondino makes his first public dissection of a human subject.

1316.	City surgeon at Lübeck at 16 marks ($4) per annum. Mondino's "Anathomia" written.	1346.	Clement VI charters University of Valladolid ("studium generale," 1418). Cannon used at battle of Crécy.
1317.	John XXII issues bull *Spondent pariter* against abuses of alchemy.	1347.	Clement VI charters University of Prague as a "studium generale."
1318.	University of Treviso chartered by Frederick the Fair.		Pembroke Hall (Cambridge) founded.
1319.	First criminal prosecution for body-snatching.	1348.	Board of Health and quarantine (*quaranta giorni*) established at Venice.
1320	University of Florence founded.	1348–1350.	Black Death.
1321.	John XXII issues bull establishing medical school at Perugia.		Guy de Chauliac succors plague-stricken at Avignon.
1326.	John XXII issues bull *Super illius specula* against practice of magic.	1349.	Clement VI charters University of Florence as "studium generale."
		1350.	Trinity Hall (Cambridge) founded.
1328.	City Physician at Strassburg.	1354.	Pedro IV founds University of Huesca.
1330.	Invention of gunpowder.	1355.	Charles IV charters University of Arezzo (1215) as "studium generale."
1331.	First mention of firearms by Muratori.	1357.	Charles IV charters University of Siena (1241) as a "studium generale."
1332.	John XXII charters University of Cahors as a "studium generale."		
1333.	Public medico-botanical garden at Venice.	1360.	Innocent VI recognizes University of Bologna as a "studium generale."
1336–1453.	Hundred Years' War.		
1338.	Exodus of students to Pisa.	1361.	University of Pavia chartered by Charles IV.
1339.	Benedict XII charters University of Grenoble as a "studium generale."	1363.	Guy de Chauliac completes his "Chirurgia magna."
1340.	14,000 students at Oxford.	1364.	Casimir the Great charters University of Cracow.
1343.	Clement VI charters University of Pisa as "studium generale."		Duke Rudolph IV founds University of Vienna.
1345.	First apothecary shop in London.	1365.	University of Orange founded by Charles IV.

43

674   HISTORY OF MEDICINE

1367. University of Fünfkirchen founded by King Louis of Hungary.
1370. John of Arderne writes surgical treatises.
1374. City ordinance of Reggio against the plague.
Return of Popes to Rome.
1376. Board of medical examiners in London.
1379. Clement VII charters Universities of Erfurt and Perpignan.
1385. Urban VI charters University of Heidelberg as a "studium generale."
1388. Urban VI charters University of Cologne as a "studium generale."
Salaried city veterinarian at Ulm.
1389. Urban VI recharters University of Erfurt.
1391. Boniface IX charters University of Ferrara as a "studium generale."
University of Lerida permitted to dissect a body every three years.
1399. Beginning of "Acta Facultatis Medicæ Viennensis" (May 6).
1402. Boniface IX charters University of Würzburg.
1404. University of Turin founded.
First public dissection at Vienna (February 12).
1406. Emperor Wenzel makes surgery respectable in Germany.
1409. Alexander V charters University of Leipzig as a "studium generale" (September 9).
Studium generale at Aix in Provence.
Insane asylum at Seville.
1410. Insane asylum at Padua.

1411. University of St. Andrews founded by Bishop Henry Wardlaw.
1412. University of Turin founded by Counts of Savoy (refounded, 1431).
1419. Martin V charters University of Rostock.
1422. University of Parma founded.
1425. Insane asylum at Saragossa.
1426. University of Louvain founded.
1431. Charles VII founds University of Poitiers (chartered by Eugenius IV).
1437. Eugenius IV charters University of Caën.
1441. University of Bordeaux founded.
1445. Alphonso of Aragon charters University of Catania.
1448. Invention of printing.
1450. Cardinal Cusanus suggests timing the pulse and weighing blood and urine.
Nicholas V founds University of Barcelona.
University of Treves founded (academic sessions, 1473).
1452. Barber surgeons of Hamburg (Meister Bartscheerer) incorporated.
University of Valence founded.
Ratisbon ordinance for midwives (Regensburger Hebammenbuch).
1453. Fall of Constantinople (end of Byzantine Empire).
University of Glasgow founded as a "studium generale."

1455.	University of Freiburg founded by Albrecht VI (first session, 1460).	1474.	University of Saragossa founded.
1456.	University of Greifswald founded by Bull of Calixtus III. Ospedale maggiore at Milan.	1475.	Sixtus IV charters University of Copenhagen (opened, 1479).
1457.	Purgation-Calendar printed by Guttenburg (first medical publication).	1476.	Saliceto's "Cyrurgia" printed. Saliceto describes renal dropsy. Sixtus IV charters University of Mainz.
1459.	Pius II founds University of Ingolstadt (academic instruction, 1472).	1477.	Universities of Tübingen and Upsala founded.
1460.	University of Basel founded by citizens of Basel. Heinrich von Pfolspeundt writes treatise on surgery.	1478.	First edition of Celsus printed at Florence. First edition of Ketham's "Fasciculus medicinæ" printed. Mondino's "Anathomia" printed at Leipzig. Spanish Inquisition.
1462.	Bloodletting-Calendar printed at Mainz.	1479.	First edition of Avicenna printed.
1463.	Pius II charters University of Nantes.	1480.	Latin text of "Regimen Sanitatis" printed.
1465.	Paul II charters Universities at Bourges and Budapest.	1484.	Innocent VIII authorizes burning of witches in bull *Summis desiderantes*.
1469–71.	Ferrari da Grado's "Practica" printed.	1486.	First Latin edition of Rhazes printed.
1470.	Medical treatises by Valescus de Taranta, Jacopo de Dondis and Matthæus Sylvaticus printed.		English epidemic of sweating-sickness.
		1489.	168 bath houses at Ulm. "Malleus malleficarum" (Witches' Codex) of Jacob Sprenger printed.
1471.	Treatises by Mesue and Nicolaus Salernitatus (Antidotarium) printed.	1490.	University of Heidelberg moves to Speyer on account of plague.
1472.	University of Ingolstadt opened. Hochenburg *Regimen sanitatis* (German text) printed. Bagellardo's treatise on pediatrics printed.		Theodoric describes soporific potion used in surgery.
		1491.	Hortus sanitatis printed.
		1492.	Discovery of America.
1473.	Simone de Cordo's "Synonyma" printed (first medical dictionary).		John of Gaddesden's "Rosa anglica" printed. Nicholas Leonicenus corrects botanical errors in Pliny.

1493.   Paracelsus born.
          Smallpox in Germany.
1494.   University of Aberdeen
          founded.
          First Aldine e d i t i o n
          printed.
1495.   Maximilian I issues Edict
          against   Blasphemers
          (first mention of syph-
          ilis).
1496.   Albert Dürer's drawing
          of a syphilitic printed.
1496–1500. European pandemic of
          syphilis.
1497.   Aldine edition of Theo-
          phrastus printed.
1499.   University of Alcala
          founded.
          Johann Peyligk publishes
          anatomical drawings.
1500.   Jacob Nufer performs
          first Cæsarean section
          on living subject.
          B e r e n g a r i o da Carpi
          treats syphilis w i t h
          mercurial inunctions.
1501.   Alexander VI charters
          University of Valencia.
          Magnus Hundt's "An-
          thropologium"   pub-
          lished.
          Morbus Hungaricus pan-
          demic in Europe.
1502.   Maximilian I constitutes
          University of Witten-
          berg as a "studium
          generale" (July 6).
1504.   University of Santiago
          (Spain) founded.
1505.   Royal College of Surgeons
          of Edinburgh founded.
          Julius II charters Univer-
          sity of Seville.
1506.   University of Frankfort
          on the Oder founded by
          bull of Julius II.
1507.   Benivieni's collection of
          post-mortem sections
          printed.

1508.   University of Madrid
          founded.
          Guaiac wood brought
          from America.
          Jerome of Brunswick's
          Book of Wound-Sur-
          gery published.
1509–1547. Reign of Henry VIII.
1510.   Ambroïse Paré born.
          Peter Hele (Henlein) of
          Nuremberg   m a k e s
          pocket watches.
          Pandemic influenza.
1513.   Röslin's R o s e g a r t e n
          printed.
1514.   Vesalius born.
          Gunshot wounds first de-
          scribed in Vigo's "Prac-
          tica."
          Brissot opposes deriva-
          tive blood-letting.
1517.   Fugitive   anatomical
          plates published by
          Johann S c h o t t of
          Mainz.
          Gersdorff's   Field-Book
          of Wound-S u r g e r y
          published.
          Linacre's first translation
          of Galen published.
1517–21. Reformation.
1518.   Royal College of Physi-
          cians of E n g l a n d
          founded.
          Nuremberg   ordinance
          regulating sale of food.
1518–1545. Collège de France (Paris).
1519–1556. Charles V, King of Spain
          and Emperor of Ger-
          many.
1519–1522. Magellan   circumnavi-
          gates the globe.
1519.   Friesen's "Spiegl der
          Artzny" and "Synon-
          ima" published.
1521.   Veithes, a Hamburg phy-
          sician, burned for de-
          livering a woman in la-
          bor.

1521–1523. Berengario da Carpi publishes anatomical treatises.

1524. Linacre foundation of medical lectures at Oxford and Cambridge.

Cortes erects first hospital in city of Mexico.

Lucas van Leyden's portrait of Ferdinand I of Spain (adenoid face).

1525. First Latin translation of Hippocrates published at Rome.

1526. Clement VII charters University of Santiago.

"Gymnasium Ægidianum" founded at Nuremberg.

First (Aldine) Greek text of Hippocrates published at Venice.

Paracelsus founds chemotherapy.

1527. University of Marburg founded (May 30) by Philip, Landgrave of Hesse (first Protestant university).

1527. Sack of Rome by Charles V (decline of Italian humanism).

1528. First Aldine edition of Paul of Ægina.

1529. Sweating sickness spreads over Europe.

1530. Fracastorius' poem on syphilis published.

Otto Brunfels publishes his atlas of plants.

Sarsaparilla introduced.

1531. Clement VII founds University of Granada.

1532. Albert Dürer's treatise on human symmetry published.

Rabelais publishes first Latin version of the aphorisms of Hippocrates.

1533. Charles V issues Constitutio Criminalis Carolina.

Buonafede holds first chair of materia medica at Padua.

Montaigne born.

1534. Aldine edition of Ætius published.

Jesuit order founded.

1535. Mariano Santo di Barletta gives first account of median lithotomy.

1536. Ambroïse Paré makes first excision of elbow-joint.

1537. Vesalius graduates at Basel.

Dryander's "Anatomia" published.

1538. Vesalius publishes his "Tabulæ anatomicæ sex."

1540. English barbers and surgeons united as "Company of the Barber Surgeons."

Statute of Henry VIII permitting four dissections annually.

Valerius Cordus discovers sulphuric ether.

Mattioli treats syphilis by internal use of mercury.

Servetus describes the pulmonary circulation.

Sebastianus Austrius publishes his pediatric treatise.

1542. Leonhard Fuchs attempts a rational botanical nomenclature.

1543. Copernicus describes revolution of planets around the sun.

Vesalius publishes the "Fabrica" (June 1) and founds modern anatomy.

English apothecaries legalized by act of Parliament.

1544.   University of Königsberg founded by Albert III (August 17).

St. Bartholomew's Hospital refounded under superintendence of Thomas Vicary.

1545.   Paré improves amputation and treatment of gunshot wounds.

Raynald translates Röslin as "The Byrth of Mankynde."

1545–1563. Council of Trent.

1546.   Valerius Cordus publishes first pharmacopœia.

Ingrassias describes stapes.

Jerome Bock's "Kräuterbuch" published.

1547.   Insane asylum of St. Mary of Bethlehem ("Bedlam") founded at London.

1548.   Charles V declares surgery honorable.

1549.   Anatomical theater at Padua.

1550.   Paré's essay on podalic version published.

Bartolommeo Maggi proves that gunshot wounds are not poisonous.

Hollerius prescribes spectacles for myopia.

1551.   Anatomical theaters at Paris and Montpellier.

1552.   Caius publishes treatise on sweating sickness.

1553.   Servetus burned.

The collection "De Balneis" published.

University of Lima founded.

1554.   Johann Lange describes chlorosis (morbus virgineus).

Jacob Rueff's midwifery (De conceptu) published.

Editio princeps of Aretæus printed at Paris.

1555   Diet of Augsburg.

Pierre Franco performs suprapubic lithotomy.

1556–1598. Philip II.

1558.   Ferdinand I charters and opens University of Jena (February 2).

Cornaro publishes treatise on personal hygiene.

1558–1603. Reign of Elizabeth.

1559.   Columbus describes the pulmonary circulation.

Caspar Stromayer's ophthalmic treatise (Sudhoff).

1560.   University of Douai (Lille) founded.

Maurolycus describes myopia, hypermetropia and the optics of the lens.

Francis Bacon born.

1561.   Fallopius publishes his "Observationes anatomicæ."

Paré founds orthopedics.

Pierre Franco's treatise on hernia published.

1562.   Witchcraft made a capital offense in England.

1562–1568. Pandemic plague.

1562–1629. Huguenot wars in France.

1563.   Witchcraft a capital crime in Scotland.

1564.   Shakespeare born.

Medical dictionaries of Stephanus and Gorræus published.

Eustachius discovers abducens nerve and suprarenal glands.

1565. Statute of Elizabeth permitting dissection of executed criminals.

Jean Nicot brings tobacco plant to France.

Johann Sturm's "Akademie" opened at Strassburg.

1567. Ulisse Aldrovandi establishes botanical garden in Bologna.

Paracelsus' account of miners' phthisis published.

1568. Constantino Varolio describes the pons Varolii.

1570. Felix Platter urges psychic treatment of the insane.

1571. Battle of Lepanto.

Francesco Bravo describes "tabardillo" (Spanish typhus).

Caroline Medico-Chirurgical Institute of Stockholm founded.

1572. Geronimo Mercuriali publishes his treatise on skin diseases.

Lead poisoning (*colica Pictonum*) in Poitou.

1573. Adam Lonitzer's ordinance for midwives (Frankfort on the Main).

1574. Gregory XIII charters University of Oviedo.

1574–1577. Pandemic plague.

1575. Universities of Leyden and Helmstädt founded.

Paré introduces massage and artificial eyes.

1576. Paracelsus publishes tract on mineral waters.

1578. Guillaume de Baillou describes whooping cough as "quinta."

William Harvey born.

Rudolph II charters University of Altorf (opened, 1580).

1580. Pandemic influenza.

Prospero Alpino introduces moxa from the Orient.

1581. Rousset's treatise on Cæsarean section published.

1582. University of Edinburgh chartered by James VI.

Augsburg "Collegium medicum" founded.

1583. George Bartisch's "Augendienst" published.

Cesalpino classifies plants in his "De plantis."

Della Porta's "Phytognomonica" published.

1583–1600. Diphtheria ("garotillo") epidemic in Spain.

1584. Sir Walter Raleigh brings curare from Guiana.

1585. Guillemeau's treatise on diseases of the eye published.

1586. University of Graz founded.

Della Porta's "Physiognomia" published.

1587. Aranzio gives first description of deformed pelvis.

1588. Defeat of Spanish Armada.

Anatomical theater at Basel.

1589. Galileo demonstrates law of falling bodies.

1589–1611. Henri IV.

1590. Invention of compound microscope by Hans and Zacharias Janssen.

José d'Acosta describes mountain sickness.

1591.   Pandemic plague.
University of Dublin (Trinity College) founded.

1593.   Marischal College (Aberdeen) founded by George Keith, Earl of Marischal.

1595.   Libavius publishes first treatise on chemistry ("Alchymia").
Quercetanus uses calomel.
City of Passau issues ordinance for midwives.

1596.   University of Cagliari (Sardinia) founded.
Harington's "Metamorphosis of Ajax" published.

1597.   Tagliacozzi publishes treatise on plastic surgery.
Codronchi's treatise on medical jurisprudence published.
Israel Spach's "Gynæcia" published.
James VI of Scotland publishes "Demonology."

1598.   Edict of Nantes.
Mercurio gives picture of the "Walcher position" in "La Comare."
Carlo Ruini publishes treatise on diseases of the horse.

1599.   Ulisse Aldrovandi's "Historia animalium" published.
Royal Faculty of Physicians and Surgeons of Glasgow established.

1600.   Queen Elizabeth charters East India Company (December 31).
Gilbert's "De magnete" published.

University of Harderwijk founded.
"Foglietti" published in Venice.

1602.   "Hamlet" produced.
Felix Platter publishes the first classification of diseases.
Fedeli publishes treatise on medical jurisprudence.

1603.   Prince Cesi founds the Accademia dei Lincei at Rome.

1604.   Johann Kepler demonstrates inversion of optic image on the retina.

1605.   Verhoeven publishes newspaper at Antwerp.

1607.   Settlement of Jamestown, Virginia (May 13).
Rudolph II charters University of Giessen (May 19).

1609.   United Netherlands.
Henry Hudson anchors "Half Moon" in New York Bay.
Kepler's "Astronomia Nova" published.
Jalap brought from Mexico.
Louise Bourgeois publishes obstetric treatise.

1610.   Galileo devises microscope.
Cristoforo Guarinoni describes gummata of the brain.
Minderer introduces ammonium acetate (spiritus Mindereri).
Rosicrucian Order founded.

1611.   Union of Brandenburg and Prussia.

Villa Real publishes account of garotillo (diphtheria).

1614. University of Groningen founded.
Rodericus à Castro publishes treatise on medical jurisprudence.

1615. *Frankfurter Postamts-zeitung* (newspaper) published.

1616. Harvey begins to lecture on the circulation of the blood.
University of Paderborn founded.
Cesare Magati treats wounds with plain water.

1617. Briggs and Napier introduce logarithms.
Guild of Apothecaries of the City of London founded.

1618. First edition of London Pharmacopœia.
Countess of Chinchon cured of malarial fever by cinchona.

1618–1648. Thirty Years War.

1619. Christoph Scheiner's "Oculus" published.

1620. Landing of the Pilgrims at Plymouth, Massachusetts (December 21).
Bacon's "Novum Organum" published.
Botanic Garden at Strassburg.
Raymund Minderer's "Medicina militaris" published.
Van Helmont teaches that a chemical substance survives in its compounds (Conservation of Matter).

1621. Universities of Strassburg and Rinteln founded by Emperor Ferdinand II.
Zacchias publishes treatise on medical jurisprudence.
Cornelius Drebbel improves the microscope.

1622 Aselli discovers the lacteal vessels.
London Weekly News published.

1622–1763. Molière.

1623. New Netherlands colonized by the Dutch.
University of Alcala moved to Madrid.
Medical Faculty added to University of Altdorf.

1625. Botanic Garden at Altdorf.

1626. Jardin des Plantes at Paris.

1628. Harvey publishes "De Motu Cordis."

1629. Botanic Garden at Jena.
Severino makes first resection of the wrist.
Petroleum described by the Franciscan friar De la Roche d'Allion.

1630. Thuillier père shows that ignis sacer (ergotism) is due to corn smut.

1631. Théophraste Renaudot edits *Gazette de France*.

1632. Gustavus Adolphus founds University of Dorpat.
Botanic Gardens at Oxford and Hampton Court.

1632–77. Spinoza.

1634. Universities of Utrecht and Sassari founded.

1635.   Richelieu founds the Académie française.

1636.   Harvard College founded by act of General Court of Massachusetts (October 28). Assembly of Virginia passes act regulating physician's fees.

1637.   Descartes shows that accommodation depends upon change in form of lens. Royal College of Physicians issues report upon public health.

1638.   Cornelius Drebbel improves the thermometer. Padre Acugna, a Portuguese monk, introduces oil of copaiva. Assembly of Maryland passes act regulating surgeon's fees.

1639.   First printing press in North America (Cambridge, Massachusetts). First hospital in Canada. Virginia Assembly passes law regulating medical practice (October 2).

1640.   Queen Christina charters University of Abo. Bay State Psalm Book published. Juan del Vigo introduces cinchona into Spain. Severino produces local anesthesia by means of snow and ice. Werner Rolfink revives dissecting ("rolfinken") in Germany.

1640–1688. The Great Elector.

1642.   Jacob Bontius describes beriberi.

1642–1649. Civil War in England.

1643.   Newton born. Torricelli constructs barometer.

1643–1715. Louis XIV.

1644.   Descartes treatise on dioptrics published. Hôtel Dieu in Montreal established. Matthew Hopkins, the witch finder.

1645.   Battle of Naseby. "Invisible Society" founded in London.

1646.   Sanctorius describes new instruments in his commentary on Avicenna. Diemerbroek publishes monograph on plague. Syphilis appears in Boston, Mass.

1647.   Pecquet discovers thoracic duct. Wirsung discovers pancreatic duct. Giles Firmin lectures on anatomy in Massachusetts.

1648.   Peace of Westphalia. University of Bamberg founded. Van Helmont's "Ortus medicinæ" published. Athanasius Kircher describes the ear trumpet. Glauber prepares fuming hydrochloric acid. Francesco Redi disproves theory of spontaneous generation.

1649.   Act regulating the practice of medicine in Massachusetts.

1649–1660. Commonwealth in England.

1650.   Glisson describes rickets.

1651. Harvey's treatise on the generation of animals published.
Highmore discovers the maxillary sinus.
Rudbeck discovers the lymphatics of the intestines.

1652. Thomas Bartholin describes the intestinal lymphatics.
Johann Hoppe describes miliary fever.
Lorenz Bausch of Erfurt founds the *Gesellschaft naturforschender Freunde*.

1653-1659. Protectorate in England.

1654. Otto von Guericke of Magdeburg invents the air-pump.
Glisson describes the capsule of the liver.
University of Herborn founded.

1654-1715. Reign of Louis XIV.

1655. University of Duisburg founded.
Scultetus publishes his "Armamentarium."

1656. Wharton's "Adenographia" published.
Rolfink shows that cataract is clouding of the lens.
Lazar houses abolished in France.

1657. Accademia del Cimento founded at Florence.
Wolfgang Hoefer describes cretinism in his "Hercules medicus."
Jan à Gehema urges that field chests of drugs be furnished armies by the state.
Comenius publishes "Orbis pictus."

1657-1669. Pandemic malarial fever.

1658. Swammerdam describes red blood-corpuscles.
Wepfer demonstrates lesion of the brain in apoplexy.
Athanasius Kircher attributes plague to a contagium animatum.

1659. Malpighi outlines lymphadenoma or Hodgkin's disease.
Diphtheria at Roxbury, Massachusetts.

1660. Schneider shows that nasal secretion does not come from pituitary body (Galen).
Willis describes puerperal fever.
Hermann Conring publishes statistical treatise (*Examen rerum publicarum*).
Malpighi discovers anastomosis between capillaries.

1660-85. Charles II.

1661. Stensen discovers duct of parotid gland.
Malpighi publishes first account of capillary system (*De pulmonibus*).
Robert Boyle defines chemical elements.
Scarlatina appears in England.

1662. Charles II charters the Royal Society.
Newton and Leibnitz originate the differential calculus.
John Graunt founds medical statistics.
Descartes publishes first treatise on physiology (*De homine*).

Lorenzo Bellini discovers excretory ducts of kidneys.

De Graaf shows that ova arise in the ovary.

Meibom discovers Meibomian glands.

1663. First hospital in American colonies (Long Island, N. Y.).

Hendrik van Roonhuyze describes operation for vesico-vaginal fistula.

Sylvius treats of digestion as a fermentation.

1664. Willis's "Cerebri anatome" published (classification of cerebral nerves).

Swammerdam discovers valves of lymphatics.

De Graaf examines pancreatic juice.

Solleysel transmits glanders from horse to horse.

De la Martinière describes gonorrheal rheumatism.

1665. Newton announces law of gravitation.

Great Plague of London.

Richard Lower transfuses blood from dog to dog.

First volume of Philosophical Transactions (Royal Society) published.

Colbert founds Académie des sciences (Paris).

University of Kiel founded by Duke Christian Albrecht of Holstein.

First number of *Journal des sçavans* published (January 5).

Malpighi discovers red blood-corpuscles.

1666. Great Fire of London.

University of Lund founded.

Malpighi's treatise on the viscera published.

Coroners appointed for each county of Maryland.

1666–1675. Smallpox in Europe.

1667. Robert Hooke describes plant cells in his "Micrographia."

Denys of Paris first transfuses blood in man.

Swammerdam describes docimasia of fetal lungs.

Hooke shows true function of lungs by artificial respiration.

Walter Needham shows that fetus is nourished by the placenta.

1668. Mayow finds "igneo-aërial spirit" (oxygen) essential for combustion and respiration.

Mauriceau's obstetric treatise published.

Yellow fever appears in New York.

1668–1672. Epidemic dysentery in England (described by Sydenham and Morton).

1669. Richard Lower's "Tractatus de corde" published.

Stensen founds stati-graphic geology (*De solido intra solidum*).

Lower shows that venous blood takes up air in the lungs.

1670. Malpighi discovers Malpighian bodies in spleen and kidneys.

Swammerdam discovers muscle-tonus.

Willis discovers sweet taste of diabetic urine ("Demedicamentorum operationibus").

Kerckring describes valvulæ conniventes of small intestine.

Physic Garden at Edinburgh.

Arsenic poisoning at Paris (St. Croix and Brinvilliers).

1671. Redi's treatise on the generation of insects published.

University of Urbino opened as a "studium generale."

1672. University of Innsbruck founded by Emperor Leopold I (Academia Leopoldina).

Le Gras introduces ipecac in Europe (mentioned by Piso, 1648).

De Graaf describes the Graafian follicles in the ovary.

1673. Malpighi describes development of the chick.

1674. Printing press at Boston, Massachusetts.

Velsch publishes monograph on Filaria medinensis.

Morel invents tourniquet for checking hemorrhage.

1675. Leeuwenhoek discovers protozoa.

Malpighi's "Anatome plantarum" published.

Sydenham describes scarlatina as it appeared in 1661–75.

1676. Richard Wiseman describes tuberculosis of joints (tumor albus).

Isaac Barlow invents repeating watch.

1677. Kaiserliche Leopoldinische Akademie der Naturforscher founded.

Johan Hamm, a pupil of Leeuwenhoek, discovers spermatozoa.

Glisson's doctrine of irritability of tissues (1662) published.

Peyer describes lymphoid follicles in small intestine.

Smallpox in Boston (Thacher's "Brief Rule" published).

1677–1681. Pandemic malarial fever in Europe.

1678. De Marchetti shows anastomosis of arterioles and veins by injection.

1679. Rivinus discovers sublingual gland.

Leeuwenhoek discovers striped muscle.

Nicholas de Blegny publishes the first medical periodical ("Nouvelles decouvertes").

Bonet's "Sepulchretum" published.

James Yonge describes flap amputation.

1680. Denis Papin constructs a miniature steam engine.

Leeuwenhoek discovers yeast plant.

Caspar Bartholin discovers excretory duct of sublingual gland.

De Marchetti performs nephrotomy for renal calculus.

Plague hospital at Magdeburg.

1680–1681. Borelli's "De motu animalium" published.
1681. Royal College of Physicians of Edinburgh founded.
Printing press at Williamsburg, Virginia.
1682. Brunner describes duodenal glands (discovered in 1672).
Nehemiah Grew's "Anatomy of Plants" published.
1682–1725. Peter the Great.
1683. University of Modena chartered by Duke Francis II of Este.
Sydenham's treatise on gout published.
Leeuwenhoek describes bacteria (with figurations).
Duverney publishes first treatise on otology.
1684. Bernier classifies races of mankind by color of the skin.
1685. Revocation of the Edict of Nantes.
Medical Faculty at the University of Edinburgh.
Printing press at Philadelphia.
Bidloo's "Anatomia" published.
Vieussens' "Nevrographia" published.
Paul Portal publishes obstetric treatise.
Prussian ordinance regulating medical fees.
1686. Sydenham describes chorea minor.
1687. Newton's "Principia" published.
Sir William Petty publishes "Essays in Political Arithmetic."
1688. Revolution in England.

1689. Richard Morton's "Phthisiologia" published.
Walter Harris publishes treatise on diseases of children.
Leeuwenhoek discovers rods in retina, and finer anatomy of cornea.
1690. Locke's "Essay on the Human Understanding" published.
"Publick Occurrences" (newspaper) published at Boston, Massachusetts.
Justine Siegemundin publishes treatise on midwifery.
Floyer counts the pulse by the watch.
1691. Clopton Havers publishes "Osteologia nova" (Haversian canals).
Autopsy of Governor Slaughter in New York.
Yellow fever in Boston.
1692. Salem Witchcraft.
Ammann teaches deafmutes.
1693. University of Halle founded.
College of William and Mary founded at Williamsburg, Virginia.
Printing press in New York.
Acoluthus of Breslau resects the lower jaw.
1694. Camerarius gives experimental proof of sexuality in plants.
1694–1778. Voltaire.
1695. Nehemiah Grew discovers magnesium sulphate in Epsom waters (Epsom salts).

1697. Anatomical theater erected in Surgeons' Hall at Edinburgh.

Pacchioni glands discovers in the dura mater.

1698. Stahl's treatise on diseases of the portal system published.

1699. History and memoirs of the French Academy of Sciences published.

Tyson's "Orang Outang" published.

Infectious diseases act in Massachusetts.

1700. Königliche Akademie der Wissenschaften founded at Berlin.

Ramazzini publishes treatise on trade diseases.

1701. Frederick, Elector of Brandenburg, crowned King of Prussia.

Yale College founded (New Haven).

Deventer's "Novum lumen" published.

Robert Houstoun taps ovarian cyst.

1701–1713. War of the Spanish Succession.

1702. University of Breslau founded by Leopold I.

Stahl states phlogiston theory.

1702–14. Reign of Queen Anne.

1703. Foundation of St. Petersburg.

House of Lords authorizes apothecaries to prescribe as well as dispense drugs.

Leeuwenhoek discovers parthenogenesis of plant lice.

1704. Valsalva publishes "De aure humana" and describes "Valsalva's method."

Dr. Eysenbarth practises as a mountebank in Germany.

1705. Robert Elliot first professor of anatomy at Edinburgh.

Brisseau and Maître Jan show that cataract is the clouded lens.

1706. First laboratory of marine zoölogy at Marseilles.

1707. Senckenburg Foundation for advancement of science.

Dionis' "Cours d' opérations de chirurgie" published.

1708. Haller born.

Influenza pandemic in Europe.

1710. Charité Hospital opened at Berlin.

Morand and Le Dran perform first exarticulation of shoulder-joint.

Anel operates for aneurysm by ligating above the sac.

Santorini's muscle in larynx discovered.

1711. John Shore invents tuning fork.

1712. Rousseau born.

Torti of Modena uses cinchona bark in pernicious malarial fever.

1713 St. Côme merged into Académie de chirurgie (Paris).

Theatrum anatomicum founded in Berlin.

Anel catheterizes lachrymal ducts.

1714. Accession of House of Hannover (England).

Fahrenheit constructs 212 degree thermometer.

G. W. von Leibnitz founds pavillion system of hospitals.

1715. J.-L. Petit differentiates between compression and concussion of the brain.

J. T. Hensing discovers phosphorus in the blood.

1716. Surgeon General appointed in German Army at 900 marks per annum.

New York City issues ordinance for midwives.

1717. Timoni has daughter inoculated against smallpox.

Hospital for infectious diseases in Boston.

1718. Theatrum anatomicum in Vienna.

Lady Mary Wortley Montague has son inoculated for smallpox.

Hoffmann's anodyne.

Edward Strother describes puerperal fever.

1719. Westminster Hospital founded.

Kaspar Neumann isolates thymol.

Morgagni describes syphilis of cerebral arteries.

Heister's surgery published.

1720. Kew Gardens opened.

1721. General Holtzendorff creates "Collegium medico-chirurgicum" at Berlin.

Philadelphia Hospital founded.

Universidad central de Venezuela founded at Caracas.

Palfyn exhibits obstetric forceps to French Academy of Surgery.

Zabdiel Boylston inoculates for smallpox in Boston (June 26).

University of Dijon founded.

Apothecaries Company of London organized.

Floyer's "Psychrolusia" published.

1723. Cheselden's treatise on lithotomy published.

Yellow-fever reaches London.

1724. Kant born.

Guyot of Versailles catheterizes the Eustachian tubes.

John Maubray gives private instruction in obstetrics in England.

A. de Moivre publishes memoir on "Annuities upon lives."

1725. Prussian edict regulating practice of medicine.

Guy's Hospital opened (January 6).

Freind's History of Physick published.

1726. Stephen Hales makes first measurement of blood-pressure.

1727. Pourfour du Petit investigates functions of cervical sympathetic.

Cheselden performs lateral operation for stone.

1728. John Hunter born.

Fauchard publishes "Le chirurgien dentiste."

Cheselden introduces operation for artificial pupil.

1729. Influenza pandemic in Europe.

1730.   Daviel improves catar-
        act operation.
        James Douglas describes
        the peritoneum.
        Gaspar Casal describes
        pellagra as "mal de la
        rosa."
        Réaumur introduces 80
        degree thermometer.
        Frobenius describes prep-
        aration of sulphuric
        ether.

1730–31. Thomas Cadwalader
        teaches anatomy in
        Philadelphia.

1731.   Friedrich Hoffmann de-
        scribes chlorosis.
        Le Dran improves
        lithotomy.

1732.   Boerhaave's "Elementa
        chemiæ" published.
        Winslow's anatomy pub-
        lished.
        Influenza pandemic in
        Europe.

1733.   St. George's Hospital
        founded at London.
        Cheselden's "Osteo-
        graphia" published.
        George Cheyne describes
        "Cheyne-Stokes respi-
        ration."
        Stephen Hales produces
        dropsy by injecting
        water into the veins.
        John Machin describes
        ichthyosis histrix in
        the Lambert family.

1734.   University of Göttingen
        founded by George II
        of England (Decem-
        ber 7).
        Friedrich Wilhelm I of
        Prussia issues first
        regulation of field
        hospitals.

1735.   Linnæus' "Systema nat-
        uræ" published.
        Werlhof describes pur-
        pura hæmorrhagica.

        Medical Society in
        Boston founded.
        Scarlatina appears in
        the United States.

1736.   Edinburgh Hospital
        founded.
        J.-L. Petit opens mastoid
        for abscess in middle
        ear.
        Haller points out func-
        tion of bile in diges-
        tion of fats.

1737.   University of Göttingen
        ("Georgia Augusta")
        formally opened (Sep-
        tember 17).
        Royal Medical Society
        of Edinburgh founded.

1738.   Haller called to Göttin-
        gen.
        Daniel Bernouilli states
        the kinetic theory of
        gases.

1739.   Special chair of mid-
        wifery in the Uni-
        versity of Edinburgh.
        F.-S. Morand makes first
        excision of hip-joint.
        Royal Swedish Academy
        of Medicine founded.

1740.   University of Pennsyl-
        vania founded as "Col-
        lege of Philadelphia."
        London Hospital founded.
        Friedrich Hoffmann de-
        scribes rubella.
        Thomas Dover invents
        "Dover's Powder."

1740–48. War of Austrian Suc-
        cession.

1740–86. Reign of Frederick the
        Great.

1741.   Chair of clinical medi-
        cine at Edinburgh.
        Süssmilch's treatise on
        vital statistics pub-
        lished.
        Archibald Cleland cathe-
        terizes Eustachian
        tube.

44

1742.   Celsius invents 100 degree thermometer.
Linnæus describes aphasia.
Pandemic influenza in Europe.

1743.   University of Erlangen chartered (February 21) and opened (November 4) by Karl VII.
American Philosophical Society founded.
University of Santiago (Chile) founded.
Stephen Hales publishes treatise on ventilation.
Frederick the Great separates main hospitals from flying ambulances.

1744.   Trembley describes regeneration of tissues in hydrozoa.
Alexander Monro publishes handbook of comparative anatomy.

1745.   Barbers separated from higher surgeons in England.
Middlesex **Hospital** founded.
Ambulatory clinic opened at Prague.
Heberden's "Antitheriaka" published (improvement of London Pharmacopœia).
C. G. Kratzenstein employs electrotherapy.
William Cooke introduces steam heating.
Antoine Deparcieux introduces idea of "mean expectation of life."

1746.   Princeton College founded.
London Lock Hospital founded.

Fauchard describes pyorrhœa alveolaris and malocclusion.

1747.   Haller's Primæ linæ physiologiæ published.

1748.   Collegium medico-chirurgicum at Dresden.
Meckel describes sphenopalatine ganglion.

1749.   Goethe born.
Medical Society in New York.
British Lying-in Hospital founded.
Senac's treatise on the heart published.
Meyer orders phthisical patients to mountains at Appenzell.
Buffon's Natural History published.

1750.   École pratique established at Paris.
City of London Lying-in Hospital founded.
Antonio Nuñez Ribero Sanchez introduces corrosive sublimate in syphilis.
Russel describes Aleppo button.
Zittmann's decoction.

1751.   Königliche Gesellschaft der Wissenschaften at Göttingen founded by Haller.
Pennsylvania Hospital founded at Philadelphia.

1752.   Haller publishes memoir on specific irritability of tissues.
Smellie's **Midwifery** published.
Pringle's treatise on camp diseases published.
Réaumur experiments on digestion in birds.

Queen Charlotte's Lying-in Hospital at London founded.

1753. Daviel publishes memoir on extraction of cataract.

Levret's "Art des Accouchemens" published.

1754. Van Swieten organizes clinical instruction in Vienna.

Watson describes scleroderma at Curzio's clinic.

Kings College (Columbia University) founded at New York.

1755. Earthquake of Lisbon.

University of Moscow founded by Czarina Elizabeth.

Zinn's atlas of the eye published.

1756. Meath Hospital, Dublin, founded.

Pfaff's treatise on dentistry published.

Nicholas André describes infraorbital neuralgia.

1756–63. Seven Years War.

1757. William Hunter describes arterio-venous aneurysm.

Lind's treatise on naval hygiene published.

1758. Return of Halley's comet (end of comet theory of disease).

De Haën employs thermometer in clinical work.

Richard Brocklesby introduces ventilated barrack hospitals (decentralization)

1759. Königliche Bayerische Akademie der Wissenschaften founded at Munich.

Wolff's "Theoria generationis" published.

Mestivier describes and operates for localized appendicitis.

John Bard operates for extra-uterine pregnancy.

Physic Garden at Kew (England).

1760. William Shippen, Jr., lectures on anatomy in Philadelphia.

Act to regulate practice of medicine in New York City.

1761. Morgagni's "De sedibus" published.

Auenbrugger's "Inventum novum" published.

Pope Clement XI gives MS. of Eustachius to Lancisi.

1762. Plenciz announces theory of contagium animatum.

Roederer and Wagler describe typhoid fever at Göttingen.

John Clayton's "Flora Virginica" published.

Shippen's private maternity hospital established at Philadelphia.

First medical library in United States (Pennsylvania Hospital).

Bilguer resects wrist.

Stoerk introduces aconite and other narcotics.

Surgical clinic opened at Lisbon.

1762–96. Reign of Catherine II of Russia.

1763. Joseph Black differentiates between specific and latent heat.

1764. Cotugno describes sciatica.

Louis introduces digital compression for hemorrhage.

First pavillion hospital at Plymouth.

1765. Medical Faculty of University of Pennsylvania founded.

Fontana publishes memoir on viper poison.

National veterinary school at Alfort (Seine).

Royal veterinary school at Dresden.

1766. Cavendish discovers hydrogen.

Desault's bandage for fractures introduced.

New Jersey State Medical Society founded.

1767. Heberden describes varicella.

Charles White resects shoulder-joint.

Influenza pandemic in Europe.

1768. Wolff's memoir on embryology of the intestines published.

Robert Whytt describes tubercular meningitis.

Heberden describes angina pectoris.

Charles White resects head of humerus.

Medical School, Kings College, New York, founded.

Lind's treatise on tropical medicine published.

1769. Cullen's Synopsis nosologiæ published.

Constitutio criminalis Theresiana (Law of torture).

Pott's treatise on fractures and dislocations published.

Medical Society of New York City, founded.

Dartmouth College founded.

1770. William Hunter founds school of anatomy in Great Windmill Street.

Rutty describes relapsing fever.

Cotugno demonstrates albumen in the urine.

William Hunter describes retroversion of the uterus.

Abbe de l'Épée invents sign language for deaf mutes.

First medical degree in United States conferred by Kings College.

Pennsylvania quarantine act.

Watt invents steam engine.

1770–71. Smallpox destroys three million people in East Indies.

1771. Priestley and Scheele isolate oxygen.

1771–8. William Hunter's treatise on the teeth published.

1772. Rutherford discovers nitrogen.

"Encyclopédie" (Diderot and d'Alembert) completed.

Priestley discovers nitrous oxide.

New Jersey act to regulate the practice of medicine.

1773. Medical Society of London founded.

First insane asylum in U. S. at Williamsburg, Virginia.

Fothergill describes facial neuralgia.

Charles White urges asepsis to prevent puerperal fever.

Jesuit order suppressed by Clement XIV.

1773–4. Revolution in Russia.

1774. William Hunter's "Anatomia uteri" published.

Benjamin Jesty vaccinates against smallpox (Gloucestershire).

Priestley discovers ammonia.

Scheele discovers chlorine.

Abraham Chovet teaches anatomy in Philadelphia.

1775. Lavoisier discovers and defines oxygen.

Pole and Dobson find grape-sugar in the urine.

John Morgan appointed Director General of American Army.

1775–83. American Revolution.

1776. Cullen's "First Lines" published.

Jasser operates successfully on the mastoid.

Scheele and Bergmann discover uric acid in vesical calculi.

Plenck's classification of skin diseases published.

Cruikshank discovers that severed nerves will grow together.

1776–1805. Scarlatina pandemic in both hemispheres.

1777. Lavoisier describes exchange of gases in respiration.

Sigault performs symphysiotomy.

John Howard's investigations of prisons and hospitals published.

School for army veterinarians at Vienna.

1778. Count Rumford investigates mechanical equivalents of heat.

C. C. von Siebold performs symphysiotomy in Germany.

John Hunter's treatise on diseases of the teeth published.

William Brown publishes first American pharmacopœia in Philadelphia.

1779. University of Palermo founded.

J. P. Frank issues first system of public hygiene (vol. i, April 24).

Bylon of Java describes dengue.

William Wright of Edinburgh introduces "Scotch douche."

Ingen Housz discovers that plants give off CO_2.

Pott describes deformity and paralysis from spinal caries.

Mesmer's memoir on animal magnetism published.

1780. University of Oxford establishes chair of clinical medicine.

University of Münster inaugurated.

Benjamin Rush describes dengue.

Chabert's memoir on animal anthrax published.

Benjamin Franklin invents bifocal lenses.

American Academy of Arts and Sciences founded at Boston.

William Shippen chosen Director General of American Army Medical Department.

1781.   Cavendish effects synthesis of water.

Kant's "Critique of Pure Reason" published.

Massachusetts Medical Society founded.

Georgetown University (D. C.) founded.

1782.   Medical Department of Harvard University founded.

University of Innsbruck reduced to a lyceum by Joseph II.

1783.   Austria separates surgeons from barbers.

Royal Society of Edinburgh publishes transactions.

1783–5. Lavoisier analyzes water and overthrows phlogiston theory.

1783.   Marschal (Strassburg) excises a prolapsed cancerous uterus.

1784.   Allgemeines Krankenhaus opened at Vienna (August 16).

Goethe discovers intermaxillary bone.

Cotugno discovers cerebro-spinal fluid.

Cavendish discovers hydrogen.

1785.   Josephinum established at Vienna.

Fowler introduces potassium arsenate (Fowler's solution).

John Hunter discovers collateral circulation and introduces proximal ligation in aneurysm.

Withering's treatise on the fox-glove published.

Charles White describes 'phlegmasia alba dolens.

Sir Gilbert Blane publishes treatise on naval medicine.

1785.   Chair of anatomy established in the University of Dublin.

University of Georgia (U. S. A.) founded.

1786.   John Hunter publishes Treatise on the Venereal Disease.

Parry describes exophthalmic goiter.

Lettsom describes drug habit and alcoholism.

P.-F. Moreau excises elbow-joint.

Fourcroy and Thouret discover adipocere.

Royal College of Physicians (London) publishes transactions.

1787.   College of Physicians of Philadelphia founded.

Mascagni publishes atlas of the lymphatics.

Guild of Bathkeepers abolished in Würzburg.

1788.   University of Louvain removed to Brussels.

Influenza pandemic in Europe.

1789.   John Hunter describes intussusception.

Matthew Baillie describes dermoid ovarian cysts.

Medical Society of Delaware founded.

Medical Society of South Carolina founded.

1789–99. French Revolution.

1790.   Royal Veterinary Schools established at Berlin and Munich.

Medical journal published in New York.

1791. Soemmerring publishes first volume of his anatomy.
University of Innsbruck restored to rank by Leopold II.
New Hampshire Medical Society founded.
Royal Veterinary College established at London.
Dr. Guillotin invents the guillotine.

1791–9. William Baynham of Virginia operates for extra-uterine pregnancy.

1792. Galvani's essay on animal electricity published.
Fodéré publishes treatise on goiter and cretinism.
Sprengel's history of medicine published.
Connecticut Medical Society founded.
Establishment of French Republic (September 21).

1793. Matthew Baillie's "Morbid Anatomy" published.
Benjamin Bell differentiates between gonorrhea and syphilis.
Matthew Carey describes yellow fever epidemic in Philadelphia.

1793–4. Reign of Terror in France.

1794. Lavoisier beheaded (May 8).
John Hunter publishes treatise on blood, inflammation, and gunshot wounds.
John Hunter describes transplantation of animal tissues.
Dalton describes color-blindness (October 31).

Scarpa's Tabulæ nevrologicæ published.
Erasmus Darwin's "Zoönomia" published.
École de sante created at Paris.
Gumpert publishes Greek text of Asclepiades.

1795. Surgeon General Görcke founds Kaiser-Wilhelm's Akademie at Berlin.
Institut de France founded.
Abernethian Society founded at London.

1796. Jenner vaccinates William Phipps (May 14).
Abernethy first ligates external iliac artery.
Wright Post successfully ligates femoral artery in America.
Société de médecine de Paris founded.
Yellow fever in Boston.

1796–1815. Napoleonic Wars.

1797. Wollaston discovers uric acid in gouty joints.
Currie publishes reports on hydrotherapy in typhoid fever.
John Rollo advocates meat diet in diabetes.
Medical Repository (New York) published.

1797–9. Yellow fever in Philadelphia.

1798. Jenner's "Inquiry" published.
Medical and Chirurgical Faculty of Maryland founded.
Imperial Medico-Military Academy founded at St. Petersburg.
John Haslam describes general paralysis.

Medical School of Dartmouth College organized.

Gas lighting introduced.

1798–1821. Willan's treatise on skin diseases published.

1799. De Carro introduces Jennerian vaccination on the continent and in Asia.

Matthew Ballie describes endocarditis.

Anderson's College Medical School established at Glasgow.

United States Congress passes quarantine act.

1799–1804. Napoleon First Consul.

1800. Royal College of Surgeons (London) chartered.

Bichat's "Traité des membranes" published.

Sir Humphry Davy discovers anesthetic effect of laughing gas.

Benjamin Waterhouse introduces Jennerian vaccination into America.

Cuvier's Comparative Anatomy published.

1801. Pinel publishes psychiatric treatise.

Thomas Young describes astigmatism and states undulatory theory of light.

Bichat's "Anatomie descriptive" published.

1802. Heberden's "Commentaries" published.

Conseil général de Santé founded in France.

Bichat's "Anatomie générale" published.

London Fever Hospital established.

1803. Anatomical and pharmaceutical societies founded in Paris.

Otto describes hemophilia.

1804. Universities of Kasan and Charkov founded by Alexander I.

Dalton states atomic theory.

Scarpa describes arteriosclerosis.

Royal London Ophthalmic Hospital founded.

Philadelphia Medical Museum published.

1804–15. Napoleon Emperor of France.

1805. Battle of Trafalgar.

Sertürner isolates morphine.

Vieussieux describes cerebro-spinal meningitis.

Chicago Hospital for Women and Children founded.

1806. End of Holy Roman Empire.

1807. Compulsory vaccination introduced into Bavaria and Hesse.

University of Altdorf united to Erlangen.

College of Medicine of Maryland founded at Baltimore.

1808. Universities of Lyons and Clermont-Ferrand founded.

Physikalisch-medizinische Sozietät founded at Erlangen.

Swedish Medical Society founded.

Medical Faculty at Rio de Janeiro founded.

Badham publishes treatise on bronchitis.

1809. University of Berlin founded by Friedrich Wilhelm III of Prussia.

McDowell performs ovariotomy.

Allen Burns describes endocarditis.

Soemmerring invents electric telegraph.

French Hospital founded at New York.

1810. Gall and Spurzhein publish treatise on the nervous system.

Hildenbrand publishes account of typhus and typhoid fever.

Wells describes rheumatism of the heart.

Marzari attributes pellagra to corn.

1811. University of Christiania founded.

Napoleon abolishes University of Salerno (November 29).

Sir Charles Bell describes functions of spinal nerve roots.

Massachusetts General Hospital (Boston) established.

1812. University of Genoa founded.

Parkinson describes perforative appendicitis.

Legallois describes action of vagus on respiration.

Academy of Natural Sciences founded at Philadelphia.

Bellevue Hospital (New York) established.

1813. Sutton differentiates delirium tremens from phrenitis.

Ling introduces Swedish movements.

1814. Royal Hospital for Diseases of the Chest (London) founded.

1815. German Confederation. Battle of Waterloo.

University of Wittenberg removed to Halle.

Laënnec discovers mediate auscultation (May 1).

Lisfranc performs exarticulation of tarsometatarsal joint.

Special chair of midwifery in Glasgow University.

1816. University of Ghent founded.

Delpech performs subcutaneous tenotomy.

Royal Ear Hospital (London) founded.

1816-30. Pandemic of cholera.

1817. University of Liége founded.

Friedrich Wilhelms Institut established at Berlin.

Parkinson describes paralysis agitans.

John King publishes book on extra-uterine pregnancy.

Sir Astley Cooper ligates abdominal aorta.

1818. University of Bonn founded by Friedrich Wilhelm III of Prussia.

Sir Humphry Davy introduces safety lamp for coal-miners.

De Riemer introduces frozen sections.

Valentine Mott successfully ligates the innominate artery.

Pelletier and Caventou isolate strychnine.

1819. University of St. Petersburg founded by Alexander I.

Steamship crosses Atlantic Ocean.

John Bostock describes hay fever.

Pelletier and Caventou isolate quinine.

Medical Society of District of Columbia founded.

1820. Académie de médécine founded at Paris.

1821. Itard's treatise on otology published.

McGill College and University founded at Montreal.

Philadelphia College of Pharmacy founded.

1822. Magendie demonstrates Bell's law of the spinal nerve roots.

British Association for the Advancement of Science founded.

Gesellschaft deutscher Naturforscher und Aerzte founded.

James Jackson describes alcoholic neuritis.

1823. Purkinje investigates finger-prints.

Chevreul investigates animal fats.

1824. Flourens publishes work on cerebral physiology.

Prout investigates acidity of gastric juice.

Sadi Carnot states the second law of thermodynamics.

1825. University of Virginia founded.

Jefferson Medical College established at Philadelphia.

Bouillaud describes and localizes aphasia.

Short introduces oleum tiglii from India.

1826. University of Munich founded (by removal of University of Ingolstadt from Landshut).

University of Åbo (1640) moved to Helsingfors.

Laënnec gives classical description of bronchitis and other thoracic diseases.

Dupuytren describes congenital dislocation of the hip-joint.

Calmeil describes general paralysis.

1827. Lord Lister born (April 5).

Von Baer discovers mammalian ovum.

Richard Bright describes essential nephritis.

Adams describes heart-block.

1828. Wöhler describes artificial synthesis of urea from ammonium cyanate.

Piorry introduces pleximeter.

Hodgkin describes aortic retroversion.

1829. Louis Braille introduces printing for the blind.

Benjamin Babington describes his "glottiscope."

1830. J. J. Lister perfects achromatic microscope.

Steinheim describes tetany.

Kopp describes thymus-death.

Priessnitz founds hydropathic establishment.

1830. Reign of Louis Phillipe.

1831. Guthrie, Liebig and Soubeiran discover chloroform.

1832. Universities of Zürich and Kiev founded.

British Medical Association founded.

Faraday describes galvanic and magnetic induction.

Anatomy Act passed in England.

Hodgkin describes lymph-adenoma.

Corrigan describes aortic insufficiency.

Boston Lying-in Hospital founded.

Liebig discovers chloral.

1833.   Johannes Müller's treatise on physiology published.

Marshall Hall investigates reflex action.

William Beaumont publishes experiments on digestion.

Geiger and Hesse isolate atropin.

Lobstein describes osteopsathyrosis.

1834.   Universities of Bern and Brussels founded.

Royal Statistical Society of London founded.

Dumas obtains and names pure chloroform.

Tulane University of New Orleans founded.

1835.   Louis founds medical statistics.

Malcolmson describes beri-beri.

Cruveilhier describes disseminated sclerosis.

Musée Dupuytren founded.

1836.   Weber brothers investigate physiology of locomotion.

Schwann discovers pepsin.

Marsh's test for arsenic introduced.

University of London founded.

Richard Bright describes acute yellow atrophy of the liver.

1837.   Gerhard differentiates between typhus and typhoid fevers.

Colles states law of maternal immunity in syphilis.

Jacob Henle describes epithelial tissues.

Schönlein describes peliosis rheumatica.

Rush Medical College (Chicago) founded.

K. k. Gesellschaft der Aerzte founded at Vienna.

1838.   University of Messina founded.

Schleiden describes plant cells.

Ehrenberg publishes treatise on infusoria.

Johannes Müller's treatise on tumors published.

Mettauer successfully operates for vesico-vaginal fistula.

Royal Orthopædic Hospital founded.

1839.   Schwann publishes treatise on the cell theory.

Skoda's treatise on percussion and auscultation published.

First volume of Littre's Hippocrates published.

Rowland Hill introduces postage stamps.

1840   Jacob Heine describes infantile poliomyelitis.

Basedow describes exophthalmic goiter.

1841.   Henle's "Allgemeine Anatomie" published.

1842   J. R. Mayer states law of Conservation of Energy.

Long operates with ether anesthesia.

Wöhler describes synthesis of hippuric from benzoic acid.

Dieffenbach publishes treatise on strabismus.

1843.   O. W. Holmes points out contagiousness of puerperal fever.

Carl Ludwig investigates mechanism of urinary secretion.

Küchler introduces test-types.

Simpson, Huguier and Kiwisch introduce uterine sound.

Société de chirurgie founded at Paris.

1844.   Rokitansky demonstrates tubercular nature of Pott's disease.

New York Pathological Society founded.

1845.   Virchow shows that embolism is the cause of pyemia.

Virchow and Hughes Bennett describe leukemia.

Andrew Buchanan investigates coagulation of the blood.

Langenbeck detects actinomyces.

Francis Rynd (Dublin) employs hypodermic injections for relief of pain.

1846.   Weber brothers discover inhibitory effect of vagus nerve.

Morton introduces ether anesthesia.

Kölliker describes smooth muscle.

Marion Sims invents vaginal speculum.

Claude Bernard discovers digestive function of pancreas.

Stokes describes heart-block.

Smithsonian Institution of Washington founded.

1847.   Helmholtz publishes treatise on Conservation of Energy.

Sir J. Y. Simpson introduces chloroform anesthesia in obstetrics.

Semmelweis discovers cause of puerperal fever.

Carl Ludwig invents kymograph.

Gerlach injects capillaries with carmine stain.

American Medical Association founded.

Royal Academy of Sciences founded at Vienna.

New York Academy of Medicine founded.

O. W. Holmes appointed Parkman professor of anatomy at Harvard.

1848.   Helmholtz locates source of animal heat in the muscles.

Claude Bernard discovers glycogenic function of the liver.

Du Bois Reymond publishes treatise on animal electricity.

Société de biologie founded at Paris.

American Association for the Advancement of Science founded.

English Act creating general and local boards of health passed.

1848–52.   Second French Republic.

1849.   Addison describes pernicious anemia and suprarenal disease.

Claude Bernard produces diabetes by puncture of the fourth ventricle.

Marion Sims operates for vesico-vaginal fistula.

J. K. Mitchell publishes treatise on cryptogamous origin of malarial fever.

Millon introduces reagent for proteins.

Hutchinson invents spirometer.

University of Wisconsin founded.

1850. Helmholtz measures the velocity of the nerve current.

Waller states law of degeneration of spinal nerves.

Daniel Drake publishes treatise on diseases of the Mississippi Valley.

William Detmold (New York) opens abscess of the brain.

1851. Helmholtz invents ophthalmoscope.

Claude Bernard explains vasomotor function of sympathetic nerves.

Ludwig and Rahn investigate nerves of salivary secretion.

Falret describes circular insanity.

Nélaton describes pelvic hematocele.

1852. Pravaz introduces hypodermic syringe.

International Congress of Hygiene at Brussels.

Kölliker's treatise on histology published.

Pirogoff employs frozen sections in his "Anatome topographica."

1852–70. Second Empire in France.

1853. Marion Sims publishes treatise on vesicovaginal fistula.

Cohn demonstrates vegetable nature of bacteria.

Gilman Kimball excises uterus for fibromyoma.

1853–6. Crimean War: Florence Nightingale.

1854. Graefe founds Archiv für Ophthalmologie.

University of Marseilles founded.

Virchow describes neuroglia.

Claude Bernard discovers function of vaso-dilator nerves.

Hermann Brehmer opens hospital for phthisis at Görbersdorf.

1855. Manuel Garcia introduces laryngoscope.

Addison publishes memoir on diseases of the suprarenal capsules.

Marion Sims founds Hospital for Women's Diseases (New York City).

Graefe introduces iridectomy.

Paris Exposition.

1856. Sir W. H. Perkin (1838–1907) obtains aniline dyes (coal-tar products).

Panum investigates chemical products of putrefaction.

Casper's treatise on medical jurisprudence published.

1857. Graefe introduces operation for strabismus.

Bouchut performs intubation of the larynx.

University of Chicago founded.

1858.   Pathological Society of Philadelphia founded.
Virchow's "Cellularpathologie" published.
Claude Bernard discovers vaso-constrictor and vaso-dilator nerves.
Niemann isolates cocaine in Wöhler's laboratory.
Pettenkofer proves that solid walls are permeable to air.
Kekulé shows quadrivalence of carbon atom.

1859.   Darwin's Origin of Species published.
Kirchhoff and Bunsen discover spectrum analysis.
Graefe describes retinal embolism.
Landry describes acute ascending paralysis.
Pflüger publishes memoir on electrotonus.
Florence Nightingale publishes "Notes on Nursing."

1860.   Lemaire points out antiseptic properties of carbolic acid.
Czermak introduces rhinoscopy.
Donders introduces cylindrical and prismatic spectacles in astigmatism.
Zenker describes trichinosis.
Ménière describes aural vertigo.
Berliner medicinische Gesellschaft founded.
University of California founded.

1861.   Ernst Brand introduces hydrotherapy in typhoid fever.
Pasteur discovers anaërobic bacteria.

E. B. Wollcott (Milwaukee) first excises renal tumor.
Max Schultze defines protoplasm and cell.
Broca discovers speech center in the brain.

1861–65.   Civil War in the United States.

1862.   Raynaud describes symmetrical gangrene.
Donders publishes studies on astigmatism and presbyopia.
V. von Bruns performs first laryngeal operation with laryngoscope.
Winternitz and Oppolzer found first hydropathic establishment at Vienna.

1863.   Helmholtz's "Tonempfindungen" published.
Voit and Pettenkofer publish investigations of metabolism in respiration.
William Banting publishes "Letter on Corpulence."
Pasteur investigates silkworm disease.

1864.   Donders publishes treatise on anomalies of accommodation and refraction.
Traube investigates pathology of fever.
Parkes' Manual of Practical Hygiene published.
Geneva Convention.
Le Verrier founds Association française pour l'avancement des sciences.

1865.   University of Odessa founded.
Cornell University (New York) founded.

Gregor Mendel publishes memoir on plant hybridity.

Villemin demonstrates infectiousness of tuberculosis.

1866. Seven Weeks' (Austro-Prussian) War.

Voit establishes first hygienic laboratory in Munich.

Ludwig and Cyon investigate the vasomotor nerves.

Marion Sims publishes Clinical Notes on Uterine Surgery.

Graefe describes sympathetic ophthalmia.

1867. Lister introduces antiseptic surgery.

Helmholtz publishes treatise on physiological optics.

Kussmaul introduces intubation of the stomach.

Moritz Traube devises semi-permeable membranes.

First International Medical Congress at Paris.

Opening of Suez Canal and of Pacific Railway.

1868. University of Tokyo founded.

Haeckel's "Natürliche Schöpfungsgeschichte" published.

Meyer of Copenhagen describes adenoid vegetations.

1869. University of Warsaw founded.

Esmarch introduces first aid bandage.

Virchow urges medical inspection of schools.

Goltz investigates nerve centers in the frog.

Gustav Simon excises kidney.

Oscar Liebriech demonstrates hypnotic effect of chloral hydrate.

American Journal of Obstetrics founded.

Torture abolished in Canton of Zug (Switzerland).

1870. Fritsch and Hitzig investigate localization of functions of brain.

Thomas performs vaginal ovariotomy.

Saemisch describes serpiginous ulcer of the cornea.

1870-71. Franco-Prussian War (test of vaccination).

1871. Establishment of German Empire and French Republic.

Darwin's "Descent of Man" published.

Weigert stains bacteria with carmine.

English Local Government Board created.

1872. University of Strassburg reopened.

University of Adelaide (Australia) founded.

Abbe introduces oil immersion lenses.

Battey performs normal ovariotomy.

Noeggerath describes effects of latent gonorrhea in women.

Infant life protection act passed in England.

1873. University of Geneva founded.

Obermeier discovers spirillum of relapsing fever.

Esmarch introduces hemostatic bandage.

Gull describes myxedema.

Billroth excises the larynx.

Schwartze and Eysell devise mastoid operation.

Cuignet introduces retinoscopy.

Canalization of Berlin begun.

Revaccination compulsory in Germany.

1874. Cholera conference in Vienna.

International postal service.

Loi Roussel enacted for the protection of infants (France).

Ehrlich introduces dried blood smears and improves stain methods.

Kahlbaum describes katatonia.

Willy Kühne discovers trypsin.

1875. Universities of Lemberg and Czernowitz founded.

Landois discovers hemolysis from transfusion of alien blood.

Sir Thomas Barlow describes infantile scurvy.

Lösch observes parasitic amebæ in dysentery.

Weir Mitchell introduces rest cure.

Meat inspection compulsory in Germany.

Public Health Act in England.

Boston Medical Library founded.

1876. Imperial Board of Health founded at Berlin (April 31).

Royal Sanitary Institute founded (London).

Johns Hopkins University founded.

Royal Academy of Medicine founded at Rome.

Physiological Society of London founded.

International Hygienic Congress at Brussels.

Sayre introduces gypsum corset for spinal deformities.

Kolbe isolates salicylic acid.

Lombroso publishes treatise on criminal man.

Paquelin cautery introduced.

Porro introduces Cæsarean section with excision of adnexa.

Koch grows anthrax bacilli on artificial media.

Peter Dettweiler treats consumptives at Falkenstein by rest cure in open air.

University of Amsterdam founded.

1877. Pasteur discovers bacillus of **malignant** edema.

Ernst von Bergmann introduces corrosive sublimate antisepsis.

Bezold describes mastoiditis.

1877–8. Russo-Turkish War.

1878. Koch discovers causes of traumatic infections.

W. A. Freund excises cancerous uterus.

International Congress of Hygiene at Paris.

1879. Neisser discovers gonococcus.

Nitze introduces cystoscopy.

German food law passed.

1880.   Pasteur isolates strep-
         tococcus and staphylo-
         coccus.
         Eberth isolates typhoid
         bacillus.
         Sandström describes
         parathyroid gland.
         Balfour's Embryology
         published.
         Mosetig Moorhof intro-
         duces iodine in surgery.
1881.   Laveran discovers para-
         site of malarial fever.
         Billroth resects the pylorus
         Czerny describes vaginal
         excision of uterine tu-
         mors.
         Hahn performs nephro-
         pexy.
         Wölfler introduces gas-
         tro-enterostomy.
         Medin discovers epidemic
         nature of poliomyelitis.
         Koch introduces plate
         cultures.
1882.   Koch discovers tubercle
         bacillus.
         Löffler discovers bacillus
         of glanders.
         Walther Flemming in-
         vestigates cell division.
         Max Sänger improves
         Cæsarean section.
         Langenbuch excises the
         gall-bladder.
1883.   Edwin Klebs discovers
         diphtheria bacillus.
         Pasteur vaccinates
         against anthrax.
         Unna introduces ichthyol.
         Lawson Tait operates for
         extra-uterine preg-
         nancy.
1884.   Koch discovers cholera
         bacillus (February 2).
         Nicolaier discovers teta-
         nus bacillus.
         Credé introduces silver
         nitrate instillations for
         infantile conjunctivitis.

          Ludwig Knorr prepares
            antipyrine.
          Baumann discovers sul-
            phonal.
          Carl Koller employs co-
            caine in eye surgery.
1885.   O'Dwyer improves intu-
            bation of the larynx.
          Weismann publishes me-
            moir on continuity of
            the germ plasm.
          Ewald and Boas intro-
            duce test-breakfasts.
          Weigert introduces he-
            matoxylin staining of
            nerve-fibers.
1886.   Escherich discovers Bacil-
            lus coli.
          Von Bergmann intro-
            duces steam sterili-
            zation in surgery.
          Fitz describes pathology
            of appendicitis.
          Marie describes acrome-
            galy as connected with
            the pituitary body.
          Marcel von Nencki intro-
            duces salol.
          Soxhlet introduces steril-
            ized milk for nutrition
            of infants.
          Cahn and Hepp intro-
            duce acetanilide (Ger-
            hardt, 1843).
1887.   Clark University founded
            (Worcester, Mass.).
          Bruce discovers bacillus
            of Malta fever.
          Weichselbaum discovers
            meningococcus.
          D'Arsonval introduces
            high frequency cur-
            rents.
          Howard Kelly performs
            hysterorrhaphy.
          Gowers and Horsley
            operate on the spinal
            cord.
          Sloane Maternity Hospi-
            tal (New York) opened.

45

1888. University of Tomsk founded.
Institut Pasteur founded.
Roux and Yersin investigate the toxins of diphtheria.
Nuttall discovers the bactericidal powers of blood-serum.

1889. Johns Hopkins Hospital and Hamburg-Eppendorff Hospitals opened.
Buchner discovers alexins (protective bodies).
Von Mering and Minkowski produce experimental pancreatic diabetes.
Infectious diseases notification act in England.
Behring discovers antitoxins.

1890. University of Lausanne founded.
Imperial Institute of Experimental Medicine founded at St. Petersburg.
Behring treats diphtheria with antitoxin.
Koch introduces tuberculin.
Infectious Diseases Prevention Act in England.
Bowditch demonstrates non-fatigability of nerve.
Weigert stains neuroglia with methyl violet.

1891. Institute for Infectious Diseases opened at Berlin under Koch.
Lister Institute for Preventive Medicine (London) founded.
Waldeyer founds neuron theory.
Quincke introduces lumbar puncture.

1892. Hygienic Institute at Hamburg opened.
Wistar Institute of Anatomy and Biology (1808) incorporated.
Halsted successfully ligates subclavian artery.
Kossel and Neumann discover pentose.
Cholera epidemic in Hamburg.

1893. Röntgen discovers X-rays.
Smith and Kilbourne demonstrate transmission of parasitic diseases by arthropoda.
Gilbert discovers para-colon and paratyphoid bacilli.
Finsen light introduced.
International Cholera Conference in Dresden.

1894. Kitasato and Yersin discover plague bacillus.
Kirstein devises direct laryngoscopy.
Schleich introduces infiltration anesthesia.
Local Government Act in England.

1895. Pfeiffer discovers bacteriolysis.
Nobel prizes introduced.
Wilhelm His reforms anatomical nomenclature.

1896. Max Gruber discovers bacterial agglutination.
Murphy produces successful circular anastomosis of blood-vessels.
Dibdin and Schweder introduce biological purification of sewage.
Widal and Sicard introduce agglutination test for typhoid fever.

1897. Shiga discovers dysentery bacillus.

Emil Fischer synthetizes caffeine, theobromine, xanthin, guanin and adenin.

Bordet discovers bacterial hemolysis.

1898. Institute for Experimental Therapy established at Frankfort.

Killian introduces direct bronchoscopy.

Löffler and Frosch investigate filterable viruses.

Radium discovered by the Curies.

Dreser introduces heroine.

Emil Fischer isolates the purin nucleus of uric acid compounds.

Looss demonstrates transmission of hook-worm infection.

Theobald Smith differentiates between bovine and human tubercle bacilli.

1899. Reed and Carroll establish transmission of yellow fever by mosquitoes.

Jacques Loeb produces chemical activation of sea urchin egg.

Ehrlich's Institute for Experimental Therapy founded at Frankfort.

Liverpool and London schools of tropical medicine founded.

1900. Robert Gersuny introduces paraffin injections.

Gärtner introduces tonometer.

Widal and Ravaut introduce cytodiagnosis.

Wertheim introduces radical operation for uterine cancer.

1901. De Vries states mutation theory.

Uhlenhuth introduces precipitin test for blood stains (Bordet, 1898).

Dutton and Ford discover parasite of sleeping sickness.

O. Cohnheim discovers erepsin.

Takamine isolates adrenalin.

Rockefeller Institute for Medical Research opened in New York.

Instituto Oswaldo Cruz opened at Rio de Janeiro.

"Biometrika" founded by Galton, Pearson and Weldon.

1902. Carrel introduces methods of vascular anastomosis and transplantation of tissues.

Herzog discovers site of Asclepeion at Cos.

Carnegie Institution of Washington founded.

Imperial Cancer Research Fund (England) founded.

1903. Metchnikoff inoculates higher apes with syphilis.

Emil Fischer and von Mering introduce veronal.

Bier introduces artificial hyperemia.

Einthoven invents string galvanometer.

Bruce shows that sleeping sickness is transmitted by tsetse fly.

Henry Phipps Institute for Tuberculosis opened.

1904. Atwater invents respiration calorimeter.

Sauerbruch introduces pneumatic cabinet for surgery of the chest.

1905. Schaudinn discovers parasite of syphilis.

Alfred Einhorn discovers novocaine.

Robert Koch investigates African fever.

Institut für Geschichte der Medizin (Leipzig) founded under Karl Sudhoff.

Bordet and Gengou discover bacillus of whooping-cough.

1906. Rudolf Virchow Hospital opened at Berlin (October 1).

Bárány develops theory of vestibular nystagmus

School of Tropical Medicine established at Brussels.

Nutrition Laboratory (Carnegie Institution) established at Boston.

Food and Drugs Act (U. S.) passed.

1907. Wassermann introduces sero-diagnosis of syphilis.

Von Pirquet introduces cutaneous reaction in tuberculosis.

Calmette and Wolff-Eisner introduce conjunctival reactions.

Royal Society of Medicine (London) founded.

1908. Sleeping Sickness Bureau (London) founded.

Royal Army Medical College opened at Millbank.

1909. University founded at Manila.

Förster introduces operation for locomotor ataxia.

Much introduces cobra venom reaction in insanity.

Ehrlich introduces salvarsan.

Noguchi improves the Wassermann reaction.

1910. Harrison demonstrates nerve-fiber outgrowth extravitally.

Henri and others introduce ultraviolet sterilization of water.

Flexner produces poliomyelitis experimentally.

Law against White Slave traffic (U. S.) passed.

1911. Carrel investigates extravital culture and rejuvenation of tissues.

Noguchi introduces luetin reaction.

Cushing describes dyspituitarism.

Gullstrand receives Nobel prize for optical researches.

Peytron Rous transmits sarcoma by means of a filterable virus.

1912. Bass cultivates malarial plasmodium in vitro.

Sudhoff opposes theory of American origin of syphilis.

1913. Abderhalden introduces ferment reaction for diagnosis of pregnancy and dementia præcox.

Supreme Court (U. S.) denies "rights" of individuals when inimical to public welfare.

Phipps Psychiatric Clinic (Baltimore) opened.

International Medical Congress in London.

II. BIBLIOGRAPHIC NOTES FOR COLLATERAL READING

A. HISTORIES OF MEDICINE

Of the larger works, the "Grundriss" of Johann Hermann **Baas** (1838–   ), of Worms on the Rhine, translated into English by H. E. Handerson (Cincinnati, 1889), is still in many respects the most readable because it was written by a practising physician, to suit the needs of the average reader. The earlier works of Le Clerc (1696), Freind (1725–7), Schulze (1728), Haller (1751), Blumenbach (1786), and Kurt Sprengel (1792–1803), are mainly of antiquarian interest, while the histories of Hecker (1822–9), Bostock (1834), Puccinotti (1850–66), Meryon (1861), Daremberg (1870), and Bouchut (1873) are now of a vintage that could only appeal to the special "taster." Heinrich **Haeser's** great work on the History of Medicine and Epidemic Diseases (3d ed., 1875–82) still stands out as the epoch-making monograph on the subject before the time of Baas and Neuburger. It is based upon original research and is unrivalled for erudition and accuracy. The merits of Baas's history are that he covers the whole ground in a thick, but not too long-winded, volume; that his statements of fact are all of them accurate as far as they go; that he gives a very thoroughgoing account of the different medical "theories," the condition of medicine and surgery in the different periods; and that he frequently carries his readers over many dull patches by his keen and frolicsome sense of humor. His faults are a certain diffuseness, the poor arrangement of his subject-matter, his long lists of relatively unimportant names, his failure to discriminate many things of scientific moment from things that are trivial, his whimsical tendency to wander away from his subject or to enlarge upon comic or erotic details and, finally, a curious lack of balance and proportion which, with all his glancing wit and humor, indicates, at times, an absolute contempt for the exigencies of literary style. He gives us many dates, but not always those we want, and like most medical historians Baas is at his weakest when he gets into the modern period. He cannot see the woods for the trees, dilates more upon theories than facts, is behind the times in his attitude towards the germ-theory, and has more to say about Broussais and Rasori than about Laënnec or Louis, Charcot or Pasteur. Yet no modern historian has given us a finer appreciation of the great English physicians, with whose practical aims he was evidently in cordial sympathy. Although a Rhinelander by birth, Baas represents the extreme North German or Protestant view of medical history. He is, everywhere, an essentially masculine-minded writer, hating all shams, humbuggery, frauds and superstitions. In relation to the fair sex, he is one of Vizetelly's "Teutonic lords of creation." We have not made Baas's acquaintance for long before we are made to realize that, for him, the sexes are in two opposite and opposing camps and he means to keep them there. His footnotes and marginalia, like Gibbon's, suggest a certain sympathy with tabooed subjects. Nothing delights him more than to isolate some indecorous or inconsistent trait of character and brandish it aloft in what Swinburne calls "the broad light of German laughter."

Julius **Pagel**[1] (1851–1912), of Berlin, a busy practitioner who devoted his whole life to medical history, was the author of many charming historical essays and an excellent medical chronology (1908), and published, in 1898, a one volume history of medicine in the form of lectures. This is a very readable book, the work of a broad, good-natured, tolerant spirit, but not specially remarkable for original research or display of erudition. In 1903–5, Pagel and Max Neuburger collaborated in bringing to editorial completion the *Handbuch der Geschichte der Medizin*, which was begun by Theodor Puschmann. This work, in three volumes, is the most reliable source of reference for facts, dates and bibliography after Haeser. It is written upon the coöperative plan, and, in dealing with the modern period, the editors have resorted to the usual plan of having each specialty treated separately by a particular authority. As with many books written by different authors, these special monographs have, at times, a somewhat dry, perfunctory and routine character. But the substantial merits of the Puschmann Handbuch as a reference work cannot be overestimated.

A formidable competitor of Baas's work is the recent "History of Medicine" by Pagel's pupil, Professor Max **Neuburger** of Vienna, which is

---

[1] A charming account of Pagel and his work by Drs. George Dock and M. G. Seelig of St. Louis is to be found in the Jour. Missouri State Med. Ass., St. Louis, 1910, ix, 366–369.

still coming out in parts and also in process of translation by Ernest Playfair under the direction of Sir William Osler (London, 1910). As a writer Neuburger is eloquent, often profound, sometimes florid, but a good stylist. As a scholar, he is richer, deeper and more serious than Baas, and his accounts of folk medicine and of Greek and Arabian medicine are by far the better of the two. Yet he has no saving salt of humor and often exhibits the Germanic tendency to rhapsodize and to wander off into philosophic reverie. He throws many new facts into the field, but does not always present them in a simple, direct manner. The large first volume of the English translation is printed on light-weight cloth paper, a great comfort in large-sized books. The succeeding volumes will be looked forward to with great interest by those advanced readers to whom such an elaborate work must specially, if not exclusively, appeal.

Of the smaller handbooks, Wunderlich's "Geschichte der Medizin" (1859) has never been translated and does not go beyond Schönlein's time. It was written by the hand of a master clinician, and is interesting for its anthology of illustrative excerpts, including the different classifications of disease down to the time of Schönlein. The "Medical History" of Edward T. Withington (London, 1894) is the work of a genuine scholar, written in an unusually engaging manner, with many valuable terminal notes and appendices. Unfortunately, it stops at the beginning of the nineteenth century, but it is based upon original research and there are few of the smaller sized books which convey so much accurate information. The "Epitome" of Roswell Park (1897) is the only American treatise of importance.

Léon Meunier's 'Histoire de la médecine" (Paris, 1911) has the merit of being very full on the modern period and can be recommended to anyone who wishes to see medical history through French eyes.

B. MEDICAL BIOGRAPHY

Bayle and Thillaye's "Biographie médicale" (Paris, 1855) is a sort of medical "Who's Who" up to the middle of the nineteenth century, eminently useful as far as it goes. The seven volumes by A.-J.-L. Jourdain prefixed to the "Encyclopédie des sciences médicales" (Paris, Panckoucke, 1820–25) are indispensable, containing many valuable bibliographies. August Hirsch's "Biographisches Lexikon" (6 vols., Wien u. Leipzig, 1884–8), and Pagel's "Biographisches Lexikon" of nineteenth century physicians (Berlin u. Wien, 1901), are standard modern works, which may be supplemented by the many admirable biographies of English physicians in Leslie Stephen's Dictionary of National Biography (68 vols., London, 1885–1912), by the Biographie française (46 vols., Paris, 1852–77), the Neuer Nekrolog der Deutschen (1823–52), the Biographisches Jahrbuch (1896–1911) and other reference works listed in the extensive bibliography given by Hirsch. The standard sources of American medical biography are those of James Thacher (1828) and Samuel D. Gross (1861), which are made up of extensive lives of a few men; Atkinson (1878), Stone (1894) and Watson (1896), which are good directories of contemporary names. Howard A. Kelly's Cyclopedia of American Medical Biography (Philadelphia, 1912) is the most recent work. For recent names, the various Who's Who's of different countries may be consulted. Many entertaining volumes of biographical essays have been written by G. T. Bettany (1885), Sir B. W. Richardson (1900), Victor Robinson (1912), and others. For biographies of individuals, the following are either readable or otherwise valuable for reference or for a certain perspicuity.

Acland (Sir Henry W.): Memoir by J. B. Altay, London, 1903.

Addison: Wilks & Bettany, History of Guy's Hospital, Lond., 1892, 221–234.—Guy's Hosp. Gaz., Lond., 1874, iii, 193; 201:1901, xxii, 520; port., 1 pl.

Arbuthnot: Life by G. A. Aitken, Oxford, 1892.

Arderne (John): Introduction to his "Treatises of fistula in ano" by D'Arcy Power (Early English Text Soc., No. 139, Lond., 1910).

Aretæus: Francis Adams, Preface to "The extant works [etc.], Lond., 1856, pp. v–xx.—München. med. Wchnschr., 1902, xlix, 1265–1267 (R. Kossmann).—Johns Hopkins Hosp. Bull., Balt., 1909, xx, 371–377 (E. F. Cordell).—Am. J. Clin. Med., Chicago, 1911, xvii, 1055–1058 or Pathfinders of Medicine, N. Y., 1912, 33–43 (V. Robinson).

von Arlt (C. F.): Meine Erlebnisse, Wiesbaden, 1887.

Auenbrugger: Jahresb. d. Ver. d. Aerzte in Steiermark, Graz, 1866, ii, 19–52 (Clar).—Jahresb. d. Gesellsch. f. Nat.- u. Heilk. in Dresd., 1863, 59–72.—Tr. Cong. Am. Phys. & Surg., 1891, New Haven, 1892, ii, 180 (Weir Mitchell).—Walsh: Makers of Modern Medicine, N. Y., 1907, 55–85.

Avicenna: Paris thesis (No. 182) by J. Eddé, 1889.—Johns Hopkins Hosp. Bull., Balt., 1908, xix, 157–160 (J. A. Chatard).—Arch. f. klin. Chir., Berl., 1884, xxx, 745–752 (H. Fröhlich).

von Baer: Selbstbiographie. 2. Aufl. Braunschweig, 1886.—Allg. Wien. med. Ztg., 1877, xxii, 357: 369 (Waldeyer).

Baglivi: Ztschr. f. klin. Med., Berl., 1888–9, xv, 279; 475 (M. Salomon).—München. med. Wchnschr., 1907, liv, 1241, port. (K. Sudhoff).

Bartlett (Elisha): Johns Hopkins Hosp. Bull., Balt., 1908, xix, 301–307 (W. R. Steiner).

Beaumont (William): Life and Letters by Jesse S. Myer (St. Louis, 1912). Also Physician & Surg., St. Louis, 529–574 (Osler, Vaughan, et al.).

Bell (Sir Charles): Life by A. Pichot, Par., 1858, English transl., London, 1860.—Letters, London, 1870.—Johns Hopkins Hosp. Bull., Balt., 1910, xxi, 171–182 (E. R. Corson).

Bell (John): Johns Hopkins Hosp. Bull., Balt., 1912, xxiii, 241–250 (E. R. Corson).

von Bergmann: Life by A. Buchholz. 2. Aufl., Leipz., 1911.

Bernard (Claude): Claude Bernard by Sir Michael Foster ("Masters of Medicine"), London, 1899. Claude Bernard par Georges Barral ("Bibliothèque Gilon"), Paris, 1889. Also: Gaz. d'hôp., Paris, 1879, lii, 326; 333 (E. Renan).

Bichat: Bull. soc. franç. d'hist. de méd., Par., 1902, i, 214; 261; 269; 277; 280; 285; 293; 309.—Interstate M. J., St. Louis, 1908, xv, 597; 667 (A. C. Eycleshymer).

Billings (John Shaw): Bull. N. Y. Public Library, 1913, xvii, 511–535 (S. Weir Mitchell, *et al.*).—Brit. M. J., Lond., 1913, i, 641–643 (Sir W. Osler, *et al.*).—Hospital, Lond., 1913, liii, 671–673 (Sir H. Burdett).

Billroth: Autobiography (Wien. med. Bl., 1894, xvii, 92–94) and his "Briefe" (7. Aufl., Hannover, 1906).—Berl. klin. Wchnschr., 1894, xxxi, 199–205 (J. Mikulicz); 205–207 (E. von Bergmann).—Deutsche Rundschau, Berl., 1893–4, xx, 274–277 (E. Hanslick).

du Bois Reymond (Emil): Deutsche med. Wchnschr., Leipz. u. Berl., 1897, xxiii, 17–19 (I. Munk).—Med. Chron., Manchester, 1896–7; n. s., vi, 241–250 (W. Stirling).—Nature, Lond., 1897, lv, 230 (J. Burdon Sanderson).

Bowditch (Henry Ingersoll): Life and Letters by V. Y. Bowditch, 2 vols., Bost., 1902.

Bright: Wilks & Bettany: History of Guy's Hospital, Lond., 1892, 212–221.—Johns Hopkins Hosp. Bull., Balt., 1912, xxiii, 173–186.

Broadbent (Sir William): Life by Miss E. B. Broadbent, Lond., 1909.

Broca: Rev. d'anthrop., Par., 1880, 2. s., iii, 577–608, 1 phot. & bibliog. (S. Pozzi).—Bull. Soc. d'anthrop. de Par., 1884, 3. s., vii, 921–956 (E. Dally).—J. Anthrop. Inst., Lond., 1880–81, x, 242–261, 1 phot. (E. W. Brabrook).—Saturday Lectures, Wash., 1882, 113–142 (R. Fletcher).

Brodie: Lives by H. W. Acland (Lond., 1864) and by Timothy Holmes ("Masters of Medicine"), Lond., 1897.—G. T. Bettany, Eminent Doctors, Lond., 1885, i, 286–303.

Browne (Sir Thomas): Biography by Edmund Gosse, London and New York, 1905.—Brit. M. J., Lond., 1905, ii, 993–998 (Sir W. Osler).—Med. Library & Hist. J., Brooklyn, 1905, iii, 264–275 (C. Williams).—Walter Pater, Macmillan's Mag., Lond., 1886, liv, 5–18.

Cardan (Jerome): Life by Henry Morley (2 vols., Lond., 1854) and by W. G. Waters, Lond., 1897.

Celsus: Fac. de méd. de Par. Confér. histor., 1866, 445–497 (P. Broca).—E. Littré, Médecine et Médecins, Par., 1872, 137–153.—Ann. Anat. & Surg., Brooklyn, 1882, v, 126; 177; 224; 280 (G. J. Fisher).—Glasgow M. J., 1892, xxxvii, 321–348 (J. Finlayson).—Handb. d. Gesch. d. Med., Jena, 1901–2, i, 415–443 (I. Bloch).

Cesalpinus: Arch. f. d. ges. Physiol., Bonn, 1884, xxxv, 295–390 (H. Tollin).—Proc. Charaka Club, N. Y., 1910, iii, 150–156 (J. Collins).

Charcot: N. iconog. de la Salpêtrière, Par., 1893, vi, 241–250 (Gilles de la Tourette). Inauguration du monument: *Ibid.*, 1898, xi, 401–418, port. Charcot artiste, 489–516, 6 pl.—Arch. f. exper. Path. u. Pharmakol., Leipz., 1893–4, xxxiii, pp. i–x (B. Naunyn).—Deutsche Ztschr. f. Nervenh., Leipz., 1893, iv, pp. i–xv (W. Erb).—Sitzungsb. d. phys.-med. Soc. zu Erlangen (1894), 1895, Heft 26, 1–14 (A. von Strümpell).—Wien. med. Wchnschr., 1893, xliii, 1513–1520 (S. Freud).—Johns Hopkins Hosp. Bull., Balt., 1893, iv, 87 (Sir W. Osler).—Internat. Clin.,

Phila., 1894, 4. s., i, pp. xv–xxi, port. (M. A. Starr).—Glasgow, M. J., 1893, xl, 292–298 (Jane B. Henderson).

Chovet (Abraham): Anat. Rec., Phila., 1911, v, 147–172, 2 port. (W. S. Miller).

Cohnheim: Ges. Abhandl., Berl., 1885, pp. vii–li, port. (W. Kühne).—Arch. f. exper. Path. u. Pharmakol., Leipz., 1884, xviii, 3.–4. Hft., pp. i–x (E. Klebs).

Colles: Works (Sydenham Soc., Lond., 1881), i–xvi, port. (R. McDonnell).

Cooper (Sir Astley): Life by B. B. Cooper, 2 v., London, 1843.—Guy's Hosp. Rep., Lond., 1841, vi, 229–234.—Quarterly Rev., Lond., 1843, lxxi, 529–560.—G. T. Bettany, Eminent Doctors, Lond., 1885, i, 202–226.— Wilks & Bettany: History of Guy's Hospital, Lond., 1892, 317–329.

Cordus (Valerius): E. L. Greene: Landmarks of Botanical History, Wash., 1909, i, 270–314.

Cullen: Life by J. Thomson, 2 v. Edinb., 1859.—Asclepiad, Lond., 1890, vii, 148–177, 2 port. (Sir B. W. Richardson).—New York M. J., 1897, lxvi, 689–691 (F. Staples).

Currie (James): Memoir by W. W. Currie, Lond., 1831.

Darwin: Life and Letters by F. Darwin, 2 v., N. Y., 1898.—More Letters, 2 v., London, 1903.—Life by E. B. Poulton, London, 1896. Gedenkschrift, Stuttgart, 1909.—Abernethian address by Sir T. L. Brunton, London, 1883. Pamphlets by Grant Allen (New York, 1886) and A. E. Shipley (Cambridge, 1909).—British Museum (Natural History), Special guide No. 4. Memorials, London, 1910.—Proc. Roy. Soc. Lond., 1888, xliv, pp. i–xxxv (T. H. Huxley).—Deutsche Rundschau, Berl., 1888, lvii, 229–254 (T. W. Preyer).—Proc. Am. Phil. Soc. Phila., 1909, xlviii, pp. iii–lvii (Sir J. Bryce, et al.). Pop. Sc. Monthly, N. Y., 1909, lxxiv, 315–343, 6 pl., 1 port. (H. F. Osborn).

Dieffenbach: H. Rohlfs: Gesch. d. deutsch. Med., Leipz., 1885, iv, 1–138.

Dioscorides: E. L. Greene: Landmarks of Botanical History, Wash., 1909, i, 151–155.

Donders: Life by J. Moleschott. Giessen, 1888.—Sitzungsb. d. math.-phys. Cl. d. k. bayer. Akad. d. Wissensch., München, 1889, xix, 118–124 (C. von Voit).—Ann. d'ocul., Brux., 1889, cii, 5–107, port. (J.-P. Nuel).— Arch. d'opht., Par., 1889, ix, 193–204 (E. Landolt).—Proc. Roy. Soc. Lond., 1890–91, xlix, pp. vii–xxiv, port. (W. B.).

Drake (Daniel): Memoirs by E. D. Mansfield, Cincinnati, 1851. Daniel Drake and his Followers, by Otto Juettner, Cincinnati, 1909. S. D. Gross, Lives (etc.), Phila., 1861, 614–662. Also: Jour. Am. Med. Ass., Chicago, 1895, xxv, 429–436 (W. Pepper). Also: Am. Jour. Med. Sc., Phila., 1876, n. s., lxxii, 451–452 (J. S. Billings).

Duchenne: C. Lasègue: Études méd., Par., 1884, i, 178–206.—Rev. internat. d'électrothér., Par., 1895–6, vi, 257–270 (Motet): 305–333, 1 pl., 2 port. (Inauguration du monument): 1899–1900, x, 69–90 (Brissaud). —Med. Rec., N. Y., 1908, lxxii, 50–54 (J. Collins).

Erasistratus: J. F. Hieronymus: Jena diss., 1790.—Glasgow M. J., 1893, 4. s., xxxix, 340–352 (J. Finlayson).

Esmarch: H. Rohlfs: Gesch. d. deutsch. Med., Leipz., 1885, iv, 353–411.— München. med. Wchnschr., 1893, xl, 8 (A. Hoffa).—Berl. klin. Wchnschr., 1908, xlv, 578 (A. Brer).—Ztschr. f. Krankenpflg., Berl., 1903, xxv, 91: 1908, xxx, 65.—Med. Mag., Lond., 1893–4, ii, 9–21 (Zobeltitz).

Fabry of Hilden: Deutsches Arch. f. Gesch. d. Med., Leipz., 1883, vi, 1–25 (P. Müller).—Abhandl. z. Gesch. d. Med., Bresl., 1904, Heft xiii (R. J. Schaefer).—Janus, Amst., 1910, xv, 65–72, 1 port. (R. J. Schaefer). —München. med. Wchnschr., 1910, lvii, 1401–1403, port. (K. Sudhoff). —Johns Hopkins Hosp. Bull., Balt., 1905, xvi, 7–10 (W. B. Platt).

Fayrer (Sir Joseph): Recollections of My Life. Edinb., 1900.

Foster (Sir Michael): J. Physiol., Lond., 1906–7, xxxv, 233–246 (J. N. Langley).—Publ. Med. Fac. Queen's Univ., Kingston, No. 7, 1913, 1–17 (J. G. Adami).

Fothergill: Memoirs by J. C. Lettsom, 4. ed., Lond., 1786.

Fracastorius: Life by F. O. Mencken, Leipz., 1731.—A. Rittmann. Culturgesch. Abhandl., Brünn, 1869–70, 3. Heft.—Gior. ital. di mal. ven., Milano, 1885, xx, 1–11 (Gamberini).—Proc. Charaka Club, N. Y., 1906, ii, 5–20, 3 pl. (Sir W. Osler).—Science, N. Y., 1910, n. s., xxxi, 500–502.

Frank (J. P.): Autobiography, Vienna, 1802.—K. Doll: Dr. Johann Peter Frank. Ein Lebensbild, Karlsruhe, 1910.—H. Rohlfs: Gesch. d. deutsch. Med., Stuttg., 1880, ii, 127–211.—Med. Jahrb., Wien, 1886, n. F., i, 97–116 (H. von Bamberger).—Wien. klin. Wchnschr., 1909, xxii, 1341: 1913, xxvi, 627 (M. Neuburger).

Frerichs: Arch. f. exper. Path. u. Pharmakol., Leipz., 1885, xix, pp. iii–viii (B. Naunyn).—Deutsche med. Wchnschr., Leipz. u. Berl., 1884, x, 257; 266; 279; 296; 1885: xi, 177 (E. Leyden).—Wien. med.Wchnschr., 1885, xxxv, 465; 497; 537 (E. Litten).

Gaddesden (John): Monograph by H. P. Cholmely. Oxford (Clarendon Press), 1912.

Galen: Sprengel: Beitr. z. Gesch. d. Med., Halle, 1794, i, 1. St., 117–195.— Gaz. méd. de Par., 1847, 3. s., ii, 591; 603 (C. Daremberg).—Ibid., 1858, 3. s., xiii, 43; 115; 171 (J.-E. Pétrequin).—Brit. M. J., Lond., 1892, i, 573; 730; 771 (J. Finlayson).—Middlesex Hosp. J., Lond., 1899, iii, 37–52 (Sir V. Horsley).—Arch. f. Gesch. d. Med., Leipz., 1911, v, 172–224 (T. Meyer-Steineg).

Galton (Sir Francis): Memories of my life, N. Y., 1909.—Eugenics Rev., Lond., 1911–12, iii, 1–9 (M. C.).—Nature, Lond., 1910–11, lxxxv, 440–445.—Pop. Sc. Monthly, 1911, lxxix, 171–190 (J. A. Harris).

Garth (Sir Samuel): Johns Hopkins Hosp. Bull., Balt., 1906, xvii, 1–17, port. (H. Cushing).

Goltz: Arch. f. d. ges. Physiol., Bonn, 1903, xciv, 1–64, port. (J. R. Ewald).

von Graefe (Albrecht): Life by E. Michaelis, Berl., 1877.—Ber. ü. d.Versamml. d. ophth. Gesellsch., Stuttg., 1886, xxiv, 5–52 (Donders & Helmholtz).— Ann. d'ocul., Brux., 1872, lxvii, 5–56 (Warlomont).

von Gräfe (Carl Ferdinand): H. Rohlfs: Gesch. d. deutsch. Med., Leipz., 1883, iii, 247–324.

Graves: Biography by W. Stokes in his "Studies in physiology" (etc.), Lond., 1863, pp. i–lxxxiii. Also: Med. Times & Gaz., Lond., 1853, vi, 1–5 (W. Stokes).—Med. Hist. Meath. Hosp., Dublin, 1888, 122–129, port.

Gross (S. D.): Autobiography, Phila., 1887.—Tr. Am. Surg. Ass., Phila,. 1897, xv, pp. xxxi–xlviii.—Am. J. M. Sc., Phila., 1884, n. s., lxxxviii, 293–308, port. (I. M. Hays).—Johns Hopkins Hosp. Bull., Balt., 1912, xxiii, 83–94 (C. W. G. Rohrer).

Gull (Sir William): Guy's Hosp. Rep., Lond., 1890, 3. s., xxxii, pp. xxv–xliii, port.—Wilks & Bettany. History of Guy's Hospital, Lond., 1892, 261–274.

Guy de Chauliac: Confér. Inst. Fac. de Méd. de Par., 1866, 173–208 (Follin).

Haeckel: Life by W. Bölsche (English transl. by J. McCabe, Phila.).

Hales (Stephen): Gentleman's Mag., Lond., 1764, xxxiv, 273–278 (P. Collinson).—Dict. Nat. Biog., Lond., 1890, xxiv, 32–36 (F. Darwin).—Johns Hopkins Hosp. Bull., Balt., 1904, xv, 185; 232 (P. M. Dawson).

Hall (Marshall): Memoirs by Charlotte Hall, Lond., 1861.—Lancet, Lond., 1850, ii, 120–128, port; 1857, ii, 172–175.—Dict. Nat. Biog., Lond., 1890, xxiv, 80–83 (G. T. Bettany).

Haller: Lives and Eulogies by J. G. Zimmermann (Zürich, 1755), E. G. Baldinger and C. G. Heyne (Göttingen, 1778).—T. Henry (Warrington, 1783), R. C. Stiles (New York, 1867).—A. Lissauer (Berlin, 1873). See also Denkschrift, Bern, 1877. Hallers Wohnungen (etc.), by H. Kronecker, Bern, 1908, has many interesting illustrations.—Die Bildnisse (etc.), by Artur Weese, Bern, 1909, gives all extant portraits.—Especially interesting are "Haller Redivivus" by H. Kronecker (Mitth. d. naturf. Gesellsch. in Bern (1902), 1903, 203–226) and Harvey Cushing's paper in Am. Med., Phila., 1901, ii, 542; 580. See also Deutsche med. Wchnschr., Leipz. u. Berl., 1908, xxxiv, 1813–1815 (H. Kronecker).—München. med. Wchnschr., 1908, lv, 2142 (K. Sudhoff).—Johns Hopkins Hosp. Bull., Balt., 1908, xix, 65–73 (J. C. Hemmeter). For his literary life, see Ludwig Hirzel's introduction to Haller's Gedichte, Frauenfeld, 1882.

Harington (Sir John): Johns Hopkins Hosp. Bull., Balt., 1908, xix, 285–295 (J. G. Adami).

Harvey (William): William Harvey by D'Arcy Power ("Masters of Medicine"), London, 1897.—Memorials of Harvey by J. H. Aveling, London, 1875. —Some Memoranda (etc.), by S. Weir Mitchell, New York, 1907.— Some recently discovered Letters (etc.), by S. Weir Mitchell, Philadelphia, 1912.—Notice of an Unpublished Manuscript by G. E. Paget, London, 1801. Also three addresses by T. H. Huxley in: Nature, London, 1878, xvii, 417; xviii, 146, and Pop. Sc. Monthly (Suppl.), New York, 1878, No. xi, 385–389. Also: Johns Hopkins Hosp. Bull., Baltimore, 1897, viii, 167–174 (W. K. Brooks). Also St. Barth. Hosp. Rep., London, 1887, xxiii, 1–12 (W. Munk). Also: Lancet, London, 1878, ii, 776–778, 1 pl. (Sir B. W. Richardson). Also: Asclepiad, London, 1884, i, 39–44, 1 pl. (Sir B. W. Richardson). Also Harveian orations (listed in Index Catalogue, 1901, 2. s., vi, 780).

Heberden: Essay by A. C. Buller (London, 1879).—Pettigrew, Med. Portr. Gallery, Lond., 1840, iii, No. 7, 1–18, port.—Dict. Nat. Biog., Lond., 1891, xxv, 359 (J. F. Payne).—Ztschr. f. klin. Med., Berl., 1910, lxx, 352–357 (J. Pawinski).—St. Barth. Hosp. Rep., Lond., 1911, xlvi, 1–12 (Sir D. Duckworth).

Heim (Ernst Ludwig): Life by G. W. Kessler, 2 v. Leipz., 1835.—Rohlfs: Gesch. d. deutsch. Med., Stuttg., 1875, i, 480–519.

Heister: V. Fossel: Stud. z. Gesch. d. Med., Stuttg., 1909, 111–152.

Helmholtz: Lives by L. Koenigsberger, 3 v. Brunswick, 1902 (English transl. by F. A. Welby, Oxford, 1906); and J. G. M'Kendrick, London, 1899. Bibliography by A. König, Leipzig, 1895. See, also: Aerztl. Vereinsbl. f. Deutschl., Leipz., 1894, xxiii, 553–556 (C. Ludwig).—Arch. d'opht., Par., 1894, xiv, 721–842 (E. Landolt).—Rev. scient., Par., 1897, 4. s., viii, 321; 360 (E. du Bois Reymond).—Proc. Roy. Soc. Lond., 1896, lix, pp. xvii–xxx.—J. Am. M. Ass., Chicago, 1902, xxxviii, 548–569.

van Helmont (J. B.): Studies by J. J. Loos (Heidelberg, 1807), D. H. Fraenkel (Leipzig, 1837), G. Rommelaere (Brussels, 1868).—Mém. d. concours . . . Acad. roy. de méd. de Belg., Brux., 1866, vi, 553–739 (J.-A. Mandon).—Bull. Acad. roy. de méd. de Belg., Brux., 1866, 2. s., ix, 985–1088 (Tallois).—J. hebd. de méd., Par., 1830, vi, 513–527 (E. Littré).

Henle: Life by F. R. Merkel, Braunschweig, 1909. See, also: Arch. f. mikr. Anat., Bonn, 1885–6, xxvi, pp. i–xxxii (W. Waldeyer).—Biol. Centralbl., Erlangen, 1885–6, v, 289–293 (W. Flemming).—Deutsche med. Wchnschr., Berl., 1885, xi, 463; 483 (K. Bardeleben).

Herophilus: K. F. H. Marx: Herophilus, Carlsruhe & Baden, 1838.—Glasgow M. J., 1893, 4. s., xxxix, 321–340 (J. Finlayson).

Hewson (William): Tr. Med. Soc. Lond., 1810, i, 51–63 (J. C. Lettsom).— Asclepiad, Lond., 1891, viii, 148–177 (Sir B. W. Richardson).—Dict. Nat. Biog., Lond., 1891, xxvii, 312 (J. F. Payne).

Hicks (Braxton): Select Essays (Sydenham Soc. Publ., vol. 173), Lond., 1901, 93–118, with bibliography (C. J. Cullingworth).

716   HISTORY OF MEDICINE

Hippocrates: Introduction to Emile Littré's translation, v. 1, pp. 1–554, Par., 1839.—J. E. Pétrequin: Chirurgie d'Hippocrate, 2 v., Par., 1878. Also Brit. & For. Med.-Chir. Rev., Lond., 1866, xxxviii, 483–496 (Sir T. C. Allbutt).—Glasgow M. J., 1892, xxxvii, 253–271 (J. Finlayson).—Brit. M. J., Lond., 1906, i, 571–577 (R. Caton).

His (Wilhelm): Am. J. Anat., Balt., 1904–5, iv, 139–161 (F. P. Mall).—Lancet, Lond., 1904, i, 1446–1449 (W. Stirling).—Deutsche med. Wchnschr., Leipz. u. Berl., 1904, xxx, 1438; 1469–1509 (W. Waldeyer).—Verhandl. d. naturf. Gesellsch. in Basel, 1904, 434–464, port.(J. Kollmann).

Hodgkin (Thomas): Wilks & Bettany: Hist. Guy's Hosp., Lond., 1892, 380–386.—Guy's Hosp. Rep., Lond., 1878, xxiii, 3. s., 55–127 (Sir S. Wilks).—Guy's Hosp. Gaz., Lond., 1909, xxiii, 528; 1910, xxiv, 13 (Wilks).

Holmes (O. W.): Lives by W. S. Kennedy (Bost., 1883), H. Lee (Bost., 1894) and J. T. Morse, Jr. (2 v., Boston, 1896).—Boston M. & S. J., 1894, cxxxi, 375–380, port.—Lancet, Lond., 1886, ii, 6–9 (Sir S. Wilks).—Brit. M. J., Lond., 1894, ii, 839–841 (Sir W. T. Gardner).—Johns Hopkins Hosp. Bull., Balt., 1894, v, 85–88 (Sir W. Osler).

Hoppe-Seyler: Arch. f. path. Anat. (etc.), Berl., 1895, cxlii, 386–388 (R. Virchow.—Ztschr. f. physiol. Chem., Strassb., 1895, pp. i–lxii, port. (E. Baumann & A. Kossell).

Hufeland: Life by J. I. J. Sachs, Berl., 1832. Also Med. Alm., Berl., 1837, 39–54, port.

Hunter (John): Stephen Paget, John Hunter ("Masters of Medicine"), London, 1897.—Memoirs (etc.) by J. Adams, London, 1817.—John Hunter and his Pupils by Samuel D. Gross, Philadelphia, 1881. Also Brit. Med. Jour., London, 1890, i, 738–740 (J. Finlayson); Ibid., 1899, i, 389–395 (Sir W. MacCormac); Ibid., 1886, i, 1093–1095 (Sir J. Paget). Also: Hunterian orations (listed in Index Catalogue, 1902, 2. s., vii, 483).

Hunter (William): William Hunter by R. Hingston Fox, London, 1901.

Huxham: Dict. Nat. Biog., Lond., 1891, xxviii, 363 (N. Moore).—Johns Hopkins Hosp. Bull., 1906, xvii, 308–311 (W. G. Vogeler).

Huxley: Life and Letters by L. Huxley, 2 v., Lond., 1900.—Autobiographical sketch (Hosp. Gaz., Lond., 1891, xix, 312–314).—Proc. Roy. Soc. Lond., 1896, lix, pp. xlvi–lxvi, port. (Sir M. Foster).—Dict. Nat. Biog., Suppl., Lond., 1901, iii, 22–31 (W. F. R. Weldon).—Science, N. Y., 1896, n. s., iii, 147–154 (H. F. Osborn); 253–263 (T. Gill).—Rep. Smithson. Inst., 1898–1900, Wash., 1900, 701–728 (W. K. Brooks, et al.).

Hyrtl: Deutsche med. Wchnschr., Leipz. u. Berl., 1894, xx, 619 (K. von Bardeleben).—Wien. klin. Wchnschr., 1894, vii, 549; 556; 557.—Wien. med. Wchnschr., 1894, xliv, 1337; 1406.

Jackson (James): Memoir by J. J. Putnam, Bost. & N. Y., 1905.—Boston M. & S. J., 1867–8, lxxvii, 106–109 (J. Bigelow & O. W. Holmes).

Jenner: Life by J. Baron, Lond., 1827–38.—Brit. M. J., Lond., 1894, i, 72; 1901, ii, 479; 1902, ii, 1; 1676.—J. Am. M. Ass., Chicago, 1896, xxvii, 312–317 (H. R. Storer).—New York M. J., 1902, lxxvi, 925; 978 (G. Dock).—Deutsche med. Wchnschr., 1896, xxii, 305–323 (Festnummer).

Knox (Robert): Life by H. Lonsdale, London, 1870.

Koch: Biographies by W. Becker (Berl., 1891) and K. Wezel (Berl., 1912).—Wien. klin. Wchnschr., 1903, xvi, 1377–1381 (R. Paltauf).—Deutsche med. Wchnschr., Leipz. u. Berl., 1910, xxxvi, 2321–2324 (G. Gaffky).—Johns Hopkins Hosp. Bull., Balt., 1911, xxxiii, 415–425 (W. W. Ford).—Ibid., 425–428 (S. A. Knopf).

Kölliker: Erinnerungen, Leipz., 1899.—Ztschr. f. wissensch. Zool., Leipz., 1906, lxxxiv, p. i–xxvi (Ehlers).

APPENDICES 717

Kühne (Willy): Ztschr. f. Biol., München u. Leipz., 1900, n. F., xxii, pp. i–viii (C. von Virt).—Med. Chron., Manchester, 1901, 4. s., i, 401–415, port. (W. Stirling).

Kussmaul: Jugenderinnerungen, 4. Aufl. Stuttg., 1900.—München. med. Wchnschr., 1902, xlix, 281–286, port. (L. Edinger).—Therap. d. Gegenw. Berl., 1902, n. F., iv, 289–291 (B. Naunyn).—Deutsches Arch. f. klin. Med., Leipz., 1902, lxxiii, 1–89 (W. Fleiner).

Laënnec: Life by A.-L.-J. Bayle. Par., 1826.—N. Orl. M. News & Hosp. Gaz., 1859–60, vi, 736–756 (A. Flint).—Conf. hist. Fac. de med., Par., 1866, 61–107 (Chauffard).—Wash. M. Ann., 1910–11, ix, 250–260, 1 pl.

Lamarck: Life by A. S. Packard, Lond., 1901.

Lanfranc: J. Missouri M. Ass., St. Louis, 1910–11, vii, 402–408 (F. J. Lutz).

Larrey: Johns Hopkins Hosp. Bull., Balt., 1906, xvii, 195–215 (J. C. Da Costa).

Leeuwenhoek: Asclepiad, Lond., 1885, ii, 319–346, port. (Sir B. W. Richardson).—J. Roy. Microsc. Soc., Lond., 1913, 121–135, port. (H. G. Plimmer).

Leidy (Joseph): Proc. Acad. Nat. Sc., Phila., 1891, 342–388 (H. C. Chapman). —Pop. Sc. Monthly, N. Y., 1907, lxx, 311–314, port. (W. K. Brooks).— Science, N. Y., 1913, n. s., xxxvii, 809–814 (C. S. Minot).

Lettsom: Life by T. J. Pettigrew, 3 vols., Lond., 1817.—Memoirs. Lond., 1817.—Dict. Nat. Biog., Lond., 1893, xxxiii, 134–136 (J. F. Payne).

Leyden: Lebenserinnerungen, Stuttg. u. Leipz., 1910.—Internat. Beitr. z. inn. Med., Berl., 1902, i, 1–21, port. (H. Nothnagel).—Mitt. a. d. Grenzgeb. d. Med. u. Chir., Jena, 1910, xxii, p. i–iv (B. Naunyn).— Wien. klin. Wchnschr., 1910, xxiii, 1488–1490 (R. von Jaksch).

Liebig: Life by J. Volhard. 2 vols., Leipz., 1909.—Autobiography (Chem. News, Lond., 1891, lxiii, 265–276).—Faraday lecture by A. W. von Hofmann, Lond., 1876.—Allg. Wien. med. Ztg., 1899, xliv, 481; 494; 505; 514 (G. Klemperer).

Linacre: Sir W. Osler, Thomas Linacre, Cambridge, 1908.

Linnæus: Life by Brightwell, Lond., 1858.—Album of Portraits by T. Tullberg. Stockh., 1907.—J. Am. M. Ass., Chicago, 1902, xxxix, 593–598 (L. Hektoen).—Janus, Amst., 1903, viii, 115–122 (W. Ebstein).—Med. Libr. & Histor. J., Brooklyn, 1904, ii, 173–184 (J. H. Hunt); 185–193 (A. Egdahl).

Lister (Lord): Collected Papers. Oxford, 1909, i, pp. i–xliv.—Brit. M. J., Lond., 1912, i, 397–402.—Lancet, Lond., 1912, i, 465–472.—Glasgow M. J., 1912, lxxvii, 190–196.—Clin. J., Lond., 1912–13, xli, 257–263 (Sir W. W. Cheyne).—Canad. J. M. & S., Toronto, 1912, xxx, 288–350 (Symposium).—Deutsche Ztschr. f. Chir., Leipz., 1912, cxx, 1–6 (E. Payr).

Littré: Notice by C.-A. Sainte-Beuve. Par., 1863. (Repr. from: Nouveaux lundis, v. v, p. 200.) Rev. d. deux mondes, Par., 1882, lii, 634–671 (C.-V. Daremberg).—Chron. med., Par., 1895, i, 11–16, port. (Cabanés).

Long (Crawford W.): Johns Hopkins Hosp. Bull., Balt., 1897, viii, 174–184 (H. H. Young).

Louis: Life by E.-J. Woillez. Par., 1873. Johns Hopkins Hosp. Bull., Balt., 1897, viii, 161–166 (Sir W. Osler).

Lower (Richard): "Two Oxford Physiologists" by F. Gotch. Oxford, 1908. —Sir M. Foster. Lect. Hist. Physiol., Cambridge, 1901, 181–185.

Ludwig (Carl): Memoir by J. von Kries. Freib. i. B. & Leipz., 1895.—Berl. klin. Wchnschr., 1895, xxxv, 466 (H. Kronecker).—Med. Chron., Manchester, 1895–6, n. s., iii, 178–191 (W. Stirling).—Proc. Roy. Soc. Lond., 1895–6, lix, pt. 2, pp. i–viii (Sir J. Burdon-Sanderson).

McDowell: Life by Mary Y. Ridenbaugh. N. Y., 1890.—Oration by S. D. Gross, Louisville, 1879.

Magendie: Leçon d'ouverture by Claude Bernard. Par., 1856. Éloge by P. Flourens, Par., 1858. Also: Rep. Smithson. Inst., Wash., 1866, 91–125 (Flourens).—E. Littré: Médecine et médecins, Par., 1872, 154–183.— Med. Libr. & Hist. J., Brooklyn, 1906, iv, 45; 198; 292; 364: 1907, v, 24, 2 port. (P. M. Dawson).

Malpighi: Lives by G. Atti (Bologna, 1847), E. Ferrario (Milan, 1860), U. Pizzoli (Milan, 1897).—Asclepiad, Lond., 1893, x, 385–406, port. (B. W. Richardson).—Sir M. Foster, Lect. Hist. Physiol., Cambridge, 1901, 84–120.—Johns Hopkins Hosp. Bull., Balt., 1905, xvii, 275–284 (W. G. MacCallum).

Martin (Henry Newell): Proc. Roy. Soc. Lond., 1896, lx, pp. xx–xxiii (Sir M. Foster).

Martin (Sir James Ronald): Life by Sir J. Fayrer, Lond., 1897.

Mayow (John): "Two Oxford Physiologists" by F. Gotch. Oxford, 1908.— Sir M. Foster. Lect. Hist. Physiol., Cambridge, 1901, 185–199.— Asclepiad, Lond., 1887, iv, 55–70, port. (B. W. Richardson).—Dict. Nat. Biog., Lond.,,1894, xxxvii, 175–177 (P. J. Hartog).

Mead: Memoirs by T. Lemon. Lond., 1755.—Gentlemen's Mag., Lond., 1754, xxiv, 510–515 (Mattley).—(W. McMichael and W. Munk: Gold-headed cane. Lond., 1827, 56–118.)—Asclepiad, Lond., 1888, v, 49–79, port. (B. W. Richardson).—Dict. Nat. Biog., Lond., 1894, xxxvii, 181–186 (N. Moore).

Mendel (Gregor): W. Bateson, Mendel's principles of heredity. Cambridge, 1913, 327–334, 3 port.—J. J. Walsh, Catholic churchmen in science, Phila., 1906, 195–221, port.

Mesmer: Erinnerungen by Justinus Kerner. Frankf. a. M. 1856.—F. Podmore, Mesmerism and Christian Science, Phila., 1909.—Brit. M. J., Lond., 1911, ii, 1555: 1912, i, 79; 133; 199; 249.

Mikulicz: Mitt. a. d. Grenzgeb. d. Med. u. Chir., Jena, 1907, Gedenkbd., 1–64, port. (W. Kausch).—München. med. Wchnschr., 1905, lii, 1297–1300, port. (Sauerbruch).—Wien. klin. Wchnschr., 1905, xviii, 671–674 (von Eiselsberg).

Mondeville: J. L. Pagel, Leben, Lehre, und Leistungen (etc.), Berl., 1892.— Proc. Charaka Club, N. Y., 1910, iii, 70–98, port. (A. G. Gerster).

Morgagni: Atti d. XI. Cong. med. internaz., 1894, Roma, 1895, i, 188–197 (R. Virchow).—Asclepiad, Lond., 1888, v, 147–173, port. (Sir B. W. Richardson).—J. J. Walsh, Makers of modern medicine, N. Y., 1907, 29–51.

Morgan (John): Journal of 1764, Phila., 1907.—Life by M. I. Wilbert. Phila., 1904.—Phila. J. M. & Phys. Sc., 1820, i, 439–442 (B. Rush).—Tr. Coll. Phys., Phila., 1887, centennial vol., 26–42 (W. S. W. Ruschenberger).

Morton (Richard): Med. Libr. & Hist. J., Brooklyn, 1904, ii, 1–7, port. (Sir W. Osler).

Mott (Valentine): Memoir by S. D. Gross, Phila., 1868.

Müller (Johannes): Gedächtnisrede by R. Virchow. Berl., 1858 (Transl. in Edinb. M. J., 1858, iv, 452–527).—Abhandl. d. k. Akad. d. Wissensch. zu Berl. (1859), 1860, 25–191 (E. du Bois Reymond).—Johns Hopkins Hosp. Bull., Balt., 1896, vii, 16–18 (W. B. Platt).—Messenger, N. Y., 1903, 5. s., iii, 668–693 (J. J. Walsh).

Mundinus: Notizie by V. Joppi, Udine, 1873.—Ann. Anat. & Surg., Brooklyn, N. Y., 1882, xi, 35; 71 (G. J. Fisher).—Columbus M. J., 1896, xvii, 343–357 (J. E. Pilcher).—Med. Libr. & Hist. J., Brooklyn, N. Y., 1903, i, 1–8: 1906, iv, 311–331, 4 pl. (L. S. Pilcher).

Nightingale (Florence): Life by Sarah A. Tooley. Lond., 1904.—Nutting and Dock: History of nursing, N. Y., 1912, 62–311.

North (Elisha): Johns Hopkins Hosp. Bull., Balt., 1908, xix, 301–307 (W. R. Steiner).

O'Dwyer (Joseph): Pediatrics, N. Y. & Lond., 1898, v, 95–97, port. (A. Jacobi).—J. J. Walsh. Makers of modern medicine, N. Y., 1907, 325–356.

Oken (Lorenz): Alexander Ecker, Lorenz Oken, Transl. by A. Fulk, London, 1883.

Owen: Life by R. Owen. 2 v., Lond., 1895.—Proc. Roy. Soc. Lond., 1894, lv, suppl., pp. i–xiv (W. H. F.).—Johns Hopkins Hosp. Bull., Balt., 1911, xxii, 133–137 (C. W. G. Rohrer).

Pagel (Julius): München. med. Wchnschr., 1912, lix, 425, port. (K. Sudhoff). —Klin.-therap. Wchnschr., Berl., 1912, xix, 205–208 (I. Bloch).—Arch. f. Gesch. d. Med., Leipz., 1912–13, vi, 71–79 (P. Richter).—J. Missouri M. Ass., St. Louis, 1913, ix, 366–369 (G. Dock).

Paget (Sir James): Dict. Nat. Biog., Lond., 1901, suppl. iii, 240–242 (D'A. Power).—St. Barth. Hosp. J., Lond., 1901–2, ix, 17–21 (S. Paget).— Tr. Rhode Island M. Soc., 1902, Providence, 1903, vi, 504–525 (Helen C. Putnam).

Paracelsus: Studies and biographies by: K. F. H. Marx (Göttingen, 1842), F. Mook (Würtzb., 1876), J. Ferguson (Glasg., 1877–85), F. Hartmann (Lond., 1887), E. Schubert & K. Sudhoff (Frankf. a. M., 1887–9), K. Sudhoff (Versuch, Berl., 1894–9), F. Hartmann (Leipz., 1899), H. Magnus (Breslau, 1906), E. Schlegel (München, 1908), and Anna M. Stoddart (Lond., 1911). Also: Arch. f. d. ges. Med., Jena, 1841, i, 26–43 (H. Haeser).—Cor.-Bl. f. Schweiz. Aerzte, Basel, 1905, xxxi, 438–488 (M. Roth).—Zentralbl. f. Biblioth.-Wes., Leipz., 1893, x, 316; 385; xi, 169 (K. Sudhoff).

Paré: Lives by J. F. Malgaigne (Œuvres completes, Par., 1840, i), Le Paulmier (Par., 1884), S. Paget (Lond., 1897). Also, Am. M.-Chir. Rev., Phila., 1869, v, 1059–1083 (S. D. Gross).

Parkinson: Johns Hopkins Hosp. Bull., Balt., 1912, xxiii, 33–45 (L. G. Rowntree).

Pasteur: R. Vallery-Radot. La vie de Pasteur. Paris, 1900 (English transl., 2 v., Lond., 1911).—Pasteur by Mr. and Mrs. Percy Frankland, London, 1898. Also: Rev. scient., Paris, 1895, 4. s., iv, 417–431 (Richet & Renan).—Berl. klin. Wchnschr., 1895, xxxii, 947 (R. Virchow).— Johns Hopkins Hosp. Bull., Balt., 1903, xiv, 325–334 (C. A. Herter).

Patin (Guy): Life by P. Pic, Par., 1911.

Pavy (F. W.): Guy's Hosp. Rep., Lond., 1912, lxvi, 1–23 (F. Taylor).—Sc. Progress 20. Cent., Lond., 1912.

Pepper (William): Lives by F. N. Thorpe (Phila., 1904) and J. Tyson (Phila., 1901). Also Phila. M. J., 1899, iii, 607–611 (Sir W. Osler).

Pettenkofer: Memoir by C. von Voit (München, 1902)—Berl. klin. Wchnschr., 1901, xxxviii, 268; 301; 321 (M. Rubner).

Pflüger: Memoir by M. Nussbaum. Bonn, 1909.

von Pfolspeundt (H.): Janus, Leyden, 1913, 109–119 (F. J. Lutz).

Platter: Selbstbiographie, ed. by H. Boos, Leipz., 1878.

Post (Wright): Memoir by Valentine Mott, N. Y., 1829.

Pott: Dict. Nat. Biog., Lond., 1896, xlvi, 207 (D'A. Power).—St. Barth. Hosp. Rep., Lond., 1894, xxx, 163–187 (Horder).

Power (Henry): Autobiography. (Stratford-upon-Avon, 1912.)

Priestley (Joseph): Memoirs, Northumberland, 1806. Also: Pop. Sc. Monthly, N. Y., 1875, vi, 90–107 (T. H. Huxley).

Pringle: Pettigrew: Med. Port. Gallery, Lond., 1840, ii, No. 14.—Dict. Nat. Biog., Lond., 1896, xlvi, 386 (J. F. Payne).

Purkinje: J. Am. M. Ass., Chicago, 1899, xxxii, 812–814 (R. B. Opitz).—Arch. f. Krim.-Anthrop. u. Kriminalist., Leipz., 1906, xxii, 326–335 (G. Roscher).—Valuable analysis of his works by Th. Eiselt in: Vrtljschr. f. d. prakt. Heilk., Prag, 1859, lxiii, Beil., 1–20.

Ramazzini: Franz Koelsch. Bernardino Ramazzini, Stuttgart, 1912.

Reed (Walter): Biography by H. A. Kelly, Balt., 2. ed., 1913.—J. Hyg., Cambridge, 1903, iii, 292–296, port. (G. H. F. Nuttall).—Pop. Sc. Month., N. Y., 1904, lxv, 262–268 (W. D. McCaw).

Remak (Robert): Berl. klin. Wchnschr., 1865, ii, 372.—Wien. med. Presse, 1865, xxxvii (M. Benedikt).

Renaudot (Théophraste): Life by G. Gilles de la Tourette. Par., 1884.—Albany M. Ann., 1907, xxviii, 599–623 (C. G. Cumston).

Richter (August Gottlieb): H. Rohlfs, Gesch. d. deutsch. Med., Leipz., 1883, iii, 33–172.

Ringer (Sidney): Proc. Roy. Soc., Lond., 1912, s. B., lxxxiv, pp. i–iii, port. (E. A. S.).—Biochem. J., Liverp., 1910–11, v, pp. i–xix (B. Moore).

Rokitansky: Festreden; Wien. klin. Wchnschr., 1898, xi, 559–564.—Wien. med. Presse, 1874, xv, Fest-Nummer, 1–8 (J. Schnitzler); 1878, xix, 965–974 (Arneth); 1549–1554 (T. Meynert).—Prag. med. Wchnschr., 1878, iii, 309 (E. Klebs).—Allg. Wien. med. Ztg., 1879, xxiv, 141–143 (S. Stricker).

Rush (Benjamin): (Recollections by J. C. Lettsom, Lond., 1815. Reminiscences by T. D. Mitchell, Transylvania J. Med., Lexington, Ky., 1839, xii, 92–116.—S. D. Gross. Lives, etc., Phila., 1861, 17–85, port. (S. Jackson).—Asclepiad, Lond., 1885, ii, 38–57 port. (Sir B. W. Richardson).—J. Am. M. Ass., Chicago, 1889, xiii, 330–335 (H. R. Storer).—Med.-Leg. J., N. Y., 1886–7, iv, 238–273, port. (C. K. Mills).

Sanctorius: Resoc. r. Accad. med.-chir. di Napoli (1889), 1890, xliii, 58–113 (M. Del Gaizo).—Tr. Cong. Am. Phys. & Surg., 1891, N. Haven, 1892, ii, 188–198 (Weir Mitchell).

Sanderson (Sir John Burdon): Memoir by Lady Sanderson, Oxford, 1911.

Scarpa: Discourse by S. Liberali, Treviso, 1834.—Mem. acad. de med., Par., 1838, vii, 1–28 (E. Pariset).—Asclepiad, Lond., 1886, iii, 128–148, port. (Sir B. W. Richardson).

Schönlein: Gedächtnisrede by R. Virchow. Berl., 1865.—Berl. klin. Wchnschr., 1864, i, 276–279 (C. Griesinger).—Wien. med. Wchnschr., 1864, xiv, 107 (Frerichs).—Ztschr. f. klin. Med., Berl., 1910, lxxi, 471–477 (E. Ebstein).—Arch. f. Gesch. d. Med., Leipz., 1911–12, v, 449–452 (E. Ebstein).

Schultze (Max): Arch. f. mikr. Anat., Bonn, 1874, x, pp. i–xxiii, port. (G. Schwalbe).

Schwann: Liber memorialis. Düsseldorf, 1879.—Arch. f. mikr. Anat., Bonn, 1882–3, xxi, pp. i–xlix (J. Henle); 1909, lxxiv, 469–473, port. (O. Hertwig & W. Waldeyer).—Arch. f. path. Anat. (etc.), Berl., 1882, lxxxvii, 389–392 (R. Virchow).—Ztschr. f. physiol. Chem., Strassb., 1882, vi, 280–285 (A. Kossel).—Nature, Lond., 1881–2, xxv, 321–323 (E. R. Lankester).

Semmelweis: Life by Sir J. W. Sinclair. Manchester, 1909.—Studies, by J. Bruck (Wien, 1887), J. Grosse (Leipz. & Wien, 1898) and F. Schürer von Waldheim (Wien & Leipz., 1905).—Med. Rev. of Rev., N. Y., 1912, xviii, 232–246 (V. Robinson).

Senator: Gedächtnisrede by A. Goldscheider, Berl. klin. Wchnschr., 1911, xlviii, 1961–1968. Also: München. med. Wchnschr., 1911, lviii, 1733–1735 (A. Wolff-Eisner).

Servetus: Servetus and Calvin by Robert Willis, Lond., 1877.—Johns Hopkins Hosp. Bull., Balt., 1910, xxi, 1–11, 4 pl. (Sir W. Osler).

Simpson (Sir James Y.): Lives by J. Duns (Edinb., 1873), Eva B. Simpson (Lond., 1896), and H. L. Gordon (Lond., 1897). Also Edinb. M. J., 1911, n. s., vi, Memorial No., 481–560, 9 pl.; vii, 12–17.

Sims (James Marion): "The Story of my Life" (N. Y., 1884).—"Ueber Marion Sims" by R. Olshausen (Berl., 1897).—Am. J. Obst., N. Y., 1884, xvii, 52–61, port. (P. F. Mundé).—Alabama M. & S. Age, Anniston, 1893–4, vi, 607–616 (T. A. Means).—Med. Rec., N. Y., 1894, xlvi, 705–708 (É. Souchon).—N. Orl. M. & S. J., 1895–6, n. s., xxiii, 455–460, 3 pl. (E. Souchon).—Ztschr. f. Geburtsh. u. Gynäk., Stuttg., 1913, lxxiii, 946–948 (A. Martin).

Smellie: William Smellie and his Contemporaries by John Glaister, Glasgow, 1894. Memoir in: "Works" (New Sydenham Soc., 1876, vi) by A. H. McClintock.

Soemmerring: Life by W. Stricker (Frankf. a. M., 1862).

Stensen: Opera v. I (Copenhagen, 1909).—Sir M. Foster. Lect. Hist. Physiol., Cambridge, 1901, 106–110.—Med. Libr. & Hist. J., Brooklyn, 1904, ii, 166–182, port. (F. J. Lutz).—J. J. Walsh. Catholic churchmen in science, Phila., 1906, 137–166, port.

Stokes: Life by Sir W. Stokes (Lond., 1897).—Dublin J. M. Sc., 1878, lxv, 186–200 (J. W. Moore).—Med. Hist. Meath Hosp., Dubl., 1888, 129–136, 1 pl.

Stromeyer: H. Rohlfs. Gesch. d. deutsch. Med., Leipz., 1885, iv, 139–260.—Wien. med. Wchnschr., 1876, xxxvi, 1064 (T. Billroth).

Süssmilch (J. P.): Publ. Am. Statist. Ass., Boston, 1900–1901, vii, 67–46 (F. S. Crum).

Swammerdam: Werk. v. h. Genootsch. t. Bevord. d. Nat.- Genees- en Heelk. te Amst., 1880, v, 1–64 (B. J. Stokvis). "Some Apostles of Physiology" by W. Stirling (Lond., 1902, p. 34). See, also: novel "Swammerdam" by H. Klencke, 3 v. (Leipz., 1860).

Sydenham: Life by J. F. Payne (Lond., 1900).—J. Brown "Horæ subsecivæ," Lond., 1858, 1–98.—Deutsche med. Wchnschr., Leipz., 1889, xv, 1068–1070 (Pagel).—Asclepiad, Lond., 1892, ix, 385–401, port., pl. (Sir B. W. Richardson).—Med. News, Phila., 1894, lxv, 234–236 (Sir H. Acland).

Sylvius (Franciscus): Sir M. Foster. Lect. Hist. Physiol., Cambridge, 1901, 145–173.—Johns Hopkins Hosp. Bull., Balt., 1909, xx, 329–339 (F. Baker).—Proc. Charaka Club, N. Y., 1910, iii, 14–28, 2 pl. (S. E. Jelliffe).

Syme: Memorials by R. Paterson, Edinb., 1874.

Tait (Lawson): Brit. M. J., Lond., 1899, i, 1561–1564.—J. Am. M. Assoc., Chicago, 1899, xxxiii, 875–880 (C. A. L. Reed).

Theophrastus of Eresos: E. L. Greene. Landmarks of Botanical History, Wash., 1909, i, 52–142.

Traube (Ludwig): Berl. klin. Wchnschr., 1876, xiii, 209 (R. Virchow).—Charité Ann., 1875, Berl., 1877, ii, 767–800, port. (E. Leyden).

Tronchin: Life by H. Tronchin, Par., 1906.

Trousseau: France méd., Par., 1869, xvi, 495–499 (C. Lasègue).—Gaz. d. hôp., Par., 1870, xliii, 17–19 (J. Béclard).

Venel: Zentralbl. f. chir. u. mech. Orthop., Berl., 1912, vi, 432–435 (M. Klemm).

Vesalius: Études by A. Burggraeve, Ghent, 1841.—Lives by M. Roth (Berlin, 1892) and J. M. Ball (St. Louis, 1910).—Sir M. Foster: Lectures on the History of Physiology, Cambridge, 1901, 1–24.

Virchow: Biography by W. Becher (Berl., 1891).—Briefe (Leipz., 1907).—Gedächtnisrede by W. Waldeyer (Abhandl. d. k. preuss. Akad. d. Wissensch., Berl., 1903, 1–52).—Gedächtnis-Feier. Verhandl. d. Berl.

46

722 HISTORY OF MEDICINE

Gesellsch. f. Anthrop., 1902, 311–330, port.—Arch. f. path. Anat. (etc.),
Berl., 1903, cxxi, 2–7 (F. von Recklinghausen).—Johns Hopkins Univ.
Circ., Balt., 1891, xi, 17–19 (Sir W. Osler).—Phila. M. J., 1902, x, 360
(W. H. Welch).—Science, N. Y. & Lancaster, Pa., 1902, n. s., xv, 441–
445 (F. Boas).—Virchow-Bibliographie (Berl., 1901).
Warren (John Collins): Life by E. Warren, 2 vols., Bost., 1860.
Werlhof: Opera medica Hannov., 1775, pars i, pp. i–xvii (J. E. Wichmann).—
H. Rohlfs: Gesch. d. deutsch. Med., Stuttg., 1875, i, 32–81.
White (Charles): Med. Libr. & Hist. J., Brooklyn, 1907, v, 1–18 (J. G. Adami).
Whytt (Robert): Med. Libr. & Hist. J., Brooklyn, 1904, 11, 153–165, 1 pl. (J.
Ruhräh).
Wilks (Sir Samuel): Biographical Reminiscences (Lond., 1911).—Guy's
Hosp. Gaz., Lond., 1911, xxv, 508–510, port.—Bibliography of his
writings by William Wale: Ibid., 512–520.—Brit. M. J., Lond., 1911,
ii, 1384–1390, port.—Lancet, Lond., 1911, ii, 1441–1445, port.
Wiseman (Richard): Life by Sir T. Longmore (Lond., 1891)—Sir B. W.
Richardson, Disciples of Aesculapius, Lond., 1900, i, 158–175, port.—
West. Lond. M. J., 1912, xvii, 203–205 (S. D. Clippingdale).
Wolff (Caspar Friedrich): Jenaische Ztschr. f. Med. u. Naturw., Jena, 1868,
iv, 193–220 (A. Kirchhoff).—[Woods Holl Biol. Lect., 1898]—[Sitzungsb.
d. k. preuss. Akad. d. Wissensch., 1904 (W. Waldeyer)].
Wunderlich: Arch. d. Heilk., Leipz., 1878, iv, 289–320 (O. Heubner); 321–
329 (W. Roser).
Young (Thomas): Lives by Gurney (Lond., 1831) and Peacock (Lond., 1855).
—Dict. Nat. Biog., Lond., 1900, lxiii, 393–399 (C. H. Lees).
Zacchias: V. Fossel: Stud. z. Gesch. d. Med., Stuttg., 1909, 46–110.

C. HISTORIES OF SPECIAL SUBJECTS

Alchemy (History of): K. C. Schmieder: "Geschichte der Alchemie" (Halle,
1832).—E. Berthelot: "Les origines de l'alchemie" (Paris, 1885).
Alexandrian Medicine: K. Sudhoff. "Aerztliches aus griechischen Papyrus-
Urkunden" (Leipzig, 1907).
American Medicine: Century (A) of American medicine (Phila., 1876), in
particular the critical survey by J. S. Billings (pp. 290–366).—S. D.
Gross: "History of American medical literature" (Phila., 1876).—
J. M. Toner: "Contributions" (etc.) (Washington, 1874).—F. R. Packard.
"History of Medicine in the United States" (Phila., 1901).—J. G.
Mumford: "A Narrative of Medicine in America" (Phila., 1903).—Uni-
versity M. Mag., Phila., 1897–8, x, 136–140 (Sir W. Osler).—J. Am.
M. Ass., Chicago, 1911, lviii, 437–441 (H. A. Kelly).
Anatomy (History of): Ludwig Choulant's "Geschichte und Bibliographie der
anatomischen Abbildung" (Leipzig, 1852); Hyrtl's studies of Arabic
and Hebrew terms (1879), anatomical terminology (1880) and old
German *termini technici* (1884); Robert von Töply's studies in
mediæval anatomy (Leipzig, 1898), Ludwig Hopf on the early cultural
phases (Breslau, 1904), and Karl Sudhoff on traditional (1907) and
graphic phases of anatomy (1908) are the most remarkable works in
this field. Töply's monograph in the Puschmann Handbuch (1903, ii,
155–325) is a good routine and bibliographic account of the whole subject. I. H. Chievitz's "Anatomiens Historie," in the Danish language
(Copenhagen, 1904) has many interesting illustrations. W. W.
Keen's "Sketch of the Early History of Practical Anatomy" (Philadelphia, 1874) is a valuable history of dissecting and injecting. Charles
R. Bardeen's "Anatomy in America" (Bull. Univ. Wisconsin, Madison,
1905, No. 115, 85–208) is the best account of this subject.
Anesthesia (History of): "Semi-centennial (The) of Anæsthesia" (Bost.,
1897).—Johns Hopkins Hosp. Bull., Balt., 1897, viii, 174–184 (H. H.
Young).—Century, N. Y., 1894, xlvii, 412–420 (Eve E. Simpson).

APPENDICES 723

Anglo-Saxon Medicine: O. Cockayne: "Leechdoms, wortcunning" (etc.), (3 v., Lond., 1864–6).—J. F. Payne: "English Medicine in the Anglo-Saxon Times" (Oxford, 1904).

Anthropology: "History of Anthropology" by A. C. Haddon, Lond. and N. Y., 1910.

Arabian Medicine: F. Wüstenfeld: "Geschichte der arabischen Aerzte" (etc.) (Göttingen, 1840).—Puschmann's Handbuch, Jena, 1902, i, 589–621 (Schrutz).

Art (Medicine in): The subject was opened up by Virchow in Arch. f. path. Anat. (etc.), Berl., 1861, xxii, 190; 1862, xxiii, 194; but was really the creation of Charcot and his pupils in the files of the Nouvelle Iconographie de la Salpêtrière, Par., 1888–1913 passim. The two monographs of Charcot & P. Richer on the demoniac, the deformed and the diseased in art (Par., 1887–9); P. Richer's L'art et la médecine (Par., 1902); Eugen Holländer's monographs on medicine in classical painting, caricature and plastic art (Stuttgart, 1903–12), and Robert Müllerheim's "Die Wochenstuben der Kunst" (Stuttg., 1904) are the best books on this subject. Such essays as those of J. W. Churchman on Jan Steen and Velasquez (Johns Hopkins Hosp. Bull., Balt., 1907, xvii, 480; 1911, xxii, 383) are well worth reading.

Assyro-Babylonian Medicine: F. von Oefele: "Keilschriftmedicin" (Breslau, 1902).

Bacteriology (History of): Friedrich Loeffler's "Vorlesungen" (1. Theil, Leipzig, 1887), incomplete, which may be supplemented by Müller and Prausnitz (Puschmann's Handbuch, 1905, iii, 804–852).

Bibliography (Medical): Haller's re-issue of the Boerhaave "Methodus Studii Medici" (2 vols., Amsterdam, 1751), and his bibliographies of botany (1771–2), anatomy (1774–7), surgery (1774–5) and practice of medicine 1776–8), make up the best of the 18th century contributions.—Carl Peter Callisen's "Medicinisches Schriftsteller-Lexicon" (33 vols., Copenhagen, 1830–45) is a sort of author Index-Catalogue of the latter half of the eighteenth and the first quarter of the nineteenth centuries. The earlier bibliographies of G. G. de Ploucquet (1808–9), Robert Watt (1824), James Atkinson (1834), and John Forbes (1835) are interesting. Ludwig Choulant's "Handbuch der Bücherkunde" (2. ed., Leipzig, 1840), with Julius Rosenbaum's "Additamenta" (Halle, 1842), and his "Bibliotheca medico-historica" (Leipzig, 1842), Haeser's "Bibliotheca epidemiographica" (Jena, 1843), with J. G. Thierfelder's "Additamenta" (Misna, 1843), and Rupprecht's Bibliotheca medico-chirurgica (1847 et seq.) are invaluable works of their kind. Quérard's La France littéraire (12 vols., 1827–64) and Brunet's "Manuel du libraire" (8 vols., Paris, 1860) are especially good for French medicine. Spanish medicine has been exhaustively treated in the "Historia bibliográfica" of Antonio Hernández Morejón (7 vols., Madrid, 1842–52) and the "Colección" of Miguel de la Plata y Marcos (Madrid, 1882). The most exhaustive modern bibliography of medicine is the Index-Catalogue of the Library of the Surgeon-General's Office (34 vols.,1879–1913), supplemented by the monthly "Index Medicus" (1879–99; 1903–1913). The hiatus caused by the suspension of publication of the latter journal was filled in part by the French Index Medicus (Paris, 1900–1902).

A valuable select bibliography of important scientific papers for the years 1800–1893 is the Royal Society's "Catalogue" (11 vols., London, 1867–96), and for anatomy, physiology, bacteriology, chemistry, biology and anthropology, the "International Catalogue of Scientific Literature," printed by the Royal Society (London, 1907–12). For parasitology, C. W. Stiles and A. Hassall's "Index Catalogue of Medical Zoölogy" (36 parts, Washington, 1902–12) is unique and invaluable. E. J. Waring's Bibliotheca Therapeutica (1878), Heinrich Laehr's bibliography of the literature of neurology (Berlin, 1900) and Emil Abderhalden's bibliography of alcoholism (Berlin, 1904) are in the same class.

Indispensable works for general reference in a library of large size are the Catalogues of the British Museum and of the Peabody Library of Baltimore, Maryland, Poggendorff's Handwörterbuch der Geschichte der exakten Wissenschaften (Leipzig, 1863–1904), Lorenz's Catalogue de la Librarie française (Paris, 1867–1911) and Heinsius' Allgemeine Bücherlexicon for the years 1700–1900 (36 vols., Leipzig, 1812–1911). Anonymous and pseudonymous literature is well handled in Halkett & Laing's "Dictionary" (4 vols., Edinburgh, 1882–8), William Cushing's Initials & Pseudonyms (1. & 2. series, and anonyms (1890), Barbier's Dictionnaire des ouvrages anonymes et pseudonymes (4 vols., Paris, 1822–7).

Botany (History of): E. H. F. Meyer: "Geschichte der Botanik" (4 v., Königsberg, 1854).—J. von Sachs: "Geschichte der Botanik" (München, 1875).—J. Wm. Harshberger: "The Botanists of Philadelphia" (Phila., 1899).—A. Hansen: "Die Entwicklung der Botanik" (Giessen, 1902).— E. L. Greene: "Landmarks of Botanical History" (Wash., 1909). Also: J. Am. M. Ass., Chicago, 1911, lviii, 437–441 (H. A. Kelly).

Celtic Medicine: Proc. Am. Phil. Soc., Phila., 1887, xxiv, 136–166 (J. Mooney).

Chemistry (History of): Histories by H. Kopp (Brnschwg., 1843–7, 1871–3), A. W. Hofmann (Berl., 1882), H. W. Picton (Lond., 1889), E. von Meyer (N. Y., 1891), M. M. P. Muir (N. Y., 1909), Sir E. Thorpe (2 v., Lond. & N. Y., 1909), and J. E. Brown (Lond., 1913). E. Berthelot: "La chimie au moyen âge" (Paris, 1896).—School Mines Quart., N. Y., 1905–6, xxvii, 87; 313; 388 (W. Ostwald).—Science, N. Y. & Lancaster, Pa., 1901, n. s., xiii, 803–809 (E. H. Keiser).

Chinese Medicine: August Pfizmaier's translation of the pulse-lore of Chang Ke (1866), and his essays in Sitzungsb. d. phil.-hist. Cl. d. k. Akad. d. Wissensch., Wien, 1865–6, on Chinese pathology, semeiology and toxicology. Also: Janus, Amst., 1904, ix, 103; 159; 201; 257.

Dentistry (History of): Vincenzo Guerini's History of Dentistry (Philadelphia, 1909) and the discriminating review of Ashley Denham in Proc. Roy. Soc. Med., Lond., 1908–9, ii, Odont. Sect., 71–98. Also: Geist-Jacobi's "Geschichte der Zahnheilkunde" (Tübingen, 1896).

Dermatology (History of): Handb. d. Gesch. d. Med., Jena, 1905, iii, 393–463 (I. Bloch).—Lancet, Lond., 1911, i, 1555–1560 (J. H. Sequeira).

Education (Medical): T. Puschmann, "Geschichte des medizinischen Unterrichts" (etc.) (Leipzig, 1889).—N. I. Davis, "History of medical education" (etc.) (Chicago, 1851).—A. Flexner, "Reports to the Carnegie Foundation for the Advancement of Teaching" (Bull. No. 4, 6, N. Y., 1910–12).

Egyptian Medicine: Papyros Ebers. 2 v., Leipzig, 1875, and transl. by H. Joachim (Berlin, G. Reimer, 1890).—Brugsch papyrus (Notice raisonnée, etc.), Leipzig, Hinrichs, 1863).—K. Sudhoff, Aerztliches aus griechischen Papyrus-Urkunden, Leipzig, A. J. Barth, 1907.—Prosper Alpinus, De medicina Ægyptorum, Venice, 1591.—Richard Millar, Disquisitions in the history of medicine, Edinburgh, 1811 (etc.). For an excellent résumé of Egyptian medicine, see Brit. M. J., Lond., 1893, i, 748; 1014; 1061 (J. Finlayson).

Electrotherapy (History of): Ann. d'électrobiol. (etc.), Par., 1904, vii, 129–146 (A. Tripier).

Embryology (History of): O. Hertwig: "Lehrbuch, etc." (9. Aufl. Jena, 1910, 5–58). Basel diss. by B. Bloch (1904).—W. A. Locy: "Biology and its makers" (N. Y., 1908, 195–236).—St. Louis M. Rev., 1904, xlix, 273–281 (A. C. Eycleshymer).—Pop. Sc. Month., N. Y., 1906, lxix, 1–20 (C. I. Minot). Also Introduction to: "Manual" (etc.) by F. Keibel and F. P. Mall (Phila., 1910, v. 1).

Epidemic Diseases: G. Sticker: "Abhandlungen" (etc.) (Giessen, 1908–12).— Handb. d. Gesch. d. Med., Jena, 1903, ii, 736–901 (V. Fossel).

Fees (Medical): Internat. Clin., Phila., 1910, 20. s., iv, 259–275 (J. J. Walsh).—Johns Hopkins Hosp. Bull., Balt., 1898, ix, 183–186 (C. C. Bombaugh).—France méd., Par., 1906, liii, 300–304 (C. Vidal).—J. de sc. méd. de Lille, 1905, i, 543–548 (É. Leclair).—New York M. J. (etc.), 1912, xcvi, 370–373 (J. J. Walsh).

Folk-lore (Medical): W. G. Black, "Folk-medicine" (etc.) (Lond., 1883).—M. Bartels, "Die Medicin der Naturvölker" (Leipzig, 1893).—O. von. Havorka & A. Kronfeld, "Vergleichende Volksmedizin" (etc.) (2 v., Stuttg., 1908–9).—Boston M. & S. J., 1888, cxviii, 29; 57 (J. S. Billings).

Graduation Ceremonies: Med. Libr. & Hist. J., Brooklyn, 1906, iv, 1–14 (W. W. Keen).

Greek Medicine: Chapters in Neuburger, Baas, Daremberg (etc.). Also: Handb. d. Gesch. d. Med., Jena, 1901, 153–402 (R. Fuchs). Also: C. V. Daremberg, État de la médecine entre Homère et Hippocrate, Par., 1867.—Mary Hamilton: Incubation, Lond., 1906.—Brit & For. M.-Chir. Rev., Lond., 1886, xxxvii, 170; xxxviii, 483 (T. C. Allbutt).—J. de chir. (Malgaigne), Par., 1846, iv, 332–342.—Brit. M. J., Lond., 1898, i, 1509; 1572 (R. Caton).—Boston M. & S. J., 1893, cxxviii, 129; 153 (Sir W. Osler). See also: Homeric medicine.

Gynecology (History of): Franz von Winckel's "Ueberblick" in his Handb. d. Geburtsh. (Wiesbaden, 1903, i, 1. Teil, 1: 1904, ii, 1. Teil, 1: 1906, iii, 2. Teil, 1: 1907, iii, 3. Teil, 1.) is the most exhaustive account of the whole subject. Kossmann (in the Puschmann Handbuch, 1905, iii, 953–980) gives a good short account. The essay by Handfield Jones at the beginning of Allbutt's system of Gynecology (1906) is an excellent free-hand discussion of the modern phases. The best account of American gynecology is the essay by Howard A. Kelly in the intro-duction to his "Cyclopedia of American Medical Biography" (Phila-delphia, W. B. Saunders, 1912). Stewart McKay's History of Ancient Gynæcology (1901) and Weindler's history of gynecological illustra-tion (Dresden, 1908) may also be consulted.

Hindu Medicine: A. F. R. Hoernle: The Bower Manuscript. Calcutta, 1893–8.—J. Jolly, Grundriss d. indo-arischen Philologie u. Alter-thumskunde, Strassburg, 1901, iii, Hft. 10.—Jee, A short history of Aryan medical science, London, 1896.—Puschmann's Handbuch, Jena, 1901, i, 119–152 (I. Bloch).—Guy's Hosp. Gaz., Lond., 1889, n. s., iii, 117; 145; 157 (B. D. Basu).—Proc. Charaka Club, N. Y., 1902, i, 1–28 (B. Sachs).

Histology (History of): Univ. M. Mag., Phila., 1888–9, i, 82–87 (G. A. Piersol).

Homeric Medicine: C. V. Daremberg: "La médecine dans Homère" (Paris, 1865)—H. Froelich: "Die Militärmedizin Homer's" (Stuttg., 1879)—Paris thesis by A. Floquet (1912).

Hydrotherapy: M. J. Oertel, "Geschichte der Wasserheilkunde" (etc.) (Leipz., 1835)—Handb. d. Gesch. d. Med., Jena, 1903, ii, 589–603 (von Oefele).—Boston M. & S. J., 1906, cliv, 85–91 (J. H. Pratt).

Hygiene (Public, History of): The subject has never been exhaustively treated. A glance at Professor Sudhoff's remarkable 593-page catalogue of the "Historische Abtheilung" of the Dresden Hygienic Exhibit (1911) will show its scope. Max Rubner's introduction to his "Handbuch der Hygiene" (vol. i, Leipzig, 1911) is a good historical sketch, as also Müller and Prausnitz in the Puschmann Handbuch (1905, iii, 783–852). Sir John Simon's "English Sanitary Institutions" (1890), Sir Edwin Chadwick's "The Health of Nations" (1887), "A History of Factory Legislation" by B. L. Hutchins and A. Harrison (1903), and "A Cen-tury of Public Hygiene in America" (1876) are good histories of the legislative phases.

Incunabula (Study of the): Ludwig Hain's "Repertorium" (4 vols., Stuttgart, 1826–28), with W. A. Copinger's "Supplement" to the same (3 vols.,

London, 1895–1902) is the standard catalogue, which is further supplemented by Choulant's "Handbuch der Bücherkunde" (Leipzig, 1828) and "Graphische Incunabeln" (Leipzig, 1858), the catalogue of French incunabula, by M. Pellechet, v. 1–3, Par., 1897–1909, Konrad Haebler's Spanish incunabula (Bibliografía Ibérica, Leipzig, 1903), Reichling's "Appendices" to Hain and Copinger (Munich, 1905–11), Voullième's Catalogue of the Berlin Incunabula (Leipzig, 1906), I. Collijn's catalogue of the Upsala incunabula (1907), Sudhoff's "Deutsche medizinische Inkunabeln" (Leipzig, 1908), the British Museum Catalogue of XV Century Books (London, 1908–12), K. Burger's "Nummerkonkordanz" (Leipz., 1908), Günther's "Wiegendrucke" of the Leipzig and Altenburg collections (Leipzig, 1909), W. L. Schreiber's Catalogue of 1910–11, R. A. Peddie's "Conspectus incunabulorum" (Pt. 1, London, 1910), and the "Nachträge" to Hain (Leipz., 1910), published by the Prussian "Kommission für den Gesamtkatalog der Wiegendrücke," which proposes to catalogue all the incunabula in existence. For comparing and identifying the typography of the different imprints, Konrad Haebler's "Typenrepertorium" (4 vols., Halle, 1905–10) is indispensable and invaluable.

Japanese Medicine: Y. Fujikawa's Geschichte der Medizin in Japan, Tokyo, 1911.

Jewish Medicine: Julius Preuss, Biblisch-talmudische Medizin, Berlin, 1911. Also: C. D. Spivak and F. T. Haneman in Jewish Encycl., N. Y., 1904, viii, 409–422.

King's Evil: Monograph by Raymond Crawford, Oxford, 1911. Also: Proc. Charaka Club, N. Y., 1906, ii, 58–71 (J. S. Billings).

Laboratories (Scientific): Johns Hopkins Hosp. Bull., Balt., 1896, vii, 19–24 (W. H. Welch).

Laryngology and Rhinology (History of) : Jonathan Wright's "The Nose and Throat in Medical History" is the best account in English, a very valuable and accurate work. The history by Gordon Holmes (Med. Press & Circ., London, 1885) was translated into French and German (1887). Paul Heymann's monographs in Handbuch d. Laryngol. und Rhinol., Vienna, 1896, and in the Puschmann Handbuch (1905, iii, 573–600) are worthy of note. Chauveau's "Histoire des maladies du pharynx" (1901–6) is an exhaustive work in five volumes.

Massage: Handb. d. Gesch. d. Med., Jena, 1903–5, iii, 327–340 (L. Ewer).

Medieval Medicine: Sir T. C. Allbutt: "Science and Medieval Thought" (Lond., 1901); his "Historical Relations of Medicine and Surgery" (etc.) (Lond., 1905); and his essay in Med. Chron., Manchester, 1903, 4. s., v, 1–15.—J. J. Walsh: "The Popes in Science" (N. Y., 1908) and "Catholic Churchmen in Science," 2 v., Phila., 1906–9.—Handb. d. Gesch. d. Med., Jena, 1901–2, i, 622–752 (J. Pagel)—and numerous essays by Sudhoff in his Archiv für Geschichte der Medizin, Leipzig, 1907–13, *passim*.

Nursing (History of): Mary A. Nutting & Lavinia L. Dock: "A History of Nursing" (4 v., N. Y., 1907–12).

Obstetrics (History of): Heinrich Fasbender's "Geschichte der Geburtshülfe" (Jena, 1906) is one of those extraordinarily exhaustive and accurate monographs such as only a German scholar could turn out, occupying 1028 pages of closely woven narrative, with full bibliographic data. It is the most valuable reference work. Siebold's Geschichte (2. Aufl., Tübingen, 1901–2), with the supplements on the modern period by Rudolf Dohrn (1903) and on American obstetrics by J. Whitridge Williams, is the most readable. Max Wegscheider's monograph in the Puschmann Handbuch (1905, iii, 878–952) is excellent for reference purposes. Witkowski's Histoire des accouchements (Paris, 1887) and his various monographs on the cultural aspects of pregnancy and labor, the female breast, etc., are full of curious and amusing facts.

Engelmann's "Labor among Primitive Peoples" (St. Louis, 1882) is an anthropological classic, and his historical sketch in Hirst's System of Obstetrics (1888, v. i, 17–67) is very valuable. Aveling's studies of English Midwives (1872) and of the Chamberlens (1882), Ingerslev on Röslin's Rosegarten (1902), Sinclair's life of Semmelweis (1909) and W. H. Allport's study of the seventeenth century Hebammen-bücher are, all of them, fascinating monographs showing the close relationship between obstetrics and the cultural history of mankind.

Ophthalmology (History of): Julius Hirschberg's Geschichte der Augenheil-kunde in the new edition of the Graefe-Saemisch Handbuch, *passim*, will, when completed, be the authoritative work for reading and reference. It is a wonderful monument of German thoroughness. The shorter histories of August Hirsch (Graefe-Saemisch Handbuch, 1st ed., 1877, vii, 235–554), Pansier (in the Lagrange & Valude En-cyclopédie, 1903, i, 1–86) and Horstmann (Puschmann's Handbuch d. Gesch. d. Med., 1905, iii, 489–572) are also valuable. Special studies of worth are Magnus on the history of cataract (Leipzig, 1876) and ancient ophthalmology (Breslau, 1901), Victor Deneffe on the Gallo-Roman oculists (Antwerp, 1896), Pansier (1901) and Emil Bock (1903) on the history of spectacles, and Alvin A. Hubbell on "The Development of Ophthalmology in America" (Chicago, 1908).

Otology (History of): Adam Politzer's Geschichte der Ohrenheilkunde (v. i, Stuttgart, F. Enke, 1907–13), just completed, is the authoritative and standard work. Michael Sachs in Puschmann's Handbuch (1905, iii, 464–488) gives a good shorter account.

Papal Physicians: P. Mandosius: Θέατρον (etc.), Rome, 1784.—G. Marini: Degli archiatri pontifici, 2 v. Rome, 1784.

Parasitology (History of): Arch. de parasitol., Par., 1908, xiii, 251; 1913, xv, 543 (L. Moulé).—Handb. d. Gesch. d. Med., Jena, 1903, ii, 648–665 (H. Vierordt).—Paris thesis by H. Rémignard (1902).

Pathology (History of): The best modern history is that of Hans Chiari in Puschmann's Handbuch (1903, ii, 473–559). Earlier sketches, as cited by Chiari, were given by Morgagni (1761), Rayer (Paris thesis, 1815), Cruveilhier (Ann. de l'anat. et physiol. path., Paris, 1846, i), Eugene Boeckel (N. dict. de med. et de chir. prat., Paris, 1865, ii) and Rudolf Virchow ("Hundert Jahre Pathologie," Berlin, 1895).

Pediatrics (History of): The address of Abraham Jacobi (Am. Med., Phila., 1904, viii, 795–805) and his history of American pediatrics in Arch. f. Kinderh., Stuttg., 1913 (Baginsky-Festschrift), 413–426. Also: Wolf Becher in Puschmann's Handbuch, 1905, iii, 982–1060.

Percussion and Auscultation (History of): Handb. d. Gesch. d. Med., Jena, 1903, ii, 604–611 (H. Vierordt).

Persian Medicine: A. M. Fonahn: "Zur Quellenkunde der persischen Medizin" (Leipzig, 1910).

Pharmacy (History of): Hermann Schelenz's Geschichte der Pharmacie (Berlin, 1904) and A. C. Wootton's "Chronicles of Pharmacy" (Lon-don, 1910) are the best works for reading and reference. Hermann Peters' "Aus pharmazeutischer Vorzeit in Bild und Wort" (2 vols., Berlin, 1889–91) takes up the cultural side of the subject, with many interesting pictures.

Physiology (History of): The most readable work on this subject in English is Sir Michael Foster's "Lectures on the History of Physiology" (16th–18th centuries, Cambridge, 1901), which is based upon original research and full of atmosphere and color. John Call Dalton's "Doctrines of the Circulation" (Philadelphia, 1884), William Marcet's "History of Respiration in Man" (London, 1897), Max Neuburger on the develop-ment of experimental physiology of the brain and spinal cord before the time of Flourens (Stuttgart, 1897) and William Stirling's "Some Apos-tles of Physiology" (London, 1902) are works of a similar character.

Stirling's work is a beautiful folio, filled with fine pictures of the great masters, and, like Foster's book, inspired with enthusiasm. Heinrich Boruttau's "Geschichte" (Puschmann's Handbuch, 1903, ii, 327–456) and John C. Cardwell's "Development of Animal Physiology" (Med. Library & Histor. Jour., New York, 1904–6, ii–iv, *passim*) may be consulted for the whole subject in its bibliographical relations).

Psychiatry (History of): The subject has been almost entirely in the hands of German writers. Heinrich Laehr, to begin with, has made a complete history of psychiatry in the form of a calendar, now in its fourth edition (Berlin, 1893), and is the author of an unsurpassable bibliography of the literature of psychiatry, neurology and psychology from 1459 to 1799 (Berlin, 1900). J. B. Friedreich made similar essays in the first half of the nineteenth century. For short histories of psychiatry, see the text-books of Heinroth (1818), von Feuchtersleben (1845), Flemming (1859), Leidesdorf (1865), von Krafft Ebing (1879, or 8th ed., 1903) and Schüle (1878). Also: S. Kornfeld in Puschmann's Handbuch (1905, iii, 601–728) and Th. Kirchhoff on the history of German psychiatry (Berlin, 1890).

Quackery: H. Magnus: "Das Kurpfuscherthum" (etc.) (Breslau, 1903).— Brit. M. J., Lond., 1911, i, 1250–1263.

Roman Medicine: Handb. d. Gesch. d. Med. (Puschmann), Jena, 1901–2, i, 403–414 (I. Bloch).—Brit. Med. Jour., Lond., 1909, ii, 1449; 1515; 1598 (Sir T. C. Allbutt).—M. Meyer: Theodorus Priscianus, Jena, 1909.—W. Schönack: Scribonius Largus, Jena, 1912.—A. Söllner: Vitruvius (Jena. med.-hist., Beitr., 1913, Heft 4).

Salerno (School of): Collectio Salernitana (S. De Renzi), 5 v., Naples, 1852– 9.—P. Giacosa, Magistri Salernitani (etc.), Turin, 1901.—H. E. Henderson: The School of Salernum, N. Y., 1883.—Med. Chron., Manchester, 1904–5, 4. s., viii, 67–93, 1 pl. (W. Stirling).

Shakespeare (Medicine in): J. Moyes: "Medicine & Kindred Arts" (etc.) (Glasgow, 1896).—B. R. Field: "Medical Thoughts of Shakespeare" (Easton, Pa., 1885).

Spectacles (History of): P. Pansier: "Histoire des lunettes" (Paris, 1901).— E. Bock: "Die Brille und ihre Geschichte" (Wien, 1903).

Surgery (History of): Up to the end of the 16th century, Gurlt's Geschichte der Chirurgie (1898) and Malgaigne's Histoire de chirurgie (1840) are the authoritative sources, the former unrivalled for accuracy. See also, Friedrich Helfreich in Puschmann's Handbuch (v. iii, 1–306), a valuable source of reference. The best history of the whole subject of surgery in English is that of John S. Billings, forming the introductory chapter to Dennis's system of surgery (New York, 1895, i, 1–144). It is not only wonderfully accurate in respect of facts and dates, but imbued with a genuinely critical spirit. In the same class are Sir William Fergusson's "Lectures" of 1867, and the important monograph of Sir Clifford Allbutt on "The Historical Relations of Medicine and Surgery to the End of the Sixteenth Century," the best history of medieval surgery in English. See also Zeis's history of plastic surgery (Leipzig, 1863), George Fischer on the cultural aspects of 18th century surgery (Chirurgie vor 100 Jahren, 1876) and J. S. Milne on surgical instruments (Oxford, 1897). English surgery is ably specialized in John Flint South's Memorials of the Craft of Surgery in England (1886), Sidney Young's Annals of the Barber-Surgeons of London (1890), and the interesting monographs of D'Arcy Power. German surgery may be studied in Rohlfs' "Die chirurgischen Klassiker Deutschlands" (Leipzig, 1883–5), in Georg Fischer (1876), Tillmann's "Hundert Jahre Chirurgie" (1898) and Ernst Becker's essay on old-time Hildesheimer surgeons (1902). American surgery up to 1876 is exhaustively treated by Samuel D. Gross in Am. Jour. Med. Sc., Phila., 1876, n. s., lxxi, 431–484. The essays of James Evelyn Pilcher

(Jour. Am. Med. Assoc., 1890, xiv, suppl. No. 18, 629–636) and Frederick S. Dennis (Med. Rec., N. Y., 1902, xlii, 637–648) are also valuable for reference.

Thermometry (History of): H. C. Bolton: "Evolution of the thermometer" (Easton, Pa., 1900).—F. Burckhardt: "Zur Geschichte des Thermometers" (Basel, 1902).—Mitt. z. Gesch. d. Med. u. d. Naturw., Hamb. & Leipzig, 1902, i, 5; 57; 143; 282 (E. Wohlwill).

Thibetan Medicine: H. Laufer: "Beiträge zur Kenntnis der tibetischen Medicin" (Leipz., 1900).

Variolation: Johns Hopkins Hosp. Bull., Balt., 1913, xxiv, 69–83 (A. C. Klebs). Also Reprint with extensive bibliography.

Veterinary Medicine: C. P. Lyman: "A History of veterinary medicine" (etc.) (Cambridge, Mass., 1898).—Bull. Soc. centr. de méd.-vét., Par., 1890, 7. s., vii, 519, *passim*.

Zoölogy (History of): V. Carus, Geschichte der Zoölogie, 1853.

TEST QUESTIONS

1. What medical men had to do with deciphering the Egyptian papyri?
2. What writers have attempted to classify diseases?
3. What are the best editions of Hippocrates? What is the best modern edition? Who made the first Latin translation of the Opera Omnia?
4. Explain the significance of the red and white stripes on the barber's pole.
5. Who made the first fundamental experiment on cardiac inhibition?
6. What important works of Malpighi were printed at the expense of the Royal Society?
7. Who originated the following expressions: protoplasm? eugenics? pneumothorax? phagocytosis? conservation of energy? dissipation of energy? pin-hole pupil? ægophony? metabolism (*Stoffwechsel*)? medical police? diphtheria? typhoid fever? enteric fever? tabes dorsalis? locomotor ataxia? erythromelalgia? anesthesia? opsonic index? coma vigil? internal secretions? aphasia? neurons? hormones? synapse? autonomic system? vagotonia? entelechies?
8. What was the condition of large hospitals in the eighteenth century?
9. What episode in the life of Erasistratus is given in Plutarch's Lives?
10. Name the principal Papal physicians of the sixteenth and seventeenth centuries.
11. What physiologists pushed vivisection to an extreme limit?
12. What medical reforms were made by Sydenham? Sir John Pringle? John Howard? Pinel? Louis? Graves? Semmelweis? Schönlein?
13. Who were the successive owners of the Gold-Headed Cane?
14. Who first saw bacteria under the microscope?
15. How did Descartes acquire his knowledge of anatomy?
16. What great chemical discovery was foreshadowed by John Mayow?
17. In what story does Balzac introduce Ambroïse Paré as a character?
18. Who were Ctesias? Oporinus? Cælius Aurelianus? Valerius Cordus Cesalpinus? Stannius? Caius? Scultetus? Simon Colinæus? Fracastorius? Oribasius? Sanctorius? Anutius Fœsius?
19. Who discovered the mammalian ovum? the spermatozoa? the red blood-corpuscles? the gastric juice? chyle? the cerebro-spinal fluid?
20. What important advances in medical science were made by great mathematicians?
21. What great physicians have also been great mathematical physicists and what discoveries did they make in this department of science?
22. Describe the status of anatomical teaching under the Monro dynasty in Edinburgh.
23. What treatises of Galen did Linacre translate?
24. What names are associated with the introduction of clinical thermometry?
25. What physicians have been eminent lexicographers?
26. What did Frederick the Great do for the development of medicine in Prussia?
27. Explain: archæus; embrocations; *chirurgiens de robe courte;* setons; Jesuit's bark; spagyric medicine; imposthumes; plica Polonica; temple sleep; "making medicine"; uromancy; doctores bullati; polypragmatism; judicial astrology; medical constitutions; "all or none."
28. What physician was styled "ultimus Romanorum" by Dr. Johnson?
29. Mention some physicians of the past who received very large fees.
30. What painters have represented chlorosis? bubonic plague? insanity? idiocy? leprosy? pregnancy? rhinophyma? syphilis?
31. Who discovered the pathogenic parasites of the following diseases: favus? dysentery? hook-worm infection? sleeping sickness? yaws? Texas fever?

32. Why did plastic surgery go into decline between Tagliacozzi and Dieffen-bach?
33. Who originated the following ideas: coction? healing by first intention? omne vivum ex vivo? omne vivum ex ovo? omnis cellula e cellula? omnis nucleus e nucleolo? therapia sterilisans? "nodal rhythms" in the heart?
34. Define "Burking" and give some account of its history.
35. What was the social status of the surgeon and his apprentice in the eighteenth century?
36. What physicians or medical students wrote the following poems: Hyperion? The Pleasures of Imagination? The Dispensary? Das Lied von der Glocke? The Last Leaf? The Deserted Village?
37. What is the experiment of Stannius and what is its significance?
38. What great architect illustrated Willis's treatise on the brain?
39. Who was the leading consultant in London during the period 1820–40?
40. What physicians wrote under the following pseudonyms: Jonathan Dawplucker? Richard Leander? Martinus Scriblerus? Dr. Oribasius?
41. What changes in medical practice were made by the following physicians: Brissot? Broussais? Corvisart? John Brown? Skoda? Brand of Stettin? James Mackenzie?
42. What artists are famous for their paintings of dissecting scenes in the seventeenth and eighteenth centuries?
43. What books are of fundamental importance in the history of dentistry?
44. Who introduced the following drugs: cinchona bark? calomel? strychnine? digitalis? morphine? ether? chloral? chloroform? sulphonal? veronal?
45. Who first devised an alphabet for deaf-mutes?
46. How did the "Origin of Species" influence medicine?
47. What English physicians in the eighteenth century possessed expensive museums and botanic gardens?
48. What is the earliest recorded instance of the use of iron as a tonic?
49. Name some great physicians who have been amateurs of music.
50. What modern cities have erected monuments to Servetus?
51. Name some prominent English Quaker physicians.
52. Who were the best pupils of: Boerhaave? Monro *primus?* John Hunter? Magendie? Johannes Müller? Louis? Carl Ludwig? Sir Astley Cooper? Billroth? Frerichs? Virchow? Naunyn?
53. How did Pirogoff influence Russian medicine?
54. What is the earliest reference to tracheotomy?
55. Who made the first experiment in hypnotism? Who introduced the term?
56. Give the history of podalic version from Soranus of Ephesus to Braxton Hicks.
57. What pathologists influenced the dermatological work of Robert Willan and Ferdinand von Hebra?
58. What are the leading medical names of Spain? Russia? Norway? Sweden? Denmark? Japan?
59. What were the fortunes of asepsis from Hippocrates to Lister?
60. Why did Goethe dislike Haller?
61. Who were Nicholas Culpeper? Louise Bourgeois? the Chamberlens? the Chevalier Taylor? Valentine Greatrakes? John St. John Long?
62. Who corrected the botanical errors of Pliny?
63. What were the medieval substitutes for anesthesia?
64. Explain "wound-drinks," and why were they used?
65. What is the historical significance of the equation: $NH_4CNO = CO(NH_2)_2$?
66. What great physicians have been army surgeons?
67. What army surgeons have achieved distinction in other fields of activity?
68 Imagine yourself an Arabian or Jewish physician of the 9th century A.D. What would be your probable modes of thought and procedure in handling a medical case?
69. What was the first medical tract to be printed? What was the first medical book to be printed?
70. What important work was done by the Anglo-Indian surgeons?

71. With what do you associate the following dates: 1543? 1628? 1798? 1832? 1847? 1867?
72. What did Ivan the Terrible do for Russian medicine?
73. Who made the earliest experiments in anaphylaxis, and who originated the term?
74. Contrast John and William Hunter as human characters.
75. What medical men have been prominent in combating the doctrine of spontaneous generation?
76. What opinions about medicine and the medical profession were entertained by the following celebrities: Petrarch? Molière? Montaigne? Frederick the Great? Goethe? Napoleon? Tolstoi?
77. What pathologists and surgeons have classified tumors?
78. What was the Hindu method of teaching surgical procedure?
79. How did Louis influence American medicine?
80. Who made the first botany? the first materia medica? the first formulary? the first pharmacopœia?
81. What was the difference between the "Nature-Philosophy" and "Natural History" schools of German medicine?
82. Give the history of spectacles.
83. What orthopedic procedure was practised by Avicenna?
84. Explain: bezoars; parabolani; facies Hippocratica; Bestiaries; Psora; Occam's razor; derivative blood-letting; moxa; St. Anthony's fire; Galenicals; *Bertillonage; couvade;* sympathetic powder; Daltonism; Geneva Convention; xenodochia; Baunscheidtism; Rosicrucians; phlogiston; odic force; azote; Brunonian theory; infibulation; metallic tractors; falling sickness; vomica; rhizotomi; *traité des blanches; loi Roussel.*
85. Who were the pioneers in vital statistics? Who originated medical statistics?
86. On what grounds did Lawson Tait oppose Lord Lister's teaching?
87. Who first described paralysis agitans? emphysema of the lungs? heart-block? aortic insufficiency? leukemia; syringomyelia? rheumatic gout? poliomyelitis? facial neuralgia? beri beri? ascending neuritis? hemolytic jaundice? myxedema? presbyophrenia? bubonic plague?
88. How did Ludwig come to devise his sphygmograph?
89. What American surgeons were associated with the rise of modern gynecology?
90. What light does the "Wundenmann" throw upon medieval surgery? What do you understand by "wound surgery"?
91. Who first successfully ligated the following arteries: the external iliac? the innominate? the vertebral? the subclavian? the common carotid? the femoral? the gluteal?
92. What distinguished men were victims of angina pectoris?
93. Why did Sir Charles Bell give up his surgical practice in London, and what were his subsequent experiences in Edinburgh?
94. Name eight physicians who did much to advance geology.
95. Tell what you know of the personal side of Harvey; Malpighi; Borelli; Auenbrugger; Broussais; Cullen; Abernethy; Sir Astley Cooper; Dupuytren; Aston Key; Skoda; Virchow; Pasteur; Hyrtl; Charcot.
96. What was the favorite English text-book on the practice of medicine in the first half of the nineteenth century?
97. Who devised the following procedures: frozen sections? litholapaxy? ophthalmoscopy? laryngoscopy? rhinoscopy? bronchoscopy? intra-vital staining? extra-vital tissue cultures? test-breakfasts? intubation of the larynx? symphysiotomy? rest cure? intratracheal insufflation? sterilization by ultraviolet rays? diazo reaction? fixation of the complement? deviation of the complement? suspension laryngoscopy?
98. Name some of the great medical printers of the sixteenth century.
99. With what do you associate the following localities: Cos? Epidaurus? Stagira? Monte Cassino? Great Windmill Street? Nauheim? Jullundur? Kaiserswerth? Görbersdorf? Gheel? Scutari? Saranac Lake?

100. What German writers are the leading authorities on anatomical illustration?
101. How are physicians described in the novels of Smollett? Le Sage? Dickens? Balzac? Charles Reade? Wilkie Collins?
102. What prominent physicians and surgeons have illustrated their own works?
103. Who made chemistry a quantitative science?
104. Give the history of the physiology of digestion up to the time of Beaumont.
105. Name the principal medical botanists.
106. What are the modern equivalents of: the āaã disease? morbus Hungaricus? cynanche trachealis? West Indian dry gripes? peripneumonia notha? tabes mesaraica? the vapors? the purples? Devonshire colic?
107. Give the history of the seton in medical practice.
108. Name the principal neurological discoveries of Sir Charles Bell; Romberg; Duchenne of Boulogne; Erb; Charcot; Marie; Weir Mitchell.
109. Why does the Talmud throw more light upon ancient Jewish medicine than the Bible?
110. What was Montaigne's malady and give some medical features of his "Journey into Italy."
111. Who were the discoverers of oxygen?
112. What races used the prehistoric chipped flint knife in later cultural periods and for what reason?
113. Name some celebrated persons who were victims of phthisis.
114. What physicians or students of medicine wrote the following: Essay on Human Understanding? Discours de la Méthode? The History of John Bull? Humphrey Clinker? The Good Natured Man? Elsie Venner? Ten Thousand a Year? Causeries du Lundi? Hugh Wynne? Der Geisterseher? Tom Burke of Ours? L'Abbé Tigrane? El Gran Galeoto?
115. What different maladies have been called by the name of the "English disease"?
116. What seventeenth century surgeon described a rational modern operation for vesico-vaginal fistula?
117. What medical journals were founded by Reil? Johannes Müller? Desault? Langenbeck? Virchow? Friedreich? A. von Graefe? Kölliker? Pflüger? Lombroso? Gegenbaur? Naunyn? Hoppe-Seyler? Schaudinn? Freud?
118. In what way was Swammerdam a remarkable experimental physiologist?
119. Who were Averroës? Lorenzo Bellini? Thomas Vicary? Daremberg? Zabdiel Boylston? Bilguer? Spallanzani? Willard Gibbs? Stephan Weszprémi? Wunderlich? Emile Littré? Tissot? Caspar Wistar? Venel? Henri Dunant? Oken? Florian Heller? Choulant?
120. Who introduced the idea of reflex action? Who demonstrated it experimentally?
121. What physicians signed the Declaration of Independence?
122. What was Galen's crucial experiment to demonstrate the motor power of the heart?
123. Who wrote the following works: Arcana naturæ? Biblia naturæ? De motu cordis? Les passions de l'âme? On airs, waters and places? De usu partium? Avis au peuple? Micrographia? Sepulchretum? Systema naturæ? L'homme machine? Hortus sanitatis? the Metamorphosis of Ajax? Antitheriaka? Inventum novum? Rosa Anglica?
124. What effect did the return of Halley's comet have upon medicine?
125. How did local codes of ethics originate?
126. Why is Mott's translation of Velpeau's Surgery more valuable for reference than the original?
127. What did the following politicians and publicists do for medicine: Napoleon III? Gambetta? Lord Warburton? Théophile Roussel? Sir Robert Peel?
128. What physicians opposed the persecution of witches?
129. What anatomists were accused of vivisecting human beings?
130. Give Wickersheimer's reasons for supposing that Nicolaus Praepositi is not the author of the Salernitan "Antidotarium" of 1471.

131. In respect of what pathological theories was Virchow at variance with the following authorities: Cruveilhier? Rokitansky? Hughes Bennett? Cohnheim? Charcot? Koch? Behring?
132. Who were instrumental in abolishing judicial torture?
133. What pathological lesions have been found in Egyptian mummies?
134. What diseases were originally described by: Benjamin Rush? Laënnec? Willis? Heberden? Fothergill? Aretæus? Parry? Sydenham? Virchow? F. von Hebra? Kussmaul? Hodgkin? Bright? Alibert? Sir Samuel Wilks?
135. Give the history of factory legislation in England.
136. Who first noted the third sound of the heart?
137. Discuss the following points in spelling: incunabulum; Auenbrugger or Avenbrugger; Fabry von Hilden or Fabriz von Hilden; Ketam or Ketham; Heinrich von Pfolspeundt or H. von Pfolsprundt; Richard Hela or R. Helain; Baillou (Ballonius) or Baillon; cocaine or cucaine; thyroid or thyreoid; Treponema pertenue or T. pertenuis; Leishmaniosis or Leishmaniasis.
138. What medical writers have pirated the anatomical plates of others?
139. Give the references to Cheyne-Stokes respiration before the time of Stokes.
140. What arguments have been advanced for and against the supposed American origin of syphilis?
141. What is the derivation of: Dum Dum fever? colica Pictonum? Thomsen's disease? nyctalopia? incunabula? Staffordshire knot? angula Ludovici? Hutchinson's triad? Merseburg triad? stovaine?
142. Who conceived the idea of representing embryonic relations in three dimensions?
143. Why should we not refer to a disease as a "clinical entity"?
144. What is the recent significance of the work of Gaskell and Langley on the vagus and visceral nerves?
145. Why should the date of Werlhof's description of purpura be 1735, instead of 1775, as often given?
146. How would you arrange and catalogue the books in a medical library?
147. Describe the three different first editions of Röslin's *Rosegarten*.
148. What bibliographical methods are employed in cataloguing and identifying the incunabula?
149. How does Hain differentiate between the three separate imprints of Leonicenus' tract on syphilis (1492)?
150. What medico-historical mares' nests have been disposed of by Sudhoff?

INDEX OF PERSONAL NAMES

INDEX OF SUBJECTS

48